Gastrointestinal Interventional Endoscopy

Mihir S. Wagh • Sachin B. Wani

Editors

Gastrointestinal Interventional Endoscopy

Advanced Techniques

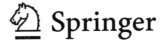 Springer

Editors
Mihir S. Wagh
Interventional Endoscopy, Division of
Gastroenterology
University of Colorado-Denver
Aurora, CO
USA

Sachin B. Wani
Interventional Endoscopy, Division of
Gastroenterology
University of Colorado-Denver
Aurora, CO
USA

Additional material to this book can be downloaded from
https://link.springer.com/book/10.1007/978-3-030-21695-5

ISBN 978-3-030-21694-8   ISBN 978-3-030-21695-5   (eBook)
https://doi.org/10.1007/978-3-030-21695-5

This Springer imprint is published by the registered company Springer Nature Switzerland AG
The registered company address is: Gewerbestrasse 11, 6330 Cham, Switzerland

To my parents, Maya and Suhas Wagh, for giving me everything.

—Mihir S. Wagh

I dedicate this book to my parents, Balkrishna and Sudha Wani, who have always inspired me to follow my own path, giving me all the opportunities I have had in my life and to whom I owe everything. To my entire family, I am grateful for all your love, encouragement, and support. To my colleagues, trainees, nurses, and mentors, I continue to learn from you every single day. Finally, to my wife, Anuja, and our twins, Kaahan and Krish, who have allowed me to pursue my dreams. I thank you for all of your sacrifices, patience, compassion, and motivation to dream big.

—Sachin B. Wani

Foreword I

Interventional endoscopy has expanded far beyond the techniques of ERCP and EUS. This outstanding text focuses on the newer procedures in interventional endoscopy that have been developed and evolved in the spaces of endoscopic resection, endoscopic bariatric therapies, per oral endoscopic myotomies, endoscopic antireflux therapies, tissue apposition, and interventional endoscopic ultrasound. My colleagues and partners, Mihir S. Wagh and Sachin B. Wani, have developed this text, with a dedication to the practice and teaching of interventional endoscopy. I have had the good fortune to directly observe their enthusiasm, teaching, and practice over the past years. For this work, they have recruited outstanding experts in this space to describe the innovations that have occurred in the past decade that have changed our approaches and expanded the minimally invasive therapies we offer our patients. While some of these techniques are being optimized, others have been established in prospective clinical trials as viable alternatives in the management of gastrointestinal disorders. Most of us enthusiastically entered this subspecialty with the intent of helping our patients with new, minimally invasive procedures. This enthusiasm continues with the development of these newer techniques and our expansion into areas that were previously not approached endoscopically. The innovation and thoughtfulness of our colleagues that practice and continue to push the boundaries of this space are impressive. The collective drive to continue to advance minimally invasive solutions to the clinical problems that we all face guarantees that some, if not all, of these techniques will be supplanted by even more novel and innovative approaches in the future. We are fortunate to view this current snapshot as the continuum of minimally invasive endoscopic care advances. The authors and editors of this text are to be commended for marking our progress to date in this comprehensive and timely work. It is a resource for practitioners and trainees alike as it nicely summarizes our current state of the practice of the newer techniques in this broadening field of interventional endoscopy.

Aurora, CO, USA   Steven A. Edmundowicz, MD, FASGE

Foreword II

Gastrointestinal (GI) endoscopy has a relatively recent history, starting in 1932 with the development of the flexible gastroscope by Schindler. Only after the introduction of the gastrocamera in 1950 by Uji and colleagues, Hischowitz invented in 1957 the first fiberscope for the upper GI tract and colon. The use of endoscopy further increased in popularity with the introduction of video endoscopes. At the same time, the first prototypes of endoscopic ultrasound (EUS) were introduced in the 1980s. EUS was initially used as a diagnostic adjunct but rapidly evolved to a therapeutic tool for various GI disorders.

In the past 10 years, GI endoscopy has seen various remarkable developments. In the following, four major developments will be highlighted.

One of these developments include endoscopic resection. It originally started with endoscopic polypectomy but soon thereafter developed further to endoscopic mucosal resection (EMR) for the removal of larger superficial lesions, followed by endoscopic submucosal dissection (ESD) for en bloc resections, and recently to endoscopic full-thickness resection (EFTR), allowing the resection of lesions that are located in the deeper layers of the GI tract.

Due to the dramatic increase in overweight and obesity in the last 10–15 years, especially in the Western world, endoscopic bariatric treatments were introduced. This initially started with minimally invasive treatments, i.e., intragastric balloon placement and aspiration therapy. Later, when endoscopic suturing devices became available, endoscopic sleeve gastroplasty was introduced.

The third development which can be considered as one of the most appealing in the last 10 years is endoscopic myotomy. It first started with a procedure developed by Dr. Haruhiro Inoue, named peroral endoscopic myotomy (POEM). This initiated several other procedures which are likewise characterized by restoring continuity in the GI tract, such as endoscopic myotomy for Zenker's diverticulum (Z-POEM), endoscopic pyloromyotomy for gastroparesis (G-POEM), and endoscopic per rectal endoscopic myotomy for Hirschsprung's disease (PREM). The technique of myotomy has also set the stage for other third-space endoscopic procedures, for example, submucosal tunneling endoscopic resection (STER).

Finally, in the mid-1990s, EUS-guided cyst gastrostomy and EUS-guided celiac plexus neurolysis shifted the perception of EUS from a purely diagnostic examination to a modality capable of performing therapeutic interventions.

Numerous advances have since been made, including EUS-directed biliary and pancreatic drainage, treatment of neoplasia, anastomosis creation, and treatment of bleeding. Most of these technologies will most likely shift several therapeutic approaches in the near future.

The editors of this book, entitled *Gastrointestinal Interventional Endoscopy: Advanced Techniques*, Drs. Mihir S. Wagh and Sachin B. Wani, are to be congratulated for their initiative to bring together a superb list of authors. This book offers an overview of therapeutic gastrointestinal endoscopy for upper and lower gastrointestinal diseases. New therapeutic techniques using advanced endoscopic devices are extensively covered. The authors are without exception experts in the field with a great store of knowledge on a wide variety of therapeutic endoscopic procedures. The book will provide a clear guidance for practicing clinicians when performing therapeutic gastrointestinal endoscopy.

Nijmegen, The Netherlands   Peter D. Siersema, MD, PhD, FASGE

Preface

It is our great pleasure to present to you this book on newer techniques in gastrointestinal interventional endoscopy. At the outset, let us start by mentioning the main reason for this endeavor. The field of interventional endoscopy is moving at a dramatically rapid pace with newer endoscopic devices and techniques emerging in the last decade. Traditionally, interventional endoscopy has included endoscopic retrograde cholangiopancreatography (ERCP) and endoscopic ultrasonography (EUS). However, the field has now expanded to more than just these procedures with the development of a new domain in endoscopy, often called "flexible endoscopic surgery." This book specifically focuses on these components of interventional endoscopy beyond ERCP and EUS. We hope that this would be the "go to" book or "textbook" for all interested in interventional endoscopy since it contains a thorough description and analysis of these newer topics.

This book is divided into six parts – Endoscopic Resection, Bariatric Endoscopy, Endoscopic Myotomy, Endoscopic Antireflux Therapies, Endoscopic Tissue Apposition, and Advances in Interventional EUS – with chapters authored by world-renowned experts in each field. We highlight indications and technical details, assess safety and efficacy, and suggest quality metrics and training pathways for these endoscopic procedures. We have included multiple illustrations, tables, and endoscopic photos and videos highlighting these topics to help the reader clearly understand key concepts and procedural details. The book is geared towards all endoscopists – gastroenterologists and surgeons, trainees, as well as seasoned practitioners – interested in this ever-evolving minimally invasive discipline.

We are grateful to our panel of distinguished contributors, national and international endoscopists from across the globe, for sharing their knowledge and experience with us. We would like to extend a special thanks to Andy Kwan and Smitha Diveshan at Springer for patiently guiding us through the publishing process.

Aurora, CO, USA

Mihir S. Wagh MD, FACG, FASGE
Sachin B. Wani MD

Contents

Contents

Part II   Bariatric Endoscopy

Part III   Endoscopic Myotomy

Part IV   Endoscopic Anti-reflux Therapies

Contributors

Seiichiro Abe Endoscopy Division, National Cancer Center Hospital, Tokyo, Japan

Barham K. Abu Dayyeh Mayo Clinic, Rochester, MN, USA

Stuart K. Amateau University of Minnesota Medical Center, Department of Medicine, Division of Gastroenterology and Hepatology, Minneapolis, MN, USA

Amol Bapaye Shivanand Desai Center for Digestive Disorders, Deenanath Mangeshkar Hospital and Research Center, Pune, India

Inmaculada Bautista-Castaño Bariatric Endoscopy Unit, Madrid Sanchinarro University Hospital, Madrid, Spain

Ciber of Obesity and Nutrition Pathophysiology (CIBEROBN), Instituto de Salud Carlos III, Madrid, Spain

Fateh Bazerbachi Department of Gastroenterology and Hepatology, Mayo Clinic, Rochester, MN, USA

Amit Bhatt Department of Gastroenterology and Hepatology, Digestive Disease and Surgery Institute, Cleveland Clinic, Cleveland, OH, USA

Michael J. Bourke Department of Gastroenterology and Hepatology, Westmead Hospital, Sydney, NSW, Australia

University of Sydney, Sydney, NSW, Australia

Olaya I. Brewer Gutierrez Johns Hopkins Medical Institution, Department of Medicine, Division of Gasroenerology and Hepatology, Baltimore, MD, USA

Bryan Brimhall Division of Gastroenterology, University of Colorado, Boulder, CO, USA

Mingyan Cai Endoscopy Center, Zhongshan Hospital of Fudan University, Shanghai, China

Kenneth J. Chang Department of Medicine, H.H. Chao Comprehensive Digestive Disease Center, University of California, Irvine Medical Center, Orange, CA, USA

Carmen Chu Division of Pancreatic-biliary Endoscopy, Institute of Digestive and Liver Care, SL Raheja Hospital, Mumbai, India

Ankit Dalal Division of Pancreatic-biliary Endoscopy, Institute of Digestive and Liver Care, SL Raheja Hospital, Mumbai, India

Division of Gastroenterology, Baldota Institute of Digestive Sciences, Mumbai, India

Vinay Dhir Division of Pancreatic-biliary Endoscopy, Institute of Digestive and Liver Care, SL Raheja Hospital, Mumbai, India

Roupen Djinbachian Division of Internal Medicine, Montreal University Hospital Center (CHUM), Montreal, Canada

Montreal University Research Center (CRCHUM), Montreal, Canada

Peter V. Draganov Division of Gastroenterology, Hepatology and Nutrition, University of Florida Health, Gainesville, FL, USA

Lorella Fanti IRCCS San Raffaele Scientific Institute, Vita-Salute San Raffaele University, Division of Gastroenterology and Gastrointestinal Endoscopy, Milano (MI), Italy

Filippo Filicori Lenox Hill Hospital-Hofstra Northwell School of Medcine, New York, NY, USA

Kyle J. Fortinsky Department of Medicine, H.H. Chao Comprehensive Digestive Disease Center, University of California, Irvine Medical Center, Orange, CA, USA

Alessandro Fugazza Digestive Endoscopy Unit, Division of Gastroenterology, Humanitas Research Hospital, Rozzano, MI, Italy

Takuji Gotoda Division of Gastroenterology and Hepatology, Department of Medicine, Nihon University School of Medicine, Tokyo, Japan

Hazem Hammad Division of Gastroenterology and Hepatology, Section of Therapeutic Endoscopy, University of Colorado Anschutz Medical Center and Veterans Affairs Eastern Colorado Health Care System, Aurora, CO, USA

Samuel Han Division of Gastroenterology and Hepatology, University of Colorado Anschutz Medical Center, Aurora, CO, USA

Juergen Hochberger Gastroenterology, GI Oncology, Interventional Endoscopy, Vivantes Klinikum im Friedrichshain, Berlin, Germany

Takao Itoi Department of Gastroenterology, The University of Tokyo, Tokyo, Japan

Vijay Kanakadandi Department of Gastroenterology and Hepatology, The University of Kansas Hospital, Kansas City, KS, USA

Calvin Jianyi Koh Division of Gastroenterology and Hepatology, National University Hospital, Singapore, Singapore

Contributors

Seiichiro Abe Endoscopy Division, National Cancer Center Hospital, Tokyo, Japan

Barham K. Abu Dayyeh Mayo Clinic, Rochester, MN, USA

Stuart K. Amateau University of Minnesota Medical Center, Department of Medicine, Division of Gastroenterology and Hepatology, Minneapolis, MN, USA

Amol Bapaye Shivanand Desai Center for Digestive Disorders, Deenanath Mangeshkar Hospital and Research Center, Pune, India

Inmaculada Bautista-Castaño Bariatric Endoscopy Unit, Madrid Sanchinarro University Hospital, Madrid, Spain

Ciber of Obesity and Nutrition Pathophysiology (CIBEROBN), Instituto de Salud Carlos III, Madrid, Spain

Fateh Bazerbachi Department of Gastroenterology and Hepatology, Mayo Clinic, Rochester, MN, USA

Amit Bhatt Department of Gastroenterology and Hepatology, Digestive Disease and Surgery Institute, Cleveland Clinic, Cleveland, OH, USA

Michael J. Bourke Department of Gastroenterology and Hepatology, Westmead Hospital, Sydney, NSW, Australia

University of Sydney, Sydney, NSW, Australia

Olaya I. Brewer Gutierrez Johns Hopkins Medical Institution, Department of Medicine, Division of Gasroenerology and Hepatology, Baltimore, MD, USA

Bryan Brimhall Division of Gastroenterology, University of Colorado, Boulder, CO, USA

Mingyan Cai Endoscopy Center, Zhongshan Hospital of Fudan University, Shanghai, China

Kenneth J. Chang Department of Medicine, H.H. Chao Comprehensive Digestive Disease Center, University of California, Irvine Medical Center, Orange, CA, USA

Carmen Chu Division of Pancreatic-biliary Endoscopy, Institute of Digestive and Liver Care, SL Raheja Hospital, Mumbai, India

Ankit Dalal Division of Pancreatic-biliary Endoscopy, Institute of Digestive and Liver Care, SL Raheja Hospital, Mumbai, India

Division of Gastroenterology, Baldota Institute of Digestive Sciences, Mumbai, India

Vinay Dhir Division of Pancreatic-biliary Endoscopy, Institute of Digestive and Liver Care, SL Raheja Hospital, Mumbai, India

Roupen Djinbachian Division of Internal Medicine, Montreal University Hospital Center (CHUM), Montreal, Canada

Montreal University Research Center (CRCHUM), Montreal, Canada

Peter V. Draganov Division of Gastroenterology, Hepatology and Nutrition, University of Florida Health, Gainesville, FL, USA

Lorella Fanti IRCCS San Raffaele Scientific Institute, Vita-Salute San Raffaele University, Division of Gastroenterology and Gastrointestinal Endoscopy, Milano (MI), Italy

Filippo Filicori Lenox Hill Hospital-Hofstra Northwell School of Medcine, New York, NY, USA

Kyle J. Fortinsky Department of Medicine, H.H. Chao Comprehensive Digestive Disease Center, University of California, Irvine Medical Center, Orange, CA, USA

Alessandro Fugazza Digestive Endoscopy Unit, Division of Gastroenterology, Humanitas Research Hospital, Rozzano, MI, Italy

Takuji Gotoda Division of Gastroenterology and Hepatology, Department of Medicine, Nihon University School of Medicine, Tokyo, Japan

Hazem Hammad Division of Gastroenterology and Hepatology, Section of Therapeutic Endoscopy, University of Colorado Anschutz Medical Center and Veterans Affairs Eastern Colorado Health Care System, Aurora, CO, USA

Samuel Han Division of Gastroenterology and Hepatology, University of Colorado Anschutz Medical Center, Aurora, CO, USA

Juergen Hochberger Gastroenterology, GI Oncology, Interventional Endoscopy, Vivantes Klinikum im Friedrichshain, Berlin, Germany

Takao Itoi Department of Gastroenterology, The University of Tokyo, Tokyo, Japan

Vijay Kanakadandi Department of Gastroenterology and Hepatology, The University of Kansas Hospital, Kansas City, KS, USA

Calvin Jianyi Koh Division of Gastroenterology and Hepatology, National University Hospital, Singapore, Singapore

Jennifer M. Kolb Division of Gastroenterology and Hepatology, University of Colorado Anschutz Medical Center, Aurora, CO, USA

Pradermchai Kongkam Pancreas Research Unit, Department of Medicine, Chulalongkorn University, Bangkok, Thailand

Gontrand Lopez-Nava Bariatric Endoscopy Unit, Madrid Sanchinarro University Hospital, Madrid, Spain

Michael X. Ma Department of Gastroenterology and Hepatology, Westmead Hospital, Sydney, NSW, Australia

Jorge D. Machicado Division of Gastroenterology and Hepatology, Mayo Clinic Health System, Eau Claire, WI, USA

Roberta Maselli Digestive Endoscopy Unit, Division of Gastroenterology, Humanitas Research Hospital, Rozzano, MI, Italy

Amit Maydeo Baldota Institute of Digestive Sciences, Global Hospital, Mumbai, India

Giorgia Mazzoleni IRCCS San Raffaele Scientific Institute, Vita-Salute San Raffaele University, Division of Gastroenterology and Gastrointestinal Endoscopy, Milano (MI), Italy

Volker Meves Gastroenterology, Klinikum Oldenburg AöR, Oldenburg, Germany

Chetan Mittal Division of Gastroenterology, University of Colorado-Denver, Aurora, CO, USA

Zaheer Nabi Department of Gastroenterology, Asian Institute of Gastroenterology, Hyderabad, India

Vikneswaran Namasivayam Department of Gastroenterology and Hepatology, Singapore General Hospital, Singapore, Singapore

Duke NUS Medical School, Singapore, Singapore

Yong Loo Lin School of Medicine, National University of Singapore, Singapore, Singapore

Mojtaba S. Olyaee Department of Gastroenterology and Hepatology, The University of Kansas Hospital, Kansas City, KS, USA

Marie Ooi Department of Gastroenterology, Royal Adelaide Hospital, Adelaide, SA, Australia

John E. Pandolfino Division of Gastroenterology, Department of Medicine, Northwestern University's Feinberg School of Medicine, Chicago, IL, USA

Lady Katherine Mejía Pérez Department of Internal Medicine, Cleveland Clinic, Cleveland, OH, USA

Amit Rastogi Department of Gastroenterology and Hepatology, The University of Kansas Hospital, Kansas City, KS, USA

D. Nageshwar Reddy Asian Institute of Gastroenterology, Hyderabad, India

Alessandro Repici Digestive Endoscopy Unit, Division of Gastroenterology, Humanitas Research Hospital, Rozzano, MI, Italy
Humanitas University, Rozzano, MI, Italy

Rommel Romano Department of Medicine, University of Santo Tomas Hospital, Manila, Philippines

Marvin Ryou Harvard Medical School, Boston, MA, USA
Brigham and Women's Hospital, Division of Gastroenterology, Hepatology, and Endoscopy, Boston, MA, USA

Yutaka Saito National Cancer Center Hospital, Endoscopy Division, Endoscopy Center, Tokyo, Japan

Jason B. Samarasena Department of Medicine – Gastroenterology, University of California, Irvine Medical Center, Orange, CA, USA

Fayez Sarkis Department of Gastroenterology and Hepatology, The University of Kansas Hospital, Kansas City, KS, USA

Raja Siva Department of Thoracic and Cardiovascular Surgery, Cleveland Clinic Foundation, Cleveland, OH, USA

Andrew C. Storm Department of Gastroenterology and Hepatology, Mayo Clinic, Rochester, MN, USA

Daniel S. Strand Division of Gastroenterology and Hepatology, University of Virginia Health System, Charlottesville, VA, USA

Shelby Sullivan University of Colorado School of Medicine, Aurora, CO, USA

Lee L. Swanström Division of Gastrointestinal and Minimally Invasive Surgery, The Oregon Clinic, Portland, OR, USA

Anthony Yuen Bun Teoh Department of Surgery, Prince of Wales Hospital, The Chinese University of Hong Kong, Shatin, Hong Kong SAR

Pier Alberto Testoni IRCCS San Raffaele Scientific Institute, Vita-Salute San Raffaele University, Division of Gastroenterology and Gastrointestinal Endoscopy, Milano (MI), Italy

Sabrina Gloria Giulia Testoni IRCCS San Raffaele Scientific Institute, Vita-Salute San Raffaele University, Division of Gastroenterology and Gastrointestinal Endoscopy, Milano (MI), Italy

Joseph Rayfield Triggs Section of Gastroenterology and Hepatology in the Department of Medicine, Northwestern Feinberg School of Medicine, Chicago, IL, USA

Eric J. Vargas Department of Gastroenterology and Hepatology, Mayo Clinic, Rochester, MN, USA

John Vargo Department of Gastroenterology and Hepatology, Digestive Disease and Surgery Institute, Cleveland Clinic, Cleveland, OH, USA

Daniel von Renteln Montreal University Research Center (CRCHUM), Montreal, Canada

Division of Gastroenterology, Montreal University Hospital Center (CHUM), Montreal, Canada

Mihir S. Wagh Interventional Endoscopy, Division of Gastroenterology, University of Colorado-Denver, Aurora, CO, USA

Andrew Y. Wang Section of Interventional Endoscopy, Division of Gastroenterology and Hepatology, University of Virginia Health System, Charlottesville, VA, USA

Thomas J. Wang Massachusetts General Hospital, Department of Medicine, Boston, MA, USA

Harvard Medical School, Boston, MA, USA

Sachin B. Wani Interventional Endoscopy, Division of Gastroenterology, University of Colorado-Denver, Aurora, CO, USA

Kenjiro Yamamoto Department of Gastroenterology, The University of Tokyo, Tokyo, Japan

Dennis Yang Division of Gastroenterology, Hepatology and Nutrition, University of Florida, Gainesville, FL, USA

Pinghong Zhou Endoscopy Center, Zhongshan Hospital of Fudan University, Shanghai, China

Part I

Endoscopic Resection

Endoscopic Lesion Recognition and Advanced Imaging Modalities

Jorge D. Machicado, Jennifer M. Kolb, and Sachin B. Wani

Introduction

The field of gastrointestinal endoscopy has evolved in the last 50 years as a consequence of significant advances in engineering, physics, chemistry, and molecular biology among others. One of the most important goals of endoscopy is in detecting and characterizing premalignant or early neoplastic lesions that may be suitable for curative therapies. The explosive growth of optical, cross-sectional, and molecular methods allows us to recognize subtle lesions that may have been missed, in addition to predicting histology and guiding endoscopic therapy.

The development of fiber-optic technology was a determinant step that permitted the introduction of flexible gastrointestinal endoscopes in 1957, which replaced the old, rigid, and semiflexible endoscopes [1]. Conventional video endoscopy was then developed in 1993 by using charge-coupled devices (CCDs), which enabled visualization of real-time imaging on a monitor [2]. During the last decade, developments in video endoscopy resolution and monitor definition have led to the introduction of high-definition white light endoscopy (HDWLE), which is now considered as the standard of care [3].

Despite these tremendous advancements in video endoscopy, subtle lesions can still be missed. Thus, other optical, cross-sectional, and molecular methods have rapidly evolved as an adjunct to HDWLE. Optical technologies such as conventional and virtual chromoendoscopy have been available in clinical practice for several years. In contrast, cross-sectional methods with the ability to provide real-time histology images such as confocal laser endomicroscopy (CLE), optical coherence tomography (OCT), and volumetric laser endomicroscopy (VLE) are still being evaluated, not yet available to most endoscopists, and hence not ready for routine clinical use. Most recently, molecular imaging has emerged to detect specific targets and guide individualized treatments, but it is at early stages and only available for research purposes. In this chapter, we will review each of these advanced imaging modalities (AIMs) and their applicability in recognizing different gastrointestinal lesions in clinical practice.

J. D. Machicado
Division of Gastroenterology and Hepatology, Mayo Clinic Health System, Eau Claire, WI, USA

J. M. Kolb
Division of Gastroenterology and Hepatology, University of Colorado Anschutz Medical Center, Aurora, CO, USA

S. B. Wani (✉)
Interventional Endoscopy, Division of Gastroenterology,
University of Colorado-Denver, Aurora, CO, USA

© Springer Nature Switzerland AG 2020
M. S. Wagh, S. B. Wani (eds.), *Gastrointestinal Interventional Endoscopy*,
https://doi.org/10.1007/978-3-030-21695-5_1

Table 1.1 Pros and cons of different advanced imaging modalities

Advanced imaging modality	Pros	Cons
Conventional chromoendoscopy	Detailed surface pit pattern Useful for dysplasia detection in IBD	Adds time and cost (dyes) Potential risks with vital stains Lack of validated classification systems Evaluation limited to the mucosa
Virtual chromoendoscopy	Detailed surface pit and vascular pattern Easy and cheap on/off button Validated classification systems Useful for neoplasia detection in Barrett's esophagus, stomach lesions, and colon polyps Useful for colon polyp characterization	Evaluation limited to the mucosa Interpretation requires training
Autofluorescence imaging (AFI)	Imaging at greater depth	Low specificity, high false positive rates Low resolution Requires special equipment
Confocal laser endomicroscopy (CLE)	High resolution Visualization of mucosa at cellular level, allows in vivo histology	Time consuming, costly Typically requires probes (pCLE) Requires IV contrast agents Evaluation limited to the mucosa
Optical coherence tomography (OCT)/ volumetric laser endomicroscopy (VLE)	Visualization of mucosa and submucosa at cellular level VLE can mark abnormal area	Low resolution Requires special equipment, costly Requires training
Molecular imaging	High specificity	Adds time and cost Requires special equipment Not available for routine clinical use

Description of Technologies

Table 1.1 summarizes the pros and cons related to the use of each advanced imaging technology in clinical practice.

White Light Endoscopy (WLE): Standard vs. High Definition

Equipment required for video endoscopy includes a video processor, a light source, the endoscope, and a monitor. An external xenon light source provides the full spectrum of visible white light which travels through fiber-optic glass bundles and is emitted through a lens at the end of the endoscope [4]. Light is reflected off the mucosa, through the objective lens of the endoscope, and reaches the photosensitive surface of the CCD – a small chip in the endoscope tip that senses an image. The CCD captures the image and transmits the charge through electrical wires to the video processor, where a digital image is produced. The initial standard-definition (SD) endoscopes were equipped with 410,000 pixel CCD that provided a digital image that was 640 (width) by 480 (height) [5]. Soon after came the realization that image quality was largely dependent on resolution, which is a function of CCD pixel density.

HDWLE uses smaller chips that produce images with a resolution of more than a million pixels and that are displayed in monitors with either 4:3 or 5:4 aspect ratios and at least 650 pixels in height [6]. In order to truly capture HD images, all of the endoscopy equipment must be HD compatible (endoscope, CCD, processor, monitor, and transmission cables). HD monitors can display progressive images where lines are scanned consecutively and the images painted 60 times per second, which produces fewer artifacts for moving objects. Optical magnification with HD endoscopy can provide images up to 150 times the original size with preserved resolution. This function can be activated with a button in newer endoscopes through a system called near focus, which modifies a mechanical movable lens at the tip of the endoscope [7].

Conventional Chromoendoscopy

This type of AIM enhances the GI mucosa with topically applied dyes to outline lesion borders, highlight surface changes, and delineate mucosal depth. Several methods of dye application are employed depending on the target surface area. For focal suspicious lesions, a 60 mL syringe of diluted dye can be pushed through the instrument channel of the endoscope, and the target area is then examined closely. In cases targeting a larger area of tissue, such as patients with inflammatory bowel disease, a more efficient method for delivering dye is through the water jet irrigation system after mixing 250 mL of normal saline with dye in various concentrations [8]. Each dye has distinct chemical properties designed for different clinical applications.

Methylene blue is a vital dye that is absorbed by the epithelial cells of the small intestine (e.g., intestinal metaplasia, IM) and colonic crypts. Absorption generally occurs within 1 minute of topical application, and the effect remains for up to 20 minutes. Whereas "normal" mucosa will soak up the dye color, neoplastic or inflamed mucosa will absorb little or no dye. Thus, a brighter and unstained area is a clue for pathology. Lugol's solution is another vital dye used mostly for screening of esophageal squamous cell cancer in high-risk populations. Suspicious areas more likely to harbor high-grade intraepithelial neoplasia appear as well-demarcated unstained regions of >5 mm, often termed the "pink color sign" as these areas retain a pink mucosal hue in contrast to the iodine-stained surrounding mucosa (Fig. 1.1) [9]. Other but less used vital dyes include crystal violet and cresyl violet.

Non-vital dyes are applied to the surface and provide contrast but without being absorbed by the epithelial cells. Indigo carmine is one of the most commonly used non-vital dyes. It collects in the pits and grooves of the mucosa, thereby enhancing visualization of mucosal structures, surface topography, lesion depth, and borders. Acetic acid is a weak acid that induces a chemical reaction in the mucosa with a goal of delineating epithelial structures. Endoscopic delivery of ace-

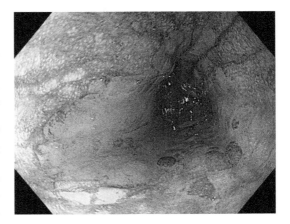

Fig. 1.1 Squamous cell dysplasia with chromoendoscopy using Lugol's solution (unstained areas representing areas of dysplasia)

tic acid through a spray catheter temporarily alters the structure of surface epithelial glycoproteins, which lasts for 2–3 minutes [10]. The unbuffered acid facilitates disruption of disulfide and hydrogen bonds, provokes deacetylation, and in turn denatures the proteins. Repeat application of acetic acid may be necessary to sustain the effect.

Virtual Chromoendoscopy

Virtual chromoendoscopy uses optical lenses and digital processing programs to achieve similar results as conventional chromoendoscopy but with the ease of only pressing a button. The most widely used of these systems is narrow band imaging (NBI, Olympus), which is based on the optical phenomenon that the depth of light penetration into tissue depends on the wavelength; the shorter the wavelength, the more superficial the penetration. In WLE, light at wavelengths 400–700 nm illuminates the surface mucosa and reproduces all images in their natural color. NBI applies an optical filter in real time using a red-green-blue illumination system at a narrower range of 400–540 nm designed to match hemoglobin absorption [11]. This allows structures with high hemoglobin content to appear dark (surface capillaries, brown; submucosal vessels, cyan) which provides a contrast to the surrounding mucosa that reflects the light.

Other systems use the full spectrum of white light to capture images and then perform post-imaging processing. The Fujinon Intelligent Chromoendoscopy (FICE) (Fujinon Inc., Japan) system applies software-based technology to modify images captured through the standard endoscopic video processor [12]. The algorithm selectively enhances specific light wavelengths and creates a reconstructed FICE image. A similar technology is iScan (Pentax, Japan), which uses a digital post-processing system to reconstitute an image [13]. The endoscopist can switch between surface, color, or tone enhancement modes by pressing a button to improve visualization of specific features. Another modality is called blue laser imaging (BLI) or Lasero (Fujinon), which uses a two-laser system. BLI was created in response to the limitations of FICE and NBI as a way to combine the strengths of each individual technology [14]. The limited-wavelength blue laser highlights the mucosal vasculature (similar to NBI), while the second laser induces fluorescent light to illuminate the target.

Autofluorescence Imaging (AFI)

This is a technology dependent on endogenous fluorophores within the GI mucosa, the most important of which is collagen. Fluorophores are naturally occurring substances that absorb energy from short-wavelength light (blue) and in turn emit longer-wavelength light (fluorescent). The patterns of fluorescence vary based on the metabolic activity, blood flow, and biochemical characteristics of the tissue, which can be abnormal with neoplasia and inflammation. Endoscopes with AFI capability have a rotating filter in front of the light source that delivers narrow-spectrum blue light (390–470 nm) alternating with green light (540–560 nm) [15]. There is an additional interference filter whereby only fluorescent and green light are filtered through the CCD to be processed. In the resulting image, normal tissue appears green, and abnormal mucosa appears dark reddish purple in color.

Confocal Laser Endomicroscopy (CLE)

This technology is based on light microscopy, but requires contrast agents administered intravenously (fluorescein) or topically (fluorescein or acriflavine hydrochloride). A laser is then focused by an objective lens to illuminate a single point in the focal plane. Light reflected back from that focal point will converge through a pinhole to the detector [16]. Light that comes from outside the focal point will be scattered and not collected. When the detector processes the light, a high-resolution image at a gray scale will be created showing cellular structures from the mucosal layer (250 um), but not deeper structures. Confocal imaging can be endoscopy based (eCLE) or probe based (pCLE) [17]. Probes are designed to pass through the endoscope working channel toward the target tissue in the biliary tree, upper GI tract, or lower GI tract.

Optical Coherence Tomography (OCT) and Volumetric Laser Endomicroscopy (VLE)

OCT is a disposable probe-based system where long wavelengths of light are used to penetrate into areas of interest and create cross-sectional images [18]. This is similar to endoscopic ultrasound, but infrared light is used instead of acoustic waves to create high-resolution images. A single light source emits two beams, one that is directed at the target tissue and the other to a reference mirror. Light is reflected from both sources and then combined again at a detector to produce interference, which is measured and translated into an image.

VLE uses technology similar to OCT, where rapid scanning facilitates capture of images at a depth of 3 mm with resolution to 10 mm [19]. It is designed for use within a circumferential lumen such as the esophagus. A balloon is passed through the instrument channel and inflated. Then an optical probe is passed through the balloon. The balloon is rotated 360 degrees as the probe is pulled back slightly. The probe VLE has the potential to quickly and effectively image large areas in short periods of time (the entire 6 cm length of the balloon in 90 seconds).

Molecular Imaging

Molecular imaging is an innovative technology where targeted probes are directed to specific molecules in the GI tract. A molecular probe can be designed using a peptide, antibody, nanoparticle, or other molecules [20]. Peptides are the most commonly described probes in molecular endoscopy as they offer certain advantages. They are small for mucosal penetration, are safe, have low immunogenicity, and are relatively easy and inexpensive to mass-produce. The peptide is isolated using a bacteriophage library and then labeled to a fluorophore to be applied topically during endoscopy using a spray catheter. Use of a multimodal video endoscope provides images using a special fluorescent and reflectance filter [21]. This technology has the potential for more accurate in vivo diagnosis and prediction of patients with higher risk of progression into neoplasia before morphologic changes even develop.

Endoscopic Evaluation of the Upper GI Tract

Barrett's Esophagus, Dysplasia, and Esophageal Adenocarcinoma

Rationale and Limitations of Surveillance Endoscopy

The global incidence of esophageal adenocarcinoma (EAC) is 0.7/100,000 person years and has significantly increased in Europe, Australia, and the United States in the last four decades [22, 23]. Most cases of EAC are diagnosed at advanced stages, which is associated with dismal survival and poor quality of life [24]. Barrett's esophagus (BE) or intestinal metaplasia (IM) of the esophagus is the precursor lesion for EAC and can be detected endoscopically in the presence of salmon-colored mucosa extending more than 1 cm proximal to the gastroesophageal junction with confirmed IM on biopsies [25].

Progression of BE to EAC involves a series of pathologic changes from non-dysplastic BE (NDBE) to low-grade dysplasia (LGD), high-grade dysplasia (HGD), and finally EAC [26]. Thus, endoscopic surveillance with targeted biopsies of visible lesions and four-quadrant random biopsies every 1–2 cm (Seattle biopsy protocol) is endorsed by international society guidelines to detect dysplasia or EAC at earlier stages, receive curative therapy, and enhance survival [25, 27–30]. Moreover, this approach can help identify patients with neoplastic lesions who are amenable to endoscopic eradication therapies (EETs) in lieu of surgery or chemoradiation. However, this approach has several limitations including sampling errors (focal distribution of neoplasia and surveillance biopsies sample only 5% of the Barrett's segment), limited reliability of histologic interpretation of dysplasia, and the associated costs, time, and labor, which may explain why community endoscopists do not adhere to the Seattle biopsy protocol [31, 32]. In addition, visible lesions can be easily missed because they are often small and focally distributed.

Endoscopic Inspection of BE

The endoscopist should inspect the Barrett's segment in a systematic fashion to maximize detection of visible lesions which can harbor dysplasia or early cancer. Careful evaluation of BE with HDWLE is recommended as the minimum standard to maximize detection of visible lesions [27, 33]. However, there are no randomized clinical trials directly comparing HDWLE with standard WLE for detection of visible lesions in BE, and this recommendation is inferred from several other studies [34, 35]. Longer inspection time, along with careful and organized BE inspection, may be associated with higher number of lesions detected and increased diagnosis of HGD/EAC [33]. Careful endoscopic examination can reassure detection of >80% of lesions with HGD/EAC [36].

The following recommendations can be considered to ensure high-quality care. First, consider the use of a transparent distal attachment cap on the tip of the endoscope to facilitate endoscopic view especially in patients with BE-related neoplasia. Second, clean the mucosa by using the water jet channel and carefully suctioning the fluid with minimal mucosal trauma. Third, inspect the suspected BE by varying insufflation and desufflation to detect subtle surface irregularities. Fourth, inspect the distal Barrett's segment in a retrograde view. Fifth, describe the location of the diaphragmatic hiatus, gastroesophageal junction, and squamocolumnar junction, as well as the extent of BE including circumferential and maximal segment length using the Prague classification [37]. After adequate inspection of BE, biopsies can then be performed. Biopsies should be avoided in normal or irregular Z line to avoid overdiagnosis of BE in patients who in fact have IM of the cardia which is not associated with EAC and in areas of erosive esophagitis until optimizing antireflux therapy, as reparative changes from active esophagitis can be difficult to distinguish from dysplasia.

Uniform Evaluation of Visible Lesions

Subtle mucosal abnormalities, such as ulceration, erosion, plaque, nodule, stricture, or other luminal irregularities in the Barrett's segment, should be sampled separately, as there is an association of such lesions with underlying dysplasia and cancer [38]. These mucosal abnormalities should undergo endoscopic mucosal resection (EMR), as this provides a better sample for pathologic review and changes the histopathologic diagnosis in approximately 30–50% of patients, compared with biopsies [39, 40]. Moreover, EMR of suspicious esophageal lesions represents a quality indicator of EET of BE, both as a diagnostic (to determine the T-stage and/or grade of dysplasia) and therapeutic maneuver [35]. Chapter 3 of this book offers further details regarding esophageal EMR techniques.

The Paris classification provides a grading system for visible mucosal lesions, which facilitates uniform communication among clinicians [41]. Visible lesions are described as follows: protruded lesions, 0-Ip (pedunculated) or 0-Is (sessile); and flat lesions, 0-IIa (superficially elevated), 0-IIb (flat), 0-IIc (superficially depressed), and 0-III (excavated). Lesions classified as 0-Is, 0-IIc, and 0-III are most likely to harbor invasive cancer, whereas 0-IIa and 0-IIb are likely associated with early neoplasia (Fig. 1.2) [27]. The length of the lesion should be reported using the

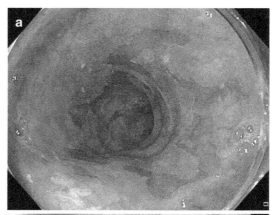
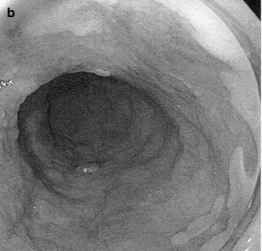
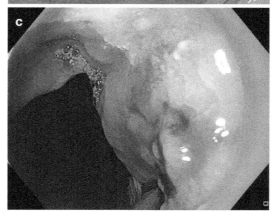

Fig. 1.2 Description of visible lesions in Barrett's esophagus using the Paris classification. (**a**) Flat Barrett's esophagus without visible lesions. (**b**) Paris IIa diffuse nodularity within Barrett's segment. (**c**) Paris IIa and IIc lesion within Barrett's segment

Table 1.2 Quality indicators for endoscopic eradication therapy (EET) in Barrett's esophagus (BE) and suggested median threshold benchmark

Type	Metric	Threshold
Pre-procedure	The rate at which the reading is made by a GI pathologist or confirmed by a second pathologist before EET is begun for patients in whom a diagnosis of dysplasia has been made	90%
	Centers in which EET is performed should have available HDWLE and expertise in mucosal ablation and EMR techniques	NA
	The rate at which documentation of a discussion of the risks, benefits, and alternatives to EET is obtained from the patient prior to treatment	>98%
Intra-procedure	The rate at which landmarks and length of BE are documented (e.g., Prague grading system) in patients with BE before EET	90%
	The rate at which the presence or absence of visible lesions is reported in patients with BE referred for EET	90%
	The rate at which the BE segment is inspected by using HDWLE	95%
	The rate at which complete endoscopic resection (en bloc resection or piecemeal) is performed in patients with BE with visible lesions	90%
	The rate at which a defined interval for subsequent EET is documented for patients undergoing EET who have not yet achieved complete eradication of intestinal metaplasia	90%
	The rate at which complete eradication of dysplasia is achieved by 18 months in patients with BE-related dysplasia or intramucosal cancer referred for EET	80%
	The rate at which complete eradication of intestinal metaplasia is achieved by 18 months in patients with BE-related dysplasia and intramucosal cancer referred for EET	70%
Post-procedure	The rate at which a recommendation is documented for endoscopic surveillance at a defined interval for patients who achieve complete eradication of intestinal metaplasia	90%
	The rate at which biopsies of any visible mucosal abnormalities are performed during endoscopic surveillance after EET	95%
	The rate at which an antireflux regimen is recommended after EET	90%
	The rate at which adverse events are being tracked and documented in individuals after EET	90%

proximal and distal margin of the lesion in relation to the endoscope distance from the incisors. The circumferential involvement should be reported using the lateral margins of the lesion relative to the clock position and with the endoscope in the neutral position.

Quality Indicators of Endoscopic Surveillance

Defining quality indicators may help to ensure the delivery of high-quality care. In this era of value-based and quality-based healthcare, the development of quality indicators that benchmark performance is critical. Thus, a recent study used a methodologically rigorous process to develop valid quality indicators for EET in the management of patients with BE-related neoplasia. The valid quality indicators were categorized into pre-procedure, intra-procedure, and post-

procedure quality indicators. The performance threshold for each of these metrics can be found in Table 1.2.

Advanced Imaging Modalities (AIMs) to Enhance Surveillance

Several AIMs have been investigated to overcome some of the limitations of current surveillance practices of BE with WLE. A Preservation and Incorporation of Valuable Endoscopic Innovations (PIVI) statement from the American Society of Gastrointestinal Endoscopy (ASGE) has outlined thresholds for performing AIMs during endoscopic surveillance of BE [42]. To eliminate random biopsies, an AIM with target biopsies should have the following characteristics: (1) per-patient sensitivity of $\geq 90\%$ and a negative predictive value of $\geq 98\%$ for detecting HGD/EAC, compared with the current standard protocol, and (2) specificity of ≥80% to allow a reduction in the number of biopsies compared with biopsies obtained using the Seattle protocol. A recent meta-analysis demonstrated that only experts in the field of BE meet these thresholds with acetic acid chromoendoscopy, NBI, and eCLE [43]. Thus, AIMs should not yet replace surveillance endoscopy with random biopsies in non-expert hands. However, AIMs can increase the diagnostic yield for identification of HGD/EAC if added to the Seattle protocol, as recently demonstrated in a meta-analysis with 34% and 35% incremental yield of HGD/EAC with virtual and conventional chromoendoscopy, respectively [44]. In head-to-head studies, both chromoendoscopy modalities have demonstrated comparable detection of HGD/EAC [34, 45].

Virtual Chromoendoscopy

The majority of studies evaluating virtual chromoendoscopy in BE have used NBI. In the largest international crossover RCT to date comparing NBI with HDWLE, there was significantly higher detection of dysplasia (30 vs. 21%) with NBI [46]. Several classification patterns (Kansas [47], Amsterdam [48], Nottingham [49]) have been proposed to predict histopathology based on NBI surface patterns, but the proposed criteria are complex, and validation studies had disappointing results. An international working group recently developed a simple and internally validated system to identify dysplasia and EAC in patients with BE based on NBI results [50]. This system, known as the BING criteria, can classify BE with >90% accuracy and a high inter-observer agreement. Regular mucosal patterns were defined as circular, ridged/villous, or tubular patterns; and irregular mucosa was marked by absent or irregular surface patterns. Regular vascular patterns were defined by blood vessels situated regularly along or between mucosal ridges and/or those showing normal, long, branching patterns; irregular vascular patterns were marked by focally or diffusely distributed vessels not following the normal architecture of the mucosa (Fig. 1.3). Additional studies are needed with BLI, FICE, and iScan to assess their utility and interpretation.

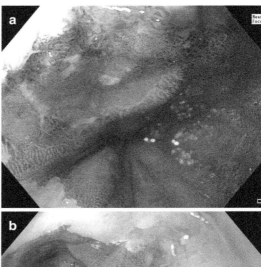
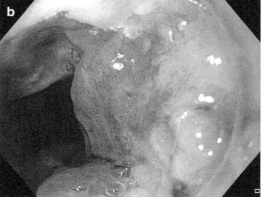

Fig. 1.3 Abnormal NBI pattern of visible lesions in Barrett's esophagus. (**a**) Paris IIa and IIc lesion with abnormal NBI pattern from 9 to 1 o'clock position and with normal NBI pattern from 1 to 9 o'clock position. (**b**) Paris Is lesion in the GE junction with abnormal NBI pattern

Conventional Chromoendoscopy

The dyes most commonly used for conventional chromoendoscopy in BE are acetic acid and methylene blue. No standardized classification criteria have been established for any dye. In the meta-analysis by Thosani et al., acetic acid chromoendoscopy was found to meet the thresholds established by the ASGE PIVI (sensitivity, 97%; negative predictive value, 98%; and specificity, 85%) and can be used in clinical practice at least by experts [43]. In contrast, methylene blue chromoendoscopy fails to meet these thresholds (sensitivity, 64%; negative predictive value, 70%; and specificity, 96%) and does not increase the diagnostic yield over random biopsies for the detection of HGD/cancer [43, 51]. Furthermore, the safety of methylene blue has been questioned as one study suggested that it can cause induce oxidative damage to DNA when photosensitized with light [52]. Acetic acid causes disruption of the columnar mucosal barrier in minutes, leading to whitening of the tissue with vascular congestion and accentuation of the villi and mucosal pattern when the acid reaches the stroma. The whitening effect in dysplastic areas is lost earlier than in the surrounding mucosa, which helps identify neoplastic areas.

Role of AFI, CLE, VLE, and OCT

Other AIMs have been investigated, but none appear to be ready for clinical application at the present time [53]. AFI is limited by its high false positive rate, fair to moderate inter-observer agreement, and minimal incremental diagnostic yield over the Seattle protocol [54]. CLE has the potential to confirm a real-time diagnosis of neoplasia without the need for histology, which could lead to immediate endoscopic therapy without biopsies, such as same-session EMR or ablative therapy. Use of eCLE meets the ASGE PIVI thresholds but is no longer commercially available, while pCLE does not meet these thresholds [43]. A meta-analysis recently showed that VLE is associated with a marginal increase in detection of HGD/cancer and has very high rates of false positive results [55]. However, OCT and VLE can evaluate epithelial thickness and buried glands, which can predict prolonged or failed ablation, and be useful in post-endoscopic ablation surveillance [56, 57]. The clinical applicability of these AIMs needs to be better defined before recommending their routine use in surveillance of BE.

Gastric Intestinal Metaplasia, Dysplasia, and Cancer

Rationale of Screening and Surveillance

Gastric cancer (GC) is one of the most frequent and lethal malignancies worldwide. The introduction of universal screening in Korea and Japan is associated with earlier GC diagnosis and lower cancer-related mortality [58–60]. Thus, universal screening is warranted in individuals from high-incidence countries, but is more selective in low-incidence countries based on demographic data and *Helicobacter pylori* status [61]. This translates in higher rates of early GC diagnosis – lesion confined to the mucosa or submucosa – in countries with national screening programs compared to Western countries (60 vs. 20%), which can be safely treated by mucosal or submucosal endoscopic resection [62, 63].

Compared with noninvasive tests, endoscopy is the best and most cost-effective screening modality to detect precancerous lesions and GC [64]. The development of intestinal-type GC is preceded by a cascade of several precancerous events that range from non-atrophic gastritis, multifocal atrophic gastritis (AG), IM, dysplasia, and ultimately GC [65]. Management and surveillance intervals are determined based on the individual histologic risk of progression into GC. A population study from the Netherlands illustrated this by showing an annual incidence of GC of 0.2% for AG, 0.3% for IM, 0.6% for mild-moderate dysplasia, and 6% for severe dysplasia [66]. The risk of GC with AG and IM can then be further stratified based upon location, severity, and extension of the lesion. Patients with widespread atrophy or IM pose high risk of cancer and require endoscopic surveillance every 3 years. Patients with LGD should be followed every 12 months, while those with HGD should be followed every 6 months or have the lesion resected [67].

Endoscopic Evaluation of Stomach Lesions

Endoscopic findings suggestive of superficial lesions such as light changes in color (redness or pale faded), irregularities of mucosal folds, absence of submucosal vessel pattern, and spontaneous bleeding should be carefully examined (Fig. 1.4a) [68]. Well-demarcated border or irregularity in color/surface pattern is more suggestive of malignant lesions. However, the sensitivity of WLE for identifying GC is ~80% and can miss

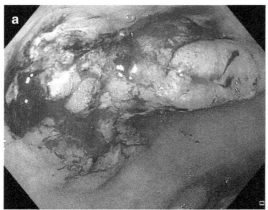

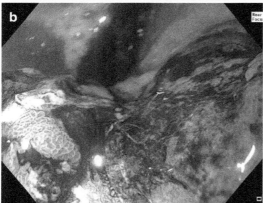

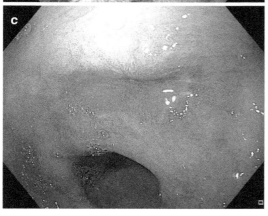

Fig. 1.4 Representative endoscopic images of gastric neoplasia. (**a**) Paris Is and IIc friable gastric mass. (**b**) Ulcerated gastric mass with abnormal NBI pattern. (**c**) Chromoendoscopy with methylene blue determining outer margins of early gastric cancer that was ultimately resected

small or flat lesions [68]. If endoscopic examination is normal, at least five nontargeted biopsies should be obtained according to the Sydney system in the antrum (×2), incisura angularis

(×1), and body (×2) [69]. Biopsy specimens should be submitted in separate jars labeled by region of the stomach sampled. This protocol is sensitive for detection of atrophic gastritis and intestinal metaplasia when performed in high-risk populations [70].

Role of Virtual and Conventional Chromoendoscopy

After recognition of suspicious lesions with WLE, virtual and conventional chromoendoscopy help in lesion characterization and highlight lesion outer margins (Fig. 1.4b, c). Diagnostic accuracy of NBI is maximized with magnifying endoscopy, by analyzing the microvascular and microsurface patterns separately. In a recent meta-analysis of 14 studies, magnifying NBI showed high sensitivity (86%) and specificity (96%) for detection of early GC [71]. This showed to be especially helpful for depressed or small lesions ≤10 mm in size, which can be more accurate than with conventional chromoendoscopy [71, 72]. Magnifying NBI can also delineate the lateral margins of a lesion even when conventional chromoendoscopy is not able to determine the margins [73]. Further research is needed to establish a standard NBI classification system to reduce various biases and improve its diagnostic accuracy in the assessment of gastric lesions. For example, fine network patterns with abundant microvessels connected one to another are characteristic of adenocarcinoma, and a corkscrew pattern with tortuous isolated microvessels is characteristic of poorly differentiated adenocarcinoma. Conventional chromoendoscopy with indigo carmine and acetic acid has been used in clinical practice for evaluation of gastric lesions, but delineation of margins is not superior to NBI.

Role of AFI and CLE

The role of other AIMs has not been fully established in the screening or surveillance of GC. AFI has limited clinical value due to its high false positive rate and low specificity. CLE has shown encouraging results for the in vivo diagnosis of premalignant lesions and early gastric cancer [74].

Duodenal Adenomas and Cancer

Rationale for Screening and Surveillance

Duodenal cancer is rare among all GI malignancies. For several years, it has been recognized that this malignancy arises from an adenoma-to-carcinoma pathway similar to colorectal cancer (CRC) [75]. Duodenal adenomas should be categorized as being ampullary or non-ampullary and as sporadic or arising in the context of familial adenomatous polyposis (FAP). The lifetime risk of duodenal cancer in patients with FAP is 5–10%, while in the general population, it ranges from 0.01% to 0.04% [76]. In addition, duodenal adenomas are diagnosed in up to 90% of FAP patients, can be multiple, and involve the ampulla. Thus, endoscopic screening and surveillance are recommended in FAP patients [77].

Endoscopic Evaluation

Endoscopic evaluation should be performed using a distal attachment cap and often requires a duodenoscope to definitively determine lesion relationship to the major and minor papilla. Morphologic features including the size of the lesion, number of folds affected, percent of circumference involved, and Paris classification should be determined to decide on management (surveillance, endoscopic resection, or surgery) (Fig. 1.5a, b).

The Spigelman staging system is widely used to evaluate the severity of duodenal polyposis and consists of a five-grade scale (0 to IV) based on polyp burden (number, size, histologic type, and degree of dysplasia) [78]. The 10-year risk of cancer can be as high as 36% for Spigelman stage IV disease, but much lower (≤2%) for lower stages [79]. Thus, endoscopic staging helps to determine the surveillance and treatment strategies for FAP patients with duodenal adenomas [77].

Diagnosis of adenoma with HDWLE and forceps biopsies is highly sensitive (>90%), but the sensitivity for detection of adenocarcinoma is lower, and biopsies can miss up to 30% of ampullary cancers [80, 81]. Cancer should be suspected in the presence of irregular margins,

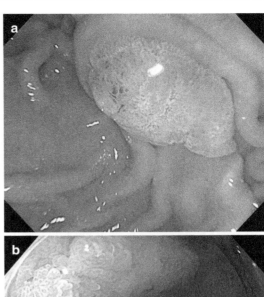

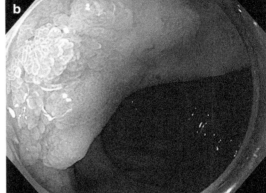

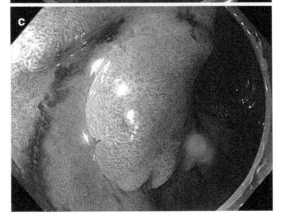

Fig. 1.5 Duodenal lesions. (**a**) Ampullary adenoma examined with duodenoscope. (**b**) Large duodenal adenoma in the second portion of the duodenum using forward view endoscope and a distal attachment cap. (**c**) Representative image of duodenal adenoma using NBI

ulceration, friability, or induration. Polyps larger than 1 cm have also been associated with advanced histology.

Role of Advanced Imaging Modalities

NBI is helpful for detection of duodenal adenomas. Predictive features of adenoma include the presence of dense white villi, large duodenal villi, leaf-shaped villi, or irregular vascular pattern (Fig. 1.5c) [81, 82]. Conventional chromoendoscopy has not been well studied for duodenal adenomas, but could be used if NBI or virtual chromoendoscopy is not available [83]. Two studies have demonstrated that real-time readings provided with pCLE have a high degree of diagnostic value when histology is used as the gold standard and may have higher sensitivity than NBI [83, 84]. Endoscopic ultrasound and endoscopic retrograde cholangiopancreatography can assess if ampullary adenomas have intraductal extension, which could preclude ampullectomy.

Recognition of Lesions in the Lower GI Tract

Colon Polyps and Colorectal Cancer

Rationale for Screening and Surveillance of Colorectal Cancer

Colorectal cancer (CRC) is the third most common cancer in men and women [85]. Colon polyps are the precursor lesion and progress to cancer via the adenoma-carcinoma sequence (adenoma) or the serrated pathway (sessile serrated adenoma (SSA) or traditional serrated adenoma) [86]. With the implementation of CRC screening programs and polypectomy, the incidence and mortality of CRC have declined [87–90]. Therefore, endoscopic detection, diagnosis, and adequate resection of polyps are critical steps for prevention of CRC. Colonoscopy techniques to improve adenoma detection rates go beyond the aims of this chapter, but use of virtual or conventional chromoendoscopy does not seem to reduce missed polyp rates compared with WLE [91, 92].

Histologic Prediction of Polyps During Colonoscopy

After a polyp is found during colonoscopy, careful evaluation and classification can help histologic prediction. Diminutive polyps (≤5 mm) represent 70–80% of all resected polyps, approximately 50% are adenomas, and rarely harbor advanced histology such as villous features and HGD (1.1–3.4%) or cancer (0–0.08%) [93–95]. If diminutive polyp histology can be determined optically in real time without the expense of pathologic examination, significant cost reduction can be achieved without compromising clinical decision-making or quality.

Optical histologic diagnosis of diminutive polyps has led to the proposal of a "resect and discard" strategy for diminutive polyps determined to be adenomatous and a "do not resect" strategy if characterized as non-adenomatous. An ASGE PIVI statement has proposed thresholds that are needed to be met to follow these strategies: (1) For diminutive rectosigmoid non-adenomatous polyps to not be removed, the negative predictive value for adenoma should be greater than 90%. (2) For any type of diminutive polyps to be resected and discarded, there should be correct predication of surveillance interval accuracy greater than 90% [96].

Role of Advanced Imaging Modalities for Histologic Prediction of Colonic Lesions

Optical diagnosis cannot be achieved by the sole use of HDWLE. Adenomas have reddish appearance, while hyperplastic polyps are whiter. Sessile serrated adenomas (SSAs) are often flat, larger in size, covered by a mucus cap, and surrounded by a rim of debris, display a lacy vessel pattern, and have indistinct borders. There is strong evidence that discrimination between adenomatous and serrated polyps can be improved with conventional or virtual chromoendoscopy [97]. NBI has been extensively studied, and in expert hands it can meet the thresholds proposed by the ASGE PIVI statement [97, 98]. NBI-assisted optical diagnosis by non-experts has shown equivocal results in comparison to the PIVI thresholds and cannot currently be recommended for routine use outside of expert centers [95, 99]. Other virtual chromoendoscopy technologies such as iScan and FICE have also shown high reliability for optical diagnosis

[100]. Diagnostic accuracy with CLE appears to be as good as with NBI, but unsatisfactory with AFI [100].

Several classification systems have been developed for the assessment of colon polyps with NBI and chromoendoscopy (Table 1.3 and Fig. 1.6). The Kudo classification was the first to be developed and helps making in vivo histologic diagnosis of polyps based on surface pit pattern [101]. Pit patterns can be grouped into three basic types: (1) Kudo I and II have round/stellar pits and represent non-neoplastic lesions; (2) Kudo IIIs, IIIL, IV, and selected cases of Vi correspond to adenomas and cancers with superficial submucosal invasion (SMI) that are endoscopically treatable; and (3) Kudo Vn and some Vi harbor cancer with SMI and are not amenable for endoscopic resection. The NBI International Colorectal Endoscopic (NICE) classification gives a simplified and standardized system for optical diagnosis of polyps based on lesion color, surface pit pattern, and vascular pattern [102]. NICE type I is found with hyperplastic polyps and SSAs, type II in adenomas, and type III in CRC with SMI. In the most recent Workgroup serrAted polypS and Polyposis (WASP) classification system, an additional category is created to differentiate hyperplastic polyps and SSAs, due to the higher malignant potential for SSAs [103].

Endoscopic Prediction of Invasive Cancer and Determination of Resectability

Because of the unique absence of lymphatics in the colonic mucosa, CRC is defined as invasion of dysplastic cells in the submucosa (SMI), and lesions confined to the mucosa are better named LGD or HGD instead of "carcinoma in situ" or "intramucosal adenocarcinoma" [104]. Endoscopic resection is adequate for lesions with LGD or HGD, but lesions with SMI are associated with 1–16% risk of lymphovascular invasion (LVI), and further stratification is needed to determine if endoscopic

Table 1.3 Kudo, NICE, and WASP classification of colon polyps

Histology	Kudo pit pattern	NICE[a]	WASP[b]
Normal	**Type I** Round		
Hyperplastic	**Type II** Star-like, papillary	**Type I** *Color* Same or lighter relative to background *Vessels* None or isolated lacy vessels coursing across lesion *Surface pattern* Dark or white spots of uniform size or homogenous absence of pattern	**Sessile serrated adenoma** *If >2 features:* 1. Cloud-like surface 2. Indistinct borders 3. Irregular shape 4. Dark spots inside crypts
Adenoma	**Type III** Tubular/roundish IIIS small IIIL large	**Type II** *Color* Browner than background *Vessels* Brown vessels surrounding white structures	
	Type IV Gyrus-like, branched	*Surface pattern* Oval, tubular, or branched white structures surrounded by brown vessels	
Deep submucosal invasive cancer	**Type V** Vi irregular Vn non-structural	**Type III** *Color* Brown to dark brown relative to background *Vessels* Areas with distorted or missing vessels *Surface pattern* Amorphous or absent surface pattern	

[a]NICE – NBI International Colorectal Endoscopic classification system
[b]WASP – Workgroup serrAted polypS and Polyposis

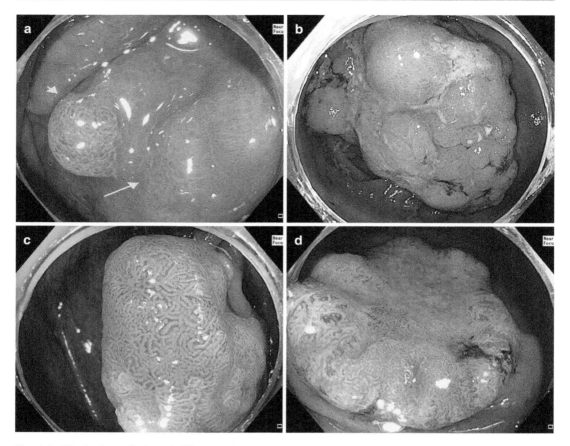

Fig. 1.6 Histologic prediction of different colon types. (**a**) Paris Is and IIb polyp, with Kudo II and IV pattern consistent with simultaneous serrated and tubulovillous histology. (**b**) Laterally spreading tumor with Kudo IIIs pattern consistent with tubular adenoma. (**c**) Kudo IV pattern consistent with tubulovillous histology. (**d**) Paris Is-IIc laterally spreading non granular tumor, with Kudo V and NICE III pattern. These features predicted submucosal invasion and endoscopic unresectability

resection is the adequate therapy [105]. Lesions with low-risk features such as superficial SMI (depth < 1 mm), well-differentiated tumor grade, and absence of LVI can be adequately treated endoscopically.

Real-time endoscopic prediction of SMI risk is essential before endoscopic resection is attempted [106]. The Paris classification of superficial neoplasia should be used for morphologic classification. Flat or sessile lesions larger than 10 mm can be designated as laterally spreading lesions (LSL) and can then be further categorized based on their surface topography into granular (G), nongranular (NG), or mixed morphologies. Focal interrogation of the pit pattern and vascular patterns with virtual or conventional chromoendoscopy is critical to further assess their risk of deep SMI. Factors associated with SMI include Kudo pit pattern V, NICE III pattern, a depressed component (0-IIc), rectosigmoid location, 0-Is or 0-IIa + Is Paris classification, nongranular surface morphology, and increasing size [107, 108]. The "non-lifting sign" is also associated with SMI but can also be found in submucosal fibrosis from prior biopsies or polypectomy attempts [109].

Colorectal Dysplasia and Cancer in Inflammatory Bowel Disease

Rationale for Dysplasia Surveillance

Patients with inflammatory bowel disease (IBD) have twofold higher risk of developing CRC compared with the general population [110].

Chronic inflammation, free radicals, and cytokines lead to genetic alterations and eventually dysplasia, which can then transition to CRC in IBD patients [111]. Thus, clinical practice guidelines recommended dysplasia surveillance to prevent CRC in patients with left-sided or extensive ulcerative colitis (UC) and for colonic Crohn's disease (CD) [112]. The efficacy of this approach has not been studied in clinical trials, but several population and observational studies have demonstrated reduction in cancer development and death associated with CRC in patients undergoing endoscopic surveillance [113–115].

Endoscopic Surveillance with High-Definition Endoscopy

Detection of dysplasia in IBD patients traditionally relied on WLE and extensive random biopsies (four every 10 cm) to identify invisible dysplasia [112]. The principle for this strategy was that dysplasia was often not accompanied by visible mucosal abnormalities during the fiberoptic endoscopy era. However, this has been increasingly disputed, and a systematic review revealed that in IBD patients with dysplasia, 80% are visible with standard WLE and 90% are visible with HDWLE or chromoendoscopy [116]. In addition, random biopsies are time consuming, distracting, expensive, and low yield – 1 episode of dysplasia detected for every 1505 random biopsies [117]. For these reasons, a targeted biopsy strategy has been developed and has been found to be superior to random biopsies for detection of neoplasia [118]. Despite these data, random biopsies have not yet been abandoned, and future studies should evaluate the incremental yield to targeted biopsies for dysplasia detection.

Recently, an international multidisciplinary group of 21 experts developed a consensus document aimed to optimize strategies for detection of dysplasia in IBD patients [116]. One of the key recommendations of this paramount document is to perform HDWLE instead of standard WLE for dysplasia surveillance of IBD patients. This is based on results from a retrospective observational study that found dysplasia to be found twice in patients undergoing HDWLE compared with those having standard WLE [3].

Uniform Terminology of Dysplasia

The SCENIC consensus also proposes that the terms dysplasia-associated lesion or mass (DALM) and adenoma-like lesion or mass (ALM) should no longer be used, and instead dysplasia should be described as visible or invisible. Visible lesions can be described using the Paris classification. Lesion margins should also be carefully examined. Dysplasia identified on random biopsies without a visible lesion should be defined as invisible dysplasia. Polypoid dysplastic lesions that occur proximal to areas affected by inflammation can be assumed to be sporadic adenomas.

Conventional Chromoendoscopy for IBD Surveillance

Another key recommendation of the SCENIC consensus is to use conventional chromoendoscopy rather than standard-definition WLE for surveillance of IBD patients [116]. A recent systematic review of randomized controlled trials recently confirmed this statement and showed that conventional chromoendoscopy identifies more patients with dysplasia compared to standard WLE [119]. This meta-analysis also showed that conventional chromoendoscopy was not superior to HDWLE or NBI. This has also been suggested in a recent randomized controlled trial, which showed that HDWLE and virtual chromoendoscopy in expert hands are not inferior to conventional chromoendoscopy for detection of dysplasia or cancer [120]. A large "real-life" retrospective cohort also recently showed that implementation of conventional chromoendoscopy in clinical practice does not increase dysplasia detection compared with WLE with targeted and random biopsies [121]. Thus, there is still debate whether conventional chromoendoscopy should be adopted in all surveillance colonoscopies for IBD patients as it adds time and costs, and requires additional endoscopic training.

When conventional chromoendoscopy is used, visible lesions should be categorized using the crypt architecture with the Kudo pit pattern classification (Fig. 1.7). The two main stains are indigo carmine and methylene blue. Pancolonic rather than local staining is recommended, using

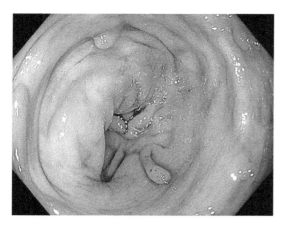

Fig. 1.7 Chromoendoscopy in IBD. Chromoendoscopy with methylene blue in a patient with well-controlled pan-ulcerative colitis, showing pseudopolyposis with Kudo I pattern

a spasmolytic if needed during withdrawal, excluding patients with active disease or inadequate bowel preparation. Pancolonic staining involves circumferential application of 250 mL of diluted dye (indigo carmine 0.3–0.1% or methylene blue 0.4–0.1%) throughout the colon after cecal intubation, using the water pump irrigation system or a spray catheter. Once a suspicious lesion is identified, approximately 30 mL of a more concentrated dye (indigo carmine 0.13% or methylene blue 0.2%) should be sprayed directly from a 60 mL syringe through the biopsy channel [116].

Virtual Chromoendoscopy and Other Technologies

NBI has not been shown to improve dysplasia detection compared with standard WLE, HDWLE, or conventional chromoendoscopy and is not recommended for surveillance of IBD patients [116]. Current endomicroscopic tools allow precise prediction of neoplasia on IBD by obtaining optical biopsies in real time, but several barriers limit their routine use in clinical practice [122]. The use of full-spectrum endoscopy (FUSE), a novel technology that incorporates two additional lateral cameras for 330° panoramic views, and stool DNA analysis, appear as promising tools for dysplasia detection in IBD patients but are not yet ready for clinical use [123, 124].

Training in AIMS

Medical societies have started to move away from a fixed time-based training to a system of competency-based education. This is structured on different assumptions: (1) people learn in different ways; (2) learners achieve competency at different rates; and (3) competency must be assessed against a fixed criterion rather than comparison against the performance of other learners or experts. Competency-based education of AIMs should be incorporated in gastroenterology fellowship training and needs development for those gastroenterologists already in practice. Training in AIMs can be obtained through classroom training programs or self-directed computer-based training modules [125]. A large body of evidence suggests that the use of these training methods in ex vivo and in vivo performance can lead trainees and academic or community endoscopists to meet the thresholds set forth by the ASGE for characterizing colon polyps with NBI examination [95, 126, 127]. These training methods are only moderately accurate among trainees for detecting neoplasia in BE with NBI [128]. Data for other AIMs is very limited to absent [129]. Future studies should assess training methods and learning curves needed to reach competency of individual AIMs in neoplasia detection and lesion characterization in the esophagus, stomach, duodenum, and colon. In the meantime, these training methods, in addition to image/video atlases, endoscopy simulators, and skill maintenance programs, should be used for motivated endoscopists.

Future Directions and Conclusions

The field of gastrointestinal endoscopy has evolved since the introduction of video endoscopy 25 years ago, with development of several advanced imaging modalities and other technologies that allow better lesion recognition and characterization. Future studies should focus on cost-effectiveness, training, and competency in the use of AIMs. The role of newer technologies such as autofluorescence, CLE, OCT, and VLE still needs to be better determined before adoption in clinical practice. In the near future, molecular imaging may allow for more accurate in vivo diagnosis and prediction of patients with higher risk of progression into neoplasia before morphologic changes develop.

References

1. Hirschowitz BI, Peters CW, Curtiss LE. Preliminary report on a long fiberscope for examination of stomach and duodenum. Med Bull (Ann Arbor). 1957;23:178–80.
2. Catalano MF, Van Dam J, Bedford R, et al. Preliminary evaluation of the prototype stereoscopic endoscope: precise three-dimensional measurement system. Gastrointest Endosc. 1993;39:23–8.
3. Subramanian V, Ragunath K. Advanced endoscopic imaging: a review of commercially available technologies. Clin Gastroenterol Hepatol. 2014;12:368–76.e1.
4. Waye JD, Aisenberg J, Rubin PH. Practical colonoscopy. 1st ed. Wiley-Blackwell: Oxford, UK; 2013.
5. Udagawa T, Amano M, Okada F. Development of magnifying video endoscopies with high resolution. Dig Endosc. 2001;13:163–9.
6. Committee AT, Kwon RS, Adler DG, et al. High-resolution and high-magnification endoscopes. Gastrointest Endosc. 2009;69:399–407.
7. Committee AT. High-definition and high-magnification endoscopes. Gastrointest Endosc. 2014;80:919–27.
8. Kaltenbach T, Shergill AK, Wallace MB. How to obtain and use chromoendoscopy dyes for surveillance colonoscopy in inflammatory bowel disease: a technical guide. Gastrointest Endosc. 2017;86:949–51.
9. Shimizu Y, Takahashi M, Mizushima T, et al. Chromoendoscopy with iodine staining, as well as narrow-band imaging, is still useful and reliable for screening of early esophageal squamous cell carcinoma. Am J Gastroenterol. 2015;110:193–4.
10. Lambert R, Rey JF, Sankaranarayanan R. Magnification and chromoscopy with the acetic acid test. Endoscopy. 2003;35:437–45.
11. Mizuno H, Gono K, Takehana S, et al. Narrow band imaging technique. Tech Gastrointest Endosc. 2003;5:78–81.
12. Pohl J, May A, Rabenstein T, et al. Computed virtual chromoendoscopy: a new tool for enhancing tissue surface structures. Endoscopy. 2007;39:80–3.
13. Kodashima S. Novel image-enhanced endoscopy with i-scan technology. World J Gastroenterol. 2010;16:1043.
14. Osawa H, Yamamoto H. Present and future status of flexible spectral imaging color enhancement and blue laser imaging technology. Dig Endosc. 2014;26(Suppl 1):105–15.
15. Committee AT, Song LM, Banerjee S, et al. Autofluorescence imaging. Gastrointest Endosc. 2011;73:647–50.
16. Wang TD. Confocal microscopy from the bench to the bedside. Gastrointest Endosc. 2005;62:696–7.
17. Committee AT. Confocal laser endomicroscopy. Gastrointest Endosc. 2014;80:928–38.
18. Kiesslich R, Goetz M, Hoffman A, et al. New imaging techniques and opportunities in endoscopy. Nat Rev Gastroenterol Hepatol. 2011;8:547–53.
19. Committee AT. Enhanced imaging in the GI tract: spectroscopy and optical coherence tomography. Gastrointest Endosc. 2013;78:568–73.
20. Goetz M, Wang TD. Molecular imaging in gastrointestinal endoscopy. Gastroenterology. 2010;138:828–33.e1.
21. Joshi BP, Pant A, Duan X, et al. Multimodal video colonoscope for targeted wide-field detection of nonpolypoid colorectal neoplasia. Gastroenterology. 2016;150:1084–6.
22. Arnold M, Soerjomataram I, Ferlay J, et al. Global incidence of oesophageal cancer by histological subtype in 2012. Gut. 2015;64:381–7.
23. Rustgi AK, El-Serag HB. Esophageal carcinoma. N Engl J Med. 2014;371:2499–509.
24. Pennathur A, Gibson MK, Jobe BA, et al. Oesophageal carcinoma. Lancet. 2013;381:400–12.
25. Shaheen NJ, Falk GW, Iyer PG, et al. ACG clinical guideline: diagnosis and management of Barrett's esophagus. Am J Gastroenterol. 2016;111:30–50; quiz 51.
26. Cameron AJ, Carpenter HA. Barrett's esophagus, high-grade dysplasia, and early adenocarcinoma: a pathological study. Am J Gastroenterol. 1997;92:586–91.
27. Fitzgerald RC, di Pietro M, Ragunath K, et al. British Society of Gastroenterology guidelines on the diagnosis and management of Barrett's oesophagus. Gut. 2014;63:7–42.
28. Weusten B, Bisschops R, Coron E, et al. Endoscopic management of Barrett's esophagus: European Society of Gastrointestinal Endoscopy (ESGE) Position Statement. Endoscopy. 2017;49:191–8.
29. Verbeek RE, Leenders M, Ten Kate FJ, et al. Surveillance of Barrett's esophagus and mortality from esophageal adenocarcinoma: a population-based cohort study. Am J Gastroenterol. 2014;109:1215–22.
30. Spechler SJ, Sharma P, Souza RF, et al. American Gastroenterological Association technical review on the management of Barrett's esophagus. Gastroenterology. 2011;140:e18–52; quiz e13
31. Abrams JA, Kapel RC, Lindberg GM, et al. Adherence to biopsy guidelines for Barrett's esophagus surveillance in the community setting in the United States. Clin Gastroenterol Hepatol. 2009;7:736–42.. quiz 710

32. Wani S, Mathur SC, Curvers WL, et al. Greater interobserver agreement by endoscopic mucosal resection than biopsy samples in Barrett's dysplasia. Clin Gastroenterol Hepatol. 2010;8:783–8.

33. Bennett C, Vakil N, Bergman J, et al. Consensus statements for management of Barrett's dysplasia and early-stage esophageal adenocarcinoma, based on a Delphi process. Gastroenterology. 2012;143:336–46.

34. Kara MA, Peters FP, Rosmolen WD, et al. High-resolution endoscopy plus chromoendoscopy or narrow-band imaging in Barrett's esophagus: a prospective randomized crossover study. Endoscopy. 2005;37:929–36.

35. Wani S, Muthusamy VR, Shaheen NJ, et al. Development of quality indicators for endoscopic eradication therapies in Barrett's esophagus: the TREAT-BE (Treatment With Resection and Endoscopic Ablation Techniques for Barrett's Esophagus) consortium. Am J Gastroenterol. 2017;112:1032–48.

36. Boerwinkel DF, Swager A, Curvers WL, et al. The clinical consequences of advanced imaging techniques in Barrett's esophagus. Gastroenterology. 2014;146:622–629.e4.

37. Sharma P, Dent J, Armstrong D, et al. The development and validation of an endoscopic grading system for Barrett's esophagus: the Prague C & M criteria. Gastroenterology. 2006;131:1392–9.

38. Reid BJ, Blount PL, Feng Z, et al. Optimizing endoscopic biopsy detection of early cancers in Barrett's high-grade dysplasia. Am J Gastroenterol. 2000;95:3089–96.

39. Moss A, Bourke MJ, Hourigan LF, et al. Endoscopic resection for Barrett's high-grade dysplasia and early esophageal adenocarcinoma: an essential staging procedure with long-term therapeutic benefit. Am J Gastroenterol. 2010;105:1276–83.

40. Wani S, Abrams J, Edmundowicz SA, et al. Endoscopic mucosal resection results in change of histologic diagnosis in Barrett's esophagus patients with visible and flat neoplasia: a multicenter cohort study. Dig Dis Sci. 2013;58:1703–9.

41. Paris Workshop on Columnar Metaplasia in the Esophagus and the Esophagogastric Junction, Paris, France, December 11–12 2004. Endoscopy 2005;37:879–920.

42. Sharma P, Savides TJ, Canto MI, et al. The American Society for Gastrointestinal Endoscopy PIVI (Preservation and Incorporation of Valuable Endoscopic Innovations) on imaging in Barrett's esophagus. Gastrointest Endosc. 2012;76:252–4.

43. Committee AT, Thosani N, Abu Dayyeh BK, et al. ASGE Technology Committee systematic review and meta-analysis assessing the ASGE Preservation and Incorporation of Valuable Endoscopic Innovations thresholds for adopting real-time imaging-assisted endoscopic targeted biopsy during endoscopic surveillance of Barrett's esophagus. Gastrointest Endosc. 2016;83:684–98.e7.

44. Qumseya BJ, Wang H, Badie N, et al. Advanced imaging technologies increase detection of dysplasia and neoplasia in patients with Barrett's esophagus: a meta-analysis and systematic review. Clin Gastroenterol Hepatol. 2013;11:1562–70.e1–2.

45. Hoffman A, Korczynski O, Tresch A, et al. Acetic acid compared with i-scan imaging for detecting Barrett's esophagus: a randomized, comparative trial. Gastrointest Endosc. 2014;79:46–54.

46. Sharma P, Hawes RH, Bansal A, et al. Standard endoscopy with random biopsies versus narrow band imaging targeted biopsies in Barrett's oesophagus: a prospective, international, randomised controlled trial. Gut. 2013;62:15–21.

47. Sharma P, Bansal A, Mathur S, et al. The utility of a novel narrow band imaging endoscopy system in patients with Barrett's esophagus. Gastrointest Endosc. 2006;64:167–75.

48. Kara MA, Ennahachi M, Fockens P, et al. Detection and classification of the mucosal and vascular patterns (mucosal morphology) in Barrett's esophagus by using narrow band imaging. Gastrointest Endosc. 2006;64:155–66.

49. Singh R, Anagnostopoulos GK, Yao K, et al. Narrow-band imaging with magnification in Barrett's esophagus: validation of a simplified grading system of mucosal morphology patterns against histology. Endoscopy. 2008;40:457–63.

50. Sharma P, Bergman JJ, Goda K, et al. Development and validation of a classification system to identify high-grade dysplasia and esophageal adenocarcinoma in Barrett's esophagus using narrow-band imaging. Gastroenterology. 2016;150:591–8.

51. Ngamruengphong S, Sharma VK, Das A. Diagnostic yield of methylene blue chromoendoscopy for detecting specialized intestinal metaplasia and dysplasia in Barrett's esophagus: a meta-analysis. Gastrointest Endosc. 2009;69:1021–8.

52. Olliver JR, Wild CP, Sahay P, et al. Chromoendoscopy with methylene blue and associated DNA damage in Barrett's oesophagus. Lancet. 2003;362:373–4.

53. Wani S, Gaddam S. Editorial: best practices in surveillance of Barrett's esophagus. Am J Gastroenterol. 2017;112:1056–60.

54. Muthusamy VR, Kim S, Wallace MB. Advanced imaging in Barrett's esophagus. Gastroenterol Clin North Am. 2015;44:439–58.

55. Qumseya BJ, Gendy S, Qumsiyeh Y, et al. Marginal increase in dysplasia detection and very high false positive rate for volumetric laser endomicroscopy in Barrett's esophagus: systemic review and meta-analysis. Gastrointest Endosc. 2017;85:AB554.

56. Tsai TH, Zhou C, Tao YK, et al. Structural markers observed with endoscopic 3-dimensional optical coherence tomography correlating with Barrett's esophagus radiofrequency ablation treatment response (with videos). Gastrointest Endosc. 2012;76:1104–12.

57. Adler DC, Zhou C, Tsai TH, et al. Three-dimensional optical coherence tomography of Barrett's esopha-

gus and buried glands beneath neosquamous epithelium following radiofrequency ablation. Endoscopy. 2009;41:773–6.

58. Nagata T, Ikeda M, Nakayama F. Changing state of gastric cancer in Japan. Histologic perspective of the past 76 years. Am J Surg. 1983;145:226–33.

59. Hamashima C, Ogoshi K, Okamoto M, et al. A community-based, case-control study evaluating mortality reduction from gastric cancer by endoscopic screening in Japan. PLoS One. 2013;8:e79088.

60. Jun JK, Choi KS, Lee HY, et al. Effectiveness of the Korean National Cancer Screening Program in Reducing Gastric Cancer Mortality. Gastroenterology. 2017;152:1319–1328.e7.

61. Lin JT. Screening of gastric cancer: who, when, and how. Clin Gastroenterol Hepatol. 2014;12:135–8.

62. Noguchi Y, Yoshikawa T, Tsuburaya A, et al. Is gastric carcinoma different between Japan and the United States? Cancer. 2000;89:2237–46.

63. Pyo JH, Lee H, Min BH, et al. Long-term outcome of endoscopic resection vs. surgery for early gastric cancer: a non-inferiority-matched cohort study. Am J Gastroenterol. 2016;111:240–9.

64. Tashiro A, Sano M, Kinameri K, et al. Comparing mass screening techniques for gastric cancer in Japan. World J Gastroenterol. 2006;12:4873–4.

65. Correa P. Human gastric carcinogenesis: a multistep and multifactorial process – First American Cancer Society Award Lecture on Cancer Epidemiology and Prevention. Cancer Res. 1992;52:6735–40.

66. de Vries AC, van Grieken NC, Looman CW, et al. Gastric cancer risk in patients with premalignant gastric lesions: a nationwide cohort study in the Netherlands. Gastroenterology. 2008;134:945–52.

67. Dinis-Ribeiro M, Areia M, de Vries AC, et al. Management of precancerous conditions and lesions in the stomach (MAPS): guideline from the European Society of Gastrointestinal Endoscopy (ESGE), European Helicobacter Study Group (EHSG), European Society of Pathology (ESP), and the Sociedade Portuguesa de Endoscopia Digestiva (SPED). Endoscopy. 2012;44:74–94.

68. Kim GH, Liang PS, Bang SJ, et al. Screening and surveillance for gastric cancer in the United States: is it needed? Gastrointest Endosc. 2016;84:18–28.

69. Dixon MF, Genta RM, Yardley JH, et al. Classification and grading of gastritis. The updated Sydney System. International Workshop on the Histopathology of Gastritis, Houston 1994. Am J Surg Pathol. 1996;20:1161–81.

70. Guarner J, Herrera-Goepfert R, Mohar A, et al. Diagnostic yield of gastric biopsy specimens when screening for preneoplastic lesions. Hum Pathol. 2003;34:28–31.

71. Hu YY, Lian QW, Lin ZH, et al. Diagnostic performance of magnifying narrow-band imaging for early gastric cancer: a meta-analysis. World J Gastroenterol. 2015;21:7884–94.

72. Fujiwara S, Yao K, Nagahama T, et al. Can we accurately diagnose minute gastric cancers (</=5 mm)? Chromoendoscopy (CE) vs magnifying endoscopy with narrow band imaging (M-NBI). Gastric Cancer. 2015;18:590–6.

73. Nagahama T, Yao K, Maki S, et al. Usefulness of magnifying endoscopy with narrow-band imaging for determining the horizontal extent of early gastric cancer when there is an unclear margin by chromoendoscopy (with video). Gastrointest Endosc. 2011;74:1259–67.

74. Li WB, Zuo XL, Li CQ, et al. Diagnostic value of confocal laser endomicroscopy for gastric superficial cancerous lesions. Gut. 2011;60:299–306.

75. Spigelman AD, Talbot IC, Penna C, et al. Evidence for adenoma-carcinoma sequence in the duodenum of patients with familial adenomatous polyposis. The Leeds Castle Polyposis Group (Upper Gastrointestinal Committee). J Clin Pathol. 1994;47:709–10.

76. Brosens LA, Keller JJ, Offerhaus GJ, et al. Prevention and management of duodenal polyps in familial adenomatous polyposis. Gut. 2005;54:1034–43.

77. Syngal S, Brand RE, Church JM, et al. ACG clinical guideline: genetic testing and management of hereditary gastrointestinal cancer syndromes. Am J Gastroenterol. 2015;110:223–62; quiz 263

78. Spigelman AD, Williams CB, Talbot IC, et al. Upper gastrointestinal cancer in patients with familial adenomatous polyposis. Lancet. 1989;2:783–5.

79. Groves CJ, Saunders BP, Spigelman AD, et al. Duodenal cancer in patients with familial adenomatous polyposis (FAP): results of a 10 year prospective study. Gut. 2002;50:636–41.

80. Sauvanet A, Chapuis O, Hammel P, et al. Are endoscopic procedures able to predict the benignity of ampullary tumors? Am J Surg. 1997;174:355–8.

81. Lopez-Ceron M, van den Broek FJ, Mathus-Vliegen EM, et al. The role of high-resolution endoscopy and narrow-band imaging in the evaluation of upper GI neoplasia in familial adenomatous polyposis. Gastrointest Endosc. 2013;77:542–50.

82. Uchiyama Y, Imazu H, Kakutani H, et al. New approach to diagnosing ampullary tumors by magnifying endoscopy combined with a narrow-band imaging system. J Gastroenterol. 2006;41:483–90.

83. Kiesslich R, Mergener K, Naumann C, et al. Value of chromoendoscopy and magnification endoscopy in the evaluation of duodenal abnormalities: a prospective, randomized comparison. Endoscopy. 2003;35:559–63.

84. Shahid MW, Buchner A, Gomez V, et al. Diagnostic accuracy of probe-based confocal laser endomicroscopy and narrow band imaging in detection of dysplasia in duodenal polyps. J Clin Gastroenterol. 2012;46:382–9.

85. Society AC. Cancer facts & figures. Am Cancer Soc. 2012;

86. Noffsinger AE. Serrated polyps and colorectal cancer: new pathway to malignancy. Annu Rev Pathol. 2009;4:343–64.

87. Rex DK, Boland CR, Dominitz JA, et al. Colorectal cancer screening: recommendations for physicians and patients from the U.S. Multi-Society Task Force on Colorectal Cancer. Gastroenterology. 2017;153:307–23.

88. Winawer SJ, Zauber AG, Ho MN, et al. Prevention of colorectal cancer by colonoscopic polypectomy. The National Polyp Study Workgroup. N Engl J Med. 1993;329:1977–81.

89. Holme O, Loberg M, Kalager M, et al. Effect of flexible sigmoidoscopy screening on colorectal cancer incidence and mortality: a randomized clinical trial. JAMA. 2014;312:606–15.

90. Schoen RE, Pinsky PF, Weissfeld JL, et al. Colorectal-cancer incidence and mortality with screening flexible sigmoidoscopy. N Engl J Med. 2012;366:2345–57.

91. Kahi CJ, Anderson JC, Waxman I, et al. High-definition chromocolonoscopy vs. high-definition white light colonoscopy for average-risk colorectal cancer screening. Am J Gastroenterol. 2010;105:1301–7.

92. Dinesen L, Chua TJ, Kaffes AJ. Meta-analysis of narrow-band imaging versus conventional colonoscopy for adenoma detection. Gastrointest Endosc. 2012;75:604–11.

93. Butterly LF, Chase MP, Pohl H, et al. Prevalence of clinically important histology in small adenomas. Clin Gastroenterol Hepatol. 2006;4:343–8.

94. Lieberman D, Moravec M, Holub J, et al. Polyp size and advanced histology in patients undergoing colonoscopy screening: implications for CT colonography. Gastroenterology. 2008;135:1100–5.

95. Patel SG, Schoenfeld P, Kim HM, et al. Real-time characterization of diminutive colorectal polyp histology using narrow-band imaging: implications for the resect and discard strategy. Gastroenterology. 2016;150:406–18.

96. Rex DK, Kahi C, O'Brien M, et al. The American Society for Gastrointestinal Endoscopy PIVI (Preservation and Incorporation of Valuable Endoscopic Innovations) on real-time endoscopic assessment of the histology of diminutive colorectal polyps. Gastrointest Endosc. 2011;73:419–22.

97. Committee AT, Abu Dayyeh BK, Thosani N, et al. ASGE Technology Committee systematic review and meta-analysis assessing the ASGE PIVI thresholds for adopting real-time endoscopic assessment of the histology of diminutive colorectal polyps. Gastrointest Endosc. 2015;81:502.e1–16.

98. McGill SK, Evangelou E, Ioannidis JP, et al. Narrow band imaging to differentiate neoplastic and non-neoplastic colorectal polyps in real time: a meta-analysis of diagnostic operating characteristics. Gut. 2013;62:1704–13.

99. Rees CJ, Rajasekhar PT, Wilson A, et al. Narrow band imaging optical diagnosis of small colorectal polyps in routine clinical practice: the Detect Inspect Characterise Resect and Discard 2 (DISCARD 2) study. Gut. 2017;66:887–95.

100. Wanders LK, East JE, Uitentuis SE, et al. Diagnostic performance of narrowed spectrum endoscopy, autofluorescence imaging, and confocal laser endomicroscopy for optical diagnosis of colonic polyps: a meta-analysis. Lancet Oncol. 2013;14:1337–47.

101. Kudo S, Hirota S, Nakajima T, et al. Colorectal tumours and pit pattern. J Clin Pathol. 1994;47:880–5.

102. Tanaka S, Sano Y. Aim to unify the narrow band imaging (NBI) magnifying classification for colorectal tumors: current status in Japan from a summary of the consensus symposium in the 79th Annual Meeting of the Japan Gastroenterological Endoscopy Society. Dig Endosc. 2011;23(Suppl 1):131–9.

103. IJspeert JE, Bastiaansen BA, van Leerdam ME, et al. Development and validation of the WASP classification system for optical diagnosis of adenomas, hyperplastic polyps and sessile serrated adenomas/polyps. Gut. 2016;65:963–70.

104. Rex DK, Hassan C, Bourke MJ. The colonoscopist's guide to the vocabulary of colorectal neoplasia: histology, morphology, and management. Gastrointest Endosc. 2017;86:253–63.

105. Bosch SL, Teerenstra S, de Wilt JH, et al. Predicting lymph node metastasis in pT1 colorectal cancer: a systematic review of risk factors providing rationale for therapy decisions. Endoscopy. 2013;45:827–34.

106. Moss A, Bourke MJ, Williams SJ, et al. Endoscopic mucosal resection outcomes and prediction of submucosal cancer from advanced colonic mucosal neoplasia. Gastroenterology. 2011;140:1909–18.

107. Hayashi N, Tanaka S, Hewett DG, et al. Endoscopic prediction of deep submucosal invasive carcinoma: validation of the narrow-band imaging international colorectal endoscopic (NICE) classification. Gastrointest Endosc. 2013;78:625–32.

108. Burgess NG, Hourigan LF, Zanati SA, et al. Risk stratification for covert invasive cancer among patients referred for colonic endoscopic mucosal resection: a large multicenter cohort. Gastroenterology. 2017;153:732–742.e1.

109. Uno Y, Munakata A. The non-lifting sign of invasive colon cancer. Gastrointest Endosc. 1994;40:485–9.

110. Jess T, Rungoe C, Peyrin-Biroulet L. Risk of colorectal cancer in patients with ulcerative colitis: a meta-analysis of population-based cohort studies. Clin Gastroenterol Hepatol. 2012;10:639–45.

111. Foersch S, Neurath MF. Colitis-associated neoplasia: molecular basis and clinical translation. Cell Mol Life Sci. 2014;71:3523–35.

112. Farraye FA, Odze RD, Eaden J, et al. AGA medical position statement on the diagnosis and management of colorectal neoplasia in inflammatory bowel disease. Gastroenterology. 2010;138:738–45.

113. Bye WA, Nguyen TM, Parker CE, et al. Strategies for detecting colon cancer in patients with inflammatory bowel disease. Cochrane Database Syst Rev. 2017;9:CD000279.

114. Ananthakrishnan AN, Cagan A, Cai T, et al. Colonoscopy is associated with a reduced risk for

colon cancer and mortality in patients with inflammatory bowel diseases. Clin Gastroenterol Hepatol. 2015;13:322–329.e1.

115. Choi CH, Rutter MD, Askari A, et al. Forty-year analysis of colonoscopic surveillance program for neoplasia in ulcerative colitis: an updated overview. Am J Gastroenterol. 2015;110:1022–34.

116. Laine L, Kaltenbach T, Barkun A, et al. SCENIC international consensus statement on surveillance and management of dysplasia in inflammatory bowel disease. Gastroenterology. 2015;148:639–651.e28.

117. East JE. Colonoscopic cancer surveillance in inflammatory bowel disease: what's new beyond random biopsy? Clin Endosc. 2012;45:274–7.

118. Gasia MF, Ghosh S, Panaccione R, et al. Targeted biopsies identify larger proportions of patients with colonic neoplasia undergoing high-definition colonoscopy, dye chromoendoscopy, or electronic virtual chromoendoscopy. Clin Gastroenterol Hepatol. 2016;14:704–12.e4.

119. Iannone A, Ruospo M, Wong G, et al. Chromoendoscopy for surveillance in ulcerative colitis and Crohn's disease: a systematic review of randomized trials. Clin Gastroenterol Hepatol. 2017;15:1684–1697.e11.

120. Iacucci M, Kaplan GG, Panaccione R, et al. A randomized trial comparing high definition colonoscopy alone with high definition dye spraying and electronic virtual chromoendoscopy for detection of colonic neoplastic lesions during IBD surveillance colonoscopy. Am J Gastroenterol. 2017;113:225–34.

121. Mooiweer E, van der Meulen-de Jong AE, Ponsioen CY, et al. Chromoendoscopy for surveillance in inflammatory bowel disease does not increase neoplasia detection compared with conventional colonoscopy with random biopsies: results from a large retrospective study. Am J Gastroenterol. 2015;110:1014–21.

122. Rasmussen DN, Karstensen JG, Riis LB, et al. Confocal laser Endomicroscopy in inflammatory bowel disease – a systematic review. J Crohns Colitis. 2015;9:1152–9.

123. Leong RW, Ooi M, Corte C, et al. Full-spectrum endoscopy improves surveillance for dysplasia in patients with inflammatory bowel diseases. Gastroenterology. 2017;152:1337–1344.e3.

124. Kisiel JB, Konijeti GG, Piscitello AJ, et al. Stool DNA analysis is cost-effective for colorectal cancer surveillance in patients with ulcerative colitis. Clin Gastroenterol Hepatol. 2016;14: 1778–1787.e8.

125. Gupta N, Brill JV, Canto M, et al. AGA white paper: training and implementation of endoscopic image enhancement technologies. Clin Gastroenterol Hepatol. 2017;15:820–6.

126. Patel SG, Rastogi A, Austin G, et al. Gastroenterology trainees can easily learn histologic characterization of diminutive colorectal polyps with narrow band imaging. Clin Gastroenterol Hepatol. 2013;11:997–1003.e1.

127. Rastogi A, Rao DS, Gupta N, et al. Impact of a computer-based teaching module on characterization of diminutive colon polyps by using narrow-band imaging by non-experts in academic and community practice: a video-based study. Gastrointest Endosc. 2014;79:390–8.

128. Daly C, Vennalaganti P, Soudagar S, et al. Randomized controlled trial of self-directed versus in-classroom teaching of narrow-band imaging for diagnosis of Barrett's esophagus-associated neoplasia. Gastrointest Endosc. 2016;83:101–6.

129. Rzouq F, Vennalaganti P, Pakseresht K, et al. In-class didactic versus self-directed teaching of the probe-based confocal laser endomicroscopy (pCLE) criteria for Barrett's esophagus. Endoscopy. 2016;48:123–7.

Samuel Han and Hazem Hammad

Introduction

Endoscopic mucosal resection (EMR) represents a widely used technique that allows for complete en bloc resection of lesions as large as 20 mm in diameter. It can be used in larger lesions via piecemeal resection and provides a diagnostic, therapeutic, and prognostic option for lesions throughout the gastrointestinal tract. The advantages of EMR include its relative simplicity, safety, and ability to obtain large samples in comparison to forceps biopsies [1]. It is a relatively quick procedure and can provide diagnostic information regarding the depth of invasion, degree of tumor differentiation, as well as presence or absence of lymphovascular invasion. The disadvantages of EMR include a higher

Electronic Supplementary Material The online version of this chapter (https://doi.org/10.1007/978-3-030-21695-5_2) contains supplementary material, which is available to authorized users.

S. Han
Division of Gastroenterology and Hepatology, University of Colorado Anschutz Medical Center, Aurora, CO, USA

H. Hammad (✉)
Division of Gastroenterology and Hepatology, Section of Therapeutic Endoscopy, University of Colorado Anschutz Medical Center and Veterans Affairs Eastern Colorado Health Care System, Aurora, CO, USA
e-mail: Hazem.Hammad@ucdenver.edu

recurrence rate and lower rate of en bloc resection in comparison to endoscopic submucosal dissection (ESD) [2, 3]. Additionally, while it does allow for piecemeal resection of large lesions, piecemeal resection does not allow for assessment of negative lateral margins, and cautery effects from repeated resections can hinder adequate histological evaluation [4, 5].

Historically, the concept of EMR was originally described in 1973, but became more popular in the 1980s, particularly in the management of colonic lesions [6, 7]. Inoue first performed an esophageal EMR in 1990 in Japan, and it was gradually incorporated into clinical practice in the West shortly thereafter [8]. This chapter will focus on the role of EMR in the esophagus, discuss its indications, technical details, safety, and efficacy, and comment on future directions, quality metrics, and training pathways.

Indications

Barrett's Esophagus and Esophageal Adenocarcinoma

In the West, EMR is primarily used in the esophagus for the diagnosis and treatment of Barrett's esophagus-related neoplasia (Figs. 2.1 and 2.2), a well-established precursor lesion for esophageal adenocarcinoma (EAC) [9, 10]. From a diagnostic perspective, EMR is recommended for all

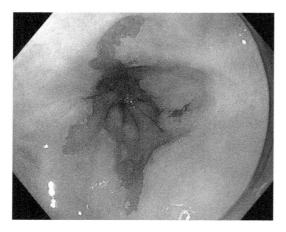

Fig. 2.1 Example of Barrett's esophagus using high-definition white-light endoscopy

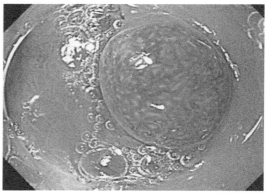

Fig. 2.3 Visible lesion under white-light endoscopy using near focus

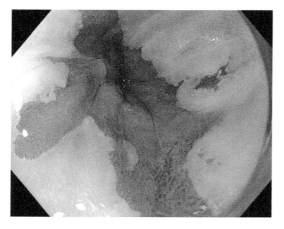

Fig. 2.2 Example of Barrett's esophagus under narrow-band imaging (NBI)

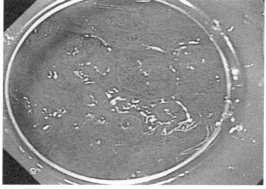

Fig. 2.4 Example of nodularity under white-light endoscopy

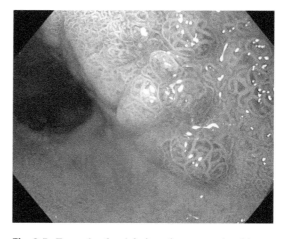

visible and nodular lesions (no matter how subtle) (Figs. 2.3, 2.4, and 2.5) in patients with Barrett's esophagus (BE) to determine the true histopathologic diagnosis [11–13]. Biopsy alone has been shown to frequently misdiagnose the true grade of dysplasia within a lesion, and studies have demonstrated that EMR will change the diagnosis in up to 30–40% of patients with early neoplasia [14–18]. Furthermore, EMR significantly increases the interobserver agreement between pathologists in the diagnosis of dysplasia compared to biopsy [19]. Given that accurate assessment of the grade of dysplasia is a critical step in determining the appropriate management step, EMR plays a critical role in the

Fig. 2.5 Example of nodularity using narrow-band imaging (NBI) with near focus

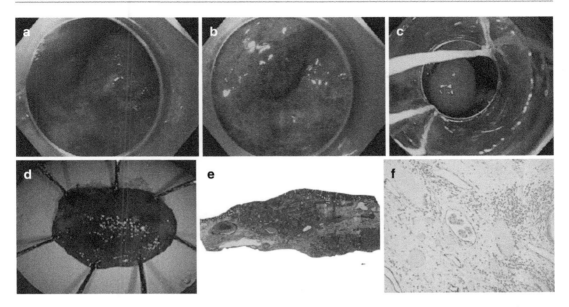

Fig. 2.6 EMR for diagnosis and management of nodular Barrett's. Footnote: (**a**) Nodular lesion under white-light endoscopy. (**b**) Nodular lesion under NBI. (**c**) Ligation-assisted EMR of nodular lesion. (**d**) Resection specimen. (**e**) Low-magnification histology demonstrating intramucosal carcinoma. (**f**) Lymphovascular invasion by intramucosal carcinoma

management of this patient population (see Fig. 2.6 for a full depiction of the use of EMR in Barrett's).

From a resection standpoint, EMR only allows for local removal of a lesion, highlighting the importance of proper selection of patients. Specifically in terms of BE, only patients with high-grade dysplasia or EAC limited to the mucosa (M1, confined to the epithelium; M2, confined to the lamina propria; or M3, invading the muscularis mucosae) with minimal risk of lymph node metastasis should be referred for EMR. The risk of lymph node metastasis for tumors limited to the mucosa has been reported as 0–3% [20].

Contention lies in EAC with submucosal involvement as esophagectomy has been considered the standard of care for quite some time given the high risk of lymph node involvement, but as will be discussed later in this chapter, certain superficial submucosal cancers may be amenable to EMR.

Currently, under the National Comprehensive Cancer Network guidelines, endoscopic therapy is recommended for patients with lesions limited to the epithelium (Tis or HGD), lamina propria, or muscularis mucosa (T1a). Endoscopic therapy can also be considered for lesions involving the superficial submucosa (T1b) – in lieu of esophagectomy – in the absence of lymph node metastasis, lymphovascular invasion, or poorly differentiated tumors. Discussion with the surgeon regarding the risk of esophagectomy vs. the risk of lymph node metastasis should also be undertaken [21]. The American Society for Gastrointestinal Endoscopy (ASGE) guidelines, for comparison, recommend endoscopic resection of all visible lesions (strong recommendation, moderate quality of evidence) while recommending against surgery in patients with high-grade dysplasia/intramucosal carcinoma (strong recommendation, very low quality of evidence) [22].

Squamous Cell Carcinoma

Esophageal EMR was one of the first endoscopic techniques described in removing early squamous cell carcinomas (SCCs) in the esophagus [23]. EMR remains a popular treatment option for SCC that is confined to the mucosa, which requires early detection given the ease of metastatic spread of SCC owing to the relatively thin wall of the esophagus as well as its rich lymphatic network. More common in Asia, it is associated with a poor prognosis, and EMR is indicated in SCC M1 and M2 lesions (confined to the epithelium or lamina propria) [24]. In M3 (invading the muscularis mucosae) or SM1 (invasion to the superficial third of the submucosa) lesions, EMR can be considered if there is no evidence of lymph node involvement. Similarly, ESD has shown complete resection rates of 78–100% of M1 and M2 lesions with low recurrence rates (0–2.6%), but like EMR is generally not utilized in SCC lesions with lymphovascular invasion or submucosal invasion >200 μm [25].

While ESD is not the focus of this chapter, it is important to note when comparing EMR to ESD in esophageal mucosal cancers 20 mm or less, ESD has been found to provide an en bloc resection rate of 100%, whereas for EMR it was 87% (cap assisted) and 71% (two-channel technique) [26, 27]. The curative resection rate for ESD was also 97%, significantly higher than either EMR technique (71% for cap and 46% for two-channel). Therefore, the European Society of Gastrointestinal Endoscopy (ESGE) recommends ESD as the preferred method of endoscopic resection of esophageal squamous cell carcinoma (ESCC) given the higher en bloc resection rate and superior histological assessment [28]. EMR can be used for lesions smaller than 10 mm if en bloc resection can be assured. For early EAC and HGD, EMR is still the mainstay method of endoscopic resection; but ESD can be considered for lesions larger than 15 mm, poorly lifting tumors, and lesions with high-risk features for submucosal invasion.

The National Comprehensive Cancer Network guidelines recommend endoscopic therapy for patients with lesions limited to the epithelium (Tis or HGD), lamina propria, or muscularis mucosa (T1a). For patients with T1b lesions, esophagectomy is recommended [21].

EMR Technique in the Esophagus

At its core, EMR involves the removal of a lesion using a snare, with or without electrocoagulation (Table 2.1). There have been a variety of techniques that have been developed for resection of esophageal lesions, accounting for the relatively flat nature of many of these lesions. Prior to EMR, our practice is to thoroughly visualize the lesion using high-definition white-light endoscopy (WLE) and narrow-band imaging (NBI). While using virtual chromoendoscopy, we then mark the boundaries of the target lesion, usually 3–5 mm from the lesion border (Fig. 2.7), using various modalities of coagulation such as argon plasma coagulation (APC) or simply using a snare tip with soft coagulation. We recommend these markers, particularly in lesions requiring multiple resections, owing to the difficulty of recognizing the margins of the lesion during the actual resection given the effect of coagulation, bleeding, and submucosal injection in obscuring the working field. After the resection, confirming resection of the entire lesion is done by ensuring that all markers are no longer visible. It is important to note that the ASGE recommends against routine complete endoscopic resection of the entire Barrett's segment, but instead supporting resection of the visible lesion followed by ablation of the remaining

Table 2.1 Steps for esophageal endoscopic mucosal resection

1. Visual inspection of lesion using high-definition white-light endoscopy and narrow-band imaging
2. Marking of borders of lesions (with snare tip or argon plasma coagulation) under visualization with WLE or narrow-band imaging
3. Resection of lesion Injection assisted: Submucosal injection for lifting of target area, followed by snare resection Ligation assisted: Band ligation of target area followed by snare resection Cap assisted: Submucosal injection followed by suctioning of target area inside cap, followed by enclosing the snare and then resection
4. Thorough inspection of resection site to ensure no residual tissue, bleeding, or deep injury/perforation
5. Treatment of any bleeding sites or closure of defects if needed
6. Pinning of specimen onto Styrofoam board

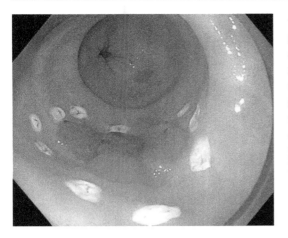

Fig. 2.7 Example of using coagulation markers to mark boundaries of visible lesion

Barrett's segment [22]. Should the segment of Barrett's contain diffusely nodular BE, however, we will perform EMR of the entire segment.

Injection-Assisted EMR

The original technique for EMR incorporates the use of solution injection into the submucosal space below the lesion to effectively create a safety barrier for resection. This injection creates a "lifting" and separation of the lesion from the underlying muscularis propria, which facilitates snaring of the intended target. Furthermore, this injection minimizes damage from electrocautery or physical forces to the muscularis propria and therefore minimizes the risk of perforation. While saline was first used as the injection solution, a wide variety of injection solutions (particularly viscous solutions) have been developed to facilitate lifting owing to the quick dissipation of saline into the adjacent space [29]. While not comprehensive, other commonly utilized solutions include dextrose 50% (an inexpensive, easily available hypertonic solution), succinylated gelatin (clear, inexpensive, safe colloid solution), hydroxyethyl starch (safe and inexpensive solution which can maintain submucosal lifting longer than saline), sodium hyaluronate (a highly viscoelastic but expensive solution), hydroxypropyl methylcellulose (HPMC, a readily available and

viscoelastic solution), and hyaluronic acid (HA, a glycosaminoglycan with high viscosity that is expensive) [30]. Additionally, dilute epinephrine (typically 1:100,000) can be added into the injection solution to reduce the bleeding during the resection which helps maintain better visualization throughout the procedure. Varying amounts of injection solution can be added at the endoscopist's discretion depending on the size of the lesion.

Ligation-Assisted EMR (Video Included)

Perhaps the simplest and most widely used of the EMR techniques, ligation-assisted EMR, also known as multiband mucosectomy (MBM), involves the use of a band ligation device [31, 32]. Similar to an esophageal varices banding device, a band ligation system includes a distal attachment cap for the endoscope with a trigger cord and control handle that goes through the working channel. This transparent cap contains six rubber bands, and once the ligation cap is maneuvered to be directly over the desired lesion, the lesion is suctioned into the cap using the endoscope's suction system. A single band is then released with clockwise rotation of the control handle, with a distinct releasing sensation felt by the endoscopist signaling deployment of the band (Fig. 2.8). This band will help create a

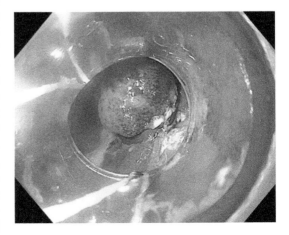

Fig. 2.8 Ligation-assisted endoscopic mucosal resection

pseudopolyp, and submucosal injection is not routinely required as the esophageal muscle layer retracts when ligated by the rubber band. An electrocautery snare can then be inserted through the working channel to cut the lesion either above or below the rubber band (Figs. 2.9 and 2.10). Piecemeal resection for larger lesions can be performed by repeating this process until complete resection is performed. The most commonly used ligation devices for this technique are the Duette Multi-Band Mucosectomy Kit (Fig. 2.11, Cook Medical, Winston-Salem, NC, USA) which incorporates a 7 Fr hexagonal snare and the Captivator EMR Device (Boston Scientific, Natick, MA, USA) which also utilizes a 7 Fr

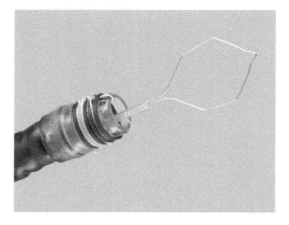

Fig. 2.11 Duette Multi-Band Mucosectomy Kit (Cook Medical, USA)

hexagonal snare. There is no consensus on the type, and settings of diathermy used for resection are widely variable in practice. In our practice, we mostly use blended current using Endo Cut Q (effect 3, cut duration 1, cut interval 6) and forced coagulation (effect 2, 50 watts).

Cap-Assisted EMR

In this technique, a transparent cap is attached to the distal end of the endoscope with a variety of caps available, with either a straight or oblique shape (Fig. 2.12). A submucosal injection is often used to create a cushion and aid in suctioning. A crescent-shaped electrocautery snare is passed through the biopsy channel and opened inside the cap. The snare is then positioned within the internal circumferential ridge at the tip of the cap. Once the snare is in good position, the cap is placed over the lesion, followed by suctioning of the lesion into the cap. Once complete suctioning of the lesion into the cap is achieved, the snare is closed with electrocoagulation, effectively removing the lesion. Piecemeal resection can be used for larger lesions by repeating this process until the entire lesion is resected (Fig. 2.13).

Once EMR is performed, the specimen is typically pinned down using thin pins on a Styrofoam board. This pinning helps preserve the orientation of the specimen for accurate histologic

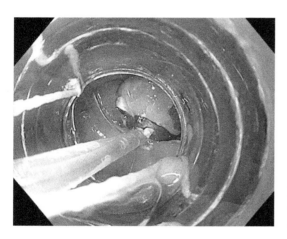

Fig. 2.9 Snare used underneath rubber band

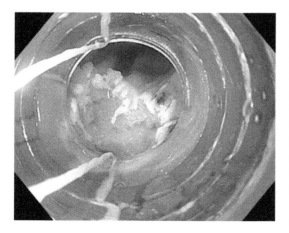

Fig. 2.10 Mucosal defect after ligation-assisted resection

Fig. 2.12 Cap-assisted resection kit displaying oblique cap (Olympus, Japan)

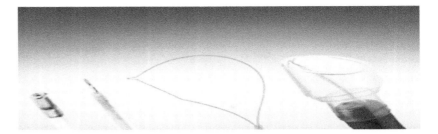

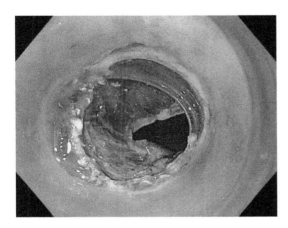

Fig. 2.13 Mucosal defect after piecemeal cap-assisted endoscopic mucosal resection

analysis and is crucial for determining the depth of invasion and whether negative horizontal and vertical margins have been obtained [33].

Safety and Efficacy

EMR used for the indications previously described is an effective, safe, and durable therapy [34–37]. EMR has been widely studied in the management of Barrett's esophagus patients with high-grade dysplasia and intramucosal EAC. Pech et al. evaluated 1000 patients who received EMR for Barrett's-associated mucosal adenocarcinomas using the cap-assisted and ligation-assisted techniques and found that complete remission was achieved in 96.3% of patients with only 2 deaths related to the cancer during a mean follow-up period of 56.6 months [37]. Major adverse events such as bleeding and perforation occurred in 1.5% of patients, and all adverse events were able to be managed endoscopically. Similarly, in the EURO-II

trial, Phoa et al. found that EMR followed by radio-frequency ablation (RFA) resulted in complete eradication of intestinal metaplasia (CE-IM) and neoplasia (CE-N) rates of 87% and 92%, respectively, in patients with high-grade dysplasia or EAC. In terms of high-grade dysplasia, a meta-analysis by Tomizawa et al. compiled data on studies where EMR was used on the entire Barrett's segment [38]. Reporting on 8 studies involving 676 patients, CE-IM and CE-N occurred in 85% and 96.6% of patients, respectively. Furthermore, Haidry et al. examined long-term outcomes from a UK registry of 500 patients with Barrett's-associated neoplasia, finding a significant increase in CE-IM (56–83%) and CE-N (77–92%) with an increase in EMR (48–60%) for visible lesions [39]. Given the high stricture rate (37.4%) of circumferential EMR, ablation methods such as radiofrequency ablation (RFA) are most frequently used in the management of flat (non-nodular) high-grade dysplasia, but EMR still plays an important diagnostic and therapeutic role in the management of nodular lesions, which may harbor areas of high-grade dysplasia or adenocarcinoma.

In terms of SCCs, Yamashina et al. examined 402 patients with mucosal and submucosal SCC who were treated endoscopically at a single center, of which 194 patients received EMR (median lesion size of 20 mm) as their resection method (208 patients received ESD) [40]. All patients had complete local remission for all lesions after a single procedure. During a mean follow-up period of 50 months, 5-year survival rates of 90.5%, 71.1%, and 70.8% were found for SCC limited to the epithelium/lamina propria, muscularis mucosa, and submucosa, respectively. Cumulative 5-year metastasis rates were 0.4%, 8.7%, 7.7%, and 36.2% for tumors limited to the epithelium/lamina propria and muscularis mucosa and with submucosal invasion to 0.2 mm and submucosal invasion more than 0.2 mm, respectively. Adverse events included perforation (0.2%), bleeding (0.2%), and strictures (13.2%). Yoshii et al. retrospectively examined 44 patients who underwent EMR for T1a (54.6%) and T1b (45.4%) SCC [41]. Within a median follow-up period of 51 months, two patients (4.5%) died from primary SCC, while four patients (9.7%) developed lymph node metastases. Adverse events included perforation (2.2%) and strictures (20%). Extrapolating from this data, it appears that EMR for SCC is safe and effective when limited to use in superficial lesions and can be considered for submucosal use if patients are not candidates for esophagectomy or unwilling to undergo surgical options.

The variety of EMR techniques prompts the question as to which technique is more effective. In terms of Barrett's-associated neoplasia, ligation-assisted EMR has become the more popular method, while in early squamous cell neoplasia, cap resection represents the most widely used technique. As mentioned above, the cap-assisted method is more technically demanding, particularly with piecemeal resections as submucosal lift-ing and repositioning of the snare is required for each resection. Zhang et al. performed a randomized controlled trial comparing the two methods ($n = 42$ in both groups) for squamous cell neoplasia and found that while complete endoscopic resection was achieved in all lesions, the procedure time was significantly shorter with the ligation method (11 vs. 22 minutes) and associated costs were lower in the ligation method [31]. Pouw et al. also compared the two methods in a randomized controlled trial for resection of high-grade dysplasia and intramucosal EAC, finding that ligation-assisted EMR was faster (34 minutes vs. 50 minutes) and cheaper (€240 vs. €322) with no significant difference in depth of resection [42]. Thus, ligation-assisted EMR appears to be quicker and easier, but selection of the EMR technique will rest on the preference of each endoscopist.

An alternative technique to EMR is ESD, which was originally designed for gastric lesions, but can be used for esophageal lesions as well. While this technique will be described in detail in other chapters, ESD utilizes an endoscopic knife to create a circumferential incision after submucosal injection to allow for an en bloc resection (Fig. 2.14) [1, 43–45].

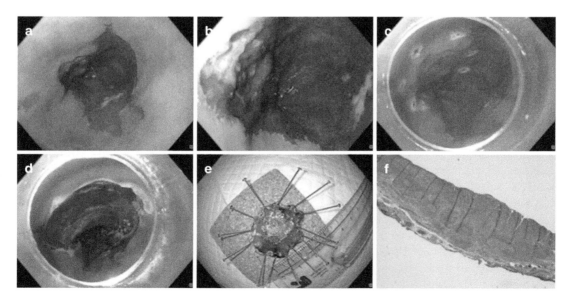

Fig. 2.14 ESD for large nodularity in Barrett's esophagus. Footnote: (**a**) Nodular lesion under white-light endoscopy from 9 to 12 o'clock. (**b**) Nodular lesion under NBI. (**c**) Thermal marking around the lesion. (**d**) Mucosal defect after ESD. (**e**) Resection specimen. (**f**) Low-magnification histology demonstrating intramucosal carcinoma

Few studies have compared ESD with EMR directly, but a randomized trial by Terheggen et al. compared the efficacy and safety of ESD ($n = 20$) and EMR ($n = 20$) in patients with Barrett's-associated neoplasia [46]. Although the ESD group did have a higher rate of margin-free resection, there was no difference in complete remission from neoplasia at 3 months, and a recurrent case of esophageal adenocarcinoma was seen once in the ESD group. As expected, ESD was also significantly longer than EMR (54 minutes vs. 22 minutes); and the only cases of perforation occurred in the ESD group ($n = 2$), although this was not statistically significant. Guo et al. performed a meta-analysis comparing both procedures for superficial esophageal cancers (total of 8 studies involving 1080 patients, all in Asia) and found that while ESD had a higher en bloc and curative resection rate, it also had a higher operative time and perforation rate with no differences in stricture and bleeding rates [44]. Therefore, individual expertise in each procedure will likely play a significant role in determining which technique to use in the treatment of superficial esophageal lesions.

Adverse Events

Adverse events from EMR include both acute and long-term adverse events. Acute complications most commonly involve pain and bleeding, the latter of which can be seen in 5.8–12% of patients [5, 47]. Perforation, while more serious, is rare and occurs in 1.8–2.3% of patients [5]. The major long-term complication of EMR is the development of strictures, which can occur from 12.2% to 38% of patients, particularly in those with circumferential resection. The main risk factors for stricture formation after EMR have been found to include large mucosal resections and resection of multiple lesions [48]. Heavy smoking may also predispose patients toward stricture formation after EMR [49].

While pain is typically mild and self-resolving, bleeding can be either immediate or delayed. Immediate bleeding can be controlled with standard techniques such as coagulation via Coagrasper (Olympus, Tokyo, Japan) or with hemostatic clips. Delayed bleeding, which can manifest as hematemesis or melena, can occur up to 30 days after the procedure and may require repeat endoscopy with use of the same hemostasis techniques mentioned above. Perforation, depending on the extent, may be able to be treated conservatively via endoscopic closure using standard endoclips or an Over-The-Scope-Clip (OTSC, Ovesco Medical, Tübingen, Germany) or endoscopic suturing (Apollo Endosurgery Inc., Austin, TX). Larger defects or delayed perforations may require surgical intervention.

Most strictures can be managed via serial dilations should the patient become symptomatic. In their single-center study, Konda et al. examined complete EMR in 107 patients with Barrett's-associated neoplasia predominantly using the cap-assisted technique and found that 37.8% of patients developed a symptomatic esophageal stricture requiring a mean number of 2.3 dilations [50]. Dilation can be done via either balloon or Savary dilators (Cook Medical, Winston-Salem, NC, USA), and injection of triamcinolone can be used for recurrent strictures [51]. See Figs. 2.15, 2.16, and 2.17.

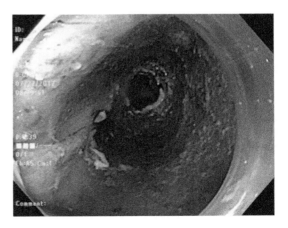

Fig. 2.15 Circumferential EMR for Barrett's-associated neoplasia

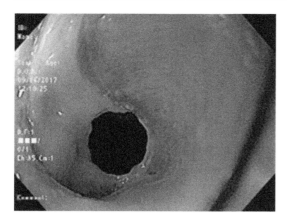

Fig. 2.16 Severe stricture after circumferential EMR

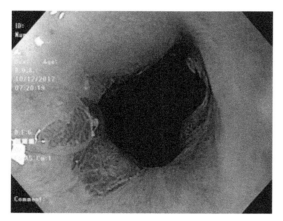

Fig. 2.17 Improvement in stricture after serial balloon dilations [3]

Future Directions

The appropriate management of EAC with submucosal invasion represents a point of controversy in the field of endoscopic resection. Several studies have examined patients who received EMR for T1b (submucosal invasion) esophageal adenocarcinomas with low-risk features (macroscopically flat or polypoid, invasion to the upper one-third of the submucosa, no lymphovascular invasion, and well to moderate tumor differentiation) and have found that recurrence rates range from 9% to 28% [52–55]. More studies will be needed to identify such patients with so-called "low-risk" submucosal adenocarcinoma who can be treated with endoscopic resection, but at this stage, surgical

esophagectomy remains the standard of care for such patients [56].

While EMR is typically used in resecting neoplasms confined to the mucosal layer, it can be used for tumors that arise from the submucosal layer and are less than 10 mm in size. Choi et al. demonstrated that in rectal carcinoid tumors, which have a low frequency of metastasis and typically invade the submucosa, ligation-assisted EMR was as effective as ESD in complete resection with no difference in recurrent rates [57]. Applying this to the esophagus, Hong et al. found 100% en bloc resection rates in esophageal submucosal tumors <10 mm in size (consisting of granular cell tumors, leiomyomas, and lipomas; see Figs. 2.18, 2.19, and 2.20) with the main complications being chest pain and heartburn [58]. Taking this data into account, EMR of

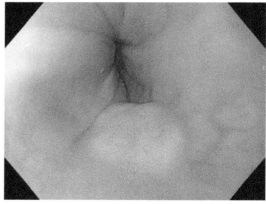

Fig. 2.18 Granular cell tumor of the esophagus

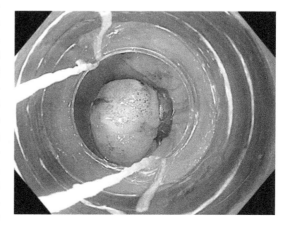

Fig. 2.19 EMR of granular cell tumor

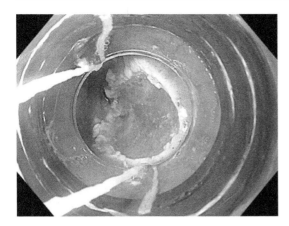

Fig. 2.20 Mucosal defect after EMR of granular cell tumor

submucosal tumors in the esophagus may be safe and effective for small lesions, but future prospective trials will be needed before EMR can be recommended in this setting.

The field of endoscopy has seen enormous advancement in technology and techniques, and assuredly, more innovations will be made to the field of EMR. Recently FDA approved, the EndoRotor (Interscope Medical, Worcester, MA, USA) represents a through-the-scope EMR system that can be used to aid EMR [59]. Consisting of a dual-cannula system, the EndoRotor has an outer cannula that helps suction tissue into the inner cannula which rotates at 1000 or 1700 rpm to cut the tissue. The suction system then draws the specimen into the tissue collection trap. By using rotation forces as opposed to heat or cautery, there is no cauterization artifact; and the suction system pulls in mucosa rather than muscle layer, reducing the risk of perforation. This can be particularly useful during piecemeal resection when lateral margins may be difficult to remove completely via traditional EMR. Nevertheless, innovations such as this system will need prospective human trials before their clinical use becomes standardized.

Quality Metrics

As healthcare systems become increasingly more focused on delivering value-based care, the development of quality metrics or indicators becomes crucial, particularly in procedure-based services, such as in gastroenterology. Quality metrics represent benchmarks of performance and often represent the ratio between the incidence of correct performance and the opportunity for correct performance [60, 61]. While no specific quality metrics have been established thus far for EMR, several important documents endorsed by the American Gastroenterological Association (AGA), American Society for Gastrointestinal Endoscopy (ASGE), and American College of Gastroenterology (ACG) regarding quality indicators in Barrett's esophagus can help guide the development of quality metrics in EMR [62–64]. In terms of pre-procedure quality metrics, for patients where a diagnosis of dysplasia has been made, the rate at which a GI fellowship-trained pathologist or a second pathologist confirms the diagnosis should be documented. All centers where endoscopic eradication therapy (EET) is performed for Barrett's should have expertise in endoscopic mucosal resection techniques; and the rate of documentation of the risks, benefits, and alternatives to EMR should be recorded. In terms of intra-procedure quality metrics, the rate at which EMR is performed for patients with visible lesions and the rate at which CE-IM or CE-N is achieved after EMR should be documented. Lastly, in terms of post-procedure quality metrics, the rate at which adverse events after EMR are documented should be noted.

Training

There currently exists a lack of standardized training for EMR for gastroenterologists. In the United States, EMR is typically learned during an advanced endoscopy fellowship which occurs after a standard gastroenterology fellowship training program. Additionally, the ASGE currently offers the Skills, Training, Assessment, and Reinforcement (STAR) certificate program consisting of online instructional videos followed by a hands-on workshop at a specialized training center. Van Vilsteren et al. performed a prospective study involving 6 endoscopists performing their first 20 EMR procedures in the esophagus under a structured training program [65]. This program consisted of four trimonthly 1-day courses with lecture, live demonstrations, hands-on training with anesthetized pigs, and one-on-one hands-on training. In the 120 EMR cases, 6 perforations occurred (5%) with 1 perforation requiring esophagectomy, and 11 cases (9.2%) had bleeding, all of which were able to be controlled endoscopically. Based on this study, performing 20 EMR procedures was deemed to be insufficient for competency in EMR; and a follow-up article delineated the top 10 tips for learning EMR:

1. Allow time for inspection and use a high-definition endoscope.
2. Create a pre-procedural plan by placing thermal markings.
3. Know the management of bleeding.
4. Optimize the endoscopic view by repeatedly cleaning out the stomach and target area.
5. Use an endoscope with water jet function during resection.
6. Always perform a test suction.
7. Keep instruments close to the tip.
8. Lift edges in piecemeal endoscopic cap resections.
9. Know the management of perforation.
10. Pin specimens down [66].

From these studies, there is support for structured one-on-one training as well as the incorporation of surgical colleagues given the perforation risk and possible need for subsequent surgical treatment based on histological assessment [67]. Furthermore, training should involve a thorough understanding of the indications of EMR as well as the ability to decipher which lesions may be more amenable to ESD or surgery [68]. Knowledge in managing adverse events is crucial as well, and continuing education through conferences and multidisciplinary meetings can only aid endoscopists in their training.

Conclusion

EMR is a widely used endoscopic technique in the esophagus that has been shown to be effective, safe, and durable in the management of Barrett's-associated neoplasia as well as early superficial squamous cell carcinoma. It plays an important role in both diagnostic and therapeutic purposes and remains a crucial skill for the interventional endoscopist.

References

1. Belghazi K, Bergman J, Pouw RE. Management of nodular neoplasia in Barrett's esophagus: endoscopic mucosal resection and endoscopic submucosal dissection. Gastrointest Endosc Clin N Am. 2017;27(3):461–70.
2. Iizuka T, Kikuchi D, Hoteya S, Nakamura M, Yamashita S, Mitani T, et al. Clinical advantage of endoscopic submucosal dissection over endoscopic mucosal resection for early mesopharyngeal and hypopharyngeal cancers. Endoscopy. 2011;43(10):839–43.
3. Ishihara R, Iishi H, Uedo N, Takeuchi Y, Yamamoto S, Yamada T, et al. Comparison of EMR and endoscopic submucosal dissection for en bloc resection of early esophageal cancers in Japan. Gastrointest Endosc. 2008;68(6):1066–72.
4. Balmadrid B, Hwang JH. Endoscopic resection of gastric and esophageal cancer. Gastroenterol Rep. 2015;3(4):330–8.
5. Barnes JA, Willingham FF. Endoscopic management of early esophageal cancer. J Clin Gastroenterol. 2015;49(8):638–46.
6. Deyhle P, Jenny S, Fumagalli I. Endoscopic polypectomy in the proximal colon. A diagnostic, therapeutic (and preventive?) intervention. Dtsch Med Wochenschr. 1973;98(5):219–20.
7. Nishizawa T, Yahagi N. Endoscopic mucosal resection and endoscopic submucosal dissection: technique and new directions. Curr Opin Gastroenterol. 2017;33(5):315–9.
8. Inoue H, Endo M. Endoscopic esophageal mucosal resection using a transparent tube. Surg Endosc. 1990;4(4):198–201.
9. Wani S, Falk GW, Post J, Yerian L, Hall M, Wang A, et al. Risk factors for progression of low-grade dysplasia in patients with Barrett's esophagus. Gastroenterology. 2011;141(4):1179–86, 86.e1
10. Kestens C, Offerhaus GJ, van Baal JW, Siersema PD. Patients with Barrett's esophagus and persistent low-grade dysplasia have an increased risk for high-grade dysplasia and cancer. Clin Gastroenterol Hepatol. 2016;14(7):956–62.e1.
11. Shaheen NJ, Falk GW, Iyer PG, Gerson LB. ACG clinical guideline: diagnosis and management of Barrett's esophagus. Am J Gastroenterol. 2016;111(1):30–50; quiz 1
12. Evans JA, Early DS, Fukami N, Ben-Menachem T, Chandrasekhara V, Chathadi KV, et al. The role of endoscopy in Barrett's esophagus and other premalignant conditions of the esophagus. Gastrointest Endosc. 2012;76(6):1087–94.

13. Wani S, Qumseya B, Sultan S, Agrawal D, Chandrashekara V, Harnke B, et al. Endoscopic eradication therapy for patients with Barrett's esophagus-associated dysplasia and intramucosal cancer. Gastrointest Endosc. 2018;87:907.

14. Peters FP, Brakenhoff KP, Curvers WL, Rosmolen WD, Fockens P, ten Kate FJ, et al. Histologic evaluation of resection specimens obtained at 293 endoscopic resections in Barrett's esophagus. Gastrointest Endosc. 2008;67(4):604–9.

15. Larghi A, Lightdale CJ, Memeo L, Bhagat G, Okpara N, Rotterdam H. EUS followed by EMR for staging of high-grade dysplasia and early cancer in Barrett's esophagus. Gastrointest Endosc. 2005;62(1):16–23.

16. Moss A, Bourke MJ, Hourigan LF, Gupta S, Williams SJ, Tran K, et al. Endoscopic resection for Barrett's high-grade dysplasia and early esophageal adenocarcinoma: an essential staging procedure with long-term therapeutic benefit. Am J Gastroenterol. 2010;105(6):1276–83.

17. Chennat J, Konda VJ, Ross AS, de Tejada AH, Noffsinger A, Hart J, et al. Complete Barrett's eradication endoscopic mucosal resection: an effective treatment modality for high-grade dysplasia and intramucosal carcinoma – an American single-center experience. Am J Gastroenterol. 2009;104(11):2684–92.

18. Wani S, Abrams J, Edmundowicz SA, Gaddam S, Hovis CE, Green D, et al. Endoscopic mucosal resection results in change of histologic diagnosis in Barrett's esophagus patients with visible and flat neoplasia: a multicenter cohort study. Dig Dis Sci. 2013;58(6):1703–9.

19. Wani S, Mathur SC, Curvers WL, Singh V, Alvarez Herrero L, Hall SB, et al. Greater interobserver agreement by endoscopic mucosal resection than biopsy samples in Barrett's dysplasia. Clin Gastroenterol Hepatol. 2010;8(9):783–8.

20. Dunbar KB, Spechler SJ. The risk of lymph-node metastases in patients with high-grade dysplasia or intramucosal carcinoma in Barrett's esophagus: a systematic review. Am J Gastroenterol. 2012;107(6):850–62.. quiz 63

21. Panel NG. Esophageal and esophagogastric junction cancers. NCCN Clinical Practice Guidelines in Oncology [Internet]. 2017 November 19th, 2017; 4.2017. Available from: https://oncolife.com.ua/doc/nccn/Esophageal_and_Esophagogastric_Junction_Cancers.pdf.

22. Wani S, Qumseya B, Sultan S, Agrawal D, Chandrasekhara V, Harnke B, et al. Endoscopic eradication therapy for patients with Barrett's esophagus-associated dysplasia and intramucosal cancer. Gastrointest Endosc. 2018;87(4):907–31.e9.

23. Inoue H, Takeshita K, Hori H, Muraoka Y, Yoneshima H, Endo M. Endoscopic mucosal resection with a cap-fitted panendoscope for esophagus, stomach, and colon mucosal lesions. Gastrointest Endosc. 1993;39(1):58–62.

24. Yip HC, Chiu PW. Endoscopic diagnosis and management of early squamous cell carcinoma of esophagus. J Thorac Dis. 2017;9(Suppl 8):S689–s96.

25. Aadam AA, Abe S. Endoscopic submucosal dissection for superficial esophageal cancer. Dis Esophagus. 2018;31(7).

26. Ono S, Fujishiro M, Niimi K, Goto O, Kodashima S, Yamamichi N, et al. Long-term outcomes of endoscopic submucosal dissection for superficial esophageal squamous cell neoplasms. Gastrointest Endosc. 2009;70(5):860–6.

27. Takahashi H, Arimura Y, Masao H, Okahara S, Tanuma T, Kodaira J, et al. Endoscopic submucosal dissection is superior to conventional endoscopic resection as a curative treatment for early squamous cell carcinoma of the esophagus (with video). Gastrointest Endosc. 2010;72(2):255–64, 64.e1–2

28. Pimentel-Nunes P, Dinis-Ribeiro M, Ponchon T, Repici A, Vieth M, De Ceglie A, et al. Endoscopic submucosal dissection: European Society of Gastrointestinal Endoscopy (ESGE) Guideline. Endoscopy. 2015;47(9):829–54.

29. Ning B, Abdelfatah MM, Othman MO. Endoscopic submucosal dissection and endoscopic mucosal resection for early stage esophageal cancer. Ann Cardiothorac Surg. 2017;6(2):88–98.

30. Yandrapu H, Desai M, Siddique S, Vennalganti P, Vennalaganti S, Parasa S, et al. Normal saline solution versus other viscous solutions for submucosal injection during endoscopic mucosal resection: a systematic review and meta-analysis. Gastrointest Endosc. 2017;85(4):693–9.

31. Zhang YM, Boerwinkel DF, Qin X, He S, Xue L, Weusten BL, et al. A randomized trial comparing multiband mucosectomy and cap-assisted endoscopic resection for endoscopic piecemeal resection of early squamous neoplasia of the esophagus. Endoscopy. 2016;48(4):330–8.

32. Schlottmann F, Patti MG, Shaheen NJ. Endoscopic treatment of high-grade dysplasia and early esophageal cancer. World J Surg. 2017;41(7):1705–11.

33. Kim SH, Choi HS, Chun HJ, Yoo IK, Lee JM, Kim ES, et al. A novel fixation method for variable-sized endoscopic submucosal dissection specimens: an in vitro animal experiment. PLoS One. 2016;11(1).

34. Pech O, Behrens A, May A, Nachbar L, Gossner L, Rabenstein T, et al. Long-term results and risk factor analysis for recurrence after curative endoscopic therapy in 349 patients with high-grade intraepithelial neoplasia and mucosal adenocarcinoma in Barrett's oesophagus. Gut. 2008;57(9):1200–6.

35. Smith I, Kahaleh M. Endoscopic versus surgical therapy for Barrett's esophagus neoplasia. Expert Rev Gastroenterol Hepatol. 2015;9(1):31–5.

36. Ell C, May A, Gossner L, Pech O, Gunter E, Mayer G, et al. Endoscopic mucosal resection of early cancer and high-grade dysplasia in Barrett's esophagus. Gastroenterology. 2000;118(4):670–7.

37. Pech O, May A, Manner H, Behrens A, Pohl J, Weferling M, et al. Long-term efficacy and safety of endoscopic resection for patients with mucosal adenocarcinoma of the esophagus. Gastroenterology. 2014;146(3):652–60.e1.

38. Tomizawa Y, Konda VJ, Coronel E, Chapman CG, Siddiqui UD. Efficacy, durability, and safety of complete endoscopic mucosal resection of Barrett esophagus: a systematic review and meta-analysis. J Clin Gastroenterol. 2018;52:210–6.

39. Haidry RJ, Butt MA, Dunn JM, Gupta A, Lipman G, Smart HL, et al. Improvement over time in outcomes for patients undergoing endoscopic therapy for Barrett's oesophagus-related neoplasia: 6-year experience from the first 500 patients treated in the UK patient registry. Gut. 2015;64(8):1192–9.

40. Yamashina T, Ishihara R, Nagai K, Matsuura N, Matsui F, Ito T, et al. Long-term outcome and metastatic risk after endoscopic resection of superficial esophageal squamous cell carcinoma. Am J Gastroenterol. 2013;108(4):544–51.

41. Yoshii T, Ohkawa S, Tamai S, Kameda Y. Clinical outcome of endoscopic mucosal resection for esophageal squamous cell cancer invading muscularis mucosa and submucosal layer. Dis Esophagus. 2013;26(5):496–502.

42. Pouw RE, van Vilsteren FG, Peters FP, Alvarez Herrero L, Ten Kate FJ, Visser M, et al. Randomized trial on endoscopic resection-cap versus multiband mucosectomy for piecemeal endoscopic resection of early Barrett's neoplasia. Gastrointest Endosc. 2011;74(1):35–43.

43. Shimizu Y, Takahashi M, Yoshida T, Ono S, Mabe K, Kato M, et al. Endoscopic resection (endoscopic mucosal resection/ endoscopic submucosal dissection) for superficial esophageal squamous cell carcinoma: current status of various techniques. Dig Endosc. 2013;25(Suppl 1):13–9.

44. Guo HM, Zhang XQ, Chen M, Huang SL, Zou XP. Endoscopic submucosal dissection vs endoscopic mucosal resection for superficial esophageal cancer. World J Gastroenterol. 2014;20(18):5540–7.

45. Hammad H, Kaltenbach T, Soetikno R. Endoscopic submucosal dissection for malignant esophageal lesions. Curr Gastroenterol Rep. 2014;16(5):386.

46. Terheggen G, Horn EM, Vieth M, Gabbert H, Enderle M, Neugebauer A, et al. A randomised trial of endoscopic submucosal dissection versus endoscopic mucosal resection for early Barrett's neoplasia. Gut. 2017;66(5):783–93.

47. Isomoto H, Yamaguchi N, Minami H, Nakao K. Management of complications associated with endoscopic submucosal dissection/ endoscopic mucosal resection for esophageal cancer. Dig Endosc. 2013;25(Suppl 1):29–38.

48. Qumseya B, Panossian AM, Rizk C, Cangemi D, Wolfsen C, Raimondo M, et al. Predictors of esophageal stricture formation post endoscopic mucosal resection. Clin Endosc. 2014;47(2):155–61.

49. Lewis JJ, Rubenstein JH, Singal AG, Elmunzer BJ, Kwon RS, Piraka CR. Factors associated with esophageal stricture formation after endoscopic mucosal resection for neoplastic Barrett's esophagus. Gastrointest Endosc. 2011;74(4):753–60.

50. Konda VJ, Gonzalez Haba Ruiz M, Koons A, Hart J, Xiao SY, Siddiqui UD, et al. Complete endoscopic mucosal resection is effective and durable treatment for Barrett's-associated neoplasia. Clin Gastroenterol Hepatol. 2014;12(12):2002–10.e1–2.

51. Hashimoto S, Kobayashi M, Takeuchi M, Sato Y, Narisawa R, Aoyagi Y. The efficacy of endoscopic triamcinolone injection for the prevention of esophageal stricture after endoscopic submucosal dissection. Gastrointest Endosc. 2011;74(6):1389–93.

52. Manner H, May A, Pech O, Gossner L, Rabenstein T, Gunter E, et al. Early Barrett's carcinoma with "low-risk" submucosal invasion: long-term results of endoscopic resection with a curative intent. Am J Gastroenterol. 2008;103(10):2589–97.

53. Alvarez Herrero L, Pouw RE, van Vilsteren FG, ten Kate FJ, Visser M, van Berge Henegouwen MI, et al. Risk of lymph node metastasis associated with deeper invasion by early adenocarcinoma of the esophagus and cardia: study based on endoscopic resection specimens. Endoscopy. 2010;42(12):1030–6.

54. Tian J, Prasad GA, Lutzke LS, Lewis JT, Wang KK. Outcomes of T1b esophageal adenocarcinoma patients. Gastrointest Endosc. 2011;74(6):1201–6.

55. Ballard DD, Choksi N, Lin J, Choi EY, Elmunzer BJ, Appelman H, et al. Outcomes of submucosal (T1b) esophageal adenocarcinomas removed by endoscopic mucosal resection. World J Gastrointest Endosc. 2016;8(20):763–9.

56. Watson TJ. Esophagectomy for superficial esophageal neoplasia. Gastrointest Endosc Clin N Am. 2017;27(3):531–46.

57. Choi CW, Kang DH, Kim HW, Park SB, Jo WS, Song GA, et al. Comparison of endoscopic resection therapies for rectal carcinoid tumor: endoscopic submucosal dissection versus endoscopic mucosal resection using band ligation. J Clin Gastroenterol. 2013;47(5):432–6.

58. Hong JB, Choi CW, Kim HW, Kang DH, Park SB, Kim SJ, et al. Endoscopic resection using band ligation for esophageal SMT in less than 10 mm. World J Gastroenterol. 2015;21(10):2982–7.

59. Hollerbach S, Wellmann A, Meier P, Ryan J, Franco R, Koehler P. The EndoRotor((R)): endoscopic mucosal resection system for non-thermal and rapid removal of esophageal, gastric, and colonic lesions: initial experience in live animals. Endosc Int Open. 2016;4(4):E475–9.

60. Petersen BT. Quality assurance for endoscopists. Best Pract Res Clin Gastroenterol. 2011;25(3):349–60.

61. Rizk MK, Sawhney MS, Cohen J, Pike IM, Adler DG, Dominitz JA, et al. Quality indicators common to all GI endoscopic procedures. Am J Gastroenterol. 2015;110(1):48–59.

62. Wani S, Muthusamy VR, Shaheen NJ, Yadlapati R, Wilson R, Abrams JA, et al. Development of quality indicators for endoscopic eradication therapies in Barrett's esophagus: the TREAT-BE (Treatment

with Resection and Endoscopic Ablation Techniques for Barrett's Esophagus) Consortium. Gastrointest Endosc. 2017;86(1):1–17.e3.

63. Wani S, Muthusamy VR, Shaheen NJ, Yadlapati R, Wilson R, Abrams JA, et al. Development of quality indicators for endoscopic eradication therapies in Barrett's esophagus: the TREAT-BE (Treatment With Resection and Endoscopic Ablation Techniques for Barrett's Esophagus) Consortium. Am J Gastroenterol. 2017;112(7):1032–48.

64. Sharma P, Katzka DA, Gupta N, Ajani J, Buttar N, Chak A, et al. Quality indicators for the management of Barrett's esophagus, dysplasia, and esophageal adenocarcinoma: international consensus recommendations from the American Gastroenterological Association symposium. Gastroenterology. 2015; 149(6):1599–606.

65. van Vilsteren FG, Pouw RE, Herrero LA, Peters FP, Bisschops R, Houben M, et al. Learning to perform endoscopic resection of esophageal neoplasia is associated with significant complications even within a structured training program. Endoscopy. 2012;44(1):4–12.

66. van Vilsteren FG, Pouw RE, Alvarez Herrero L, Bisschops R, Houben M, Peters FT, et al. Learning endoscopic resection in the esophagus. Endoscopy. 2015;47(11):972–9.

67. Mannath J, Ragunath K. A one-to-one training program would be valuable in learning how to perform esophageal endoscopic mucosal resection. Endoscopy. 2012;44(6):632; author reply 3

68. Feurer ME, Draganov PV. Training for advanced endoscopic procedures. Best Pract Res Clin Gastroenterol. 2016;30(3):397–408.

Gastric and Duodenal Endoscopic Mucosal Resection

Rommel Romano and Pradermchai Kongkam

Introduction

Endoscopic mucosal resection (EMR), previously known as mucosectomy, is a minimally invasive procedure currently being recommended as treatment for early malignant lesions of the gastrointestinal tract [1]. Endoscopic removal of tumors has been reported as early as 1973 when polypectomy was performed using electrocautery [2], but EMR for early gastric cancer was pioneered by the Japanese in 1983 [3]. The techniques and devices used for EMR have come a long way since Tada's strip biopsy using saline injection into the mucosa [4], but this method is still being used up to this day. This chapter will focus on EMR for gastric and duodenal lesions. This chapter will focus on the following domains: (i) indications, (ii) endoscopic techniques, (iii) contraindications, (iv) benefits and clinical outcomes, and (v) adverse events associated with EMR.

R. Romano
Department of Medicine, University of Santo Tomas Hospital, Manila, Philippines

P. Kongkam (✉)
Pancreas Research Unit, Department of Medicine, Chulalongkorn University, Bangkok, Thailand
e-mail: kongkam@homail.com

Clinical Indications

This treatment option for GI malignancy is enticing, but meticulous selection of patients must be done before considering EMR. Because this technique should be utilized to remove mucosal lesions, this technique should be limited to lesions that are within the mucosal layer (lesions that do not breach the muscularis mucosa). A review by Soetikno and colleagues published in 2003 [5] acknowledged the importance of the estimation of depth of the lesion, as well as the limitations of the technology they were using at the time. In the current ASGE technical review [1], EMR is a treatment option for the definitive management of premalignant and early-stage (T1N0) malignant lesions and should not be performed in lesions which are deeper than the mucosa. The Japanese gastric cancer treatment guidelines [6] state that lesions that are amenable to endoscopic resection are those with no evidence of lymph node or vascular involvement and well-differentiated T1a lesions not bigger than 3 cm if with ulcerations or more than 2 cm in size without ulceration. If the lesion is undifferentiated, it may still be resected endoscopically if it is non-ulcerative and not larger than 2 cm. These guidelines, however, recommend the performance of endoscopic submucosal dissection (ESD) over EMR to avoid incomplete resection.

The non-lifting sign, which is a predictor of depth of invasion of the tumor [7, 8], is useful in

© Springer Nature Switzerland AG 2020
M. S. Wagh, S. B. Wani (eds.), *Gastrointestinal Interventional Endoscopy*,
https://doi.org/10.1007/978-3-030-21695-5_3

determining whether or not a lesion is amenable to EMR. Failure of a lesion to completely lift after submucosal injection, unless thought to be secondary to fibrosis from a previous biopsy, usually means that the tumor has invaded deep into the submucosa or beyond. Endoscopic ultrasound (EUS) is currently the best diagnostic tool for locoregional staging. While some authors will point out that nodal metastases are better diagnosed with cross-sectional imaging, it cannot be contested that EUS is better in T staging, especially in small gastric tumors, which becomes more relevant because it is concerned more about tumor depth than size. However, the best diagnostic approach is a combination of these imaging modalities.

Recently, endoscopic methods like high-resolution magnification and mucosal enhancement technologies are increasingly used to identify suitable lesions for EMR. Clinical application of such endoscopic image technologies to determine depth of lesions before the removal procedure will be discussed in other chapters.

Endoscopic Techniques

Injection Assisted

As previously mentioned, submucosal normal saline injection was the first technique employed to perform EMR. Several solutions are now being used as "lifting" agents, but the idea remains the same: an endoscopic needle is passed through the working channel and directed onto multiple points surrounding the area in question to provide a cushion between the mucosal lesion and the deeper submucosa to facilitate an easier and safer endoscopic resection. At this day, en bloc resection of lesion is preferred over piecemeal resection, if possible.

Normal saline is still very commonly used as a lifting solution, but the main problem is that the cushion it provides usually subsides within a few minutes. Other solutions being used are 3.75% NaCl, 20% dextrose water, glycerin-fructose solution, and sodium hyaluronate [9]. Yamamoto has shown that a 0.4% hyaluronic acid solution provides a longer-lasting cushion which results in significantly steeper lifts and less reinjections

[10]. In a systematic review of literature, however, Ferreira et al. have found that sodium hyaluronate solutions clinically perform just as well as normal saline and may not be cost-effective [11].

Device Assisted

Several devices are developed to make EMR easier. Probably the most common of these devices is the cap or hood, which is a transparent plastic extension fitted onto the tip of the endoscope for the purpose of applying suction and lifting the mucosa with the lesion while being able to easily apply a cutting or ligating tool no different with the principle of endoscopic band ligation. Cap-assisted endoscopic mucosal resection (EMRC) or endoscopic aspiration mucosectomy (EAM) begins with marking the border of the lesion with an electrocautery device followed by injection of the lifting solution into the submucosa to raise the lesion. A cap is then fitted onto the scope tip, and a snare is opened and positioned in a groove within the cap. The cap is then positioned over the raised lesion where suction is applied retracting the mucosa toward the tip of the scope within the cap where the snare is used to guillotine the mucosa using electrocautery.

Ligation-assisted EMR is similar to cap-assisted EMR. But as the name implies, this method is similar to what is done during variceal endoscopic band ligation. A cap is fitted onto the tip of the endoscope and positioned over the mucosa of the lesion. The mucosa is lifted by suction into the cap without the need for submucosal injection. After deployment of the ligator, a pseudopolyp is then produced, and resection of the mucosa will be completed by a snare with electrocautery just like a standard snare polypectomy.

Underwater EMR

First described in 2012 by Binmoeller [12], underwater EMR (UEMR) is more commonly used for endoscopic resection of large colorectal lesions [13–16]. There is a report from 2014 about the performance of UEMR for removal of large duodenal adenomas [17]. The rationale of performing EMR underwater is the muscularis propria floats into the bowel lumen without the compression effect of air allowing it to be static independent of the changes of the mucosa and submucosa, even during peristaltic contractions [16]. This means that submucosal injection is not necessary before resection with a snare. Since this technique is usually employed in large lesions, as well as lesions in which prior EMR failed to achieve complete resection [1], the lesion is usually removed in a piecemeal fashion. A low-profile cap is likewise attached onto the tip of the endoscope similar to cap-assisted EMR, but its purpose is to facilitate visualization of the lesion rather than providing room for mucosa that is being "lifted" toward the endoscope.

Contraindications

The obvious clinical contraindication of performing EMR is the presence of a more advanced tumor. The lesions that are amenable to this procedure have been discussed above, and those that are more advanced than the aforementioned lesions are therefore not good candidates for EMR. Procedural contraindications to other endoscopic procedures also apply to EMR.

Clinical Outcomes

Long-term results of endoscopic resection of early gastric cancer in carefully selected patients show that complete remission is achieved by endoscopic therapy in 97% of patients over one to three endoscopic therapy sessions spread in an average of 3.5 months [18]. In an earlier trial, the complete remission rate was 89% and required one to four endoscopy sessions [19]. However, despite this good numbers, the fact remains that despite en bloc resection, it does not eliminate the possibility of metachronous or synchronous lesions, which can be present in about 3.2% and 35%, respectively [20, 21]. Also, the local recurrence post-endoscopic treatment is 4.1%, with only one of those patients needing a repeat endoscopic resection [21].

Adverse Events

In general, the most common complication of EMR is bleeding, which occurs in an average of 10% of cases [1]. The risk of bleeding increases with the size of the tumor being resected, from 4% on subcentimeter lesions to 32% on lesions larger than 3 cm [19]. However, the risk of bleeding from gastric and duodenal EMR ranges from 0% to 16% [1, 22], and the risk of delayed bleeding is 5% [22]. Perforation is the most serious complication of endoscopic mucosal resection. Perforation risk in gastric and duodenal EMR is about 1% and 2%, respectively [23, 24].

Conclusions

As with any advanced endoscopic technique, the risk of adverse events is inversely related to endoscopist experience. It is therefore recommended that these techniques be performed by expert endoscopists with an equally experienced endoscopy team or a novice therapeutic endoscopist under close supervision by an expert until the learning curve is overcome.

References

1. ASGE Technology Committee, Hwang JH, Konda V, et al. Endoscopic mucosal resection. Gastrointest Endosc. 2015;82:215–26.
2. Deyhle P, Largiadèr F, Jenny S, et al. A method for endoscopic electroresection of sessile colonic polyps. Endoscopy. 1973;5:38–40.
3. Inoue H, Tani M, Nagai K, et al. Treatment of esophageal and gastric tumors. Endoscopy. 1999;31:47–55.
4. Tada M, Shimada M, Murakami F, et al. Development of strip-off biopsy. Gastroenterol Endosc. 1984;26:833–9.
5. Soetikno RM, Gotoda T, Nakanishi Y, et al. Endoscopic mucosal resection. Gastrointest Endosc. 2003;57:567–79.
6. Japanese Gastric Cancer Association. Japanese gastric cancer treatment guidelines 2014 (ver. 4). Gastric Cancer. 2017;20:1–19.
7. Kato H, Haga S, Endo S, et al. Lifting of lesions during endoscopic mucosal resection (EMR) of early colorectal cancer: implications for the assessment of resectability. Endoscopy. 2001;33:568–73.
8. Ishiguro A, Uno Y, Ishiguro Y, et al. Correlation of lifting versus non-lifting and microscopic depth

of invasion in early colorectal cancer. Gastrointest Endosc. 1999;50:329–33.

9. Fujishiro M, Yahagi N, Kashimura K, et al. Comparison of various submucosal injection solutions for maintaining mucosal elevation during endoscopic mucosal resection. Endoscopy. 2004;36:579–83.

10. Yamamoto H, Yahagi N, Oyama T, et al. Usefulness and safety of 0.4% sodium hyaluronate solution as a submucosal fluid "cushion" in endoscopic resection for gastric neoplasms: a prospective multicenter trial. Gastrointest Endosc. 2008;67:830–9.

11. Ferreira AO, Moleiro J, Torres J, et al. Solutions for submucosal injection in endoscopic resection: a systematic review and meta-analysis. Endosc Int Open. 2016;4:E1–E16.

12. Binmoeller KF, Weilert F, Shah J, et al. "Underwater" EMR without submucosal injection for large sessile colorectal polyps (with video). Gastrointest Endosc. 2012;75:1086–91.

13. Binmoeller KF, Hamerski CM, Shah JN, et al. Attempted underwater en bloc resection for large (2-4 cm) colorectal laterally spreading tumors (with video). Gastrointest Endosc. 2015;81:713–8.

14. Uedo N, Nemeth A, Johansson GW, et al. Underwater endoscopic mucosal resection of large colorectal lesions. Endoscopy. 2015;47:172–4.

15. Curcio G, Granata A, Ligresti D, et al. Underwater colorectal EMR: remodeling endoscopic mucosal resection. Gastrointest Endosc. 2015;81:1238–42.

16. Amato A, Radaelli F, Spinzi G. Underwater endoscopic mucosal resection: the third way for en bloc resection of colonic lesions? United European Gastroenterol J. 2016;4:595–8.

17. Flynn MM, Wang AY. Underwater endoscopic mucosal resection of large duodenal adenomas (video). Video J Encyclopedia GI Endosc. 2014;2:84–6.

18. Manner H, Rabenstein T, May A, et al. Long-term results of endoscopic resection in early gastric cancer: the Western experience. Am J Gastroenterol. 2009;104:566–73.

19. Ahmad NA, Kochman ML, Long WB, et al. Efficacy, safety, and clinical outcomes of endoscopic mucosal resection: a study of 101 cases. Gastrointest Endosc. 2002;55:390–6.

20. Oka S, Tanaka S, Kaneko I, et al. Advantage of endoscopic submucosal dissection compared with EMR for early gastric cancer. Gastrointest Endosc. 2006;64:877–83.

21. Ono H. Endoscopic mucosal resection for treatment of early gastric cancer. Gut. 2001;48:225–9.

22. Okano A, Hajiro K, Takakuwa H, et al. Predictors of bleeding after endoscopic mucosal resection of gastric tumors. Gastrointest Endosc. 2003;57:687–90.

23. Park Y-M, Cho E, Kang H-Y, et al. The effectiveness and safety of endoscopic submucosal dissection compared with endoscopic mucosal resection for early gastric cancer: a systematic review and metaanalysis. Surg Endosc. 2011;25:2666–77.

24. Fanning SB, Bourke MJ, Williams SJ, et al. Giant laterally spreading tumors of the duodenum: endoscopic resection outcomes, limitations, and caveats. Gastrointest Endosc. 2012;75:805–12.

A Pragmatic Approach to Complex Colon Polyps

4

Michael X. Ma and Michael J. Bourke

Abbreviations

CAST	Cold-forceps avulsion with adjuvant snare tip soft coagulation
CSP	Cold snare polypectomy
CSPEB	Clinically significant post-endoscopy bleeding
DMI	Deep mural injury
EMR	Endoscopic mucosal resection
ER	Endoscopic resection
ESD	Endoscopic submucosal dissection
FICE	Flexible spectral imaging colour enhancement
GIT	Gastrointestinal tract
ICV	Ileocaecal valve
IPB	Intra-procedural bleeding
LSL	Laterally spreading lesion
MP	Muscularis propria
NBI	Narrow band imaging
NICE	NBI International Colorectal Endoscopic
OR	Odds ratio
SMF	Submucosal fibrosis
SMI	Submucosal invasion
SSP	Sessile serrated polyp
STSC	Snare tip soft coagulation
TS	Target sign
TSC	Topical submucosal chromoendoscopy
TTS	Through the scope
UEMR	Underwater endoscopic mucosal resection
WLE	White light endoscopy

Electronic Supplementary Material The online version of this chapter (https://doi.org/10.1007/978-3-030-21695-5_4) contains supplementary material, which is available to authorized users.

M. X. Ma
Department of Gastroenterology and Hepatology, Westmead Hospital, Sydney, NSW, Australia

M. J. Bourke (✉)
Department of Gastroenterology and Hepatology, Westmead Hospital, Sydney, NSW, Australia

University of Sydney, Sydney, NSW, Australia
e-mail: michael@citywestgastro.com.au

Introduction

Endoscopic resection (ER) is the accepted first-line treatment for large laterally spreading lesions (LSLs) and other complex polyps of the colorectum. ER includes conventional polypectomy as well as endoscopic mucosal resection (EMR) and endoscopic submucosal dissection (ESD). Injection-assisted EMR was first introduced in 1955 for rigid sigmoidoscopy and later adapted for flexible colonoscopy in 1973 [1, 2]. ESD was first conceptually described in Japan in 1988 as a technique to treat early gastric cancer [3] and is now also widely used to treat early neoplastic lesions in the colorectum and esophagus. As will be discussed, ER of early gastrointestinal tract

© Springer Nature Switzerland AG 2020
M. S. Wagh, S. B. Wani (eds.), *Gastrointestinal Interventional Endoscopy*,
https://doi.org/10.1007/978-3-030-21695-5_4

(GIT) neoplasms is highly efficacious and holds morbidity and cost advantages over surgery [4, 5].

EMR is suitable for the vast majority of colorectal lesions, although for lesions ≥20 mm with suspected superficial submucosal invasion (SMI), resection by ESD is recommended as en bloc resection provides more meaningful local histological staging information and is potentially curative. This advantage of ESD however is offset by it being more technically demanding and requiring longer procedural duration with increased procedural risk than EMR [6]. Therefore, the decision to perform EMR or ESD for any lesion is best individualised based upon careful initial endoscopic assessment to stratify its risk of SMI and endoscopist experience and always within the context of the patient's overall health and comorbidities.

Lesion Assessment

Careful endoscopic assessment of every lesion should be performed prior to undertaking ER, noting in particular its size, peripheral extent and margins, relation to surrounding anatomical structures, and likelihood of harbouring SMI. Good bowel cleansing is essential, and patients should be advised to carefully complete a split preparation prior to their procedure. Any residual stool in the colon not only presents a barrier to lesion assessment but may also be hazardous in case of complications such as perforation.

Although larger LSLs are technically more demanding to remove, lesion size per se is becoming less problematic for ER, especially for expert endoscopists. Even near-circumferential and circumferential LSLs can be endoscopically resected, by following a systematic approach and meticulous technique [7, 8]. Nonetheless, accurate and adequate assessment of each LSL before commencing ER allows the endoscopist to estimate the duration of the procedure and anticipate any difficulties or requirement for any ancillary devices to complete the procedure.

The peripheral extent of most LSLs can be adequately assessed using white light endoscopy (WLE) with current high-definition endoscopes,

and its accurate determination helps to plan ER. Endoscopic image enhancement technologies such as narrow band imaging (NBI, Olympus, Tokyo, Japan), flexible spectral imaging colour enhancement (FICE, Fujifilm, Tokyo, Japan), or chromoendoscopy may assist when WLE is equivocal and may be particularly useful for flat LSLs or larger sessile serrated polyps (SSPs). Inclusion of dye such as methylene blue or indigo carmine within the submucosal injectate may also assist to delineate normal colonic mucosa from adenomatous tissue once it has been lifted.

Stratifying Risk of Submucosal Invasion

The risk of SMI within an LSL can be accurately determined by assessment of its morphological features and surface pit pattern. Invasion into the submucosa is associated with risk of lymph node metastasis, and this risk directly correlates with the depth of SMI. For example, for colonic lesions, invasion into the superficial third of the submucosa (sm1) has 3% risk of nodal metastases, whereas invasion into the deepest third of the submucosa (sm3) has 25% risk of nodal metastases [9]. Given the risk of nodal metastases, particularly for lesions that are sm2 (middle third of submucosa) or sm3, a therapeutic outcome from ER of lesions with SMI is generally not possible, and these patients are best referred for surgical resection. An exception could be when only superficial SMI exists (<1000 μm or sm1) in an elderly or comorbid patient, where the risks of surgery may outweigh the relatively low risk of lymph node metastasis.

Morphological Classification

Large colonic polyps are morphologically classified according to the Paris classification (Fig. 4.1) [10]. The broad categories are sessile (0-Is, protruded or polypoid morphology), non-polypoid (0-IIa, slightly elevated; 0-IIb, flat; or 0-IIc, slightly depressed) or excavated (0-III). Non-polypoid, slightly elevated lesions (0-IIa) and polypoid (0-Is) lesions can be further

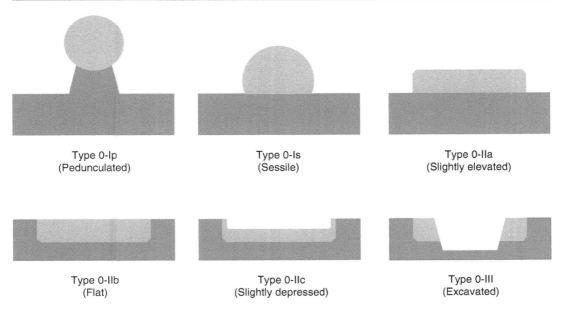

Fig. 4.1   Paris endoscopic classification of superficial neoplastic colorectal lesions

morphologically categorised as granular (a 'bubbly' surface contour akin to that of a bowl of Rice Bubbles cereal) or non-granular (a relatively smooth and firm surface contour).

Such morphological classifications serve not only to standardise descriptions of LSLs but also convey important information regarding SMI risk within the LSL. For example, data from a large, prospective multicentre cohort study showed granular 0-IIa LSLs harbour a very low risk of SMI (approximately 1%), granular 0-IIa + Is LSLs harbour an intermediate risk of SMI (approximately 7%) and non-granular 0-Is LSLs harbour a high risk of SMI (approximately 15%) [5, 11]. Figure 4.2 summarises the risk of SMI within LSLs according to their morphology and location within the colon [11].

Surface Assessment

Assessment of a lesion's surface pit pattern using the Kudo classification may distinguish non-neoplastic from neoplastic polyps [12]. This classification was originally developed using chromoendoscopy and magnifying colonoscopy, but its principles can also be applied using high-definition colonoscopes with magnification and NBI or FICE. According to this classification,

Kudo type I appear as roundish pits; Kudo type II are stellar or papillary pits; Kudo type III-S are small, roundish, tubular pits (smaller than type I) and Kudo type III-L are roundish, tubular pits (larger than type I); Kudo type IV are branch-like or gyrus pits; Kudo type Vi are irregular pits; and Kudo type Vn are non-structural pits with an amorphous structure.

Polyps with type I or II pits are considered benign (e.g. normal, hyperplastic or inflammatory), whereas polyps with type III are usually tubular adenomas, type IV usually contain villous histology, type Vi are indicative of superficial SMI and type Vn are associated with deep SMI. For the purpose of determining suitability of ER, it is important to exclude the presence of any type V pit pattern, although diminutive focal SMI may sometimes still be present within an LSL with a seemingly intact surface pit pattern. Other classification systems that assess surface vascular pattern (Sano and NBI International Colorectal Endoscopic [NICE] classification) [13, 14] are also validated to assess the histology of colorectal polyps.

Taken together, stratification of SMI risk within an LSL is best determined by assessing both its surface pit pattern and gross morphology.

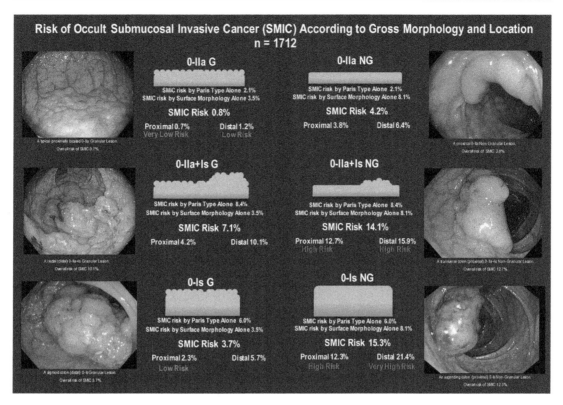

Fig. 4.2 Risk of occult SMI in LSLs according to morphology and location. (Adapted from Burgess et al. *Gastroenterology* 153(3), 2017; 732–742.e1)

This is supported by findings from a recent large prospective multicentre study of 2277 LSLs of ≥20 mm size, where particular features that should alert endoscopists to an increased risk of covert SMI included recto-sigmoid located LSLs (odds ratio [OR] 1.91), lesions with Paris 0-IIc and 0-Is morphologies (OR 1.80 and OR 2.73, respectively), non-granular surface morphology (OR 2.80), increasing lesion size (OR 1.12 per 10 mm increase) and Kudo pit pattern V (OR 14.2) [11].

Lesion Biopsy

Routine lesion biopsy to determine its histology and/or exclude presence of SMI prior to ER is generally discouraged. Lesion biopsy, particularly over flat (0-IIa or 0-IIb) areas, may cause significant submucosal fibrosis (SMF). This can hinder adequate expansion of the submucosal space following injection and impede subsequent

ER. Biopsies from 0-Is nodules, which are more likely to harbour SMI, may result in less SMF; but this has not been confirmed in any large study. Nonetheless, biopsies are prone to sampling error, as they are not representative of an entire lesion and therefore may potentially underestimate its histological grade. As such, lesions without obvious SMI after careful endoscopic assessment are best referred for ER without biopsy. However, if SMI is suspected, targeted biopsies to confirm invasive disease can be considered prior to further management.

Endoscopic Mucosal Resection

EMR is the recommended first-line therapy for colorectal LSLs ≥20 mm in size (Figs. 4.2 and 4.3). On an intention-to-treat basis within tertiary centres, EMR was technically successful for

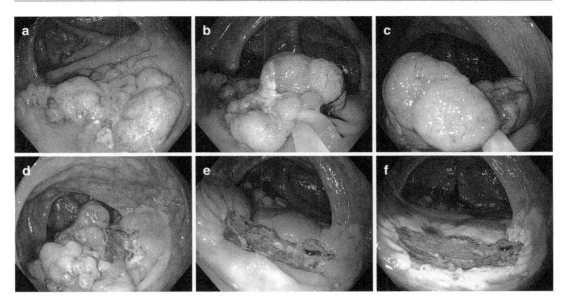

Fig. 4.3 EMR of 40 mm LSL in the proximal ascending colon. (**a**) A granular, Kudo IV, 40 mm Paris 0-IIa + Is LSL in the proximal ascending colon. The lesion is in the dependant side, and the patient is repositioned to improve access. (**b**) Submucosal injection with formation of a fluid cushion beneath the lesion. (**c**) Snare resection of the 0-Is component is performed to allow access to the remaining lesion. (**d**) Piecemeal resection proceeds progressively from one side of the lesion to the other. (**e**) Completion of EMR with blue-stained submucosal tissue indicating absence of deep injury. A non-bleeding arteriole is visible within the resection defect and does not require prophylactic treatment. (**f**) Snare tip soft coagulation applied to resection margins. This has been shown to reduce adenomatous recurrence

>95% of lesions with >90% avoiding surgery on long-term follow-up [5, 15]. Large prospective studies have also demonstrated the safety of EMR [5, 16]. Economic modelling studies have shown EMR treatment of LSLs is significantly more cost-effective compared with surgery, saving between 7000 and 13,000 USD per patient with reduction in hospitalisation length of stay by 2.8 days [4, 17]. Nonetheless, every case should be assessed based on the risks and benefits of resection and in the context of a patient's overall health and comorbidities. The following paragraphs discuss the technique of EMR, emphasising several key technical aspects that have been shown to improve complete resection, reduce recurrence and lower rates of adverse events.

Patient Preparation

All patients need to be consented to the procedure and informed of its risks and treatment alternatives. Referrals should include description of the lesion size, location and Paris morphology including colour images. The endoscopist should be aware of a patient's full medical history and medication list, in particular any regular antithrombotic agents. We suggest that all antiplatelet agents, including aspirin, be withheld for 7 days so that their effects are not active at the time of ER. Similarly, anticoagulants should also be withheld for sufficient duration, but this period varies according to medication and the patient's renal function. Endoscopists should refer to published guidelines [18, 19] or seek the opinion of a haematologist if unsure. Temporary cessation of these medications may substantially increase the risk of thrombosis, and some cases (e.g. recent coronary stent or significant thromboembolism) are best discussed with the patients' treating specialty physician before proceeding.

Once the lesion is located at colonoscopy, it should be positioned at 6 o'clock, ideally on the non-dependant side of the lumen. Correct positioning is important as this avoids obscuration of the working field by luminal contents, optimises access and minimises extra-luminal contamination in the event of a perforation. Carbon dioxide is routinely used for insufflation in all endoscopic procedures and has been shown to significantly reduce post-procedural admissions for pain after EMR [20]. Lastly, for polyps in difficult positions (e.g. ileocaecal valve, extending over folds or flexures), multiple patient position changes and use of a short distal attachment cap may assist access, positioning and resection of the lesion. Use of an adult colonoscope where possible may help reduce procedure time as its larger working channel (3.7 mm) compared with a paediatric colonoscope (3.2 mm) allows more specimens to be suctioned directly into a polyp trap, rather than requiring retrieval using a net. However, for difficult-to-access positions, especially where retroflexion views are required, the increased flexibility of the paediatric colonoscope may be advantageous.

Submucosal Injectate and Snares

The submucosal injectate includes a colloidal solution, epinephrine diluted to 1:100,000 and an inert dye (80 mg indigo carmine or 20 mg methylene blue per 500 mL solution). Fluid injection into the submucosa creates a cushion between the mucosal polyp and muscularis propria (MP). This reduces the risk of entrapment of deeper tissues by the snare, thereby avoiding deep mural injury (DMI) after resection. Use of colloid solutions such as succinylated gelatin (Gelofusine; Braun, Melsungen, Germany) is preferred as it is associated with reduced number of injections and resections and procedural duration compared with normal saline [21]. Diluted epinephrine reduces intra-procedural bleeding (IPB) and delays dispersion of the submucosal injectate, but does not alter the incidence of clinically significant post-procedural bleeding (CSPEB) [22]. The inert dye is avid for the submucosal connective tissue, which facilitates identification of lesion margins and the resection plane.

Snares of different sizes, shapes and wire types are often required to complete EMR. Specific snares perform better in different situations, influenced by factors such as lesion size, location and morphology. Stiff spiral or braided snares (0.48 mm thickness wire of 15, 20 and 25 mm diameter) are designed to increase tissue capture and are suited for piecemeal EMR. In most cases, the 15 mm snare provides adequate balance of efficacy and safety, but the choice of snare is usually a personal preference. Small, thin-wire snares (0.3 mm thickness wire of 10 mm diameter) are useful for difficult-to-remove tissue (e.g. peri-appendiceal or submucosal fibrosis) as well as small residual tissue within and at the margin of the EMR defect.

Resection Technique

Submucosal Injection

The needle tip should be primed with submucosal injectate, be placed tangentially to the lesion and be touching but not penetrating the mucosa. Begin by asking the assistant to commence injection whilst simultaneously penetrating the needle tip into the submucosa. The correct plane is confirmed by immediate elevation of the polyp, indicating expansion of the submucosa (Video 4.1). Injection and resection is best commenced in the most difficult-to-access aspect of the LSL. Generally, this is the caecal side of the LSL that is behind or below a mucosal fold. By first elevating this side, the lesion is moved toward the scope aiding its access and resection. Sometimes, retroflexion of the scope, particularly for LSLs located in the right colon, may assist injection and elevation of its difficult-to-access side.

Submucosal injection is performed using a dynamic technique by simultaneously pulling back slightly on the injection catheter and gentle rotation of the colonoscope with slow upward tip deflection whilst keeping the needle tip within the submucosa. This method ensures a more even distribution of the injectate into the submucosa and also allows the endoscopist to manipulate the direction of lift to move difficult-to-reach parts of an LSL into a more accessible location. Endoscopists should be wary to avoid over-injection as excessive tension within the fluid cushion may hinder visualisation and prevent adequate tissue capture by the snare.

Poor lesion elevation may be due to SMF or deep SMI. SMF may result from previous biopsy or ER attempts, reaction to submucosal injection of tattoo particles or prolapse of a large sessile (Paris 0-Is) lesion over a flexure [23]. When SMF is present, a 'jet sign', where a jet of fluid exits the lesion at high pressure during injection, or 'canyoning effect', where the centre of the lesion remains fixed in its original position but the peripheries elevate, may occur [5, 23]. Inadequate elevation may also result from transmural injection. When this is suspected, gently pull back the needle, whilst continuing injection will assist locating the submucosal plane. Conversely, superficial injection into only the mucosa will result in the immediate appearance of a superficial blue bleb without lesion elevation. In the setting of invasive disease, complete absence of lesion elevation typically only occurs when there is deep SMI with resulting obliteration of the submucosa by tumour infiltration.

Snare Resection

Correct snare placement is essential to ensuring effective resection and procedural safety. As mentioned, the lesion should be first optimally orientated, at 6 o'clock on the endoscopic view. Begin resection on one side of the lesion (usually the most difficult-to-access side) and systematically perform piecemeal resection across the lesion, aiming to resect the lesion in as few pieces as possible. LSLs ≤20 mm are best removed en bloc if safe to do so, as such a specimen improves histological assessment and is associated with less recurrence compared with piecemeal resection.

Open the snare fully over the lesion, taking care to align it along the same plane as the tissue. Then angle down firmly with the up-down dial onto the fluid cushion while gently aspirating gas. The aspiration of gas reduces colonic wall tension and allows the tissue to 'fall' into the opened snare. When closing the snare over the edge of a lesion, aim to include a 2–3 mm rim of normal mucosa to ensure complete resection and avoid small residual islands of adenoma at the margins (Video 4.1). Once adequately positioned, gradually close the snare whilst anchoring the catheter into the mucosa. Tight closure of the snare helps to exclude MP from the tissue within the snare. Concern for premature resection is not required as it is generally not possible to transect

tissue of more than 10 mm with a braided or spiral snare without the use of diathermy.

It is recommended that the endoscopist take control of the snare for tissue transection as sensory feedback provides information regarding the safety and efficacy of excision. Safe tissue capture is confirmed by three manoeuvres:

- Mobility: movement of the snare catheter quickly back and forth should result in independent and free movement of the tissue relative to the underlying colonic wall.
- Degree of closure: the snare should close fully (a distance of no more than 1 cm between thumb and fingers). If the endoscopist is unsure, the snare can be partially opened and tented into the lumen to allow any inadvertently captured MP to drop away, before repeating snare closure.
- Transection speed: transection should occur quickly. The snare is kept tightly closed while the foot pedal is depressed in short pulses. Usually one to three pulses are sufficient to transect the polyp tissue. A longer transection raises concern of MP entrapment, SMF or SMI.

Microprocessor-controlled electrosurgery is essential for safe and effective EMR. The microprocessor senses tissue impedance and adjusts power output in order to avoid deep tissue injury. Fractionated current that alternates cutting and coagulating cycles is preferred (e.g. Endo Cut mode Q, effect 3, cut duration 1, cut interval 6; ERBE, Tübingen, Germany). Low-voltage coagulation (Soft Coag, effect 4, maximum 80 W; ERBE, Tübingen, Germany) may be used for coagulation of bleeding vessels using the tip of the snare by gently placing this over any points of bleeding (STSC, snare tip soft coagulation) (Video 4.2). Following resection, adequate irrigation of the mucosal defect allows assessment for residual adenomatous tissue and evidence of DMI and assists identification and control of IPB.

The edge of the defect is used as a guide for the next resection. The inside edge of the snare should be aligned along the defect margin, the snare placed over an area of adenoma, and the steps of tissue capture as outlined above repeated. Using the defect edge as the starting point for the subsequent piecemeal resection allows for a systematic approach to EMR (Video 4.3). This method also reduces the risk of adenoma islands forming with the defect, which can be difficult to completely remove, especially when they are small. STSC is then performed by gently touching the snare tip to the EMR margin following completion of resection and has been shown to reduce adenomatous recurrence at the EMR scar from 21% to 6% at first surveillance colonoscopy (RR 0.28, $P < 0.001$) without an increase in incidence of delayed bleeding or perforation (Video 4.5) [24].

Lastly, LSLs containing a nodule (e.g. Paris 0-IIa + Is lesions) are best treated by first removing the 0-IIa component, followed by resection of the 0-Is component in one piece. The 0-Is component should be submitted separately for histological assessment as these are more likely to harbour SMI. Lesions other than those definitely located within the caecum, adjacent to the ileocaecal valve or in the low rectum, with suspicion of harbouring SMI, should have two to three endoscopic tattoos placed at different points 2–3 cm distal to the resection site [23]. The tattoo serves to assist localisation at surgery or identification of the post-EMR scar for surveillance purposes.

Aftercare

Patients undergoing advanced ER should be closely observed following their procedure. A two-stage management algorithm as shown in Fig. 4.4 is

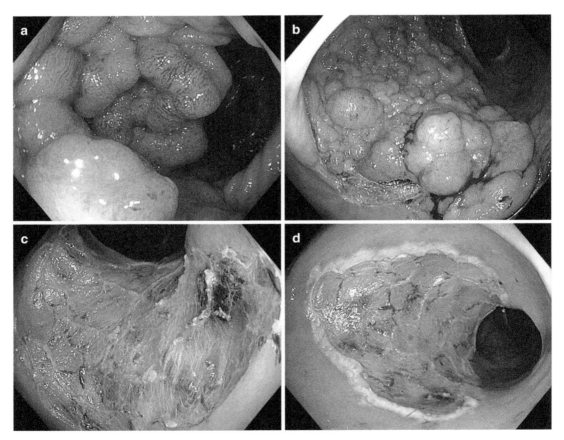

Fig. 4.4 EMR of 60 mm LSL from the descending colon. (**a**) 60 mm granular, Paris 0-IIa, Kudo IV LSL in the descending colon. (**b**) Injection and resection of the lesion is commenced at one side of the lesion and progresses toward the other. (**c**) Completed EMR with homogeneous blue matt appearance of dye-stained submucosa indicating absence of DMI. (**d**) Snare tip soft coagulation is applied to the resection margins to treat any nonvisible residual adenoma and reduce risk of adenomatous recurrence

suggested. Patient discomfort and abnormalities in vital signs may herald perforation or significant bleeding and necessitate immediate medical assessment. Most abdominal pain due to benign causes will be responsive to simple analgesia such as intravenous acetaminophen. CT abdomen should be obtained for pain that persists or if associated with clinical signs of peritonitis.

Patients who appear well and are asymptomatic with normal vital signs after a period of observation can be moved to second-stage recovery. Following a successful trial of clear liquids

and period of observation, patients may be discharged home on the same day with instructions to represent to the hospital should they develop symptoms of rectal bleeding, fevers or abdominal pain. Those who become unwell during the period of observation are admitted and further investigations organised. A suggested management algorithm of patients following complex colorectal ER is shown in Fig. 4.5.

Repeat colonoscopy is advised following the index procedure to assess presence of residual or recurrent adenoma. Typically, guidelines suggest

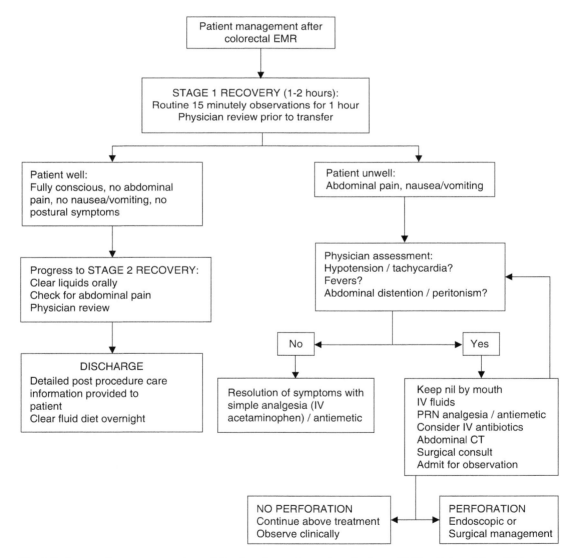

Fig. 4.5 Suggested management scheme following advanced resection of colorectal LSLs. (Adapted from Klein A and Bourke MJ *Gastroenterology Clinics of North America* 2015)

that this be performed at 4–6 months, although recent evidence from prospective multicentre data suggests LSLs <40 mm, without IPB nor high-grade dysplasia, have a 91% negative predictive value for residual or recurrent adenoma at first surveillance colonoscopy [25]. For lesions satisfying all these criteria, first surveillance colonoscopy could be delayed until 18 months after index EMR; otherwise, colonoscopy should be performed after 4–6 months.

Variant Techniques

Piecemeal Cold Snare Polypectomy

The main disadvantage to ER using electrosurgery is the risk of delayed bleeding and perforation. Cold snare polypectomy (CSP) is not associated with these risks, but this technique can only resect small polyps (≤10 mm) en bloc. For larger polyps, utilisation of CSP in a piecemeal fashion with or without submucosal injection has the potential to achieve complete excision whilst mitigating many of the adverse events of EMR. The data is so far limited, but available studies of piecemeal CSP for selected sessile adenomatous and serrated polyps 10–19 mm in size show good clinical efficacy with very few significant adverse events, and larger, prospective and comparative studies are awaited [26, 27].

Underwater EMR

Underwater EMR (UEMR) is performed in a decompressed colonic segment devoid of insufflated air, in which water is infused to assist visualisation. Submucosal injection to lift polyps is not required in this setting as the MP layer remains both circular and distant from the mucosal and submucosal layers, which 'float' within the lumen. As such, large pieces of dysplastic mucosal tissue can be removed by snare resection and electrosurgery. Since its first description in 2012, multiple studies have reported its efficacy and safety. Recently, a retrospective comparative study found UEMR was associated with higher rates of complete macroscopic resection and lower recurrence at first surveillance colonoscopy and required fewer procedures to reach curative resection compared with conventional EMR [28]. However, these findings have not been validated in a randomised controlled trial, and it remains an alternate technique to conventional EMR, for which a broader and more robust evidence base is available.

Polyps for Special Considerations

LSLs in the Anorectum

Unlike elsewhere in the colon, lymphovascular drainage of the distal rectum within 5 cm of the anal verge and the anus enters directly into the systemic circulation, bypassing the reticuloendothelial system of the portal system which has a major role in sequestering enteric pathogens. As a result, resection of LSL located in the anorectum is associated with significant bacteraemia, and prophylactic intravenous antibiotics are recommended for EMR of larger LSLs (≥30 mm). In addition, somatic sensation supplies the dentate line, and addition of a long-acting local anaesthetic such as ropivacaine 0.5–0.75% to the submucosal injectate is effective for post-procedural analgesia [29]. In this setting, cardiac monitoring by electrocardiography is required. Lastly, haemorrhoidal vessels are thick walled and are resistant to snare entrapment as long as there's adequate submucosal lift and generally present no additional bleeding risk during EMR [29].

Peri-appendiceal and Ileocaecal Valve LSLs

EMR of LSLs involving the appendiceal orifice is challenging but can generally be successfully completed provided that <50% of the valve circumference is involved and the proximal (deep) margin within the appendix is adequately visualised. A small (10 mm), stiff thin-wire snare is useful for removing adenomatous tissue from within the orifice. ER around and within the appendiceal orifice may precipitate appendicitis, and administration of a prophylactic intra-procedural intravenous antibiotic effective against enteric pathogens followed by a short 5–7-day oral course should be considered.

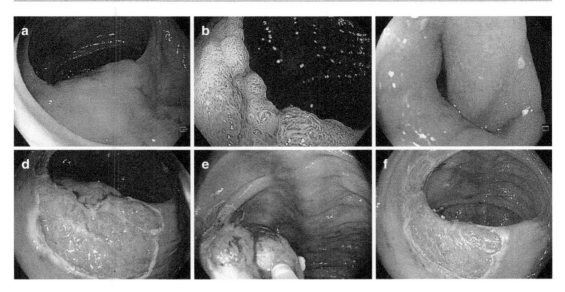

Fig. 4.6 EMR of LSL over ileocaecal valve. (**a**) 30 mm Paris 0-IIa LSL over ICV. On white light endoscopy, the lesion is not easily discerned. (**b**) Obvious Kudo type IV pit pattern is seen under NBI magnification. (**c**) The lesion does not extend into the terminal ileum. (**d**) Piecemeal resection reveals adipose tissue within the submucosa, characteristic of EMR over the ICV. The central portion is initially resistant to snare capture, likely related to submucosal fibrosis. (**e**) This area is injected and resected. (**f**) The final defect with LSL completely removed. EMR endoscopic mucosal resection, ICV ileocaecal valve, LSL laterally spreading lesion, NBI narrow band imaging

EMR of LSLs involving the ileocaecal valve (ICV) has higher risk of failure (OR 3.38, 95% CI 1.2–9.52, $P = 0.021$) [5]. Lesion access can be improved by use of a transparent distal cap attached to a paediatric colonoscope, which is preferable over an adult scope in this setting due to its smaller retroflexion radius, which may assist access to the inferior lip, and better overall manoeuvrability. The cap helps to deflect mucosal folds, stabilise the endoscope and visualise the distal ileum and ICV lips. Extensive proximal extension of adenomatous tissue into the narrow terminal ileum and LSLs that involve both the superior and inferior lips is challenging for complete EMR [30]. The EMR technique of LSLs involving the ICV is similar to that used in other colonic locations, albeit with a few notable adaptions. A small (10 mm), stiff thin-wire snare is preferred when working with the distal ileum due to space constraints. Submucosal injection should be conservative as excessive amounts can hamper endoscopic visualisation and lesion access. Careful attention should be paid to the anterior and posterior angles of the ICV, where residual tissue can be missed [30]. Lastly, the ICV submucosa is relatively adipose, and commonly underlying fat is exposed following resection, but is not necessarily a sign of deeper injury (Fig. 4.6).

Large Pedunculated Polyps

Pedunculated polyps account for a third of all colonic polyps. Many are larger than 10 mm and typically contain a feeding vessel within its stalk. Complete resection of a pedunculated polyp is achieved by transection of its pedicle. This minimises the risk of perforation, but risks bleeding from the feeding vessel, which can be severe. An increased risk of bleeding is associated with stalk thickness ≥5 mm, polyp head ≥20 mm in size, right colonic location and presence of malignancy [31]. The risk of delayed bleeding following resection of pedunculated polyps can be reduced by mechanical prophylaxis with clips and/or nylon loops applied to the stalk, with or without pre-injection with diluted (1:10,000) adrenaline [32, 33]. Following satisfactory ligation of the stalk, snare resection above the point of ligation with blended or coagulation current is performed. Pure cutting current should be avoided as this is associated with an increased risk of immediate bleeding.

Lesions Previously Attempted for Resection

Previous attempts at resection or aggressive biopsies can cause significant SMF, which hinders safe and effective EMR. For such lesions, where possible, careful submucosal lift should be attempted, starting injection and resection away from any sites of obvious fibrosis to assist finding the right submucosal plane. Small, stiff thin-wire snares are preferable. When fibrosis prevents snare capture of adenomatous tissue, cold-forceps avulsion with adjuvant snare tip soft coagulation (CAST) (Soft Coag, effect 4, maximum 80 W; ERBE, Tübingen, Germany) to the avulsed area is an effective technique to remove small residual islands (Video 4.4) [34]. Following this approach, a type II–V DMI (see below section on 'perforation') may result within the resection defect that is best treated by application of through-the-scope (TTS) clips to this area to prevent delayed perforation. A recent prospective multicentre observational study also showed that two-stage EMR performed by tertiary centre endoscopists is a safe and effective salvage therapy after a failed single session, with 84% technical success and 82% of patients avoiding surgery on long-term follow-up using this approach [35].

Managing Adverse Events

The most frequent adverse events occurring after EMR are bleeding and perforation. Of these, bleeding is the most common and can occur during the procedure or be delayed for up to 2 weeks. Severity can range from self-limited oozing to brisk arterial bleeding, although endoscopic haemostasis can be achieved in most instances.

Intra-procedural Bleeding

Intra-procedural bleeding, defined as bleeding that lasts for longer than 60 seconds or that requires endoscopic intervention, occurs in up to 11% of cases and is associated with increasing lesion size (OR 1.24/10 mm), Paris 0-IIa + Is lesion morphology (OR 2.12), lesions with tubulovillous or villous histology (OR 1.84) and endoscopy centres that perform fewer than 75 EMRs per year (OR 3.78) [22]. Most cases of IPB are controllable endoscopically, although difficult-to-control bleeding prolongs the procedure and is associated with increased adenomatous recurrence (OR 1.68) [22].

IPB can be effectively treated by thermal modalities, and use of a voltage-limited microprocessor-controlled current helps to avoid deep thermal injury. STSC is an effective and safe technique to control IPB arising from small arterioles or veins. It is performed by protruding the snare tip 2–3 mm beyond the catheter, followed by application of coagulating current (Soft Coag, effect 4, 80 W; ERBE, Tübingen, Germany) whilst gently touching the tip directly onto the bleeding vessel. Irrigating the defect with the foot pump clears the field and localises the point of bleeding and may also have a tamponade effect through expansion of fluid into the submucosa. In the minority of cases where STSC does not achieve haemostasis, additional treatment of the bleeding vessel with coagulating forceps (Soft Coag, effect 4, 80 W; ERBE, Tübingen, Germany) or TTS clips may be used. Injection of dilute adrenaline may be used for initial haemostasis, but should be used with another modality such as thermal ablation or mechanical haemostasis [23].

Delayed Bleeding

Delayed bleeding (also termed clinically significant post-endoscopic bleeding [CSPEB]) is defined as any bleeding occurring up to 30 days after EMR, resulting in emergency room presentation, hospitalisation or re-intervention. Based on data from a large multicentre study, the incidence of CSPEB is 6.2%, with increased risk associated with proximal colon location (OR 3.72), use of an electrosurgical current not controlled by a microprocessor (OR 2.03) and IPB (OR 2.16) [22]. Lesion size and patient comorbidities did not appear to predict CSPEB [22].

Most cases of CSPEB resolve spontaneously without need for intervention. Need for intervention is associated with hourly or more frequent

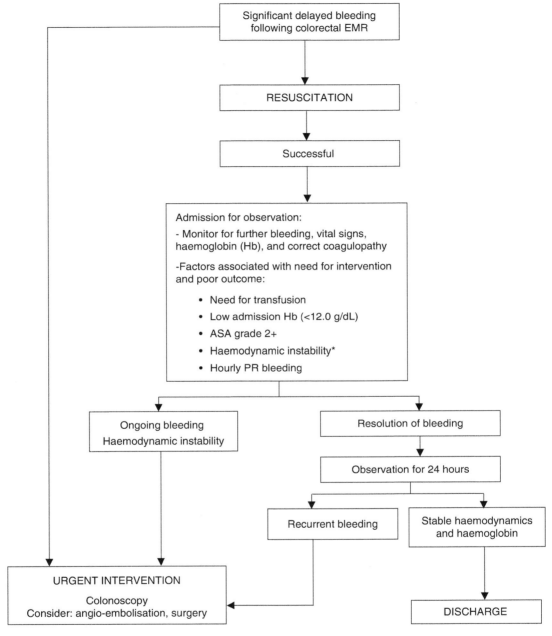

Fig. 4.7 Management algorithm for clinically significant post-EMR bleeding. *Haemodynamic instability defined as heart rate ≥100/min, systolic blood pressure ≤100 mmHg or orthostatic decrease in SBP ≥20 mmHg. (Adapted from Burgess NB, Metz AJ, Williams SJ et al. *Clin Gastro Hep* 2014)

haematochezia (OR 36.7), American Society of Anesthesiologists grade ≥ 2 (OR 20.1) and need for transfusion (OR 18.7). These factors form the basis of an algorithm to manage post-EMR CSPEB (Fig. 4.7) [36]. Prophylactic coagulation to non-bleeding vessels within the resection defect does not significantly decrease the incidence of CSPEB after EMR [37]. Closure of resection defects with clips may reduce the risk of CSPEB, particularly for proximal and larger

LSLs, although prospective, randomised data supporting a benefit of this practice are pending [38].

Perforation

The incidence of perforation related to colonic EMR of LSLs is 1–2% [5]. Early identification and management of perforation after EMR reduces both the need for surgery and mortality, with high effectiveness of endoscopic closure. Perforation is one of five categories of endoscopically identifiable MP injuries, classified as deep mural injury (DMI) (Table 4.1) [39]. The DMI classification standardises description of colonic wall injury with prognostic implications (Fig. 4.8). Type I DMI represents exposed but uninjured MP fibres and requires no treatment. In type II DMI, the distinction between submucosa and MP is unclear, often due to poorly staining SMF. As deep injury cannot be excluded, this area should be prophylactically clipped, even if no obvious defect target sign (type III DMI, Fig. 4.9) is present [40]. In type III, IV and V DMI, the injured MP is represented by concentric white rings within the MP and should always be promptly closed by clips to avoid extension of injury or contamination.

Endoscopically subtle MP injury is probably responsible for some cases of delayed perforations. In situations with poor staining of the resection defect, assessment of this area by topical irrigation of the injection solution using the injection catheter with needle retracted (topical submucosal chromoendoscopy, TSC) can reveal either uninjured submucosa or MP injury [41]. The submucosal fibres avidly take up the dye, and the resulting blue matt appearance reassures that no MP injury has occurred. Conversely, any exposed MP fibres will not take up the dye, and non-staining areas after TSC suggest deep injury and should be prophylactically treated by application of TTS clips.

TTS clips have been shown to have similar tensile strength to surgical sutures and are ideal for closure of ER-related perforations (Video 4.6). The principles and techniques of perforation closure with clips involve the following:

- Minimising gas insufflation to reduce tension on the defect. Administer anti-peristaltic agents to prevent peristalsis from contaminating the site.
- Keep the working field clean by positioning the patient so fluid pools away from the defect.
- Remove adenomatous tissue adjacent to the defect if possible before placement of clips for DMI types II and III. Prompt closure takes precedence in obvious perforations (DMI types IV and V).
- MP wounds are generally aligned perpendicular to the long axis of the colon. The sequence of clip placement is best progressed from left to right to maintain access. Gravity should also be considered, and it is best to avoid placing a clip where it will fall across the working field.
- The first clip can be placed just beyond the defect to elevate the bowel wall and facilitate subsequent clip placement. First, suction the mucosa into the open clip making sure to have the defect in the centre pivot of the clip, followed by gentle pressure from the clip against the mucosa. With further suction, the lumen is deflated, and the clip is closed. Confirm adequate convergence of the defect edges within the clip on re-insufflation, before deploying the clip.
- Endoscopic closure of perforations by suture devices is also feasible, although this technique requires endoscope exchange and reinsertion, risking extra-luminal contamination

Table 4.1 Sydney classification of deep mural injury (DMI) following EMR

Type I	MP visible, but no mechanical injury. May have minimal thermal injury
Type II	Focal or generalised loss of the submucosal plane raising concern for MP injury or rendering the MP defect uninterpretable
Type III	MP injured, target or mirror target identified
Type IV	Hole within a white cautery ring, no observed contamination
Type V	Hole within a white cautery ring, observed contamination

EMR endoscopic mucosal resection, *MP* muscularis propria

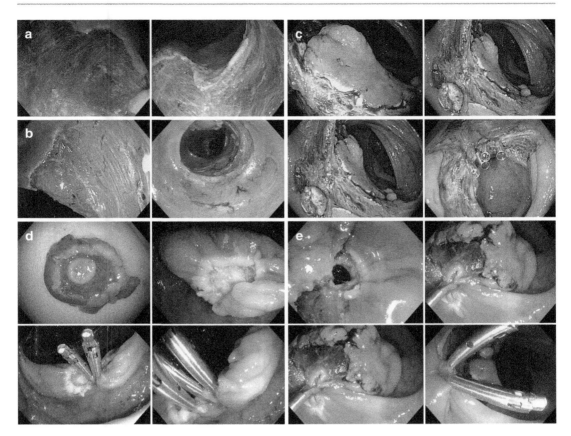

Fig. 4.8 Examples of deep mural injury and their management following EMR. (**a**) (two images, top left): type 0. This is a normal finding. The submucosa is homogeneously stained with blue dye, without exposure of the MP. Vessels may be seen within or upon the blue layer. (**b**) (two images, top left): type I. The submucosa has been deeply resected, revealing the underlying parallel striations of muscle in the MP. The MP generally does not stain well with dye and has a whiter appearance. There is no risk of delayed perforation. (**c**) (four images, top right): type II. Focal area of poor staining within the centre of the defect. It is usually due to submucosal fibrosis. However, as this area cannot be adequately interrogated for MP injury, prophylactic closure with TTS clips is recommended. (**d**) (four images, lower left): type III. The specimen TS (first image) is characterised by a whitish circle of resected MP on the transected surface of the specimen surrounded by a web of blue-stained submucosal tissue and encircled by white cauterised mucosa. This is an endoscopic marker of partial- or full-thickness MP injury. Patients with TS should be promptly managed by endoscopically placed clips and usually do not require operative management. (**e**) (four images, lower right): type IV. An obvious perforation is demonstrated. Full-thickness excision of MP has occurred without faecal contamination. These defects should be promptly closed to avoid peritoneal contamination. EMR endoscopic mucosal resection, MP muscularis propria, TS target sign, TTS through the scope. (Adapted from Ma MX, Bourke MJ, *Best Prac Res Clin Gastroenterol* 2016)

in the process, and is probably best suited to large gaping perforations where clips are less likely to be effective.

Patients who are clinically well without signs of peritonitis following treatment of DMI types II–III can be safely discharged on the same day as their procedure. Extra-luminal gas seen on abdominal CT without intraperitoneal fluid after satisfactory closure of a non-contaminated intra-procedural perforation in a well patient generally has a good prognosis. However, the presence of extra-luminal fluid is a much more serious situation that requires careful ongoing clinical review and surgical consultation.

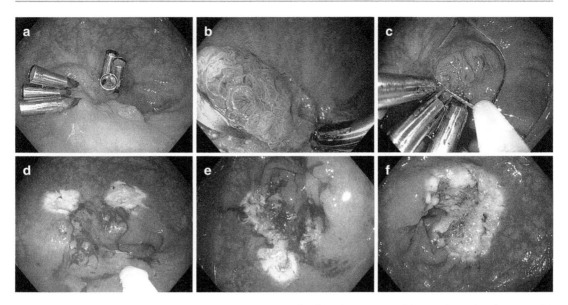

Fig. 4.9 Endoscopic treatment of small adenomatous recurrence. (**a**, **b**) Small area of adenomatous recurrence at the site of previous EMR viewed under white light and NBI. (**c**) A 10 mm stiff thin-wire snare is used to resect the adenomatous tissue using forced coagulation. (**d**) The clips have been removed by traction using the snare. (**e**) Visible areas of adenoma unable to be captured by the snare are resected using cold-forceps biopsy resulting in some superficial bleeding. (**f**) The cold-forceps biopsied area is then treated using snare tip soft coagulation

Post-polypectomy Electrocoagulation Syndrome and Delayed Perforation

Post-polypectomy electrocoagulation syndrome (PPES) occurs as a result of transmural thermal injury to the bowel wall, with associated serosal inflammation and localised peritonitis. Patients usually present hours to days after colonic ER with fever, localised signs of peritonitis, raised inflammatory markers and absence of perforation on radiological imaging. The incidence of PPES is about 0.5% with risk factors including ER in the right colon, polyp size ≥20 mm, hypertension and lesions with a non-polypoidal morphology [31]. The risk of PPES can be reduced by minimising transmission of electrocoagulation current to the submucosal layers of the bowel wall, e.g. by adequate submucosal injection and tenting of the snared lesion into the colonic lumen before resection by diathermy. Treatment is conservative with intravenous fluids, antibiotics and bowel rest.

Delayed perforation fortunately is rare and, like PPES, may result from electrocoagulation-related thermal injury or subtle, unrecognised MP injury. Most cases present within 24 hours of ER, but can occur up to a week later. When suspected, urgent CT abdomen is required to establish the diagnosis and evaluate extent of peritonitis. As delayed perforations are associated with a high rate of faecal peritonitis, surgery is often required although primary repair by laparoscopy may be possible if tissue appear healthy. Otherwise, faecal diversion by colostomy or ileostomy may be required [31].

Endoscopic Submucosal Dissection

ESD is a controlled endoscopic knife-based method to dissect LSLs from the submucosal space above a dye-stained fluid cushion (Fig. 4.10). Large series evaluating ESD vs. EMR for the treatment of colorectal LSLs show a higher rate of en bloc resection (84–95%) and lower local recurrence (0–2%) in favour of ESD [42, 43]. However, the advantages of colorectal ESD over EMR come at the cost of increased procedural duration (mean weighted difference 1.76; 95% CI 0.60–2.92) and higher rate of perforation (OR 4.09) [6].

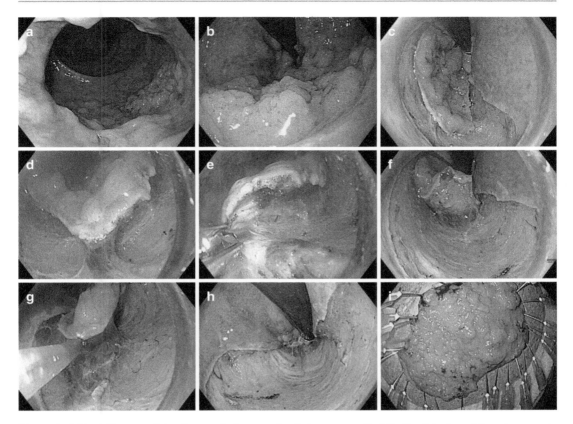

Fig. 4.10 ESD of 50 mm traditional serrated adenoma of the rectum. (**a**, **b**) Forward and retroflexion views of lesion. (**c**) The lesion margins have been incised. (**d**) A large submucosal vessel is encountered during dissection. (**e**) The vessel is prophylactically treated with the coagulating grasper. (**f**, **g**) Further injection of the submucosa to complete dissection. (**h**, **i**) The resection defect showing visible but uninjured MP fibres, with pinned specimen. ESD endoscopic submucosal dissection, MP muscularis propria

ESD is preferred for lesions with an increased likelihood of superficial SMI, particularly those ≥20 mm in size; however, these lesions are uncommon and were found in only 3.7% of 2000 LSLs treated by EMR in a large Western multicentre prospective study [11]. The study showed that although most LSLs are effectively treated by EMR, as most adenomatous recurrence was small and endoscopically treatable (Fig. 4.9), ESD remains a very useful procedure for carefully selected lesions. For superficially invasive lesions, ESD has curative potential with reduced morbidity compared with surgery and is particularly relevant in the rectum. As ESD expertise and availability increases, good immediate and long-term outcomes following colorectal ESD have been reported even from lower-volume centres [44].

Resection Technique

A variety of endoscopic knives are available for ESD, and the choice is usually a personal preference of the endoscopist. Certain knives may be more advantageous in particular situations, although few comparative studies are currently available. Some knives, e.g. HybridKnife (ERBE, Tübingen, Germany) and DualKnife J (Olympus, Tokyo, Japan), have both cutting and injection capabilities, thereby minimising instrument exchange and reducing procedure time. A clear cap attached to the distal end of the scope is used to assist access to the submucosa and its controlled dissection. A colonoscope is used for most cases, although gastroscopes may be advantageous for rectal ESD, particularly distal lesions where a more acute angle of scope retroflexion can assist dissection near the anal verge.

The peripheral extent of colorectal LSLs is usually easily discerned endoscopically (in contrast to gastric or oesophageal lesions), and marking of the lesion peripheries generally is not required. The patient is preferably positioned with the lesion in a non-dependant position, so that gravity assists dissection by aiding its separation from the submucosa. This also helps to avoid contamination of the working field in the event of bleeding or perforation. The constituents in the injectate for ESD are similar to those used for EMR, except that the dye used is diluted to a quarter concentration, to improve visibility of the submucosal fibres during dissection.

Following creation of the submucosal fluid cushion, a circumferential mucosal incision is made using the ESD knife, with a 3–4 mm margin of normal mucosa. A suggested electrosurgical setting is Endo Cut Q (effect 3, cut duration 3, cut interval 3; ERBE VIO300D, Tübingen, Germany). In particular, it is important to note where the fluid pools in the lumen relative to the lesion. The mucosal edge of the lesion adjacent to the fluid pool is definitively incised early during the procedure as access to this side will be impeded once the lesion 'flips' over with progression of dissection due to gravity. The endoscopist should continually check the plane of dissection throughout the procedure and particularly be aware of the MP at all times. Correct orientation allows dissection to occur along one submucosal plane, increasing en bloc resection whilst reducing the risk of inadvertent DMI.

As dissection progresses, it is important to avoid bleeding as blood inhibits visualisation and impedes subsequent injection and expansion of the submucosa and treatment of bleeding prolongs the procedure. Different electrosurgical settings may optimise dissection depending on the submucosal vascularity. A suggested setting is Dry Cut (effect 2, 50 W; ERBE VIO300D, Tübingen, Germany) for routine submucosal dissection. For more vascular areas that contain minute vessels, a setting with increased coagulation is preferred such as Swift Coag (effect 3, 30 W; ERBE VIO300D, Tübingen, Germany).

Visible vessels are best treated prophylactically with the knife tip (small vessels) or coagulation grasper (moderate vessels, arterioles) using soft coagulation (effect 4, 80 W; ERBE VIO300D, Tübingen, Germany), before dissection with the knife. For larger vessels traversing the submucosal dissection field, prophylactic application of a haemostatic clip prior to vessel coagulation and dissection may be required.

A more recently utilised variant of rectal ESD involves making an initial submucosal tunnel in an anal-oral direction below the lesion, followed by resection of the tunnel walls to completely remove the lesion [45, 46]. This technique was first described for en bloc resection of large oesophageal neoplastic lesions. Compared with routine ESD, endoscopic tunnel dissection has a number of potential advantages including improved visualisation of the submucosa and slower dissipation of the fluid cushion. This aids better identification of the MP and submucosal vessels to achieve high R0 resection and lower complication rates such as perforation and bleeding. Additional research on this new technique, including larger comparative studies with conventional methods, is awaited before its adoption into mainstream ESD practice.

Managing Adverse Events

Bleeding

Bleeding after colorectal ESD occurs in 0.5–9.6% of cases, and overall the risk appears to be lower compared with EMR (OR 0.85, 95% CI 0.45–1.60) [47]. Focal bleeding from small arterioles during dissection can be treated by soft coagulation (effect 4, 80 W; ERBE VIO300D, Tübingen, Germany) delivered through the retracted knife tip and is usually sufficient to achieve haemostasis. Persistent bleeding may require haemostasis using the coagulation grasper. The vessel is grasped and gently tented away from the MP and adjacent submucosa. Satisfactory mechanical tamponade of the vessel is indicated by cessation of bleeding and can be confirmed by briefly flushing the area with the foot pump whilst holding the vessel with the grasper. The vessel is then obliterated using soft coagulation (effect 4, 80 W; ERBE VIO300D, Tübingen, Germany). Bleeding that persists despite these interventions may require mechanical haemostasis using a TTS clip, but this may hinder access to further submucosal dissection.

Post-ESD bleeding typically occurs from one of the many feeding arteries to the artificial ulcer floor of the resected specimen. Risk factors for delayed bleeding after colorectal ESD include lesion size ≥30 mm, rectal location of lesions, presence of submucosal fibrosis and low-volume centres [48]. Some experts advocate prophylactic ablation of non-bleeding vessels in the post-ESD ulcer to prevent bleeding, although this practice is not scientifically proven. Delayed bleeding can usually be treated with standard endoscopic techniques, preferably with TTS clips to avoid further thermal injury to the muscle layer.

Perforation

ESD traditionally carried a higher rate of perforation compared with EMR (5–8% vs. 1.3–3.4%, respectively), although contemporary data from expert ESD centres report perforation rates as low as 1–2% [43]. Risk factors for ESD-related perforations include lesions located in the colon, larger LSL size, presence of submucosal fibrosis and endoscopist experience <50 cases [31]. Surgery related to ESD-associated complications is fortunately seldom required and was reported in only 1% in a systematic review of nearly 3000 cases with the majority of complications being endoscopically treatable [49].

Prevention of ESD-related MP injury and its management follows similar principles to those following EMR. Dissection should occur over an adequate submucosal fluid cushion with appropriate electrosurgical settings to minimise transmural transfer of energy. Following resection, the defect should be carefully inspected for exposed or damaged MP fibres and TSC applied to areas where the submucosa is not well stained with dye. Areas of non-staining after TSC and where MP injury has occurred may be prophylactically treated by TTS clips. Obvious perforations should be closed promptly, and endoscopic suturing devices have also been used with success in small numbers of patients after ESD. Endoscopic closure after delayed perforation is usually not possible due to extra-luminal soiling and associated peritonitis, and surgery is often required.

Stricturing

Extensive or circumferential LSLs are uncommonly encountered, and their removal by EMR and ESD is described [8, 50]. A unique complication arising from such ER is luminal stricturing, where the degree of circumferential involvement and longitudinal length of resection are risk factors for stenosis. This may occur in up to 50% of cases following circumferential ER. Fortunately, this stricturing is usually responsive to endoscopic therapy and may be avoided by a proactive serial prophylactic dilatation regimen following ER. In addition, topical treatment with hydrocortisone enemas may also have a role in prevention of rectal stricture formation [31].

Summary

- Endoscopic resection of complex mucosal polyps is safe, effective, cost-efficient, and considered the first-line therapy for these lesions.
- Various ER techniques for these polyps exist and are broadly categorised as EMR or ESD.
- A patient-centred approach to ER is imperative, and the decision to undertake EMR or ESD needs to be weighed against the comorbidities of the patient and should only be undertaken where a clear benefit is identified.
- Accurate and thorough endoscopic assessment of a lesion including its peripheral extent, anatomical relationships and risk of harbouring SMI should be performed for all lesions prior to ER.
- EMR is suitable for most lesions, provided the lesion does not harbour SMI.
- ESD is associated with higher en bloc resection rates, but is technically more demanding to perform, requires longer procedural duration and is associated with greater procedural risk compared with EMR.

- Lesions suspected of harbouring superficial SMI are best resected by ESD as this optimises localised histological staging and may offer a cure.
- To achieve optimal outcomes with either EMR or ESD, the endoscopist should adopt a meticulous technical approach focused toward safe and complete resection whilst being aware of all the potential complications and methods to appropriately manage these if they occur.

References

1. Rosenberg N. Submucosal saline wheal as safety factor in fulguration or rectal and sigmoidal polypi. AMA Arch Surg. 1955;70(1):120–2.
2. Deyhle P, Jenny S, Fumagalli I. Endoskopische Polypektomie im proximalen Kolon. Dtsch Med Wochenschr. 1973;98(05):219–20.
3. Hirao M, Masuda K, Asanuma T, Naka H, Noda K, Matsuura K, et al. Endoscopic resection of early gastric cancer and other tumors with local injection of hypertonic saline-epinephrine. Gastrointest Endosc. 1988;34(3):264–9.
4. Jayanna M, Burgess NG, Singh R, Hourigan LF, Brown GJ, Zanati SA, et al. Cost analysis of endoscopic mucosal resection vs surgery for large laterally spreading colorectal lesions. Clin Gastroenterol Hepatol. 2016;14(2):271–8.e1–2.
5. Moss A, Bourke MJ, Williams SJ, Hourigan LF, Brown G, Tam W, et al. Endoscopic mucosal resection outcomes and prediction of submucosal cancer from advanced colonic mucosal neoplasia. Gastroenterology. 2011;140(7):1909–18.
6. Cao Y, Liao C, Tan A, Gao Y, Mo Z, Gao F. Meta-analysis of endoscopic submucosal dissection versus endoscopic mucosal resection for tumors of the gastrointestinal tract. Endoscopy. 2009;41(9):751–7.
7. Tutticci N, Klein A, Sonson R, Bourke MJ. Endoscopic resection of subtotal or completely circumferential laterally spreading colonic adenomas: technique, caveats, and outcomes. Endoscopy. 2016;48(5):465–71.
8. Tutticci N, Sonson R, Bourke MJ. Endoscopic resection of subtotal and complete circumferential colonic advanced mucosal neoplasia. Gastrointest Endosc. 2014;80(2):340.
9. Nascimbeni R, Burgart LJ, Nivatvongs S, Larson DR. Risk of lymph node metastasis in T1 carcinoma of the colon and rectum. Dis Colon Rectum. 2002;45(2):200–6.
10. Participants in the Paris W. The Paris endoscopic classification of superficial neoplastic lesions: esophagus, stomach, and colon. Gastrointest Endosc. 2003;58(6):S3–S43.
11. Burgess NG, Hourigan LF, Zanati SA, Brown GJ, Singh R, Williams SJ, et al. Risk stratification for covert invasive cancer among patients referred for colonic endoscopic mucosal resection: a large multicenter cohort. Gastroenterology. 2017;153:732. https://doi.org/10.1053/j.gastro.2017.05.047.
12. Kudo S, Rubio CA, Teixeira CR, Kashida H, Kogure E. Pit pattern in colorectal neoplasia: endoscopic magnifying view. Endoscopy. 2001;33(4):367–73.
13. Ikematsu H, Matsuda T, Emura F, Saito Y, Uraoka T, Fu KI, et al. Efficacy of capillary pattern type IIIA/IIIB by magnifying narrow band imaging for estimating depth of invasion of early colorectal neoplasms. BMC Gastroenterol. 2010;10:33.
14. Hewett DG, Kaltenbach T, Sano Y, Tanaka S, Saunders BP, Ponchon T, et al. Validation of a simple classification system for endoscopic diagnosis of small colorectal polyps using narrow-band imaging. Gastroenterology. 2012;143(3):599–607.e1.
15. Pellise M, Burgess NG, Tutticci N, Hourigan LF, Zanati SA, Brown GJ, et al. Endoscopic mucosal resection for large serrated lesions in comparison with adenomas: a prospective multicentre study of 2000 lesions. Gut. 2017;66(4):644–53.
16. Conio M, Repici A, Demarquay JF, Blanchi S, Dumas R, Filiberti R. EMR of large sessile colorectal polyps. Gastrointest Endosc. 2004;60(2):234–41.
17. Law R, Das A, Gregory D, Komanduri S, Muthusamy R, Rastogi A, et al. Endoscopic resection is cost-effective compared with laparoscopic resection in the management of complex colon polyps: an economic analysis. Gastrointest Endosc. 2016;83(6):1248–57.
18. Acosta RD, Abraham NS, Chandrasekhara V, Chathadi KV, Early DS, Eloubeidi MA, et al. The management of antithrombotic agents for patients undergoing GI endoscopy. Gastrointest Endosc. 2016;83(1):3–16.
19. Veitch AM, Vanbiervliet G, Gershlick AH, Boustiere C, Baglin TP, Smith LA, et al. Endoscopy in patients on antiplatelet or anticoagulant therapy, including direct oral anticoagulants: British Society of Gastroenterology (BSG) and European Society of Gastrointestinal Endoscopy (ESGE) guidelines. Endoscopy. 2016;48(4):385–402.
20. Dellon ES, Hawk JS, Grimm IS, Shaheen NJ. The use of carbon dioxide for insufflation during GI endoscopy: a systematic review. Gastrointest Endosc. 2009;69(4):843–9.
21. Moss A, Bourke MJ, Metz AJ. A randomized, double-blind trial of succinylated gelatin submucosal injection for endoscopic resection of large sessile polyps of the colon. Am J Gastroenterol. 2010;105(11):2375–82.
22. Burgess NG, Metz AJ, Williams SJ, Singh R, Tam W, Hourigan LF, et al. Risk factors for intraprocedural and clinically significant delayed bleeding after wide-field endoscopic mucosal resection of large colonic lesions. Clin Gastroenterol Hepatol. 2014;12(4):651–61.e1–3.
23. Ferlitsch M, Moss A, Hassan C, Bhandari P, Dumonceau JM, Paspatis G, et al. Colorectal polypectomy and endoscopic mucosal resection

(EMR): European Society of Gastrointestinal Endoscopy (ESGE) Clinical Guideline. Endoscopy. 2017;49(3):270–97.

24. Klein A, Jayasekeran V, Hourigan LF, Tate DJ, Singh R, Brown GJ, et al. 812b A multi-center randomized control trial of thermalaablation of the margin of the post endoscopic mucosal resection (EMR) mucosal defect in the prevention of adenoma recurrence following EMR: preliminary results from the "SCAR" study. Gastroenterology. 2016;150(4):S1266–S7.

25. Tate DJ, Desomer L, Klein A, Brown G, Hourigan LF, Lee EY, et al. Adenoma recurrence after piecemeal colonic EMR is predictable: the Sydney EMR recurrence tool. Gastrointest Endosc. 2017;85(3):647–56. e6.

26. Choksi N, Elmunzer BJ, Stidham RW, Shuster D, Piraka C. Cold snare piecemeal resection of colonic and duodenal polyps >/=1 cm. Endosc Int Open. 2015;3(5):E508–13.

27. Piraka C, Saeed A, Waljee AK, Pillai A, Stidham R, Elmunzer BJ. Cold snare polypectomy for non-pedunculated colon polyps greater than 1 cm. Endosc Int Open. 2017;5(3):E184–e9.

28. Schenck RJ, Jahann DA, Patrie JT, Stelow EB, Cox DG, Uppal DS, et al. Underwater endoscopic mucosal resection is associated with fewer recurrences and earlier curative resections compared to conventional endoscopic mucosal resection for large colorectal polyps. Surg Endosc. 2017;31:4174.

29. Holt BA, Bassan MS, Sexton A, Williams SJ, Bourke MJ. Advanced mucosal neoplasia of the anorectal junction: endoscopic resection technique and outcomes (with videos). Gastrointest Endosc. 2014;79(1):119–26.

30. Nanda KS, Tutticci N, Burgess NG, Sonson R, Williams SJ, Bourke MJ. Endoscopic mucosal resection of laterally spreading lesions involving the ileocecal valve: technique, risk factors for failure, and outcomes. Endoscopy. 2015;47(8):710–8.

31. Ma MX, Bourke MJ. Complications of endoscopic polypectomy, endoscopic mucosal resection and endoscopic submucosal dissection in the colon. Best Pract Res Clin Gastroenterol. 2016;30(5):749–67.

32. Paspatis GA, Paraskeva K, Theodoropoulou A, Mathou N, Vardas E, Oustamanolakis P, et al. A prospective, randomized comparison of adrenaline injection in combination with detachable snare versus adrenaline injection alone in the prevention of postpolypectomy bleeding in large colonic polyps. Am J Gastroenterol. 2006;101(12):2805.. quiz 913

33. Kouklakis G, Mpoumponaris A, Gatopoulou A, Efraimidou E, Manolas K, Lirantzopoulos N. Endoscopic resection of large pedunculated colonic polyps and risk of postpolypectomy bleeding with adrenaline injection versus endoloop and hemoclip: a prospective, randomized study. Surg Endosc. 2009;23(12):2732–7.

34. Tate DJ, Bahin FF, Desomer L, Sidhu M, Gupta V, Bourke MJ. Cold-forceps avulsion with adjuvant snare-tip soft coagulation (CAST) is an effective and safe strategy for the management of non-lifting large laterally spreading colonic lesions. Endoscopy. 2018;50(1):52–62.

35. Tate DJ, Desomer L, Hourigan LF, Moss A, Singh R, Bourke MJ. Two-stage endoscopic mucosal resection is a safe and effective salvage therapy after a failed single-session approach. Endoscopy. 2017;49(9):888–98.

36. Burgess NG, Williams SJ, Hourigan LF, Brown GJ, Zanati SA, Singh R, et al. A management algorithm based on delayed bleeding after wide-field endoscopic mucosal resection of large colonic lesions. Clin Gastroenterol Hepatol. 2014;12(9):1525–33.

37. Bahin FF, Naidoo M, Williams SJ, Hourigan LF, Ormonde DG, Raftopoulos SC, et al. Prophylactic endoscopic coagulation to prevent bleeding after wide-field endoscopic mucosal resection of large sessile colon polyps. Clin Gastroenterol Hepatol. 2015;13(4):724–30.e1–2.

38. Liaquat H, Rohn E, Rex DK. Prophylactic clip closure reduced the risk of delayed postpolypectomy hemorrhage: experience in 277 clipped large sessile or flat colorectal lesions and 247 control lesions. Gastrointest Endosc. 2013;77(3):401–7.

39. Burgess NG, Bassan MS, McLeod D, Williams SJ, Byth K, Bourke MJ. Deep mural injury and perforation after colonic endoscopic mucosal resection: a new classification and analysis of risk factors. Gut. 2017;66(10):1779–89.

40. Swan MP, Bourke MJ, Moss A, Williams SJ, Hopper A, Metz A. The target sign: an endoscopic marker for the resection of the muscularis propria and potential perforation during colonic endoscopic mucosal resection. Gastrointest Endosc. 2011;73(1):79–85.

41. Holt BA, Jayasekeran V, Sonson R, Bourke MJ. Topical submucosal chromoendoscopy defines the level of resection in colonic EMR and may improve procedural safety (with video). Gastrointest Endosc. 2013;77(6):949–53.

42. Saito Y, Fukuzawa M, Matsuda T, Fukunaga S, Sakamoto T, Uraoka T, et al. Clinical outcome of endoscopic submucosal dissection versus endoscopic mucosal resection of large colorectal tumors as determined by curative resection. Surg Endosc. 2010;24(2):343–52.

43. Nakajima T, Saito Y, Tanaka S, Iishi H, Kudo SE, Ikematsu H, et al. Current status of endoscopic resection strategy for large, early colorectal neoplasia in Japan. Surg Endosc. 2013;27(9):3262–70.

44. Boda K, Oka S, Tanaka S, Nagata S, Kunihiro M, Kuwai T, et al. Clinical outcomes of endoscopic submucosal dissection for colorectal tumors: a large multicenter retrospective study from the Hiroshima GI Endoscopy Research Group. Gastrointest Endosc. 2018;87(3):714–22.

45. Yang JL, Gan T, Zhu LL, Wang YP, Yang L, Wu JC. Endoscopic submucosal tunnel dissection: a feasible solution for large superficial rectal neoplastic lesions. Dis Colon Rectum. 2017;60(8):866–71.

46. Pioche M, Rivory J, Lepilliez V, Saurin JC, Ponchon T, Jacques J. Tunnel-and-bridge strategy for rectal endoscopic submucosal dissection: tips to allow strong countertraction without clip and line. Endoscopy. 2017;49(S 01):E123–e4.

47. Fujiya M, Tanaka K, Dokoshi T, Tominaga M, Ueno N, Inaba Y, et al. Efficacy and adverse events of EMR and endoscopic submucosal dissection for the treatment of colon neoplasms: a meta-analysis of studies comparing EMR and endoscopic submucosal dissection. Gastrointest Endosc. 2015;81(3):583–95.

48. Saito Y, Uraoka T, Yamaguchi Y, Hotta K, Sakamoto N, Ikematsu H, et al. A prospective, multicenter study of 1111 colorectal endoscopic submucosal dissections (with video). Gastrointest Endosc. 2010;72(6):1217–25.

49. Repici A, Hassan C, De Paula Pessoa D, Pagano N, Arezzo A, Zullo A, et al. Efficacy and safety of endoscopic submucosal dissection for colorectal neoplasia: a systematic review. Endoscopy. 2012;44(2):137–50.

50. Abe S, Sakamoto T, Takamaru H, Yamada M, Nakajima T, Matsuda T, et al. Stenosis rates after endoscopic submucosal dissection of large rectal tumors involving greater than three quarters of the luminal circumference. Surg Endosc. 2016;30:5459.

Endoscopic Tools and Accessories for ESD

Calvin Jianyi Koh, Dennis Yang, and Peter V. Draganov

Introduction: Why Do We Need Specialized Devices

By definition, endoscopic mucosal resection (EMR) is performed with a snare, and therefore the size of a lesion that can be removed en bloc is typically limited to a maximum of 20 mm. Piecemeal resection of larger lesions is a major limitation of EMR. On the other hand, ESD permits the en bloc resection of lesions irrespective of size and thereby has gained traction for the management of early gastrointestinal tumors. Potential advantages of en bloc resection include provision of an optimum specimen for accurate histopathological evaluation, opportunity to provide curative resection, and low risk of recurrence.

Being a markedly different technique than EMR, many devices have been developed over the years that allow ESD to be performed safely. At the heart of the tools for ESD, the electrosurgical knife plays a key role as it is the device that allows precise cutting and dissection of the submucosal tissue planes. Furthermore, specialized longer-lasting injection solutions for submucosal layer expansion and sophisticated electrosurgical equipment have been developed over the years to aid in the efficacy, efficiency, and safety of the procedure.

This chapter outlines some of the tools of the trade for ESD focusing primarily on equipment readily available in North America [1].

A Japanese proverb goes, *A master does not choose his brush-pen*, presumably because he can produce beauty regardless of his writing tool. Similarly, while the devices and accessories for ESD have come a long way since its inception two decades ago, we are reminded that instrument design is only to facilitate effective dissection. No instrument, no matter how advanced, can replace good technique and application of sound principles.

That being said, the future development of new approaches such as robot-actuated platforms does provide an exciting horizon where the learning and performance of ESD might one day be radically transformed due to maneuverability that we have yet to witness with our current endoscopic techniques.

C. J. Koh
Division of Gastroenterology and Hepatology, National University Hospital, Singapore, Singapore

D. Yang
Division of Gastroenterology, Hepatology and Nutrition, University of Florida, Gainesville, FL, USA

P. V. Draganov (✉)
Division of Gastroenterology, Hepatology and Nutrition, University of Florida Health, Gainesville, FL, USA
e-mail: Peter.Draganov@medicine.ufl.edu

© Springer Nature Switzerland AG 2020
M. S. Wagh, S. B. Wani (eds.), *Gastrointestinal Interventional Endoscopy*,
https://doi.org/10.1007/978-3-030-21695-5_5

Mucosal Lift Solutions

For safe mucosal incision and submucosal dissection, the submucosal space has to be adequately infiltrated and expanded with a suitable solution. This initial step of ESD has a dual mechanical and visual function: expansion of the submucosal space with the solution provides a physical barrier protecting the deeper layers from thermal injury while allowing a safe margin of dissection and identification and cautery of submucosal vessels during ESD [2]. The ideal solution should be inert and safe, without toxic effects to the surrounding tissue and to not distort the resected specimen as to affect its pathological assessment. Other factors that influence selection of one solution over another include the viscosity which correlates to how hard it is to inject through a needle, as well as the height of the lift, which varies among different solutions. Finally, price and availability always remain major contributors to the choice of solution.

The initiation and maintenance of this mucosal lift can be achieved with a variety of solutions of differing characteristics as described in the following table. It is worth noting that there is no conclusive evidence to support the use of one injection fluid over another, in part due to the paucity of head-to-head trials and the heterogeneity of outcomes available in the literature. Current meta-analysis data [3] reinforce that no single solution appears to be superior over the rest when it comes to complete resection rate, post-resection bleeding, or perforation incidence [4]. Nonetheless, many centers that perform ESD favor using a viscous solution over saline for the potential increased durability of the lift.

A staining dye is routinely added to the mucosal lifting solution. Either indigo carmine or methylene blue can be admixed with the solution to obtain a light-to-medium blue color, which facilitates recognition of the submucosal space. The goal of the dye is to stain the connective tissue within the submucosal plane, yet this should not be too dark as to potentially obscure the identification of submucosal vessels during dissection.

The various characteristics of commonly used mucosal lift solutions are discussed in the following and summarized in Table 5.1.

Saline

Normal saline (0.9% NaCl) is isotonic and commonly used for most EMRs. Main advantages include familiarity and ease of use, availability, and cost-effectiveness. Normal saline is also safe to the surrounding tissue and with minimal specimen distortion on histology. The drawback of normal saline is that it diffuses quickly following initial submucosal injection, thereby requiring the need for multiple repeated injections for lift maintenance, which is not ideal for a long procedure like ESD.

Hypertonic solutions such as hypertonic saline (3.75% NaCl) as well as dextrose water have

Table 5.1 Comparative characteristics of solutions for submucosal injection

Solution	Cushion duration[a]	Cost	Viscosity (Pa.s)	Comments
Normal saline	+	+	0.0043	Cost-effective and readily available, but dissipates quickly
Hydroxypropyl methylcellulose	+++	+++	0.0022	Relatively inexpensive with a durable lift
Hydroxyethyl starch (Voluven)	+++	++	0.0026	Commonly available and has a better lift than normal saline
Hydroxyethyl starch (Hetastarch)	++	++	0.0075	Similar to Voluven
Sodium hyaluronate	+++++	+++++	0.04	Gold standard, but costly and with limited availability
Eleview	++++	++++	<0.02	New product, purpose designed for submucosal injection, costly

[a]Data suggests that although cushion duration is statistically different in normal saline compared to other injection fluids discussed here, the differences between other injection fluids (e.g., hydroxypropyl methylcellulose and sodium hyaluronate) are not statistically significant

longer-lasting submucosal fluid lift when compared to normal saline but are on the whole still generally unsatisfactory with the additive risk of tissue injury due to high osmolality. Indeed, high concentrations of saline have been shown to give rise to delayed mucosal injury.

Carbohydrate-Based Solutions

Hydroxypropyl methylcellulose (Gonak 2.5%, Akom Inc., Somerset, NJ, USA) is a water-soluble polymer derived from cellulose. This provides readily available, lower-cost viscous fluid that is safe for injection. 15 mL of 2.5% solution is typically diluted with 85 mL of normal saline to make 100 mL of injectate [5]. This preparation has been demonstrated to provide a higher and more durable lift when compared to normal saline [6] and, in a retrospective study on EMR by Bacani et al., was shown to have longer lift effect (15–20 min) compared with normal saline (2–3 min) [7].

Hydroxyethyl starch (6% Voluven, Pfizer, NY, NY, USA; Hetastarch, Hospira, Inc., Lake Forest, IL, USA) originally used as a crystalloid solution for intravascular replenishment has a similar durability to hydroxypropyl methylcellulose in animal models. In clinical use, a comparative study by Fasoulas et al. showed that hydroxyethyl starch had more durable lift, required less solution, and resulted in a faster resection time compared with

normal saline. There was no observed difference in safety or long-term outcomes in either arm [8].

Sodium Hyaluronate

The prototypical high-viscosity solution has been sodium hyaluronate (MucoUp, Boston Scientific, Tokyo, Japan), with extensive data from Japan where it is commonly used in ESDs. Not only has it been shown to provide one of the most sustainable mucosal lifts, but porcine data suggests that it also results in a steeper mucosal elevation compared with colloids or saline, which is useful in ESD as steeper borders facilitate snaring. The downside to sodium hyaluronate solutions would be the high cost of such preparations, which can come up to approximately 40 times that of carbohydrate-based solutions. Hyaluronate solutions are available in the USA in various preparations as a viscosupplement (Healon, Abbott Laboratories, Abbott Park, IL, USA; Hyalgan, Fidia Pharma USA Inc., Florham Park, NJ), but the cost is generally prohibitive for its use as a mucosal lift solution.

Eleview

Eleview (Aries Pharmaceuticals, San Diego, CA, USA) is a proprietary composition (Fig. 5.1) designed for use for submucosal lift in

Fig. 5.1 Eleview. (Photo Credit: Olympus, Olympus America, Center Valley, PA, USA)

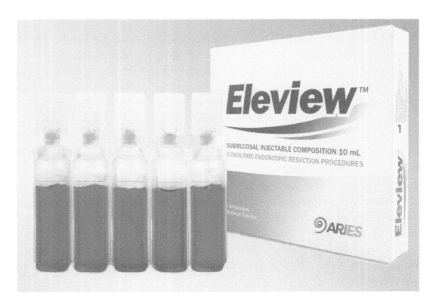

gastrointestinal endoscopic procedures and combines medium-chain triglycerides, poloxamer 188 (bulking agent), polyoxyl-15-hydroxystearate (surfactant), and methylene blue (dye) in suspension. Animal models suggests a mucosal lift superior to normal saline, and this is borne out by clinical data which suggests a small volume required per lesion as well as an overall faster resection time. As a new proprietary product, the cost of this would also be considerable.

Caps/Distal Attachments

Lack of triangulation and tissue retraction are the main drawbacks of efficient tissue dissection during ESD. To facilitate tissue retraction and visibility, a cap or distal attachment is routinely used. The distal attachment is a clear transparent hood that is affixed to the end of the endoscope, to allow it to retract folds or resected tissue to get a clear view of the resection field. It also provides firm traction to the target tissue, allowing optimal dissection [2].

The cap does slightly decrease the peripheral endoscopic visual field, but this trade-off is inevitable given the need for retraction and adequate visualization of the resection field.

The cap, being a simple plastic tube, is not difficult to manufacture; and a variety of brands and designs are available, with a straight cap being the most commonly used and widely applicable. Caps are also available with the edge being tapered like a short funnel for entering narrower spaces, as well as angle tips which have a beveled edge that offers better retraction of tissue mainly in one direction, for example, in the peroral endoscopic myotomy (POEM) procedure.

The soft distal attachment (Olympus America, Center Valley, PA, USA; Fig. 5.2) is one of the more commonly used caps and offers a drainage hole which is usually placed at 12 o' clock with respect to the screen which would allow drainage of excess fluid at the site opposite to the scope suction channel which usually comes out at 7 o' clock [5].

The short-type (ST) hood (Fujifilm America, Valhalla, NY, USA; Fig. 5.2) is a cap with a

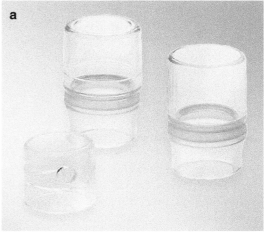

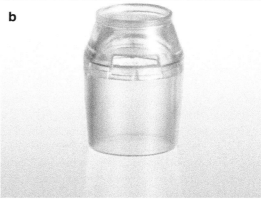

Fig. 5.2 Distal attachments used in ESD. (**a**) Olympus distal attachments. (Photo Credit: Olympus America, Center Valley, PA, USA). (**b**) Short-type (ST) hood. (Photo Credit: Fujifilm America, Valhalla, NY, USA)

tapered tip, which is useful for accessing a submucosal tunnel, such as in the POEM procedure or resections employing the tunnel technique. It also has a drain design allowing flow of fluid around the cap for better visibility.

Electrosurgical Generators and Electrical Currents

ESD requires a modern electrosurgical generator to provide the modulated current options that help deal with various phases of the resection. These produce high-frequency (>100,000 Hz) current to avoid neuromuscular depolarization, at varying energy levels to achieve tissue effects.

At slow heating of tissue at lower energy levels, the tissue gradually heats to beyond 50 °C and dries out, and this desiccation causes shrinkage of tissue resulting in a coagulation effect. Because energy transfer is lower, direct contact is required.

At rapid heating of tissue at high energy levels, water in tissue vaporizes to steam beyond 100 °C; and this vaporization disrupts cell structures, causing a cutting effect. Because the energy transfer is high, the current sparks from the electrode to the tissue, and the effect can be achieved at a very short distance from the electrode.

Generator Unit

Modern electrosurgical generators are able to alternate between the two modes and have options to have a combination of both effects, which is termed a blended current. This allows fine-tuning of the current to the stage of the procedure and greatly enhances the speed and hemostasis of the dissection. The ESGs available in the USA that are suitable for ESD are the ICC 200E, the VIO 200S and VIO 300D (ERBE USA, Marietta, GA, USA; Fig. 5.3), and the ESG 100 (Olympus America, Center Valley, PA USA).

Current Modes

The various modes of electrosurgical generators have been reviewed extensively in an ASGE review [9], and a synopsis focusing on the ERBE electrosurgical unit is outlined in Table 5.2, and these are used to discuss steps in ESD. It must be noted that some variations in the use of electrosurgical modes exist among experts, due to differences in the type of knife used, as well as some local practice differences (types of ESD performed, mucosal lift solution used, the typical amount of fibrosis encountered, etc.).

Mucosal Markings

Careful inspection is the first step to any resection to determine the edge of the lesion, also termed the demarcation line, which is the

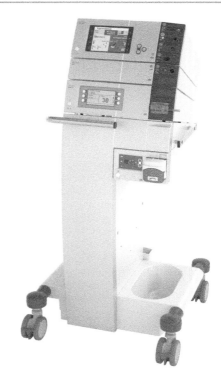

Fig. 5.3 ERBE VIO 300D generator unit. (Photo Credit: ERBE USA, Marietta, GA, USA)

junction between the lesion and the surrounding normal tissue. This is typically done with image-enhanced endoscopy (such as narrow band imaging or blue laser imaging) and chromoendoscopy employing methylene blue, indigo carmine, or, in the case of squamous lesions of the esophagus, Lugol's iodine.

Circumferential mucosal markings are typically placed for gastric and esophageal ESDs (although not always for rectal ESDs) at the start of the procedure approximately 5 mm from the demarcation line to guide subsequent injection and dissection. This key first step helps to ensure adequate lateral margin. The tissue is lightly touched with the tip of the ESD knife with soft coagulation or endo cut modes to create a visible superficial burn mark. Alternatively, argon plasma coagulation can also be used to mark the margins, but this adds additional cost and necessitates switching instruments. Use of forced coag current should be avoided because it creates extensive tissue damage which may compromise

Table 5.2 Summary of electrosurgical generator modes and utility in ESD

Mode	Features	Some uses in ESD
Endo cut	A cutting mode with alternating cut coagulation modes cycling to achieve cut and a concurrent, milder hemostatic effect	Mucosal incision Dissecting dense fibrotic tissue in the submucosal space
Dry cut	A cutting mode similar to endo cut but with enhanced coagulation, consequently with greater thermal effect	Precise submucosal dissection Mucosal incision when bleeding is a problem
Forced coagulation	A coagulation mode with high voltage	Submucosal dissection in vascular tissues
Soft coagulation	A coagulation mode with relatively low voltage. As tissue desiccates, resistance increases and the current falls, allowing the tissue to fall off with less char and controlled energy application	Hemostatic forceps Lesion marking
Swift coagulation	A coagulation mode with enhanced cutting properties. Less hemostatic than forced coagulation, but more hemostatic than dry cut (and less cutting effect)	Pinpoint hemostasis of vessels Creating a divot during coagulation
Spray coagulation	A coagulation mode with a continuous very high voltage resulting in arcing to surrounding tissue, similar to argon plasma coagulation	Non-contact hemostasis POEM procedure for ease of submucosal tunneling with concurrent non-contact hemostasis

lateral margin evaluation and can also serve as an escape point of the submucosal injectate.

Incision

Mucosal incision, both the initial incision and the circumferential incision, separates the lesion's lateral borders from the rest of the tissue and allows access to the deep submucosal space. This can be achieved with endo cut (ERBE)/pulse cut (Olympus), although dry cut or swift coagulation modes have also been deployed, depending on the knife and type of tissue dissected.

Dissection

Classically, forced coagulation has been used to dissect through the generally vascular submucosal space, particularly under a lesion with neovascularization with fine vessels; and a good coagulative effect is desirous. If the submucosa is less vascular, swift coagulation or dry cut modes can also be used, with the advantage of creating less carbonization.

Fibrotic tissue has less water content and easily carbonizes with coagulation modes; hence, careful application of a cutting mode, for example, endo cut or dry cut, should be employed because submucosal lift cannot be achieved and the margin of error above the muscularis propria is small.

Hemostasis

When it comes to hemostasis, an ounce of prevention is worth a pound of cure. Preemptively identifying and addressing vessels in the submucosal space keeps the dissection field clean and clear and eventually leads to faster resections. Every attempt should be made to effectively coagulate vessels before cutting through the area and causing active bleeding.

The general rule of thumb for vessels smaller than 1 mm would be to use the same electrosurgical knife and switch to a coagulating mode (forced coagulation, dry cut, or swift coagulation). It is worth remembering that total energy delivered is a function of both power and time, and adequate time has to be spent in the particular spot for the coagulation mode to work.

For vessels larger than 1 mm, it is often worth the while to change out to hemostatic forceps such as the Coagrasper (Olympus America, Center Valley, PA USA), grasp the vessel, and use soft coagulation to deliver a controlled burn to the target. The same is typically applied to bleeding vessels, with grasping of the bleeding spot, careful retraction to achieve gentle tenting of the spot, and application of soft coagulation until adequate hemostasis. Importantly, only soft coagulation current should be used with coagulating forceps.

For hemostasis of active bleeding during resection, the same principle applies. For low-level bleeding such as a small vessel or venous ooze, the same ESD knife can be employed with consideration to switch to a more coagulative current. For brisk bleeding, usually from a sizable artery, the coagulating forceps should be employed. As blood accumulates and obscures the endoscopic view, the earlier the bleed is dealt with, the better. The use of a through-the-scope water jet is advisable if not mandatory to flush away the blood to identify the bleeding point for effective hemostasis.

It should be emphasized that electrosurgical settings are a very important component of safe and effective ESD, yet multiple other factors contribute to the final tissue effect. Some of these factors are related to the device in use (material and thickness of the ESD knife electrode), some are related to the endoscopist technique (the speed of movement of the electrode, the amount of contact between the tissue and the electrode, the pressure applied by the electrode, the amount of time the generator stays activated), and finally some are dependent on the type of target tissue itself (water content and degree of fibrosis). Therefore, frequent change of electrosurgical unit settings is typically not needed because the endoscopist can vary many of the factors listed above. Furthermore, this complex environment highlights the fact that there is no one "best" electrosurgical unit set of settings.

ESD Knives

At the heart of the specialized instruments that make ESD possible are the ESD knives. These are essential for dissection of the submucosal plane and come in a wide variety of forms (Fig. 5.1). Categorizing them broadly by form, we have needle knives which are bare, metal fine-tip knives, insulated-tip (IT) knives which have a ceramic non-conducting tip that limits current at the very tip of the knife and mainly allows controlled dissection along the shaft, and scissor-type knives which resemble a pair of shears in design and function. These are available in various forms from different manufacturers and are elaborated in detail in the following [2] and summarized in Table 5.3.

Table 5.3 Characteristics of selected ESD tools

Type	Knife name (Model Number)	Manufacturer	Cutting knife length	Working length	Minimum channel diameter
Needle knives	DualKnife KD-650L	Olympus America, Center Valley, PA, USA	2.0 mm	1650 mm	2.8 mm
	DualKnife KD-650U	Olympus America, Center Valley, PA, USA	1.5 mm	2300 mm	2.8 mm
	HookKnife KD-620LR	Olympus America, Center Valley, PA, USA	4.5 mm	1650 mm	2.8 mm
	HookKnife KD-620UR	Olympus America, Center Valley, PA, USA	4.5 mm	2300 mm	2.8 mm
Needle knives with water jet	HybridKnife I type 20,150–261	ERBE USA, Marietta, GA, USA	2.3 mm	1900 mm	2.8 mm
	FlushKnife needle type DK2618J	Fujifilm America, Valhalla, NY, USA	1.0, 1.5, 2.0, 2.5, 3.0 mm	1800 mm	2.8 mm
	FlushKnife ball type DK2618J	Fujifilm America, Valhalla, NY, USA	1.5, 2.0, 2.5, 3.0 mm	1800 mm	2.8 mm
	DualKnife J KD-655L	Olympus America, Center Valley, PA, USA	2.0 mm	1650 mm	2.8 mm
	DualKnife J KD-655U	Olympus America, Center Valley, PA, USA	1.5 mm	2300 mm	2.8 mm
IT knives	ITknife2 KD-611L	Olympus America, Center Valley, PA, USA	4.0 mm	1650 mm	2.8 mm

(continued)

Table 5.3 (continued)

Type	Knife name (Model Number)	Manufacturer	Cutting knife length	Working length	Minimum channel diameter
	ITknife nano KD-612U	Olympus America, Center Valley, PA, USA	2.8 mm	2300 mm	2.8 mm
Scissor-type knives	Clutch cutter DP2618DT-35	Fujifilm America, Valhalla, NY, USA	3.5 mm	1800 mm	2.7 mm
	Clutch cutter DP2618DT-50	Fujifilm America, Valhalla, NY, USA	5.0 mm	1800 mm	2.7 mm
	Stag beetle knife junior MD47703W	Sumitomo Bakelite, Tokyo, Japan	3.5 mm	1950 mm	2.8 mm
	Stag beetle knife standard MD-47704	Sumitomo Bakelite, Tokyo, Japan	7.0 mm	1800 mm	2.8 mm

Needle Knife Type (DualKnife, HookKnife) (Fig. 5.4)

The needle knife is a bare-tipped metal knife of which there are several variations. The DualKnife has a retractable tip, which allows the cutting length to be adjusted to two positions – retracted and extended. This allows the knife to be used for both marking (with the tip retracted) and cutting/dissection with the tip extended.

Another knife that is commonly used particularly in areas of fibrosis is the HookKnife (Olympus America, Center Valley, PA USA). This has a distal L-shaped hook that is fully rotatable for incision and dissection and has the advantage of being able to grasp and apply traction on fibrotic tissues to reduce collateral burns.

Needle Knife Type with Injection Capabilities (Hybrid, Flush, DualKnife J Type) (Fig. 5.5)

A more recent innovation would be the addition of injection function to the tip of the needle knife, allowing it not only to cut and dissect but also to be able to inject fluid directly into the submucosal space, which previously required an instrument change to an injector needle. When combined with an injection system that can be controlled by the endoscopist via a foot pedal, this greatly reduces the reliance on assistants, who no longer have to keep switching instruments as frequently. This is also advantageous in the USA, where assistants depending on their qualification might not be credentialed to inject fluid.

The knives that are available for such use would be the HybridKnife (ERBE USA, Marietta, GA, USA), the FlushKnife (Fujifilm America, Valhalla, NY, USA), and the DualKnife J type (Olympus America, Center Valley, PA USA) which is an enhancement to the existing DualKnife with the addition of a water jet function. These knives offer improvements in speed but at greater capital investment, for example, the HybridKnife requires the accessory, the ERBE Jet, for its use.

Insulated-Tip (IT) Knives (Fig. 5.6)

Insulated-tip knives have a small non-conducting ceramic ball at the tip of the metal needle. This makes the tip theoretically less prone, but not impossible, to perforation as the cutting occurs at the side. This difference also means the maneuvering and use of the IT knives are completely different from the needle-type knives. While using needle-type knives, controlled push movements are used to dissect the submucosal plane, whereas the IT knife uses more pull or lateral dragging to achieve this cutting effect [5].

Cutting with the original IT knife was difficult to achieve at some angles. Therefore, the ITknife2 (IT2) was designed with an additional triangular electrode on the back side of the ceramic tip. This additional electrode significantly facilitates both mucosal incision and submucosal dissection. The IT2 use is limited to the stomach where there is sufficient maneuverable space and the muscle layer is robust. They are not so helpful and potentially dangerous to use

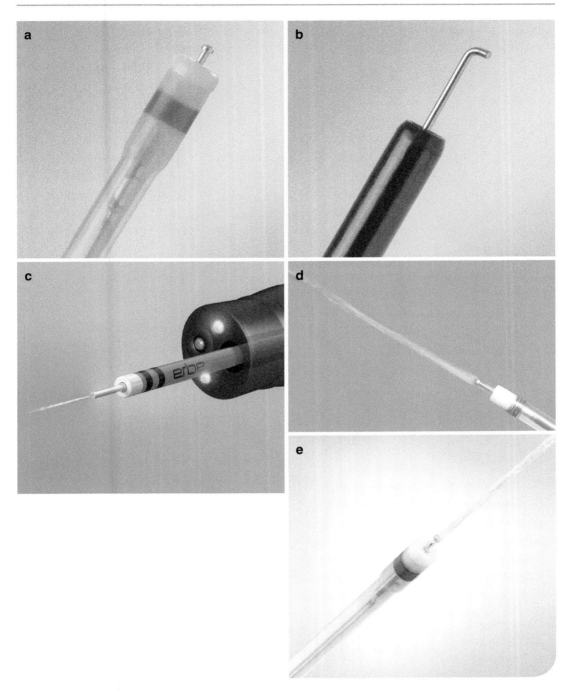

Fig. 5.4 Needle-type knives. (**a**) DualKnife. (Photo Credit: Olympus America, Center Valley, PA, USA). (**b**) HookKnife. (Photo Credit: Olympus America, Center Valley, PA, USA). (**c**) HybridKnife. (Photo Credit: ERBE USA, Marietta, GA, USA). (**d**) FlushKnife. (Photo Credit: Fujifilm America, Valhalla, NY, USA). (**e**) DualKnife J type. (Photo Credit: Olympus America, Center Valley, PA, USA)

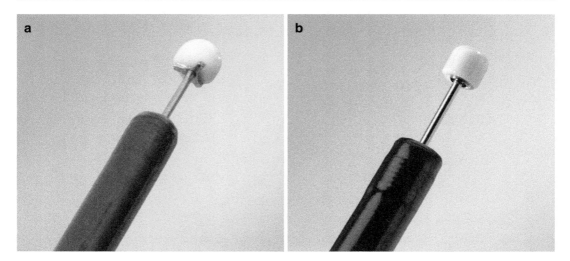

Fig. 5.5 Insulated-tip knives. (**a**) ITknife2. (Photo Credit: Olympus America, Center Valley, PA, USA). (**b**) ITknife nano. (Photo Credit: Olympus America, Center Valley, PA, USA)

Fig. 5.6 Scissor-type knives. (**a**) Clutch Cutter (Photo Credit: Fujifilm America, Valhalla, NY, USA). (**b**) Stag Beetle Knife. (Photo Credit: Olympus America, Center Valley, PA, USA)

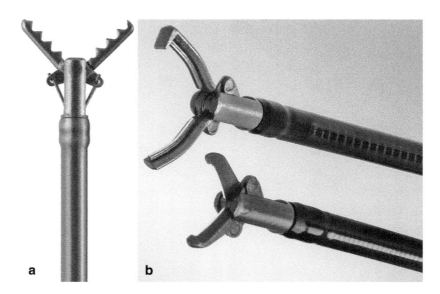

in the esophagus or in the colon. To address this technical challenge, the ITknife nano (Olympus America, Center Valley, PA, USA) is available with a smaller ceramic tip (1.7 mm vs. 2.2 mm for the ITknife2) and disk-shaped electrode (rather than triangular for the IT2).

Of note, in order to use the IT knife, an initial incision to enter the submucosal space is needed; and therefore, the use of a needle knife is still required.

Scissors Type (Clutch Cutter, Stag Beetle) (Fig. 5.6)

A relatively recent development is the partially insulated scissor-type knife device [1]. These include the Clutch Cutter (Fujifilm America, Valhalla, NY, USA) and the Stag Beetle (SB) Knife (Sumitomo Bakelite, Tokyo, Japan). These devices resemble in form and action miniature scissors with blunt blades and grasp the tissue being resected before lifting and application of electrosurgical current, which has the advantage of limiting collateral tissue injury [10]. These devices are partially insulated to concentrate the cutting energy at the scissor blades. This allows a very controlled and precise cut and may potentially be useful in situations where there is considerable inadvertent movement such as respiratory movements or motion.

Another use of the scissor-type knife would be in esophageal diverticulectomy (e.g., in Zenker's diverticulum or Killian-Jamieson diverticulum). The scissor-type knife is able to grasp and directly cut the diverticular septum – mucosa, submucosa, and muscle – in a few cuts, making this procedure technically easy and shortening procedural time considerably [11].

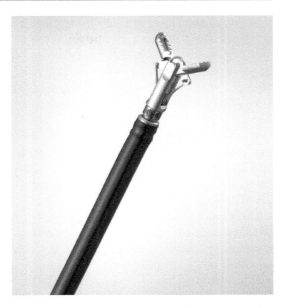

Fig. 5.7 Coagrasper. (Photo Credit: Olympus America, Center Valley, PA, USA)

Hemostasis

The submucosal dissection entails encountering blood vessels, either deliberately or inadvertently, and controlled hemostasis is vital to ensuring visibility of the resection field as well as safety in terms of reducing hemorrhage post-procedure.

ESD Knives

The first line for hemostasis, often for minor bleeding as well as prophylactic cautery of small vessels, would be using the ESD knife itself. ESD knives can, with the appropriate electrosurgical current mode, be used effectively for hemostasis. The "dual" function of the DualKnife (Olympus America, Center Valley, PA, USA) relies on the fact that when it is fully retracted, the tip of the knife that remains can be used as a targeting tool for hemostasis while minimizing the collateral burns by having minimal exposed cutting edge.

Hemostatic Forceps

As discussed above, minor bleeding during the procedure or tiny vessels <1 mm generally can be treated with the existing electrosurgical device, switching to a coagulative mode of electrosurgical current. But larger vessels or brisk (including arterial) bleeding requires the use of hemostatic forceps. The technique used would be to identify the bleeding point by using water jets to clear the residual blood, use the hemostatic forceps to grasp the vessel and surrounding tissue, tent the vessel away from deeper tissues, and apply the appropriate coagulative current, such as the soft coagulation mode. The Coagrasper (Olympus America, Center Valley, PA, USA; Fig. 5.7) is a rotatable device with effective tissue grasping that is commonly used in this setting. Other options include the Hot Biopsy Forceps (Boston Scientific, Marlborough, USA), although not its original intended use. Hemostatic forceps have been so successful that they are also increasingly being used in non-ESD bleeding situations, such as for coagulating a visible vessel on a gastric ulcer.

Clips

Although clipping during the procedure is generally difficult as it interferes with further dissection, there is a role for hemostatic clips in two situations: large-vessel hemostasis and closure of mucosal defects/tunnels (e.g., in the POEM procedure). Although large vessels are usually addressed with hemostatic forceps, clips are an option of hemostasis, where hemostatic forceps are unsuccessful, or at the end of the procedure where the resection is complete and it is desirous to avoid additional thermal injury to the base of the resection.

If clips are deployed during the dissection, clips with smaller footprint, such as the Olympus EZ Clip (Olympus America, Center Valley, PA USA), are less likely to interfere with the subsequent dissection.

Other roles where clips might be employed would be as an adjunctive tool in traction devices or perforation management which is discussed in the following.

New Developments

Traction Devices (Clip-Dental Floss Technique, Lumendi, LumenR)

As the ESD devices enter in the same axis as the endoscope, traction to achieve better exposure of the submucosal space is often difficult. One way to overcome this would be to use gravity to aid the resection, positioning the patient and cutting such that as the dissection continues, the flap hangs away from the underlying tissues. But given that this is not feasible in many cases, there has been an interest in traction devices for better exposure which would lead to safer and faster dissection.

A simple method readily applicable would be to tie a long string, usually a dental floss, to the arm of an endoclip, deploy the clip on the edge of the partially resected lesion, and apply gentle traction through the string onto the lesion. This has been shown by Suzuki et al. to achieve significantly shorter procedure times compared with standard techniques for gastric ESDs – mean of 82.2 min vs. 118.2 min [12]. Although simple to deploy, this technique still has limitations, the major one being the collinearity of the string with the scope which often means the angle of traction is far from ideal, although an improvement from gravity.

Lumendi (DiLumen, Westport, CT, USA) is an overtube with anchoring balloons proximal and distal to the scope tip that stabilizes the colonic mucosa and enhances visualization by flattening folds and straightening bends.

ORISE Tissue Retractor System (Boston Scientific, Marlborough, MA, USA) is a platform that facilitates ESD in the colon by combining an endoscopic overtube with an occluding device to stabilize a resection field in front of the scope and with independent instrument channels which allow the employment of a grasping forceps for traction of the lesion. The angle at which the instrument channels come out is more perpendicular to the plane of dissection, making it more useful in delivering appropriate traction.

Robotics-Enhanced Surgical Systems

One of the main technical limitations of ESD would be that the device motion all relies mainly on the motion of the endoscope. This results in the technique requiring a high degree of endoscopic training to develop the skill sets required and limit its generalizability. This is the challenge that robotics-enhanced platforms hope to overcome. Having two or more articulated manipulators at the end of the scope allows the scope shaft to remain steady as a stable platform from which the articulated arms triangulate to do the work of dissection and retraction. This exciting development allows ESD in locations that are challenging even for experts, due to scope limitations, for example, the gastric cardia or pyloric region. It is also hoped that this will lessen the learning curve and make ESD a more widely available technique by lowering the barrier to adoption.

Many platforms have been in development [13], but human studies have been conducted in very few, one of which would be the Master and Slave Transluminal Endoscopic Robot (MASTER) (Endomaster, Singapore) (Fig. 5.8) which showed in a small case series to be deployed in resection of early gastric neoplasia with a mean submucosal dissection time of 18.6 min [14]. The platform utilizes robotic arms

Fig. 5.8 Master and Slave Transluminal Endoscopic Robot (MASTER). (Photo Credit: Endomaster, Singapore)

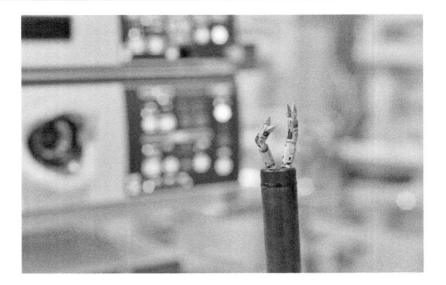

on a flexible endoscope, with the arms controlled separately by a proceduralist who sits at a separate console with actuators that transmit the controls to the robotic arms.

ESD Defect Closure or Coverage (Clips, Suturing Devices, Gel Sheets, Auto Transplants)

Small perforations during ESD are typically managed endoscopically with clips, with targeted application of standard endoclips being able to traverse the defect and achieve good closure. Should the muscularis propria defect be larger than the width of a standard clip, an Ovesco clip (Ovesco Endoscopy USA Inc., Cary, NC, USA) which is an over-the-scope clip with a larger diameter might be considered with concurrent use of the accessory Twin Grasper to grab either side of the defect and close it.

For perforations beyond reach of the over-the-scope clip, endoscopic closure might be considered by several techniques: OverStitch endoscopic suturing device (Apollo Endosurgery Inc., Austin, TX, USA) can be used to close large defects, provided there is sufficient endoscopic space to maneuver the bulky head of the device. Also described and applied is the clip and endoloop method where a double-channel therapeutic scope

is used to deploy a series of clips to anchor an endoloop around the edge of the defect, which is then closed like a purse string [15].

Although most ESD mucosal defects are not closed, there may be occasion to achieve mucosal apposition, such as in cases with submucosal tunneling like the POEM procedure or sometimes in cases with perforation or endoscopic full-thickness resections [16]. Closure of colonic mucosal ESD defects has also been shown to accelerate wound healing [16] although the clinical outcomes were unchanged.

Because of the nature of the lesions subject to ESD which can be in excess of 100 mm in length, mucosal defect closure can be a challenge with conventional endoscopic devices. Various adaptations of existing endoscopic equipment have been attempted, such as a the "loop clip" [17] which is a looped nylon string tied around one arm of the clip, allowing sequential grasping of tissue from previously deployed loop clips. Other techniques have also been reported such as double-layered clip closure [18], where the initial row of clips placed in the midline help to partially reduce the defect width, before a second series of clips placed alternating to the first series completely oppose both edges of the mucosa.

ESD defect coverage has been explored, particularly in the realm of esophageal ESDs with more than two-thirds of the lumen resected as the resultant scarring and post-procedural stenosis are problematic. Some techniques still under investigation [19] include covering the defect with a sheet of material, either a biocompatible scaffold to help re-epithelialization or an auto transplant of the patient's own cells, such as oral mucosal epithelial cell sheet transplantation [19].

Other reports of ESD defect coverage include post-procedural perforations using polyglycolic acid sheets and fibrin glue [20], where post-gastric and duodenal perforations have been described. Being a bioabsorbable scaffold that covers the defect and aids the closure of the defect by providing a scaffold, such investigational techniques hold promise in the future of endoscopic management of large perforations.

Conclusion

The development of tools and devices available to support ESD has grown rapidly in the past few years to a respectable armamentarium, and the future looks promising in terms of new platforms which enhance safety and speed as well as push the boundaries of what is resectable.

However, for most endoscopists, a sound understanding of the capabilities and limitations of existing equipment is key to performing an efficient and successful procedure. Technology and equipment might change, but the principles of dissection and a healthy respect for blood vessels in the submucosal space will be constant, regardless of the device used.

References

1. Hironori Y. Endoscopic submucosal dissection—current success and future directions. Nat Rev Gastroenterol Hepatol. 2012;9(9):519–29.
2. Fukami N. Endoscopic submucosal dissection: principles and practice. New York: Springer; 2015.
3. Zhang Yu H, Wei Feng X, Luo Chang J, Wang Xi C. Submucosal injection solution for endoscopic resection in gastrointestinal tract: a traditional and network meta-analysis. Gastroenterol Res Pract. 2015;2015:1–10.
4. Alexandre Oliveira F, Joana M, Joana T, Mario D-R. Solutions for submucosal injection in endo-

scopic resection: a systematic review and meta-analysis. Endosc Int Open. 2016;4(1):E1–E16.
5. Peter VD, Takuji G, Disaya C, Michael BW. Techniques of endoscopic submucosal dissection: application for the Western endoscopist? Gastrointest Endosc. 2013;78(5):677–88.
6. Dimitrios P, George K, Konstantinos T, George K, John GP, Spiros DL. Comparative performance of novel solutions for submucosal injection in porcine stomachs: an ex vivo study. Dig Liver Dis. 2010;42(3):226–9.
7. Christopher JB, Timothy AW, Massimo R, Mohammad AA-H, Kyung WN, Surakit P, et al. The safety and efficacy in humans of endoscopic mucosal resection with hydroxypropyl methylcellulose as compared with normal saline. Surg Endosc. 2008;22(11):2401–6.
8. Fasoulas K, Lazaraki G, Chatzimavroudis G, Paroutoglou G, Katsinelos T, Dimou E, et al. Endoscopic mucosal resection of giant laterally spreading tumors with submucosal injection of hydroxyethyl starch: comparative study with normal saline solution. Surg Laparosc Endosc Percutan Tech. 2012;22(3):272–8.
9. Committee AT, Jeffrey LT, Bradley AB, Subhas B, Shailendra SC, Klaus TG, et al. Electrosurgical generators. Gastrointest Endosc. 2013;78(2):197–208.
10. Akahoshi K, Akahane H, Motomura Y, Kubokawa M, Itaba S, Komori K, et al. A new approach: endoscopic submucosal dissection using the clutch cutter® for early stage digestive tract tumors. Digestion. 2012;85(2):80–4.
11. Goelder SK, Brueckner J, Messmann H. Endoscopic treatment of Zenker's diverticulum with the stag beetle knife (sb knife) - feasibility and follow-up. Scand J Gastroenterol. 2016;51(10):1155–8.
12. Kroh M, Reavis KM, SpringerLink (Online service). The SAGES manual operating through the endoscope. Springer Nature Switzerland AG.
13. Sho S, Takuji G, Yoshiyuki K, Shin K, Kunio I, Naoko Y-K, et al. Usefulness of a traction method using dental floss and a hemoclip for gastric endoscopic submucosal dissection: a propensity score matching analysis (with videos). Gastrointest Endosc. 2016;83(2):337–46.
14. Baldwin Po Man Y, Terence G. A technical review of flexible endoscopic multitasking platforms. Int J Surg. 2012;10(7):345–54.
15. Soo Jay P, Nageshwar R, Philip WYC, Pradeep R, Guduru VR, Zheng W, et al. Robot-assisted endoscopic submucosal dissection is effective in treating patients with early-stage gastric neoplasia. Clin Gastroenterol Hepatol. 2012;10(10):1117–21.
16. Kazuhiro Y, Seigo K, Keiichi I, Kazuki S, Hisao T. Assessment of a manipulator device for NOTES with basic surgical skill tests: a bench study. Surg Laparosc Endosc Percutan Tech. 2014;24(5):e191–5.
17. Shintaro F, Hirohito M, Hideki K, Noriko N, Tae M, Maki A, et al. Management of a large mucosal

defect after duodenal endoscopic resection. World J Gastroenterol. 2016;22(29):6595.

18. Yin Z, Xiang W, Guanying X, Yun Q, Honggang W, Li L, et al. Complete defect closure of gastric submucosal tumors with purse-string sutures. Surg Endosc. 2014;28(6):1844–51.

19. Taro O, Naoto S, Hideaki R, Takashi M, Hiroya U, Kenshi M, et al. Closure with clips to accelerate healing of mucosal defects caused by colorectal endoscopic submucosal dissection. Surg Endosc. 2016;30(10):4438–44.

20. Tanaka S, Toyonaga T, Obata D, Ishida T, Morita Y, Azuma T. Endoscopic double-layered suturing: a novel technique for closure of large mucosal defects after endoscopic mucosal resection (EMR) or endoscopic submucosal dissection (ESD). Endoscopy. 2012;44(Suppl 2):E153–4.

Esophageal ESD

Lady Katherine Mejía Pérez, Seiichiro Abe,
Raja Siva, John Vargo, and Amit Bhatt

Introduction

Esophageal cancer is the eighth most common malignancy worldwide and the sixth most common cause of cancer-related deaths [1]. It carries a dismal prognosis if not discovered early, as demonstrated by 5-year survival rates ranging from 15 to 20% [2, 3]. Squamous cell carcinoma (SCC) and esophageal adenocarcinoma (EAC) are the two main histological subtypes. Worldwide, 80–90% of cases occur in the form of squamous cell cancer [4]. However, in North America and several regions in Europe, the incidence of esophageal adenocarcinoma has increased substantially, exceeding the rates of squamous cell carcinoma [5]. This trend has coincided with a rise in the prevalence of gastroesophageal reflux and obesity [6–9].

Historically, radical esophagectomy was the standard of care for the management of esophageal cancer including early esophageal cancers and Barrett's esophagus with high-grade dysplasia (BE-HGD). While perioperative mortality rates were high in the past, advances in surgical technique and postoperative care have significantly reduced mortality to around 3.4% per the Society of Thoracic Surgery Database and to less than 1% in select high-volume centers [10]. Nevertheless, morbidity remains high at over 33% leading to the exploration of less invasive, organ-preserving options [11–14]. Endoscopic resection, namely, endoscopic mucosal resection (EMR) and endoscopic submucosal dissection (ESD), arose as a therapeutic organ-preserving alternative for superficial esophageal cancer with similar cancer-free survival rates and significantly lower morbidity rates than surgery [15–17]. ESD was initially developed in the East for removal of early gastric cancer. ESD allows en bloc resection of lesions regardless of size, location, and fibrosis [18, 19]. It emerged as a technique to improve rates of complete resection, therefore decreasing the rates of local recurrence. It also provides the most reliable histopathologic assessment for accurate staging. In esophageal cancer, the high density of submucosal lymphatics results in higher rates of lymph node involvement, even in superficial cancers such as T1b submucosal tumors, making ESD appropriate in the management of low-risk (0.6%) T1a mucosal cancers [20, 21].

L. K. Mejía Pérez
Department of Internal Medicine, Cleveland Clinic, Cleveland, OH, USA

S. Abe
Endoscopy Division, National Cancer Center Hospital, Tokyo, Japan

R. Siva
Department of Thoracic and Cardiovascular Surgery, Cleveland Clinic Foundation, Cleveland, OH, USA

J. Vargo · A. Bhatt (✉)
Department of Gastroenterology and Hepatology, Digestive Disease and Surgery Institute, Cleveland Clinic, Cleveland, OH, USA
e-mail: bhatta3@ccf.org

© Springer Nature Switzerland AG 2020
M. S. Wagh, S. B. Wani (eds.), *Gastrointestinal Interventional Endoscopy*,
https://doi.org/10.1007/978-3-030-21695-5_6

The majority of data for superficial esophageal cancer arises from Asia and Europe, where SCC is more common. Furthermore, ESD is currently the standard of care for removal of superficial esophageal SCC because of its optimal histological outcomes and better morbidity profile when compared to surgery.

For the case of high-grade dysplasia (HGD) and EAC associated with Barrett's esophagus, esophageal EMR remains the treatment of choice. It is considered safe and effective, and it is the most widely studied technique [15–17]. However, EMR can only achieve en bloc resection of lesions smaller than 15–20 mm [22, 23]. It is well known that piecemeal resection is a risk for recurrence of esophageal adenocarcinoma [24]. Along these lines, the American Society for Gastrointestinal Endoscopy (ASGE) recommends ESD for excision of lesions larger than 20 mm if expertise is available, while the European Society of Gastrointestinal Endoscopy (ESGE) recommends it for lesions larger than 15 mm, for those with scarring from fibrosis, or as a staging procedure if superficial submucosal invasion is suspected [25, 26].

Indications

ESD is indicated for resection of tumors with a negligible risk of lymph node metastasis. The accepted indications for ESD are aligned along the rates of metastasis, the available experience according to geographical distribution, and the perceived risk of the procedure.

Squamous Cell Carcinoma

The majority of data regarding this subtype comes from Asia, where experience with ESD is higher. According to the Japan Esophageal Society guidelines for treatment of esophageal cancer, endoscopic resection is absolutely indicated in lesions limited to the mucosa (T1a, m1/m2). In addition, lesions with superficial infiltration of the submucosa (T1b/SM1, m3/sm1) are a relative indication of ESD (Table 6.1) [27]. The European Society of Gastrointestinal Endoscopy (ESGE) recommends ESD as the first option for

Table 6.1 Indications for endoscopic resection (EMR/ESD) for squamous cell cancer, according to the Japan Esophageal Society [27]

	Absolute indications	Relative indications
Depth of invasion	m1, m2	m3, sm1 (≤200 μm)

EMR endoscopic mucosal resection, *ESD* endoscopic submucosal dissection

Table 6.2 Indications for ESD for high-grade dysplasia and esophageal adenocarcinoma associated with Barrett's esophagus according to the European Society of Gastrointestinal Endoscopy [25]

	Indication
Depth of invasion	sm1 (≤500 μm)
Size	>15 mm
Lifting	Poor

ESD endoscopic submucosal dissection

resection of superficial esophageal squamous cell cancers (m1 or m2). The ESGE recommends ESD over EMR due to its ability to provide en bloc resection [25].

Barrett's Esophagus and Esophageal Adenocarcinoma

Endoscopic resection is indicated for treatment of high-grade dysplasia (HGD) and esophageal adenocarcinoma (EAC) associated with Barrett's esophagus [25]. EMR is preferred for small lesions where en bloc resection can be achieved [28–32]. ESD is recommended for selected cases, such as lesions larger than 15 mm, poorly lifting tumors, and lesions at risk for submucosal invasion (Table 6.2) [25]. Regardless of the endoscopic resection technique, treatment is typically supplemented with an endoscopic ablation technique, such as radiofrequency ablation, in order to decrease the risk of metachronous lesions from the remaining Barrett's epithelium [24].

Procedure

Esophageal ESD is a technically challenging procedure because the narrow lumen of the esophagus limits endoscopic manipulation. In addition, the wall of the esophagus is thinner than that of the stomach, increasing the risk of perforation and mediastinitis [33]. Hence, to achieve successful outcomes, ESD should be performed in a high-volume, multidisciplinary center [34]. Before execution of the procedure in the esophagus, it is recommended to have performed at least 20–40 procedures in easier locations (distal stomach, rectum) [35, 36].

Equipment

ESD is performed in a stepwise manner, and different devices are specially designed to facilitate performance of each step [37]. Some of the equipment for ESD, such as endoscope, coagulation devices, and high-frequency electrogenerators, is similar to that used in standard endoscopy. Electrosurgical knives are unique to ESD. Choice of type of equipment requires special attention because of the complexity of the procedure [37]. Endoscopic tools and accessories for ESD are discussed elsewhere in this book and are not included in this chapter.

In regard to esophageal ESD, a straight soft distal attachment is preferred. As for knives for marking, circumferential incision, and submucosal dissection, the HookKnife (Olympus KD 620LR/KD 620UR, Tokyo, Japan), DualKnife (Olympus KD 650L/KD 650U, Tokyo, Japan), and FlushKnife (Fujinon Optical Co., Tokyo, Japan) knives are the only uncovered devices recommended for esophageal ESD [38]. The ITknife nano (Olympus KD 612L/U, Tokyo, Japan) and the Mucosectom2 (HOYA Pentax, Tokyo, Japan) are the insulated knives indicated for esophageal ESD [39, 40]. Additionally, Akahoshi et al. recently described the use of the Clutch Cutter (Fujifilm, Tokyo, Japan) for resection of SCC [41].

Preoperative Assessment

Precise patient selection and pre-procedural endoscopic evaluation of the lesion are vital to assess the extent and depth of tumor invasion and to recognize tumor margins [25, 38]. These will determine if the lesion is amenable for ESD. Standard use of the Paris classification to describe nodular lesions and the Prague criteria of all visible Barrett's mucosa is suggested [25]. High-resolution endoscopy is recommended for detection of neoplasia and local staging [25].

Lugol chromoendoscopy is currently the gold standard technique to evaluate esophageal squamous cell carcinoma; however, lugol staining sometimes leads to patient discomfort following the procedure [45]. Therefore, recent virtual chromoendoscopy imaging techniques have been developed, such as narrow band imaging (NBI). NBI has shown to have similar sensitivity and superior specificity when compared with chromoendoscopy to predict the depth of invasion of both Barrett's-associated neoplasia and SCC with the drawback of having a moderate interobserver agreement [46–49]. Biopsy samples of visible lesions should be obtained if malignancy is suspected [25].

High-frequency probe endoscopic ultrasound (EUS) has shown to have limited accuracy for detection of submucosal invasion in early esophageal cancer [50, 51]. However, it has been noted to be superior than computed tomography (CT) scan in assessment of nodal staging [52, 53]. Therefore, EUS is useful for locoregional staging of esophageal lesions with high risk of invasive cancer [46, 48].

Generally, monitored anesthesia care and sedation are performed for esophageal ESD. When available, general anesthesia with endotracheal intubation has the benefit of decreased risk of aspiration of secretions or blood [54].

Technique

Marking

Appropriate identification, mapping, and demarcation of the lesion are mandatory before starting the procedure [54, 55]. Circumferential marking should be carefully performed to avoid perforation of the thin wall of the esophagus. Cautery, argon plasma coagulation, or the tip of a needle-type knife can be used to mark at 3–5 mm from the edge of the lesion (Fig. 6.1).

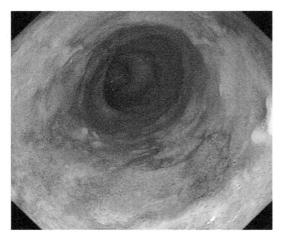

Fig. 6.1 Suspicious flat lesion involving the entire circumference of the esophagus

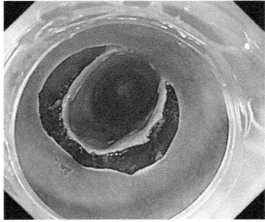

Fig. 6.3 Partial circumferential mucosal incision on the proximal side of the lesion using the DualKnife and ITknife nano

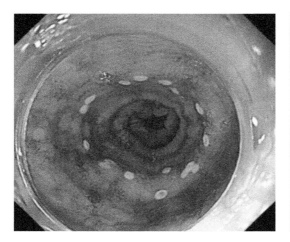

Fig. 6.2 Circumferential marking around the lesion

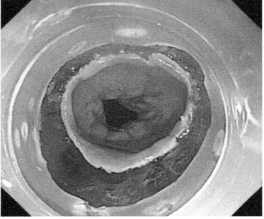

Fig. 6.4 Complete circumferential mucosal incision on the distal side of the lesion

Partial Circumferential Incision

In esophageal ESD, we prefer partial circumferential incision to prevent the escape of fluid from the submucosal layer (Figs. 6.2 and 6.3) [42]. The oral and anal incisions are made first. Mucosal incision using a FlushKnife or DualKnife along the left lateral border mucosal lesion is then performed allowing the lesion to retract away from the water pool on the gravity-dependent side. Circumferential incision of the right lateral wall is completed when approximately three-fourths of the lesion has been dissected.

Submucosal Dissection

After exposure of the submucosal layer, the lesion is then lifted with injection of a lifting solution. The submucosa can be dissected with an ITknife nano (KD 612L/U, Olympus) or HookKnife (KD 620LR/KD 620UR, Olympus) by hooking and cutting the submucosa or by contact with the tip of a DualKnife (KD 650L/KD 650U, Olympus) (Figs. 6.3 and 6.4). The Stag Beetle Knife (MD-47707; Sumitomo Bakelite Co., Ltd.) and Mucosectom2 (HOYA Pentax) have also been used for dissection.

Recently, the clip line traction method has been commonly used for submucosal dissection in esophageal ESD [56] (Figs. 6.5 and 6.6). It allows for improved exposure of submucosa allowing easier identification of the edges of exposed submucosa to direct dissection. One prospective study showed clip line traction contributed to significantly shorten the procedure time [57]. In addition,

the submucosal tunneling method is proposed to keep nice visualization of submucosal layer and submucosal fluid cushion. This technique allows for safe ESD, shortening procedure time [58]. This technique can be performed with the use of the ITknife nano device even for large esophageal cancer involving complete luminal circumference (Figs. 6.7 and 6.8) [59].

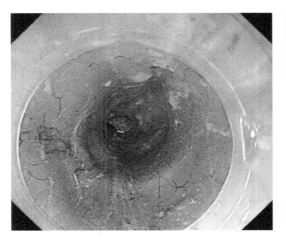

Fig. 6.5 Submucosal tunnel created starting on the proximal side using the distal cap of the scope and ITknife nano

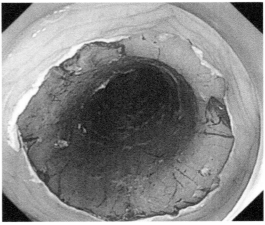

Fig. 6.7 ESD ulcer defect

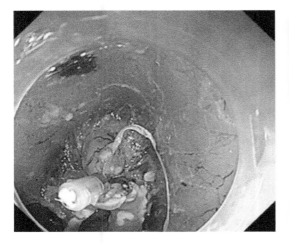

Fig. 6.6 An endoclip attached to the dental floss placed on the mucosal side of the specimen. Floss is pulled from the mouth in order to provide traction. The ITknife nano is then used to dissect the submucosa lateral to the tunnel

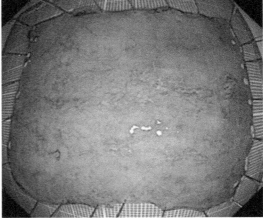

Fig. 6.8 Opened and fixed resected specimen measuring 69 × 57 mm. Histopathology revealed SCC with the deepest invasion to the muscularis mucosae, without lymphovascular involvement, and negative margins. This represented a curative endoscopic resection

Table 6.3 Histological outcomes of ESD for early esophageal neoplasia

Histological subtype	N, lesions	Procedure time range, min	En bloc resection rate, % [95% CI] (range)	R0 resection rate, % [95% CI] (range)	Curative resection rate, % [95% CI] (range)	Local recurrence rate, % [95% CI] (range)	Reference
SCC	970	24–160	99 (83.3–100)	82.8 (78–100)	75.6 (69–100)	0.3 (0–2.6)	[18, 19, 33, 42, 43, 61–64, 85, 88]
BE-HGD or EAC	524	86.4–128.5	92.9 [90.3–95.2]	74.5 [66.3–81.9]	64.9 [55.7–73.6]	0.17 [0–0.3%]	[28–30, 44, 68, 84, 96]

ESD endoscopic submucosal dissection, *SCC* squamous cell cancer, *BE* Barrett's esophagus, *HGD* high-grade dysplasia, *EAC* esophageal adenocarcinoma, *CI* confidence interval

Histological Outcomes

Superficial Squamous Cell Carcinoma

Studies for ESD of SCC have revealed en bloc resection rates of 99% (83–100%), complete resection rates of 82.8% (78–100%), curative resection rates of 75.6% (69–100%), and local recurrence rates of 0.3% (0–2.6%) [18, 19, 33, 42, 43, 60–64]. Furthermore, a meta-analysis comparing ESD and EMR for resection of early SCC showed significantly higher en bloc resection rates in the ESD group than in the EMR group regardless of lesion size (97.1% vs. 49.3%), as well as higher curative resection rates (92.3% vs. 52.7%) and lower recurrence rates (0.3% vs. 11.5%) (Table 6.3) [65].

Barrett's Esophagus-Associated High-Grade Dysplasia or Early Adenocarcinoma

A recent meta-analysis evaluated the safety and efficacy of ESD in the treatment of early BE neoplasia [66]. It included 11 studies, of which 10 were cohort studies and 1 was a randomized controlled trial. Seven studies were from Europe, 3 from Asia, and 1 from the United States. Mean lesion size was 27 mm (20.9–33.1), and average procedure time was 107.5 minutes (86.4–128.5). The pooled en bloc resection rate was 92.9% (95% confidence interval (CI), 90.3–95.2%), while the R0 and curative resection rates were 74.5% (95% CI, 66.3–81.9%) and 64.9% (95% CI, 55.7%–73.6%), respectively (Table 6.2). Interestingly, the authors found significant heterogeneity in R0 and curative resection rates [66]. Variation has been attributed to infiltrated lateral margins that were not evident before endoscopic resection, highlighting the importance of detailed pre-procedural evaluation. This meta-analysis reported highly favorable outcomes and safety profiles, comparable to those in gastric and colorectal ESD from Asia and Europe [66].

Two recent multicenter analyses demonstrated the efficacy and safety of ESD in the West for resection of BE-HGD and EAC. The multicenter retrospective analysis from five academic tertiary referral centers in the United States reported en bloc and curative resection rates of 96% and 70%, respectively. Early bleeding was noted in 6% of the patients, perforation in 2.1%, and strictures in 15% [67]. The European analysis from three centers, which included large (≥2 cm), nodular, or fibrotic lesions, revealed similar outcomes. The en bloc resection rate was 90.8% and curative resection rate 65.8%. The learning curve portraying en bloc resection revealed that it plateaued after 30 procedures, providing evidence of better outcomes with experience. Rate of bleeding was 1.4%, perforation 0%, and stricture 2.1% [68]. These findings highlight the potential role of ESD for the assessment and management of neoplastic lesions associated with BE and provide reassurance on the safety of the technique when performed by experts in high-volume centers.

Post-ESD Recommendations

Squamous Cell Cancer

The risk of lymph node metastasis in SCC lesions limited to the lamina propria is almost 0, while those invading the muscularis mucosa carry a risk of metastasis of 8–15%, and those invading the submucosal layer to 200 um or less have a risk of 11–53% [69–72]. Based on the risk of lymph node metastasis, the following post-treatment recommendations are suggested by the ESGE based on histological outcomes after ESD:

1. A resection is considered curative if en bloc R0 resection is achieved, with a depth < m2, without lymphovascular invasion [72, 73].
2. Multidisciplinary discussion is advisable in the case of an en bloc resection of a well-differentiated m3/sm1 lesion (≤200 µm) without lymphovascular invasion [69–71].
3. Further treatment, in the form of surgery or chemoradiotherapy, is recommended in case of a poorly differentiated tumor, with lymphovascular invasion, positive vertical margins, or a depth > sm2 (>200 µm) [25, 73].
4. If a positive horizontal margin is the only high-risk criteria, endoscopic surveillance and retreatment are reasonable options [33, 42, 43, 55, 74].

High-Grade Dysplasia and Esophageal Adenocarcinoma Associated with Barrett's Esophagus

A recent multicenter retrospective Japanese study found that lesions with lymphovascular involvement, poorly differentiated type, and size >30 mm were independently associated with detection of metastasis of adenocarcinoma of the esophagus. If none of these were present in mucosal and submucosal neoplasms (1–500 µm), the risk of metastasis was very low [75]. Therefore, after detailed histopathologic examination of resected ESD sample, the ESGE recommends the following:

1. A resection is considered curative if en bloc R0 resection of a mucosal lesion is achieved [29, 76].
2. A multidisciplinary discussion is advised in the case of an en bloc resection of a well-differentiated sm1 tumor (≤500 µm) without lymphovascular invasion [77].
3. Surgery is recommended if lymphovascular invasion, poorly differentiated histology, depth > 500 µm, or positive vertical margins are found [25, 29, 76].
4. Endoscopic surveillance or retreatment are recommended if horizontal margins are positive, and there are no other high-risk criteria [25, 28, 29, 76].

Surveillance After Curative ESD

Evidence for the most effective follow-up interval after esophageal ESD is lacking. However, based on the risk of recurrence rates of Barrett's-associated neoplasia after endoscopic resection that range from 11% to 30%, close endoscopic follow-up and an ablation technique are recommended after excision [78, 79]. Per experts' practice, a 3-monthly approach for 1 year, and yearly thereafter, is suggested [80]. For the case of superficial squamous cell cancer, high-resolution endoscopy and biopsies of suspicious areas at 3 and 6 months, and annually thereafter, are recommended [25].

Adverse Events

Management of the potential complications associated with ESD is vital for performing successful procedures [38]. The perceived rate of adverse events is higher for ESD when compared to EMR, because of the longer procedure times and its technically challenging nature. However, a significant difference in the complication rates has been noted only for esophageal strictures [28, 64, 74, 81]. No mortality has been observed after esophageal ESD procedures.

Bleeding

Bleeding, defined as ≥ 2 g/dL drop in hemoglobin, has been noted in 0–22.8% of esophageal ESD case series, with a mean of 2.5% [19, 28, 29, 32, 33, 42, 43, 55, 60, 61, 63, 67, 82–86]. It usually presents during the procedure or within the first 24 hours. According to a recent systematic review, bleeding was controlled conservatively in 95% of cases and required intervention in less than 10% of cases [81]. Delayed bleeding after esophageal ESD is rare, being reported in 0–5.2% of patients.

Perforation

Perforation has been noted in 0–4% of ESD procedures for resection of squamous cell carcinoma and HGD and EAC associated with BE [19, 28, 29, 32, 33, 42, 43, 55, 60, 61, 63, 67, 82–86]. Small perforations can be successfully treated with endoscopic clip placement, while large perforations may require urgent surgical intervention [25, 64]. Given the resection of the submucosa (the strength layer) in ESD and the lack of serosa in the esophagus, endoscopic salvage and, to a lesser degree, primary surgical repair of larger defects are challenging. In those patients who develop mediastinal emphysema without a recognizable perforation, it might be beneficial to provide conservative treatment [63].

Stricture

An esophageal stricture after ESD is defined as a stenosis that limits the passage of a gastroscope. It develops in 12–17% of patients [87, 88]. This complication creates additional challenges in patients who may need adjuvant therapy, such as radiotherapy, where the development of a stricture may be a relative contraindication. A circumferential extent $\geq 75\%$ of the lumen and greater invasion depth (>T1m2) have been associated with occurrence of strictures [18]. In light of its high prevalence, several interventions have been proposed to prevent this complication [89]. Currently, the first-line options are oral or locally injected steroids [89–94]. A randomized controlled trial is ongoing to rigorously evaluate the efficacy of stricture prevention in both methods [95]. Alternatives include prophylactic endoscopic balloon dilation, self-expandable metal stents, local injection of botulinum toxin, and oral tranilast [90, 96, 97]. In addition, promising approaches, including tissue-shielding resection sites with carboxymethyl cellulose, polyglycolic acid sheets followed by fibrin glue, as well as autologous cell sheet transplantation, are currently under investigation [98–103].

Future

Randomized controlled trials addressing the efficacy and safety of ESD for Barrett's HGD and EAC are needed, especially from Western endoscopists. Further investigation is needed for lifting solutions with submucosal dissecting properties that may decrease the technical difficulty of ESD, promoting its universalization. Prevention of adverse events by way of tissue-shielding techniques and endoscopic suturing is a promising field of research.

Conclusion

ESD is an established technique for treatment of early esophageal squamous cell carcinoma. Compared with EMR, ESD has higher rates of en bloc, curative, and R0 resections, resulting in lower local recurrence rates. Adoption of ESD for removal of HGD and EAC associated with Barrett's esophagus has been restricted by its technical complexity, limited training opportunities, a high risk of adverse events, long procedure times, and suboptimal reimbursement. However, promising fields include the development of techniques to prevent adverse events and decrease the technical difficulty of ESD.

References

1. Ferlay J, Soerjomataram I, Dikshit R, Eser S, Mathers C, Rebelo M, et al. Cancer incidence and mortality worldwide: sources, methods and major patterns in GLOBOCAN 2012. Int J Cancer. 2015;136(5):E359–86.
2. DeSantis CE, Lin CC, Mariotto AB, Siegel RL, Stein KD, Kramer JL, et al. Cancer treatment and survivorship statistics, 2014. CA Cancer J Clin. 2014;64(4):252–71.
3. Rustgi AK, El-Serag HB. Esophageal carcinoma. N Engl J Med. 2014;371(26):2499–509.
4. Arnold M, Soerjomataram I, Ferlay J, Forman D. Global incidence of oesophageal cancer by histological subtype in 2012. Gut. 2015;64(3):381–7.
5. Pohl H, Sirovich B, Welch HG. Esophageal adenocarcinoma incidence: are we reaching the peak? Cancer Epidemiol Biomark Prev. 2010;19(6):1468–70.
6. Devesa SS, Blot WJ, Fraumeni JF Jr. Changing patterns in the incidence of esophageal and gastric carcinoma in the United States. Cancer. 1998;83(10):2049–53.
7. Kubo A, Corley DA. Marked multi-ethnic variation of esophageal and gastric cardia carcinomas within the United States. Am J Gastroenterol. 2004;99(4):582–8.
8. Simard EP, Ward EM, Siegel R, Jemal A. Cancers with increasing incidence trends in the United States: 1999 through 2008. CA Cancer J Clin. 2012;62(2):118–28.
9. Dubecz A, Solymosi N, Stadlhuber RJ, Schweigert M, Stein HJ, Peters JH. Does the incidence of adenocarcinoma of the esophagus and gastric cardia continue to rise in the twenty-first century?- a SEER database analysis. J Gastrointest Surg 2014;18(1):124–129.
10. Raymond DP, Seder CW, Wright CD, Magee MJ, Kosinski AS, Cassivi SD, et al. Predictors of major morbidity or mortality after resection for esophageal cancer: a Society of Thoracic Surgeons General Thoracic Surgery Database Risk Adjustment Model. Ann Thorac Surg. 2016;102(1):207–14.
11. Birkmeyer JD, Stukel TA, Siewers AE, Goodney PP, Wennberg DE, Lucas FL. Surgeon volume and operative mortality in the United States. N Engl J Med. 2003;349(22):2117–27.
12. Luketich JD, Pennathur A, Awais O, Levy RM, Keeley S, Shende M, et al. Outcomes after minimally invasive esophagectomy: review of over 1000 patients. Ann Surg. 2012;256(1):95–103.
13. Orringer MB, Marshall B, Chang AC, Lee J, Pickens A, Lau CL. Two thousand transhiatal esophagectomies: changing trends, lessons learned. Ann Surg. 2007;246(3):363–72; discussion 372–4
14. Weksler B, Sullivan JL. Survival after esophagectomy: a propensity-matched study of different surgical approaches. Ann Thorac Surg. 2017;104(4):1138–46.
15. Ngamruengphong S, Wolfsen HC, Wallace MB. Survival of patients with superficial esophageal adenocarcinoma after endoscopic treatment vs surgery. Clin Gastroenterol Hepatol. 2013;11(11):1424–9.. e2; quiz e81
16. McCulloch P, Ward J, Tekkis PP, ASCOT group of surgeons, British Oesophago-Gastric Cancer Group. Mortality and morbidity in gastro-oesophageal cancer surgery: initial results of ASCOT multicentre prospective cohort study. BMJ. 2003;327(7425):1192–7.
17. Suzuki H, Oda I, Abe S, Sekiguchi M, Mori G, Nonaka S, et al. High rate of 5-year survival among patients with early gastric cancer undergoing curative endoscopic submucosal dissection. Gastric Cancer. 2016;19(1):198–205.
18. Ono S, Fujishiro M, Niimi K, Goto O, Kodashima S, Yamamichi N, et al. Long-term outcomes of endoscopic submucosal dissection for superficial esophageal squamous cell neoplasms. Gastrointest Endosc. 2009;70(5):860–6.
19. Oyama T, Tomori A, Hotta K, Morita S, Kominato K, Tanaka M, et al. Endoscopic submucosal dissection of early esophageal cancer. Clin Gastroenterol Hepatol. 2005;3(7. Suppl 1):S67–70.
20. Li Z, Rice TW, Liu X, Goldblum JR, Williams SJ, Rybicki LA, et al. Intramucosal esophageal adenocarcinoma: Primum non nocere. J Thorac Cardiovasc Surg. 2013;145(6):1519–1524.e3.
21. Raja S, Rice TW, Goldblum JR, Rybicki LA, Murthy SC, Mason DP, et al. Esophageal submucosa: the watershed for esophageal cancer. J Thorac Cardiovasc Surg. 2011;142(6):1403–11.e1.
22. Tanabe S, Koizumi W, Higuchi K, Sasaki T, Nakatani K, Hanaoka N, et al. Clinical outcomes of endoscopic oblique aspiration mucosectomy for superficial esophageal cancer. Gastrointest Endosc. 2008;67(6):814–20.
23. Katada C, Muto M, Manabe T, Ohtsu A, Yoshida S. Local recurrence of squamous-cell carcinoma of the esophagus after EMR. Gastrointest Endosc. 2005;61(2):219–25.
24. Pech O, May A, Manner H, Behrens A, Pohl J, Weferling M, et al. Long-term efficacy and safety of endoscopic resection for patients with mucosal adenocarcinoma of the esophagus. Gastroenterology. 2014;146(3):652–660.e1.
25. Pimentel-Nunes P, Dinis-Ribeiro M, Ponchon T, Repici A, Vieth M, De Ceglie A, et al. Endoscopic submucosal dissection: European Society of Gastrointestinal Endoscopy (ESGE) guideline. Endoscopy. 2015;47(9):829–54.
26. ASGE Standards of Practice Committee, Evans JA, Early DS, Chandraskhara V, Chathadi KV, Fanelli RD, et al. The role of endoscopy in the assessment and treatment of esophageal cancer. Gastrointest Endosc. 2013;77(3):328–34.
27. Kuwano H, Nishimura Y, Oyama T, Kato H, Kitagawa Y, Kusano M, et al. Guidelines for diagnosis and treatment of carcinoma of the esophagus

April 2012 edited by the Japan Esophageal Society. Esophagus. 2015;12:1–30.

28. Chevaux JB, Piessevaux H, Jouret-Mourin A, Yeung R, Danse E, Deprez PH. Clinical outcome in patients treated with endoscopic submucosal dissection for superficial Barrett's neoplasia. Endoscopy. 2015;47(2):103–12.

29. Neuhaus H, Terheggen G, Rutz EM, Vieth M, Schumacher B. Endoscopic submucosal dissection plus radiofrequency ablation of neoplastic Barrett's esophagus. Endoscopy. 2012;44(12):1105–13.

30. Kagemoto K, Oka S, Tanaka S, Miwata T, Urabe Y, Sanomura Y, et al. Clinical outcomes of endoscopic submucosal dissection for superficial Barrett's adenocarcinoma. Gastrointest Endosc. 2014;80(2):239–45.

31. Peters FP, Brakenhoff KP, Curvers WL, Rosmolen WD, ten Kate FJ, Krishnadath KK, et al. Endoscopic cap resection for treatment of early Barrett's neoplasia is safe: a prospective analysis of acute and early complications in 216 procedures. Dis Esophagus. 2007;20(6):510–5.

32. Terheggen G, Horn EM, Vieth M, Gabbert H, Enderle M, Neugebauer A, et al. A randomised trial of endoscopic submucosal dissection versus endoscopic mucosal resection for early Barrett's neoplasia. Gut. 2017;66(5):783–93.

33. Fujinami H, Hosokawa A, Ogawa K, Nishikawa J, Kajiura S, Ando T, et al. Endoscopic submucosal dissection for superficial esophageal neoplasms using the stag beetle knife. Dis Esophagus. 2014;27(1):50–4.

34. Cameron GR, Jayasekera CS, Williams R, Macrae FA, Desmond PV, Taylor AC. Detection and staging of esophageal cancers within Barrett's esophagus is improved by assessment in specialized Barrett's units. Gastrointest Endosc. 2014;80(6):971–83.e1.

35. Deprez PH, Bergman JJ, Meisner S, Ponchon T, Repici A, Dinis-Ribeiro M, et al. Current practice with endoscopic submucosal dissection in Europe: position statement from a panel of experts. Endoscopy. 2010;42(10):853–8.

36. Yamamoto S, Uedo N, Ishihara R, Kajimoto N, Ogiyama H, Fukushima Y, et al. Endoscopic submucosal dissection for early gastric cancer performed by supervised residents: assessment of feasibility and learning curve. Endoscopy. 2009;41(11):923–8.

37. ASGE Technology Committee, Maple JT, Abu Dayyeh BK, Chauhan SS, Hwang JH, Komanduri S, et al. Endoscopic submucosal dissection. Gastrointest Endosc. 2015;81(6):1311–25.

38. Bhatt A, Abe S, Kumaravel A, Vargo J, Saito Y. Indications and techniques for endoscopic submucosal dissection. Am J Gastroenterol. 2015;110(6):784–91.

39. Gotoda T, Kondo H, Ono H, Saito Y, Yamaguchi H, Saito D, et al. A new endoscopic mucosal resection procedure using an insulation-tipped electrosurgical knife for rectal flat lesions: report of two cases. Gastrointest Endosc. 1999;50(4):560–3.

40. Matsui N, Akahoshi K, Nakamura K, Ihara E, Kita H. Endoscopic submucosal dissection for removal of superficial gastrointestinal neoplasms: a technical review. World J Gastrointest Endosc. 2012;4(4):123–36.

41. Akahoshi K, Kubokawa M, Gibo J, Osada S, Tokumaru K, Shiratsuchi Y, et al. Endoscopic resection using the Clutch Cutter and a detachable snare for large pedunculated colonic polyps. Endoscopy. 2017;49(1):54–8.

42. Kawahara Y, Hori K, Takenaka R, Nasu J, Kawano S, Kita M, et al. Endoscopic submucosal dissection of esophageal cancer using the Mucosectom2 device: a feasibility study. Endoscopy. 2013;45(11):869–75.

43. Repici A, Hassan C, Carlino A, Pagano N, Zullo A, Rando G, et al. Endoscopic submucosal dissection in patients with early esophageal squamous cell carcinoma: results from a prospective Western series. Gastrointest Endosc. 2010;71(4):715–21.

44. Hobel S, Dautel P, Baumbach R, Oldhafer KJ, Stang A, Feyerabend B, et al. Single center experience of endoscopic submucosal dissection (ESD) in early Barrett's adenocarcinoma. Surg Endosc. 2015;29(6):1591–7.

45. Inoue H, Rey JF, Lightdale C. Lugol chromoendoscopy for esophageal squamous cell cancer. Endoscopy. 2001;33(1):75–9.

46. Lee CT, Chang CY, Lee YC, Tai CM, Wang WL, Tseng PH, et al. Narrow-band imaging with magnifying endoscopy for the screening of esophageal cancer in patients with primary head and neck cancers. Endoscopy. 2010;42(8):613–9.

47. Mannath J, Subramanian V, Hawkey CJ, Ragunath K. Narrow band imaging for characterization of high grade dysplasia and specialized intestinal metaplasia in Barrett's esophagus: a meta-analysis. Endoscopy. 2010;42(5):351–9.

48. Takenaka R, Kawahara Y, Okada H, Hori K, Inoue M, Kawano S, et al. Narrow-band imaging provides reliable screening for esophageal malignancy in patients with head and neck cancers. Am J Gastroenterol. 2009;104(12):2942–8.

49. Curvers WL, Bohmer CJ, Mallant-Hent RC, Naber AH, Ponsioen CI, Ragunath K, et al. Mucosal morphology in Barrett's esophagus: interobserver agreement and role of narrow band imaging. Endoscopy. 2008;40(10):799–805.

50. May A, Gunter E, Roth F, Gossner L, Stolte M, Vieth M, et al. Accuracy of staging in early oesophageal cancer using high resolution endoscopy and high resolution endosonography: a comparative, prospective, and blinded trial. Gut. 2004;53(5):634–40.

51. Larghi A, Lightdale CJ, Memeo L, Bhagat G, Okpara N, Rotterdam H. EUS followed by EMR for staging of high-grade dysplasia and early cancer in Barrett's esophagus. Gastrointest Endosc. 2005;62(1):16–23.

52. Pech O, May A, Gunter E, Gossner L, Ell C. The impact of endoscopic ultrasound and computed tomography on the TNM staging of early cancer in Barrett's esophagus. Am J Gastroenterol. 2006;101(10):2223–9.

53. Pech O, Gunter E, Dusemund F, Ell C. Value of high-frequency miniprobes and conventional radial endoscopic ultrasound in the staging of early Barrett's carcinoma. Endoscopy. 2010;42(2):98–103.

54. Kothari S, Kaul V. Endoscopic mucosal resection and endoscopic submucosal dissection for endoscopic therapy of Barrett's esophagus-related neoplasia. Gastroenterol Clin N Am. 2015;44(2):317–35.

55. Higuchi K, Tanabe S, Azuma M, Katada C, Sasaki T, Ishido K, et al. A phase II study of endoscopic submucosal dissection for superficial esophageal neoplasms (KDOG 0901). Gastrointest Endosc. 2013;78(5):704–10.

56. Oyama T. Counter traction makes endoscopic submucosal dissection easier. Clin Endosc. 2012;45(4):375–8.

57. Koike Y, Hirasawa D, Fujita N, Maeda Y, Ohira T, Harada Y, et al. Usefulness of the thread-traction method in esophageal endoscopic submucosal dissection: randomized controlled trial. Dig Endosc. 2015;27(3):303–9.

58. Huang R, Cai H, Zhao X, Lu X, Liu M, Lv W, et al. Efficacy and safety of endoscopic submucosal tunnel dissection for superficial esophageal squamous cell carcinoma: a propensity score matching analysis. Gastrointest Endosc. 2017;86:831. Available online 9 March 2017

59. Abe S, Oda I, Suzuki H, Yoshinaga S, Saito Y. Insulated tip knife tunneling technique with clip line traction for safe endoscopic submucosal dissection of large circumferential esophageal cancer. VideoGIE. 2017. Available online 30 September 2017.

60. Kanzaki H, Ishihara R, Ohta T, Nagai K, Matsui F, Yamashina T, et al. Randomized study of two endo-knives for endoscopic submucosal dissection of esophageal cancer. Am J Gastroenterol. 2013;108(8):1293–8.

61. Toyonaga T, Man-i M, East JE, Nishino E, Ono W, Hirooka T, et al. 1,635 Endoscopic submucosal dissection cases in the esophagus, stomach, and colorectum: complication rates and long-term outcomes. Surg Endosc. 2013;27(3):1000–8.

62. Yamashina T, Ishihara R, Uedo N, Nagai K, Matsui F, Kawada N, et al. Safety and curative ability of endoscopic submucosal dissection for superficial esophageal cancers at least 50 mm in diameter. Dig Endosc. 2012;24(4):220–5.

63. Takahashi H, Arimura Y, Masao H, Okahara S, Tanuma T, Kodaira J, et al. Endoscopic submucosal dissection is superior to conventional endoscopic resection as a curative treatment for early squamous cell carcinoma of the esophagus (with video). Gastrointest Endosc. 2010;72(2):255–64, 264.e1–2

64. Fujishiro M, Yahagi N, Kakushima N, Kodashima S, Muraki Y, Ono S, et al. Endoscopic submucosal dissection of esophageal squamous cell neoplasms. Clin Gastroenterol Hepatol. 2006;4(6):688–94.

65. Guo HM, Zhang XQ, Chen M, Huang SL, Zou XP. Endoscopic submucosal dissection vs endoscopic mucosal resection for superficial esophageal cancer. World J Gastroenterol. 2014;20(18):5540–7.

66. Yang D, Zou F, Xiong S, Forde JJ, Wang Y, Draganov PV. Endoscopic submucosal dissection for early Barrett's neoplasia: a meta-analysis. Gastrointest Endosc. 2017;86:600.

67. Yang D, Coman RM, Kahaleh M, Waxman I, Wang AY, Sethi A, et al. Endoscopic submucosal dissection for Barrett's early neoplasia: a multicenter study in the United States. Gastrointest Endosc. 2017;86(4):600–7.

68. Subramaniam S, Chedgy F, Longcroft-Wheaton G, Kandiah K, Maselli R, Seewald S, et al. Complex early Barrett's neoplasia at 3 Western centers: European Barrett's Endoscopic Submucosal Dissection Trial (E-BEST). Gastrointest Endosc. 2017;86(4):608–18.

69. Natsugoe S, Baba M, Yoshinaka H, Kijima F, Shimada M, Shirao K, et al. Mucosal squamous cell carcinoma of the esophagus: a clinicopathologic study of 30 cases. Oncology. 1998;55(3):235–41.

70. Tajima Y, Nakanishi Y, Tachimori Y, Kato H, Watanabe H, Yamaguchi H, et al. Significance of involvement by squamous cell carcinoma of the ducts of esophageal submucosal glands. Analysis of 201 surgically resected superficial squamous cell carcinomas. Cancer. 2000;89(2):248–54.

71. Bollschweiler E, Baldus SE, Schroder W, Prenzel K, Gutschow C, Schneider PM, et al. High rate of lymph-node metastasis in submucosal esophageal squamous-cell carcinomas and adenocarcinomas. Endoscopy. 2006;38(2):149–56.

72. Higuchi K, Koizumi W, Tanabe S, Sasaki T, Katada C, Azuma M, et al. Current management of esophageal squamous-cell carcinoma in Japan and other countries. Gastrointest Cancer Res. 2009;3(4):153–61.

73. Japan Esophageal Society. Japanese classification of esophageal cancer, 11th edition: part I. Esophagus. 2017;14(1):1–36.

74. Ishihara R, Iishi H, Takeuchi Y, Kato M, Yamamoto S, Yamamoto S, et al. Local recurrence of large squamous-cell carcinoma of the esophagus after endoscopic resection. Gastrointest Endosc. 2008;67(6):799–804.

75. Ishihara R, Oyama T, Abe S, Takahashi H, Ono H, Fujisaki J, et al. Risk of metastasis in adenocarcinoma of the esophagus: a multicenter retrospective study in a Japanese population. J Gastroenterol. 2017;52(7):800–8.

76. Yoshinaga S, Gotoda T, Kusano C, Oda I, Nakamura K, Takayanagi R. Clinical impact of endoscopic submucosal dissection for superficial adenocarcinoma

located at the esophagogastric junction. Gastrointest Endosc. 2008;67(2):202–9.

77. Manner H, May A, Pech O, Gossner L, Rabenstein T, Gunter E, et al. Early Barrett's carcinoma with "low-risk" submucosal invasion: long-term results of endoscopic resection with a curative intent. Am J Gastroenterol. 2008;103(10):2589–97.

78. Larghi A, Lightdale CJ, Ross AS, Fedi P, Hart J, Rotterdam H, et al. Long-term follow-up of complete Barrett's eradication endoscopic mucosal resection (CBE-EMR) for the treatment of high grade dysplasia and intramucosal carcinoma. Endoscopy. 2007;39(12):1086–91.

79. Fleischer DE, Overholt BF, Sharma VK, Reymunde A, Kimmey MB, Chuttani R, et al. Endoscopic radiofrequency ablation for Barrett's esophagus: 5-year outcomes from a prospective multicenter trial. Endoscopy. 2010;42(10):781–9.

80. Bedi AO, Kwon RS, Rubenstein JH, Piraka CR, Elta GH, Scheiman JM, et al. A survey of expert follow-up practices after successful endoscopic eradication therapy for Barrett's esophagus with high-grade dysplasia and intramucosal adenocarcinoma. Gastrointest Endosc. 2013;78(5):696–701.

81. Sgourakis G, Gockel I, Lang H. Endoscopic and surgical resection of T1a/T1b esophageal neoplasms: a systematic review. World J Gastroenterol. 2013;19(9):1424–37.

82. Hirasawa K, Kokawa A, Oka H, Yahara S, Sasaki T, Nozawa A, et al. Superficial adenocarcinoma of the esophagogastric junction: long-term results of endoscopic submucosal dissection. Gastrointest Endosc. 2010;72(5):960–6.

83. Ishihara R, Iishi H, Uedo N, Takeuchi Y, Yamamoto S, Yamada T, et al. Comparison of EMR and endoscopic submucosal dissection for en bloc resection of early esophageal cancers in Japan. Gastrointest Endosc. 2008;68(6):1066–72.

84. Probst A, Aust D, Markl B, Anthuber M, Messmann H. Early esophageal cancer in Europe: endoscopic treatment by endoscopic submucosal dissection. Endoscopy. 2015;47(2):113–21.

85. Yamashita T, Zeniya A, Ishii H, Tsuji T, Tsuda S, Nakane K, et al. Endoscopic mucosal resection using a cap-fitted panendoscope and endoscopic submucosal dissection as optimal endoscopic procedures for superficial esophageal carcinoma. Surg Endosc. 2011;25(8):2541–6.

86. Mochizuki Y, Saito Y, Tsujikawa T, Fujiyama Y, Andoh A. Combination of endoscopic submucosal dissection and chemoradiation therapy for superficial esophageal squamous cell carcinoma with submucosal invasion. Exp Ther Med. 2011;2(6): 1065–8.

87. Kim JS, Kim BW, Shin IS. Efficacy and safety of endoscopic submucosal dissection for superficial squamous esophageal neoplasia: a meta-analysis. Dig Dis Sci. 2014;59(8):1862–9.

88. Ono S, Fujishiro M, Niimi K, Goto O, Kodashima S, Yamamichi N, et al. Predictors of postoperative stricture after esophageal endoscopic submucosal dissection for superficial squamous cell neoplasms. Endoscopy. 2009;41(8):661–5.

89. Abe S, Iyer PG, Oda I, Kanai N, Saito Y. Approaches for stricture prevention after esophageal endoscopic resection. Gastrointest Endosc. 2017;86:779.

90. Yamaguchi N, Isomoto H, Nakayama T, Hayashi T, Nishiyama H, Ohnita K, et al. Usefulness of oral prednisolone in the treatment of esophageal stricture after endoscopic submucosal dissection for superficial esophageal squamous cell carcinoma. Gastrointest Endosc. 2011;73(6):1115–21.

91. Hashimoto S, Kobayashi M, Takeuchi M, Sato Y, Narisawa R, Aoyagi Y. The efficacy of endoscopic triamcinolone injection for the prevention of esophageal stricture after endoscopic submucosal dissection. Gastrointest Endosc. 2011;74(6):1389–93.

92. Deprez PH. Esophageal strictures after extensive endoscopic resection: hope for a better outcome? Gastrointest Endosc. 2013;78(2):258–9.

93. Bahin FF, Jayanna M, Williams SJ, Lee EY, Bourke MJ. Efficacy of viscous budesonide slurry for prevention of esophageal stricture formation after complete endoscopic mucosal resection of short-segment Barrett's neoplasia. Endoscopy. 2016;48(1):71–4.

94. Mori H, Rafiq K, Kobara H, Fujihara S, Nishiyama N, Oryuu M, et al. Steroid permeation into the artificial ulcer by combined steroid gel application and balloon dilatation: prevention of esophageal stricture. J Gastroenterol Hepatol. 2013;28(6):999–1003.

95. Mizutani T, Tanaka M, Eba J, Mizusawa J, Fukuda H, Hanaoka N, et al. A phase III study of oral steroid administration versus local steroid injection therapy for the prevention of esophageal stricture after endoscopic submucosal dissection (JCOG1217, steroid EESD P3). Jpn J Clin Oncol. 2015;45(11):1087–90.

96. Wen J, Lu Z, Linghu E, Yang Y, Yang J, Wang S, et al. Prevention of esophageal strictures after endoscopic submucosal dissection with the injection of botulinum toxin type A. Gastrointest Endosc. 2016;84(4):606–13.

97. Ezoe Y, Muto M, Horimatsu T, Morita S, Miyamoto S, Mochizuki S, et al. Efficacy of preventive endoscopic balloon dilation for esophageal stricture after endoscopic resection. J Clin Gastroenterol. 2011;45(3):222–7.

98. Iizuka T, Kikuchi D, Yamada A, Hoteya S, Kajiyama Y, Kaise M. Polyglycolic acid sheet application to prevent esophageal stricture after endoscopic submucosal dissection for esophageal squamous cell carcinoma. Endoscopy. 2015;47(4):341–4.

99. Kim YJ, Park JC, Chung H, Shin SK, Lee SK, Lee YC. Polyglycolic acid sheet application to prevent

esophageal stricture after endoscopic submucosal dissection for recurrent esophageal cancer. Endoscopy. 2016 0;48(S 01):E319–20.

100. Sakaguchi Y, Tsuji Y, Ono S, Saito I, Kataoka Y, Takahashi Y, et al. Polyglycolic acid sheets with fibrin glue can prevent esophageal stricture after endoscopic submucosal dissection. Endoscopy. 2015;47(4):336–40.

101. Lua GW, Tang J, Liu F, Li ZS. Prevention of esophageal strictures after endoscopic submucosal dissection: a promising therapy using carboxymethyl cellulose sheets. Dig Dis Sci. 2016;61(6):1763–9.

102. Takagi R, Murakami D, Kondo M, Ohki T, Sasaki R, Mizutani M, et al. Fabrication of human oral mucosal epithelial cell sheets for treatment of esophageal ulceration by endoscopic submucosal dissection. Gastrointest Endosc. 2010;72(6): 1253–9.

103. Ohki T, Yamato M, Ota M, Takagi R, Kondo M, Kanai N, et al. Application of regenerative medical technology using tissue-engineered cell sheets for endoscopic submucosal dissection of esophageal neoplasms. Dig Endosc. 2015;27(2):182–8.

Gastric ESD

7

Takuji Gotoda

Abbreviations

DFC	Dental floss and a hemoclip
EGC	Early gastric cancer
EMR	Endoscopic mucosal resection
EMRC	EMR with cap-fitted panendoscope method
EMRL	EMR using multi-band ligation
ESD	Endoscopic submucosal dissection
IT knife	Insulated-tip diathermic knife
LNM	Lymph node metastasis
QOL	Quality of life

Introduction

In the history of gastric cancer treatment, many of the cases with gastric cancer discovered in the 1970s were in the advanced stage. As represented by the Appleby operation, extended radical surgery with lymph node dissection was globally accepted as a mainstream approach to gastric cancer, even in early gastric cancer (EGC). With the widespread adoption of nationwide screening in Japan [1] and the advancement of endoscope technology in the 1980s, the number of patients diagnosed with early gastric cancer has increased.

The major advantage of endoscopic resection is the ability to provide an accurate pathological staging without precluding future surgical therapy [2, 3]. After endoscopic resection, pathological assessment of depth of cancer invasion, degree of cancer differentiation, and involvement of lymphatics or vessels allows the prediction of the risk of lymph node metastasis (LNM) [4]. The risk of LNM or distant metastasis is then weighted against the risk of surgery [5]. However, endoscopic resection which is local treatment presents important trade-offs such as less morbidity but also a higher risk of metachronous recurrence [6]. Patients' preferences and particularly fear of recurrence are an important element in choosing the optimal therapy.

Toward ESD

The first endoscopic resection was reported in colorectal polypectomy using high-frequency electric surgical unit [7]. Indeed, the first endoscopic polypectomy used to treat pedunculated or semipedunculated EGC was first described in Japan in 1974 [8].

The "strip biopsy" technique, an early method of endoscopic mucosal resection (EMR), was devised

Electronic Supplementary Material The online version of this chapter (https://doi.org/10.1007/978-3-030-21695-5_7) contains supplementary material, which is available to authorized users.

T. Gotoda (✉)
Division of Gastroenterology and Hepatology, Department of Medicine, Nihon University School of Medicine, Tokyo, Japan

in 1984 as an application of endoscopic snare polypectomy [9]. To obtain resected material with less tissue damage causing adequate pathological staging, a technique called ERHSE (endoscopic resection with local injection of hypertonic saline-epinephrine solution) was developed in 1988 [10].

EMR with cap-fitted panendoscope method (EMRC) was developed in 1992 for the resection of early esophageal cancer and directly applicable for the resection of EGC [11, 12]. The technique of EMR using ligation, which subsequently was extended to EMR using multi-band ligation (EMRL), utilizes band ligation to create a "pseudopolyp" by suctioning the lesion into the banding cap and deploying a band underneath it [13, 14]. Although the EMR technique has the advantage of being relatively simple, it cannot be used to remove lesions en bloc larger than 2 cm [15, 16]. Piecemeal resections in lesions larger than 2 cm lead to a high risk of local cancer recurrence and inadequate pathological staging [17, 18].

Insulated-tip diathermic knife (IT knife) was devised in the middle 1990s at the National Cancer Center Hospital in Japan in order to remove EGC en bloc and avoid local recurrence. IT knife has a ceramic ball tip, thus preventing it from puncturing the wall during the application of cautery and causing perforation. The knife can also be used to dissect the submucosa – leading to the name of the technique: endoscopic submucosal dissection (ESD) technique [19–21]. Complete en bloc resection regardless of tumor size, location, and/or submucosal fibrosis can be now possible [22].

Procedure of ESD for the Stomach

ESD has a higher risk of complications such as severe bleeding or perforation and still requires high endoscopic skills. In order to standardize the ESD procedure worldwide, more innovation and modification should be demanded. The traction method using dental floss and a hemoclip (DFC, any hemoclip available) for gastric ESD can make submucosal dissection easier and safer because of good visualization and tension (Fig. 7.1a–c)

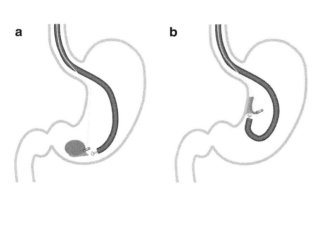
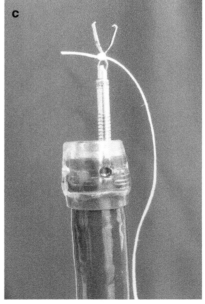

Fig. 7.1 (**a**) Schema and endoscopic view of ESD with DFC, involving an approach from the straight endoscopic position. In the lesions located in the anterior wall of the gastric antrum, the oral side of the resected mucosa is elevated by pulling the dental floss out through the mouth. (**b**) Schema and endoscopic view of ESD with DFC, involving an approach from the retroflexed endoscopic position. In lesions located in the lesser curvature of the gastric corpus, the anal side of the resected mucosa is elevated by pulling the dental floss out through the mouth. (**c**) Preparation of the DFC. A long piece of dental floss is tied to the arm of the hemoclip, and then the hemoclip tied with the dental floss is withdrawn into the transparent hood and the accessory channel of the endoscope to enable the insertion of the endoscope

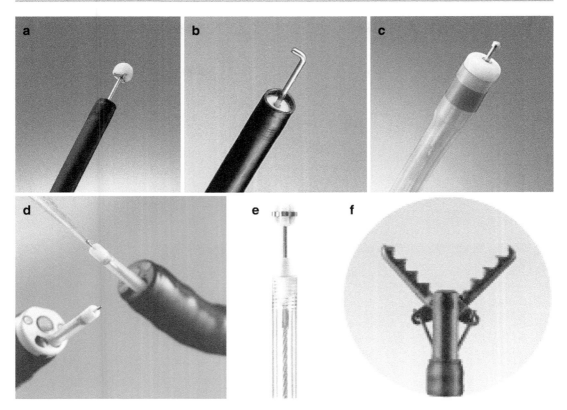

Fig. 7.2 (**a**) ITknife2 (KD-611L, Olympus Medical Systems). (**b**) HookKnife (KD-620LR, Olympus Medical Systems). (**c**) DualKnife (KD-650L, Olympus Medical Systems). (**d**) FlashKnife BT (Fujifilm Medical Co., Ltd.). (**e**) SafeKnife (DK2518DV1, Fujifilm Medical Co., Ltd.). (**f**) Clutch Cutter (DP2618DT-50-, Fujifilm Medical Co., Ltd.)

whenever we dissect submucosal layer by any ESD devices (Fig. 7.2) [23, 24]. It has been standard that several steps for ESD – marking, injecting fluid, circumferentially mucosal cutting, and submucosal dissection – are carried out by IT knife and needle-type devices in Japan [25]. However, ESD using conventional devices has its technical difficulty and requires intensive training under experts. Because these knives lack the ability to grasp the target tissue, maneuverability is often difficult under unstable conditions (like single-hand surgery). Standard gastric ESD with needle-type ESD knives is similar to ESD techniques described elsewhere in this book. Comparing those devices, Clutch Cutter is technically easier and simpler to perform (Fig. 7.3). Thus, gastric ESD using Clutch Cutter (DP2618DT-50-, Fujifilm Medical Co., Ltd.) may be acceptable in the countries with less incidence of EGC. Thus, in order to standardize gastric ESD

procedure, simple ESD with Clutch Cutter under the traction method using DFC is demonstrated in this chapter [26, 27].

Device Settings

Clutch Cutter used for gastric ESD has a 0.4 mm-wide and 5 mm-long serrated cutting edge well suited for grasping function. The outer side of the forceps is insulated so that electrosurgical current energy is concentrated at the inner closed edge of the blade. Forced coagulation mode (VIO 300D, Erbe, Tübingen, Germany; 30 W, effect 3) is used for marking, ENDO CUT Q mode (effect 1, duration 3, interval 1) is used for mucosal incision and submucosal dissection, and soft coagulation mode (100 W, effect 5) is recommended for hemostatic treatment.

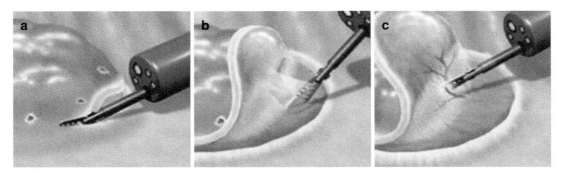

Fig. 7.3 (**a**) Mucosal cutting by Clutch Cutter surrounding marking dots after submucosal injection. (**b**) Submucosal dissection using Clutch Cutter. (**c**) Endoscopic hemostasis for small vessels by using Clutch Cutter

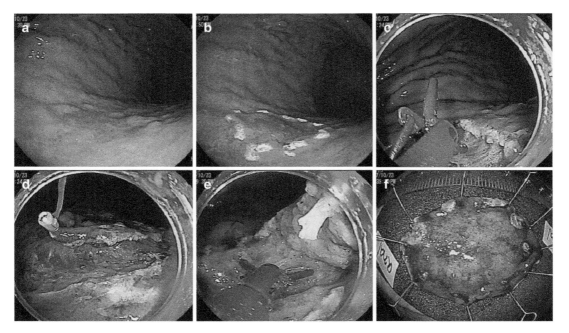

Fig. 7.4 (**a**) A shallow depressed lesion on the posterior wall of the corpus. (**b**) Marking dots by the Clutch Cutter with forced coag (50 W) 5 mm outside the lesion. (**c**) Mucosal incision using Clutch Cutter scissors allows easy incision with the rotatable device with enough grasping. (**d**) Hemoclip – tied by a dental floss – as an anchor for traction. (**e**) Visualized and safe dissection of submucosal layer using Clutch Cutter by ENDO CUT Q mode under good visualization and tension of the submucosa. (**f**) Resected material pinned on the board

A soft transparent hood (JMDN 38819001, Top Corp., Tokyo, Japan) or a small-caliber-tip transparent hood (ST hood, Fujifilm Medical Co., Ltd.) is sometimes useful to stabilize the operating field and to create countertraction for exfoliating the submucosal tissue [28].

Mucosal Cutting

Figure 7.4a shows an EGC 2 cm in size on the posterior wall of the upper corpus of the stomach. Mucosal incision is smoothly carried out on the peripheral side of the marking dots after submucosal injection with normal saline with indigo carmine dye. The Clutch Cutter is rotatable to the desired orientation (Fig. 7.4b, c). Indigo carmine is added to the submucosal injection fluid in order to better identify the blue-colored submucosal layer (with any injection needle available). Sodium hyaluronate (MucoUp, Boston Scientific, Tokyo, Japan) is also often used because of longer-lasting submucosal cushion in order to prevent perforation [29].

Submucosal Dissection

After completing the circumferential cutting, the submucosal layer underneath the lesion is directly dissected. At this step, the traction method is very useful and makes dissection easy, safe, and rapid because of good visualization (Fig. 7.4d). The hemoclip – tied by a dental floss – is anchored to a suitable site of the lesion for oral traction. The clip varies according to the location of the lesion. For lesions approached from the retroflexed endoscopy position, the clip is anchored at the anal side edge of the resected mucosa. In lesions approached from the straight endoscopy position, the clip is anchored at the oral side edge of the resected mucosa. During submucosal dissection, the anchored suture material located outside of the patient is pulled to the oral side with gentle manual traction by the operator or an assistant. Good visualization and tension of the submucosa are obtained by the resected mucosa that is turned over (Fig. 7.4e).

When a small artery and/or vein is encountered in the submucosal layer, the Clutch Cutter can first control the vessel with soft coagulation mode and after that cut it with ENDO CUT Q mode. However, do not hesitate to change Clutch Cutter to Coagrasper G (Olympus Medical Systems) which is more effective to grasp the bleeding vessel and control it.

Preparation for Pathological Staging

The importance of meticulous pathological staging after endoscopic resection cannot be overemphasized. Accurate staging can only be achieved when the specimen is properly oriented by the endoscopist or their assistant immediately after excision in the endoscopy unit prior to be immersed in formaldehyde.

Orientation of the specimen is best performed by fixing its periphery with thin needles inserted into an underlying plate of rubber or wood (Fig. 7.4f). The submucosal side of the specimen is placed in contact with the plate. After fixation, the specimen is sectioned serially at 2 mm intervals parallel to a line that includes the closest resection margin of the specimen so that both lateral and vertical margins are assessed. The depth of tumor invasion (T) is then evaluated along with the degree of differentiation and lymphovascular invasion, if any. The report must include histological type, tumor depth, size, location, and macroscopic appearance. The presence of ulceration and lymphatic and/or venous invasion and the status of the margins of resection should be reported in detail to determine the curability.

Surveillance After Gastric ESD

According to the Japanese guidelines, the curability after ESD/EMR for EGC is classified into three groups: curative resection, curative resection for expanded indication, and non-curative resection (Fig. 7.5) [30–34]. En bloc resection with no lymphovascular invasion and a negative surgical margin are required for curative resection or that for expanded indication. No additional treatment is needed in patients with curative resection.

According to the European guidelines (European Society of Gastrointestinal Endoscopy, ESGE) [35], additional treatment is also not necessary after curative resection, which is the same as in the Japanese guidelines. In the USA, the National Comprehensive Cancer Network guidelines (NCCN guidelines) regard EMR or ESD as having the potential of being therapeutic and one of the treatment options for Tis or T1a cancer ≤2 cm [36].

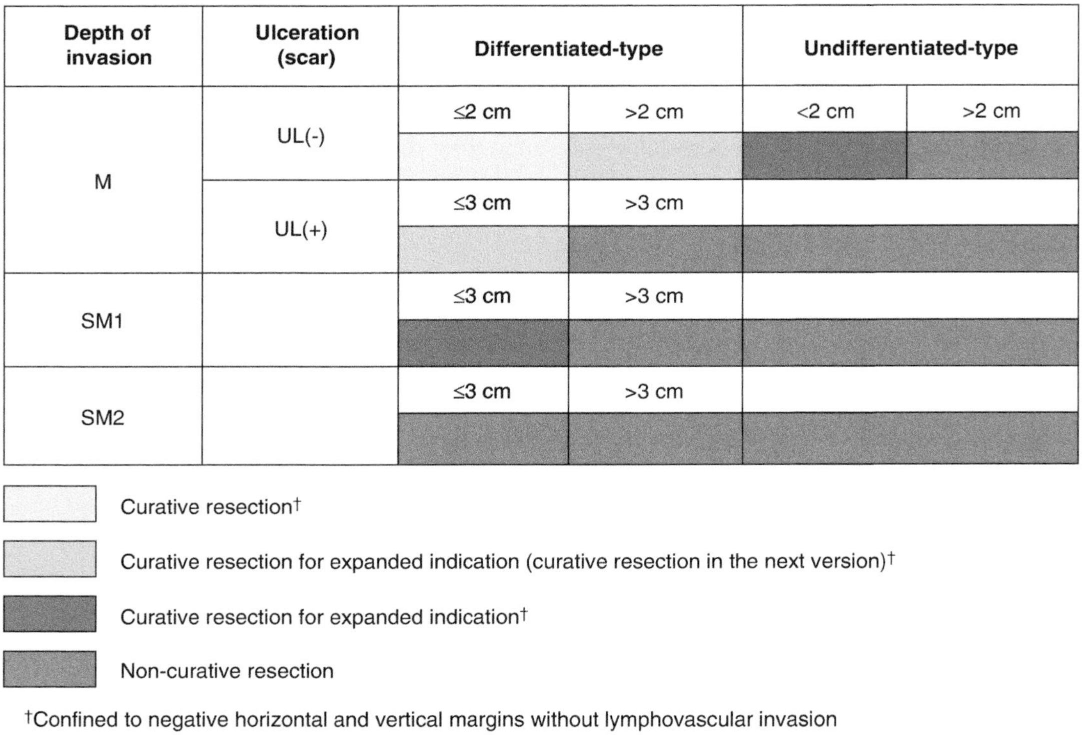

Depth of invasion	Ulceration (scar)	Differentiated-type		Undifferentiated-type	
M	UL(-)	≤2 cm	>2 cm	<2 cm	>2 cm
	UL(+)	≤3 cm	>3 cm		
SM1		≤3 cm	>3 cm		
SM2		≤3 cm	>3 cm		

☐ Curative resection[†]

☐ Curative resection for expanded indication (curative resection in the next version)[†]

☐ Curative resection for expanded indication[†]

☐ Non-curative resection

[†]Confined to negative horizontal and vertical margins without lymphovascular invasion

Fig. 7.5 The therapeutic flowchart after gastric ESD/EMR in the Japanese guidelines

After gastric ESD, attention should be focused on the development of metachronous gastric cancers. The 5-year and 10-year cumulative incidences were 9.5% and 22.7%, respectively [37]. Almost all secondary gastric cancers were treatable by ESD by the scheduled endoscopic surveillance (6–12 months) [38]. The Japanese guidelines also recommend endoscopic surveillance at intervals of 6–12 months, whereas ESGE and NCCN guidelines recommend annual endoscopy from 1 year after ESD/EMR. Thus, when complete resection could be achieved for the initial EGC, the following endoscopic surveillance is recommended after ESD/EMR (Fig. 7.6).

When the histopathological findings meet the expanded criteria, no additional treatment is needed in the Japanese guidelines (Fig. 7.5). Recently, a multicenter retrospective analysis in Japan clarified that 0.14% (6/4202) of such patients had metastatic recurrence during the median follow-up duration of 56 months after ESD [39]. Surveillance for metastatic recurrence as well as metachronous gastric can-

cer is recommended, although the risk of the former is very small. In addition to endoscopic surveillance at every 6 months in the first year and at intervals of (6–)12 months for at least 10 years after ESD/EMR, follow-up with computed tomography (CT) (or ultrasonography) is desirable at intervals of 6–12 months. Hence, patients should be explained that they have a negligible but not zero risk of metastatic recurrence after gastric ESD/ESD.

It is controversial whether the expanded criteria are applicable for European patients. For differentiated-type EGC, the ESGE recommends ESD for EGCs that meet the expanded criteria, whereas ESMO and the German Society of Gastroenterology give restrictive recommendations [40, 41], which recommend gastrectomy for cases meeting the expanded criteria. Regarding undifferentiated-type EGC, the ESGE guidelines regard ESD for the expanded criteria as an option. In such patients, the ESGE guidelines recommend that gastrectomy is always considered with the decision made on an individual basis. There has

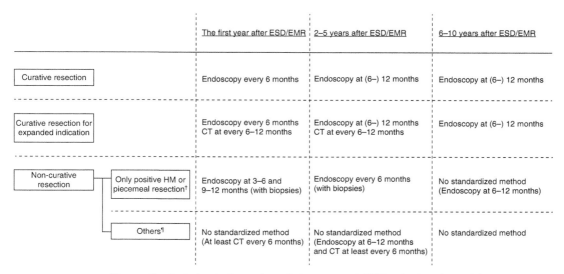

	The first year after ESD/EMR	2–5 years after ESD/EMR	6–10 years after ESD/EMR
Curative resection	Endoscopy every 6 months	Endoscopy at (6–) 12 months	Endoscopy at (6–) 12 months
Curative resection for expanded indication	Endoscopy every 6 months CT at every 6–12 months	Endoscopy at (6–) 12 months CT at every 6–12 months	Endoscopy at (6–) 12 months
Non-curative resection → Only positive HM or piecemeal resection†	Endoscopy at 3–6 and 9–12 months (with biopsies)	Endoscopy every 6 months (with biopsies)	No standardized method (Endoscopy at 6–12 months)
Others¶	No standardized method (At least CT every 6 months)	No standardized method (Endoscopy at 6–12 months and CT at least every 6 months)	No standardized method

†There are the other treatment options such as radical surgery, repeated ESD, and endoscopic coagulation.
¶The standard method is additional gastrectomy with lymph node dissection.

Fig. 7.6 The flowchart of follow-up after gastric ESD/EMR

been no report about the expanded criteria for gastric ESD/EMR in USA. As described previously, the NCCN guidelines regard EMR or ESD as one of the treatment options only for Tis or T1a cancer ≤2 cm. However, a report based on the Surveillance, Epidemiology, and End Results (SEER) database of the USA suggests the existence of different biological aggressiveness in T1a gastric cancer among racial/ethnic groups [42].

When the lesion does not meet the curative criteria, the ESD is regarded as non-curative resection. In cases of differentiated-type EGC with the only unsatisfactory curative factor of piecemeal resection or resection en bloc with a positive horizontal margin, surgical resection is not the only option because such cases have a very low risk of harboring LNM. Repeated ESD, endoscopic coagulation using a laser or argon plasma coagulator, or close observation expecting a burn effect of the initial endoscopic resection could be proposed as an alternative in such cases, with the patient's informed consent.

In the other type of non-curative resection, additional gastrectomy with lymph node dissection is recommended in the ESGE and Japanese guidelines because such lesions have the potential for LNM. When gastric ESD/EMR is performed, 17–29% of the patients do not meet the

curative criteria. However, LNM is found in only 5–10% of patients with such lesions [43]. In the clinical setting, nearly half of such patients are followed up with no additional treatment after ESD in Japan, due to the age, underlying disease, and patients' preference. Also, in Germany, 69% (27/39) of such patients were followed up with no additional treatment after non-curative resection for EGC [44].

A randomized controlled trial clarified that prophylactic eradication of *Helicobacter pylori* after ESD/EMR for EGC reduced the risk of metachronous gastric cancer to about one-third [45]. However, some studies including one randomized controlled trial revealed conflicting results [46]. Although eradication therapy is recommended in *Helicobacter pylori*-infected patients, further investigation about this issue is needed.

Future Perspective

Patients who are stratified to have no or lower risk of LNM than the risk of mortality from surgery are ideal candidates for endoscopic resection [47, 48]. Endoscopic resection allows complete pathological staging of the cancer, which is critical for determining potential for

Fig. 7.7 eCura system. "eCura system" was developed for predicting lymph node metastasis after non-curative resection for early gastric cancer. This is a seven-point scoring system with three risk categories based on five clinicopathological factors. CSS, cancer-specific survival; SM2, cancer with depth of invasion from the muscularis mucosa ≥500 μm

Risk category	Total points	Rate of LNM[†] (%)	5-year CSS (%) (in patients with no additional treatment[†])
Low-risk	0–1	2.5	99.6
Intermediate-risk	2–4	6.7	96.1
High-risk	5–7	22.7	90.1

3 points: lymphatic invasion

1 point: tumor size >30 mm, positive vertical margin, SM2, venous invasion

[†]Among patients with non-curative resection for early gastric cancer

metastasis [49]. The optimal staging method of EGC is to evaluate the pathology of en bloc resected material [50, 51].

In cancer treatment, completely curing the illness is extremely important. However, if quality of life (QOL) is impaired by procedures that are superior only in terms of reducing marginal risks, patients may have difficulties in daily life and social rehabilitation after treatment [52, 53]. The stomach not only serves as a storage compartment but also plays a role in external secretion for digestion and absorption as well as in internal secretion. Therefore, if there is no difference of curability among different treatment methods, long-term QOL should be considered seriously when we select a treatment method, especially in elderly patients [48].

Recently, a simple risk-scoring system, named eCura system, was established for stratifying the risk of LNM in such patients (Fig. 7.7) [54]. This is a seven-point scoring system with three risk categories based on five clinicopathological factors in order to predict LNM. In this system, 3 points are assigned for positive lymphatic invasion, and 1 point is assigned for tumor size of >30 mm, SM2 invasion, positive venous invasion, and positive vertical margin. The rate of LNM in the low- (0–1 point), intermediate- (2–4 points), and high-risk (5–7 points) categories was 2.5%, 6.7%, and 22.7%, respectively. In addition,

when the patients were followed up with no additional treatment after non-curative resection for EGC, 5-year cancer-specific survival (CSS) in each risk category was 99.6%, 96.1%, and 90.1%, respectively. A Japanese multicenter evaluation of laparoscopic gastrectomy (mainly distal gastrectomy) for EGC reported 5-year CSS rates of 99.8% for stage T1a disease and 98.7% for stage T1b disease [55]. Thus, although radical surgery is the standard therapy for patients with non-curative resection for EGC, the eCura system provides useful information for deciding the treatment strategy after non-curative resection for EGC, especially in elderly patients and/or those with severe comorbidities.

Medical care will always be provided with consideration of the following points: whether ESD is really minimally invasive; whether "complete" treatment attempted by physicians, such as gastrectomy, is beneficial for patients; and whether treatment that is not the best but more tolerable to the patients is an option [6].

References

1. Gotoda T, Ishikawa H, Ohnishi H, et al. Randomized controlled trial comparing gastric cancer screening by gastrointestinal X-ray with serology for Helicobacter pylori and pepsinogens followed by gastrointestinal endoscopy. Gastric Cancer. 2015;18(3):605–11.

2. Yanai H, Matsubara Y, Okamoto T, et al. Clinical impact of strip biopsy for early gastric cancer. Gastrointest Endosc. 2004;60:771–7.

3. Farrell JJ, Lauwers GY, Brugge WR. Endoscopic mucosal resection using a cap-fitted endoscope improves tissue resection and pathology interpretation: an animal study. Gastric Cancer. 2006;9:3–8.

4. Gotoda T, Sasako M, Shimoda T, et al. An evaluation of the necessity of gastrectomy with lymph node dissection for patients with submucosal Invasive gastric cancer. Br J Surg. 2001;88:444–9.

5. Etoh T, Katai H, Fukagawa T, et al. Treatment of early gastric cancer in the elderly patient: results of EMR and gastrectomy at a national referral center in Japan. Gastrointest Endosc. 2005;62:868–71.

6. Gotoda T, Yang HK. The desired balance between treatment and curability in treatment planning for early gastric cancer. Gastrointest Endosc. 2015;82(2):308–10.

7. Deyhle P, Largiader F, Jenny P. A method for endoscopic electroresection of sessile colonic polyps. Endoscopy. 1973;5:38–40.

8. Oguro Y. Endoscopic gastric polypectomy with high frequency currents. Stomach Intest (in English abstract). 1974;9:309–16.

9. Tada M, Shimada M, Murakami F, et al. Development of strip-off biopsy. Gastroenterol Endosc (in English abstract). 1984;26:833–9.

10. Hirao M, Masuda K, Asanuma T, et al. Endoscopic resection of early gastric cancer and other tumors with local injection of hypertonic saline-epinephrine. Gastrointest Endosc. 1988;34:264–9.

11. Inoue H, Endo M, Takeshita K, et al. A new simplified technique of endoscopic esophageal mucosal resection using a cap-fitted panendoscope (EMRC). Surg Endosc. 1992;6:264–5.

12. Inoue H, Takeshita K, Hori H, et al. Endoscopic mucosal resection with a cap-fitted panendoscope for esophagus, stomach, and colon mucosal lesions. Gastrointest Endosc. 1993;39:58–62.

13. Akiyama M, Ota M, Nakajima H, et al. Endoscopic mucosal resection of gastric neoplasms using a ligating device. Gastrointest Endosc. 1997;45:182–6.

14. Soehendra N, Seewald S, Groth S, et al. Use of modified multiband ligator facilitates circumferential EMR in Barrett's esophagus (with video). Gastrointest Endosc. 2006;63:847–52.

15. Korenaga D, Haraguchi M, Tsujitani S, et al. Clinicopathological features of mucosal carcinoma of the stomach with lymph node metastasis in eleven patients. Br J Surg. 1986;73:431–3.

16. Ell C, May A, Gossner L, et al. Endoscopic mucosectomy of early cancer and high-grade dysplasia in Barrett's esophagus. Gastroenterology. 2000;118:670–7.

17. Tanabe S, Koizumi W, Mitomi H, et al. Clinical outcome of endoscopic aspiration mucosectomy for early stage gastric cancer. Gastrointest Endosc. 2002;56:708–13.

18. Kim JJ, Lee JH, Jung HY, et al. EMR for early gastric cancer in Korea: a multicenter retrospective study. Gastrointest Endosc. 2007;66:693–700.

19. Ono H, Kondo H, Gotoda T, et al. Endoscopic mucosal resection for treatment of early gastric cancer. Gut. 2001;48:225–9.

20. Hosokawa K, Yoshida S. Recent advances in endoscopic mucosal resection for early gastric cancer. Jpn J Cancer Chemother (in English abstract). 1998;25:483.

21. Gotoda T, Kondo H, Ono H, et al. A new endoscopic mucosal resection (EMR) procedure using an insulation-tipped diathermic (IT) knife for rectal flat lesions. Gastrointest Endosc. 1999;50:560–3.

22. Yokoi C, Gotoda T, Oda I, et al. Endoscopic submucosal dissection (ESD) allows curative resection of local recurrent early gastric cancer after prior endoscopic mucosal resection. Gastrointest Endosc. 2006;64:212–8.

23. Suzuki S, Gotoda T, Kobayashi Y, et al. Usefulness of a traction method using dental floss and a hemoclip for gastric endoscopic submucosal dissection: a propensity score matching analysis (with videos). Gastrointest Endosc. 2016;83:337–46.

24. Yoshida M, Takizawa K, Ono H, et al. Efficacy of endoscopic submucosal dissection with dental floss clip traction for gastric epithelial neoplasia: a pilot study (with video). Surg Endosc. 2016;30(7):3100–6.

25. Gotoda T. A large endoscopic resection by endoscopic submucosal dissection (ESD) procedure. Clin Gastroenterol Hepatol. 2005;3:S71–3.

26. Akahoshi K, Motomura Y, Kubokawa M, et al. Endoscopic Submucosal Dissection for Early Gastric Cancer using the Clutch Cutter: a large single-center experience. Endosc Int Open. 2015;3(5):E432–8.

27. Han S, Hsu A, Wassef WY. An update in the endoscopic management of gastric cancer. Curr Opin Gastroenterol. 2016;32(6):492–500.

28. Yamamoto H, Kawata H, Sunada K, et al. Successful en bloc resection of large superficial tumors in the stomach and colon using sodium hyaluronate and small-caliber-tip transparent hood. Endoscopy. 2003;35:690–4.

29. Yamamoto H, Yahagi N, Oyama T, et al. Usefulness and safety of 0.4% sodium hyaluronate solution as a submucosal fluid "cushion" in endoscopic resection for gastric neoplasms: a prospective multicenter trial. Gastrointest Endosc. 2007;67:830–9.

30. Gotoda T, Yanagisawa A, Sasako M, et al. Incidence of lymph node metastasis from early gastric cancer: estimation with a large number of cases at two large centers. Gastric Cancer. 2000;3:219–25.

31. Gotoda T, Iwasaki M, Kusano C, et al. Endoscopic resection of early gastric cancer treated by guideline and expanded National Cancer Centre criteria. Br J Surg. 2010;97:868–71.

32. Hirasawa T, Gotoda T, Miyata S, et al. Incidence of lymph node metastasis and the feasibility of endoscopic resection for undifferentiated-type early gastric cancer. Gastric Cancer. 2009;12:148–52.

33. Japanese Gastric Cancer A. Japanese gastric cancer treatment guidelines 2014 (ver. 4). Gastric Cancer. 2017;20:1–19.

34. Hasuike N, Ono H, Boku N, et al. A non-randomized confirmatory trial of an expanded indication for endoscopic submucosal dissection for intestinal-type gastric cancer (cT1a): the Japan Clinical Oncology Group study (JCOG0607). Gastric Cancer. 2018;21(1):114–23.

35. Pimentel-Nunes P, Dinis-Ribeiro M, Ponchon T, et al. Endoscopic submucosal dissection: European Society of Gastrointestinal Endoscopy (ESGE) Guideline. Endoscopy. 2015;47:829–54.

36. NCCN Clinical Practice Guidelines in Oncology (NCCN Guidelines) Gastric Cancer. Version 3. 2017. https://www.nccn.org/professionals/physician_gls/pdf/gastric.pdf. Accessed 17 Sep 2017.

37. Abe S, Oda I, Suzuki H, et al. Long-term surveillance and treatment outcomes of metachronous gastric cancer occurring after curative endoscopic submucosal dissection. Endoscopy. 2015;47:1113–8.

38. Kato M, Nishida T, Yamamoto K, et al. Scheduled endoscopic surveillance controls secondary cancer after curative endoscopic resection for early gastric cancer: a multicentre retrospective cohort study by Osaka University ESD study group. Gut. 2013;62:1425–32.

39. Tanabe S, Ishido K, Matsumoto T, et al. Long-term outcomes of endoscopic submucosal dissection for early gastric cancer: a multicenter collaborative study. Gastric Cancer. 2017;20:45–52.

40. Smyth EC, Verheij M, Allum W, et al. Gastric cancer: ESMO Clinical Practice Guidelines for diagnosis, treatment and follow-up. Ann Oncol. 2016;27:v38–49.

41. Moehler M, Al-Batran SE, Andus T, et al. German S3-guideline "Diagnosis and treatment of esophagogastric cancer". Z Gastroenterol. 2011;49:461–531.

42. Choi AH, Nelson RA, Merchant SJ, et al. Rates of lymph node metastasis and survival in T1a gastric adenocarcinoma in Western populations. Gastrointest Endosc. 2016;83:1184–92.e1.

43. Hatta W, Gotoda T, Oyama T, et al. Is radical surgery necessary in all patients who do not meet the curative criteria for endoscopic submucosal dissection in early gastric cancer? A multi-center retrospective study in Japan. J Gastroenterol. 2017;52:175–84.

44. Probst A, Schneider A, Schaller T, Anthuber M, Ebigbo A, Messmann H. Endoscopic submucosal dissection for early gastric cancer: are expanded resection criteria safe for Western patients? Endoscopy. 2017;49:855–65.

45. Fukase K, Kato M, Kikuchi S, et al. Effect of eradication of Helicobacter pylori on incidence of metachronous gastric carcinoma after endoscopic resection of early gastric cancer: an open-label, randomised controlled trial. Lancet. 2008;372:392–7.

46. Choi J, Kim SG, Yoon H, et al. Eradication of Helicobacter pylori after endoscopic resection of gastric tumors does not reduce incidence of metachronous gastric carcinoma. Clin Gastroenterol Hepatol. 2014;12:793–800.e1.

47. Ludwig K, Klautke G, Bernhard J, et al. Minimally invasive and local treatment for mucosal early gastric cancer. Surg Endosc. 2005;19:1362–6.

48. Kusano C, Iwasaki M, Kaltenbach T, et al. Should elderly patients undergo additional surgery after non-curative endoscopic resection for early gastric cancer? long-term comparative outcomes. Am J Gastroenterol. 2011;106:1064–9.

49. Hull MJ, Mino-Kenudson M, Nishioka NS, et al. Endoscopic mucosal resection: an improved diagnostic procedure for early gastroesophageal epithelial neoplasms. Am J Surge Pathol. 2006;30:114–8.

50. Ahmad NA, Kochman ML, Long WB, et al. Efficacy, safety, and clinical outcomes of endoscopic mucosal resection: a study of 101 cases. Gastrointest Endosc. 2002;55:390–6.

51. Katsube T, Konno S, Hamaguchi K, et al. The efficacy of endoscopic mucosal resection in the diagnosis and treatment of group III gastric lesions. Anticancer Res. 2005;25:3513–6.

52. Fukunaga S, Nagami Y, Shiba M, et al. Long-term prognosis of expanded-indication differentiated-type early gastric cancer treated with endoscopic submucosal dissection or surgery using propensity score analysis. Gastrointest Endosc. 2017;85:143–52.

53. Choi JH, Kim ES, Lee YJ, et al. Comparison of quality of life and worry of cancer recurrence between endoscopic and surgical treatment for early gastric cancer. Gastrointest Endosc. 2015;82:299–307.

54. Hatta W, Gotoda T, Oyama T, et al. A scoring system to stratify curability after endoscopic submucosal dissection for early gastric cancer: "eCura system". Am J Gastroenterol. 2017;112(6):874–81.

55. Kitano S, Shiraishi N, Uyama I, et al. A multicenter study on oncologic outcome of laparoscopic gastrectomy for early cancer in Japan. Ann Surg. 2007;245:68–72.

Colonic ESD

Vikneswaran Namasivayam and Yutaka Saito

Introduction

Endoscopic submucosal dissection (ESD) is a specialised endoscopic resection technique that utilises an electrosurgical knife to resect superficial gastrointestinal neoplastic lesions by dissecting the submucosa. First described almost two decades ago, colorectal ESD has gained acceptance as a safe and effective mainstream therapeutic option in many parts of the world where it is available [1]. The main advantage of ESD over endoscopic mucosal resection (EMR) is it enables *en bloc* removal of lesions irrespective of lesion size. This allows for definitive histological diagnosis and staging of superficially invasive cancers that is superior to EMR and routine biopsies while also providing a

Electronic Supplementary Material The online version of this chapter (https://doi.org/10.1007/978-3-030-21695-5_8) contains supplementary material, which is available to authorized users.

V. Namasivayam
Department of Gastroenterology and Hepatology, Singapore General Hospital, Singapore, Singapore

Duke NUS Medical School, Singapore, Singapore

Yong Loo Lin School of Medicine, National University of Singapore, Singapore, Singapore
e-mail: vikneswaran.namasivayam@singhealth.com.sg

Y. Saito (✉)
National Cancer Center Hospital, Endoscopy Division, Endoscopy Center, Tokyo, Japan
e-mail: ytsaito@ncc.go.jp

treatment alternative to surgery for early cancer without the risk of lymph node metastasis.

While the basic principles of ESD are similar throughout the gastrointestinal tract, ESD in the colorectum entails several key considerations that are specific to the colon. The relatively thin colonic wall and the limited scope for manoeuvrability within the colon, the presence of semi-lunar folds, peristalsis and respiratory movements add to the technical difficulty of colorectal ESD and the associated increased procedure time and risk of perforation. Developments in endoscopic techniques and accessories that have helped to address the challenges posed by ESD in the colorectum will be further discussed in the chapter.

Indications for ESD

Endoscopic resection is indicated in superficial colorectal neoplastic lesions that are associated with a negligible risk of lymph node metastases. Lesions with histology of no poorly differentiated adenocarcinoma or mucinous adenocarcinoma, tumour budding grade I, submucosal invasion up to 1 mm and no lymphovascular invasion are associated with a very low risk of lymph node metastases and may be cured with endoscopic resection [2, 3]. While the vast majority of colorectal lesions may be resected by EMR, ESD should be considered when the likelihood of malignancy is high [4]. This is because ESD is associated with superior rates of *en bloc* resection which enables accurate histological staging and a high chance of curative resection. In contrast, EMR, when performed piecemeal, reduces the quality and reliability of histopathological assessment, in particular the lateral and vertical resection margins. Piecemeal EMR is also associated with higher local recurrence rates [5]. In addition, EMR may not be feasible in non-lifting lesions with underlying fibrosis. ESD is thus considered when the likelihood of malignancy is high; *en bloc* removal of EMR is not feasible because of lesion size (>20 mm diameter) and in non-lifting lesions

Endoscopic Diagnosis of Colorectal Cancer with Deep Submucosal Invasion

While endoscopic resection provides definitive histological assessment and adequate treatment for lesions with superficially invasive cancer,

ESD is avoided in cancers with deep submucosal invasion as they carry a significant risk of lymph node metastases. Instead lesions with deeper invasion should be sent for surgery. Hence an attempt is made to gauge the preoperative T stage as that influences subsequent treatment strategy – i.e. whether to proceed with ESD or refer for surgery if deep submucosal invasion is suspected. Although definitive T staging is ultimately based on histological assessment of the resected specimen, the depth of tumour invasion may be estimated based on the morphological features of the lesion in a high-quality endoscopic examination. Though advanced endoscopic imaging is imperfect, the presence of deep submucosal invasion may be largely predicted based on the presence of a depressed morphology, Kudo type V pit pattern, or invasive pattern (Fig. 8.1) on chromoendoscopy and type 3 pattern (JNET classification) on narrowband imaging [6, 7] (Fig. 8.2).

Furthermore, the following morphological features may provide ancillary information that

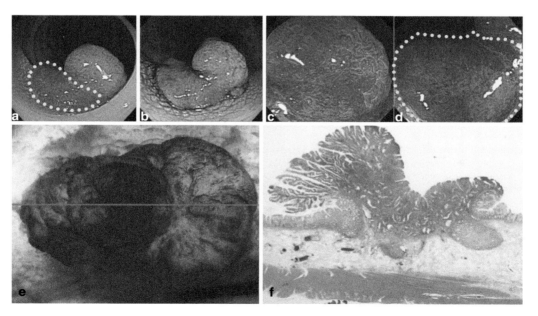

Fig. 8.1 (**a–f**) Invasive pattern. Invasive pattern is defined as irregular and distorted crypts in a demarcated area as observed in Kudo's type VN and selected cases of VI (e.g. deep submucosal invasive cancers), where surgical resection is the appropriate treatment. (**a**) The left side of this tumour is flat and depressed morphology as outlined by yellow dots. (**b**) Indigo-carmine dye spray demonstrates the tumour margin and surface structure clearly. (**c**) Crystal-violet staining of the right-side protrusion showed a regular-type IV pit pattern suggesting intramucosal

neoplasia in this protrusion. (**d**) Crystal-violet staining of the left side of this tumour revealed an irregular distorted pit pattern corresponding to the yellow dots area and diagnosed as an invasive pattern suggesting submucosal deep invasion. (**e**) A stereomicroscopic image of the surgical specimen. The protruded area is on the left side and flat/depressed area lined by yellow dots is on the right side. (**f**) Histopathology confirmed submucosal deep invasion in the area of invasive pattern and intramucosal neoplasia in the type 4 pit area

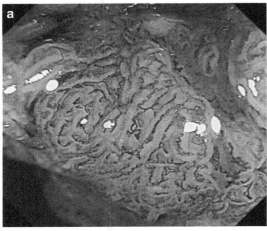 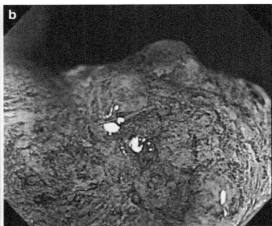

Fig. 8.2 JNET type 2B and 3. The Japan NBI Expert Team (JNET) classification consists of four categories of vessel and surface patterns – types 1, 2A, 2B and 3. Types 1, 2A, 2B and 3 correspond to histopathological findings of hyperplastic polyp/sessile serrated polyp (SSA/P), low-grade intramucosal neoplasia, high-grade intramucosal neoplasia/superficial submucosal invasive cancer and deep submucosal invasive cancer, respectively. (**a**) A slight depressed area showed an irregular vessel pattern (variable calibre and irregular distribution) and irregular surface pattern diagnosed as JNET type 2B suggesting high-grade intramucosal neoplasia or submucosal slight invasive caner. (**b**) Irregular nodular area showed loose vessel pattern and interruption of thick vessels and amorphous areas in surface pattern diagnosed as JNET type 3 suggesting deep submucosal invasive cancer. It is important to keep in mind that JNET type 2B lesions correspond to high-grade dysplasia/superficial cancer, which implies that there is a risk of SM invasion. The gold standard for differentiating SM1 and SM2 is crystal-violet staining. Therefore, pit pattern diagnosis is essential for choosing the appropriate treatment strategy for JNET type 2B lesions

suggests the presence of deep submucosal invasion – deep depression, fold convergence, irregular bottom of depression surface, chicken skin appearance, redness, expansive appearance, firm consistency, irregular surface, loss of lobulation and thick stalk (Fig. 8.3).

Biopsies should be avoided before ESD as the malignant potential is often underestimated on biopsy specimens, and biopsy-induced fibrosis within the lesion may compromise submucosal lifting, thus making ESD more difficult, especially for flat tumours.

Preparation and Setting of ESD

Sedation and Bowel Preparation

ESD is a technically challenging procedure that is associated with significantly longer procedural time than EMR which has implications for patient preparation. Colorectal ESD may be performed with conscious sedation as it allows for the patient to be repositioned during the procedure to enlist the help of gravity to achieve counter-traction of the lesion. The routine use of carbon dioxide insufflation [8] is preferred as it minimises patient discomfort associated with prolonged insufflation and reduces the risk of severe complication, such as pneumothorax or pneumoperitoneum, even when perforation has occurred. Adequate bowel preparation is essential to facilitate optimal visualisation of the lesion as well as to mitigate the risk of peritoneal contamination in the event of a perforation.

Equipment and Accessories

The tools used in ESD have evolved significantly to meet the unique challenges posed by both the procedure and the site of resection. Hence familiarity with the equipment is essential for performing ESD.

Endoscope

An endoscope with an auxiliary water channel to produce a water jet is preferred to maintain visualisation when bleeding is encountered. An endoscope with a 3.2 mm instrument channel is

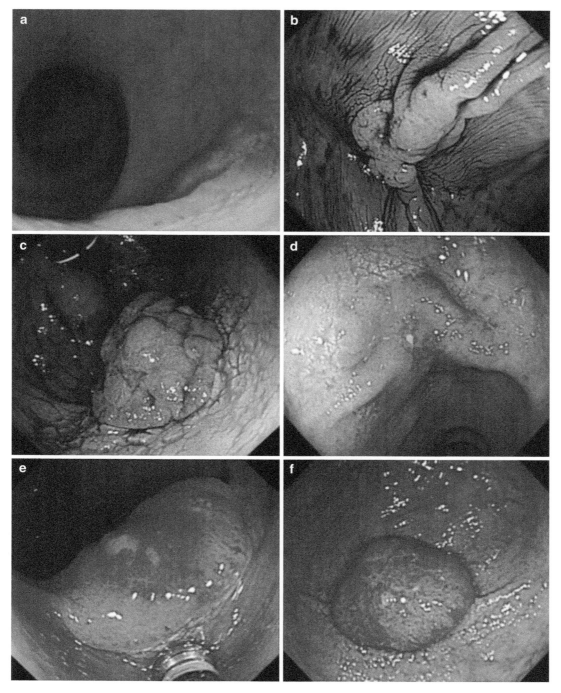

Fig. 8.3 The following morphological features may provide ancillary information that suggest the presence of deep submucosal invasion – (**a**) deep depression, (**b**) fold convergence, (**c**) irregular bottom of depression surface, (**d**) chicken skin appearance, (**e**) redness, (**f**) expansive appearance, (**g**) firm consistency, (**h**) irregular surface, (**i**) loss of lobulation and (**j**) thick stalk

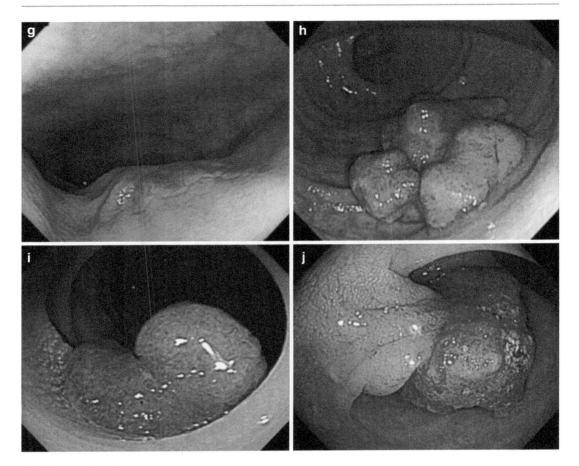

Fig. 8.3 (continued)

preferred, if available, to accommodate ESD accessories.

Carbon Dioxide Regulator

The use of carbon dioxide insufflation is preferred during ESD. CO_2 is more rapidly absorbed than nitrogen and oxygen, the main constituents of room air. Hence CO_2 insufflation gives rise to less sustained luminal insufflation, which is associated with less patient discomfort and shorter procedural time, and is safe with deep sedation [8–12]. It is also believed that rapid CO_2 reabsorption in the setting of CO_2 insufflation may reduce the likelihood of tension pneumoperitoneum following a perforation. CO_2 insufflation is generally safe in patients with pulmonary dysfunction. In patients with severe obstructive lung disease, CO_2 retention may occur with longer procedure time; hence CO_2 monitoring may be considered [13].

Electrosurgical Generators

Electrosurgical Generators (ESUs) with simple cutting and coagulation modes have been superseded by newer models that have multiple modes to be used on different lesion characteristics. These modes are specific to the manufacturer. Pure cutting and coagulation current modes are avoided due to the increased risk of bleeding and delayed perforation, respectively [14]. The newer ESUs provide a variety of electrosurgical waveforms that produce a variety of tissues effects that is useful for the various steps in ESD. The ESUs also contain microprocessors that adjust power according to tissue impedance to avoid deep tissue injury [15].

ESD Knives

Electrosurgical knives are essential tools for ESD as submucosal dissection differentiates ESD from other types of endoscopic resection. ESD knives fall into two broad categories— needle-knife and scissors type. The former can be further classified into those with a blunt tip and the tip-cutting knives [16]. The knives differ in their indication and methods of use and the endoscopist should be familiar with the use of the specific knives. These accessories and other ESD tools are described in details elsewhere in this book.

Distal Attachments and Other Counter-Traction Methods

A disposable transparent cap affixed to the distal end of the endoscope is an essential tool in ESD. It serves to provide counter-traction to maintain visualization during submucosal dissection by keeping the resected mucosal flap off the endoscope lens. Caps with holes on the side facilitate drainage of fluid and blood. Various other tools and methods have been devised to provide counter-traction though none have gained widespread use. The clip-line traction method using dental floss is useful primarily in the rectum and distal colon but less effective in the proximal colon [17, 18]. Other methods would include clip with sinker method, external grasping forceps, internal traction, double-channel scope and double-scope methods [19]. The SO clip is commercially available in Japan and is applicable to any location without the need for scope reinsertion.

The lack of a truly effective counter-traction method highlights the inherent limitation of the flexible endoscope – therapeutic accessories for an increasingly complex array of interventional procedures are delivered through an accessory channel that is also required for periodic insufflation, suction and water irrigation. Novel triangulation platforms with independent instrument channels that enable endoscopic resection to be performed with the comparative ease of laparoscopic surgery are currently under development [20, 21].

Technical Aspects of ESD

The basic steps in ESD are injecting fluid into the submucosa to elevate the tumour, incising the surrounding mucosa to gain access to the submucosa and dissecting the submucosa beneath the tumour to achieve tumour resection.

Conventional ESD Method

The conventional ESD method comprises of the following steps (Fig. 8.4):

1. Submucosal injection under the lesion and the surrounding normal mucosa
2. An initial partial mucosal incision (i.e. one-quarter of the circumference)
3. Submucosal dissection beneath the incision
4. Repeat partial mucosal incision and dissection in a segmental fashion
5. Completion of the *en bloc* resection.

Unlike gastric ESD, the perimeter of the colorectal lesion need not be marked by cautery prior to ESD as the borders of colorectal lesions are more distinct and readily identified. The lesion is lifted by injecting a submucosal injection agent to create a submucosal cushion. Suboptimal lifting may indicate either deep submucosal tumour invasion or the presence of fibrosis which in severe cases may preclude further ESD. The addition of dyes (e.g. indigo carmine) to the injectable enables clearer delineation of the submucosal plane of dissection though some experts advocate avoiding the addition of dyes to enable better visualisation of submucosal vessels during dissection.

Following lifting, a partial mucosal incision is made around the lesion to gain access to the submucosa to facilitate submucosal dissection. Instead of creating a circumferential mucosal incision, a partial marginal incision, either at the oral or anal end, is recommended before submucosal dissection is commenced. This is to ensure that the submucosal cushion is sustained without dispersion of fluid during dissection. The authors

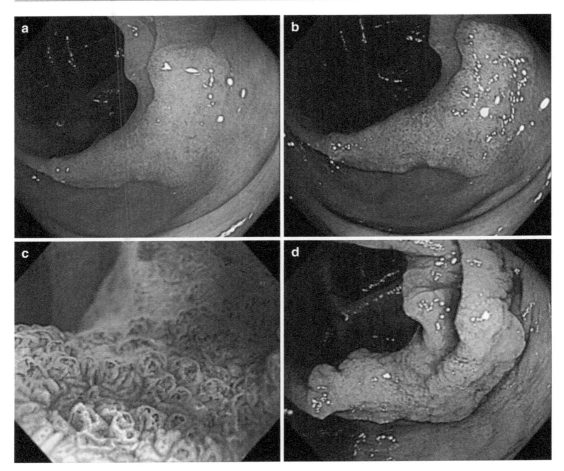

Fig. 8.4 (**A**) Diagram of conventional ESD. Before ESD, the depth of tumour invasion is estimated using a combination of magnified NBI and chromoendoscopy with indigo-carmine and crystal-violet staining for pit pattern diagnosis. (**a**) 0-IIa + IIc (laterally spreading tumour nongranular type, LST-NG) lesion in a transverse colon, and the estimated tumour size was 25 mm in diameter. Fold convergences were recognised and submucosal invasion is suspected by a conventional endoscopy. (**b**) An NBI image revealed the tumour margin clearly, and NICE classification might be type 2 suggesting an intramucosal neoplasia. (**c**) A magnified NBI revealed variable calibre and irregular distribution of vessel pattern/irregular or obscure surface pattern, therefore, diagnosed as JNET type 2B suggesting a high-grade intramucosal neoplasia or submucosal superficial invasive cancer. (**d**) An indigo-carmine dye spray revealed a tumour margin and surface structure clearly. (**e**) A magnified image after indigo-carmine spray revealed type IIIs and IIIL pit pattern in this relative depressed area. (**f–h**) After crystal-violet staining

(**f**), IIIs pit (**g**) and Vi slight irregular pit (**h**) were observed in the centre, but the area of type Vi was relatively small; therefore, a type Vi (non-invasive pattern) suggesting intramucosal or submucosal superficial invasion was diagnosed. (**B**) Diagram of conventional ESD. (**a**) A retroflexed view of a LST-NG after indigo-carmine dye spraying. A short-type ST hood (Fujifilm Medical Co.) was attached to PCF260J (Olympus Medical Co.). (**b**) After submucosal injection under the lesion and the surrounding normal mucosa, an initial partial mucosal incision (i.e. one-quarter of the circumference) is made and submucosal dissection is performed beneath the incision. (**c**) Repeat partial mucosal incision and dissection in a segmental fashion similar to pocket-creation method. (**d**) After completing 50% of the dissection, a partial marginal resection is planed from anal side using a straightforward view. (**e**) Repeat submucosal dissection. (**f, g**) Completion of the *en bloc* resection. (**h**) A resected specimen was stretched out using fine needles for detailed histopathological analysis

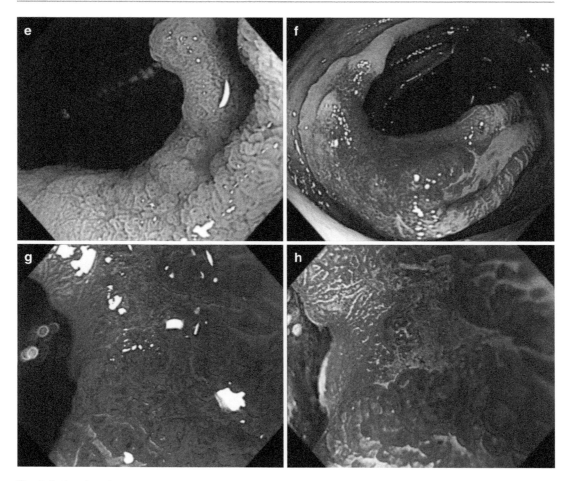

Fig. 8.4 (continued)

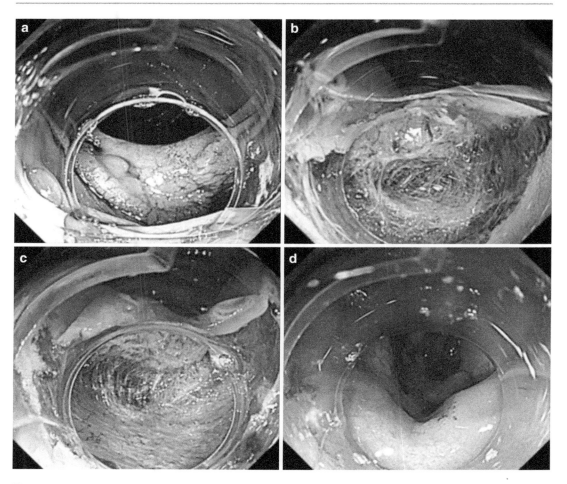

Fig. 8.4 (continued)

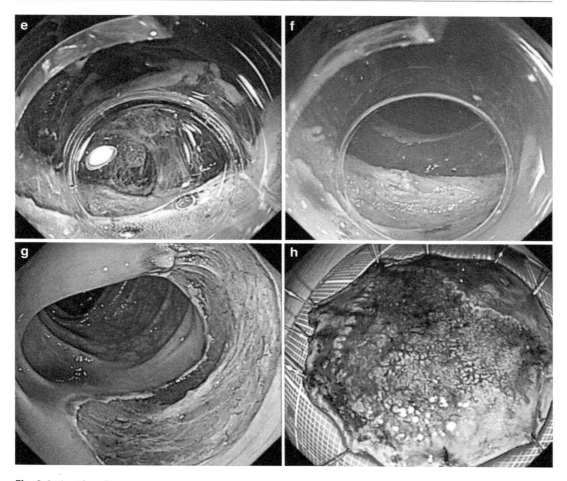

Fig. 8.4 (continued)

advocate initial submucosal dissection to be performed just beneath the mucosal layer to prevent perforation. Once the submucosal layer has opened sufficiently to allow adequate visualisation of the cutting area, dissection may be extended to the lower third of the submucosal layer. Repeated injections are made to maintain the submucosal fluid cushion to minimise the risk of perforation.

As the lesion is dissected in a segmental fashion, the position of the patient may be changed periodically to enlist the effect of gravity to achieve traction or counter-traction on the lesion. The lesion is repositioned by rotating the patient to use gravity to keep the field of vision clear of blood and water. This allows the endoscopist to have a clear field of vision and achieve traction. The use of conscious sedation in this instance facilitates changes in patient's position.

Following resection, the base of resection is examined for bleeding and perforation. Unlike gastric ESD, the routine coagulation of visible vessels following colorectal ESD is minimised to prevent thermal injury.

Pocket-Creation Method (PCM) (Fig. 8.5)

The PCM is a newer ESD technique that is based on the creation of a submucosal pocket beneath the lesion using a needle-type knife [22, 23]. It involves the following basic steps:

1. Submucosal injection
2. Creation of tunnel entry with 20 mm mucosal incision on the anal side of the lesion
3. Creation of a submucosal pocket by dissection under the lesion
4. Lateral dissection on the dependent side (i.e. closer to gravity)
5. Lateral dissection on the antigravity side (i.e. away from gravity)
6. Completion of *en bloc* resection.

The PCM offers the following potential advantages. As only a minimal incision is made to introduce the knife into the pocket for subsequent dissection, the submucosal fluid cushion is sustained during ESD with minimal dispersion of injected fluid. The position of tip of the scope is stabilised within the pocket which facilitates tissue retraction allowing for dissection to proceed tangential to the muscle layer. This may be particularly helpful in navigating dissection across semilunar folds as these substantially alter the

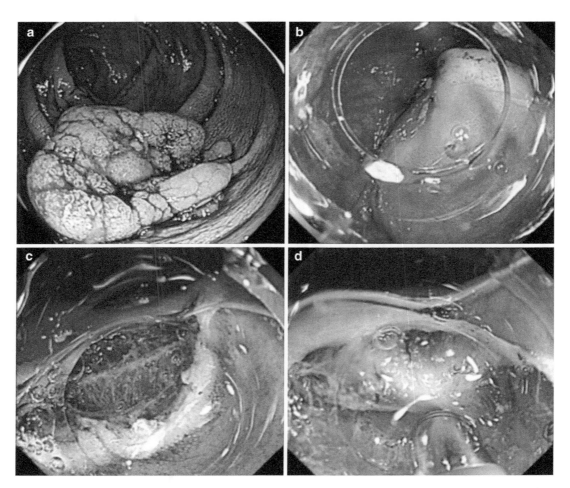

Fig. 8.5 (**A**) PCM-1. (**a**) A LST-granular (nodular mixed type) in the transverse colon. (**b**) Submucosal injection to the anal side of this tumour. (**c**) Creation of tunnel entry with 20 mm mucosal incision on the anal side of the lesion. (**d, e**) Creation of a submucosal pocket by dissection under the lesion. (**f**) Lateral dissection on the dependent side (i.e. closer to gravity). (**g**) Additional submucosal dissection using a traction by short-type ST hood (Fujifilm Medical Co.). (**h**) Lateral dissection on the antigravity side (i.e. away from gravity). (**B**) PCM-2. (**a**) Creation of a submucosal pocket by dissection using IT knife nano under the lesion. (**b, c**) Lateral dissection using IT knife nano away from gravity. (**d–f**) Completion of *en bloc* resection

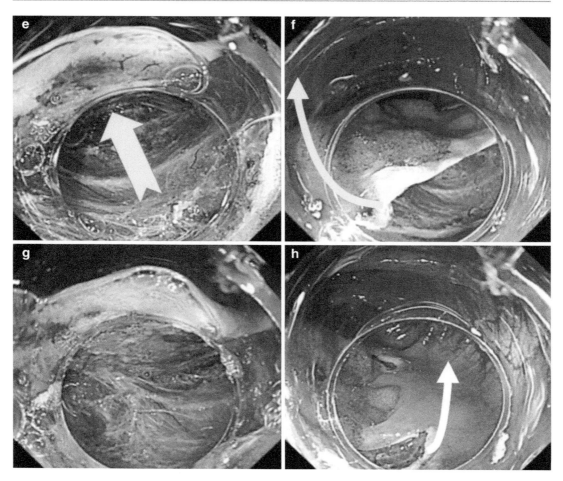

Fig. 8.5 (continued)

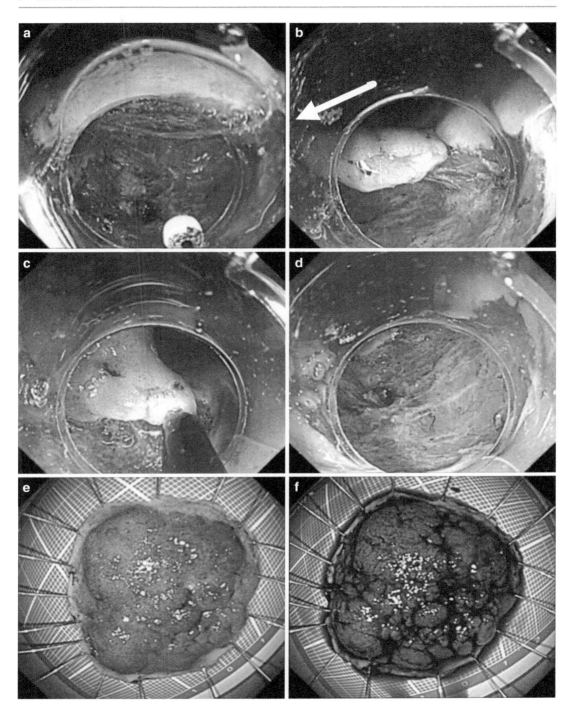

Fig. 8.5 (continued)

angle of the mucosal layer, thus predisposing to failure of *en bloc* resection and perforation [24]. Emerging data suggest PCM may be associated with higher *en bloc* resection rates and shorter procedure times compared to the conventional method although this requires confirmation from prospective trials [25].

Hybrid ESD Technique

In view of the technical difficulty of performing colorectal ESD, a hybrid EMR-ESD has been described that is characterised by a circumferential mucosal incision followed by snare resection of the lesion [26, 27]. However, compared to the conventional technique, the hybrid technique is associated with lower R0 and *en bloc* resection rates and has a similar rate of adverse events [28, 29].

Management of Complications
While ESD has been associated with a higher rate of complications than EMR, most ESD complications can be managed endoscopically, and only a small proportion of patients require surgery for complications. Hence the risk of ESD complications that require surgery is low (<1%). In addition, the risk of ESD complication for tumours larger than 20 mm in diameter may be comparable to EMR. However the complication rates are higher in Western countries compared to Asian countries (3.1% vs 0.8%) [29, 30].

Intraprocedural Bleeding

Intraprocedural bleeding is an expected occurrence during ESD. Hence its prevention and management are important aspects of performing colorectal ESD. Bleeding is often encountered during mucosal incision and submucosal dissection. This may be largely avoided by using appropriate electrosurgical settings during the pre-cut and dissection phases and coagulation of exposed vessels. Bleeding may be arrested with soft coagulation using the ESD knife and, if unsuccessful, with the use of haemostatic for-

ceps. The connective tissue surrounding the vessel is dissected to isolate the vessel. The vessel is then either hooked by the ESD knife or grasped by the haemostatic forceps and coagulation current is applied. The use of clips is avoided as it may interfere with continued dissection of the tumour. Intraprocedural bleeding may be avoided by identifying larger non-bleeding submucosal vessels during dissection and coagulating them prophylactically. Intraprocedural bleeding rarely requires surgery for haemostasis.

Delayed Bleeding

Delayed bleeding has been reported in an average 2.7% and up to 13.9% of patients [29, 31]. The risk factors for delayed bleeding include lesion size, rectal location, presence of submucosal fibrosis and low-volume centres [31, 32]. The rate of bleeding with the hybrid technique is similar to the conventional technique [29]. Delayed bleeding may be treated endoscopically with deployment of clips. The use of thermal methods is less favoured so as to avoid further thermal injury to the muscle layer.

Perforation

Perforation rates of 4 to 10% have been reported with higher-volume centres reporting lower complication rates [33–36]. More recent data report a perforation rate of 1–2%. Tumour size, location and presence of submucosal fibrosis and endoscopist inexperience (<50 cases) are risk factors for perforation [34, 37–40]. While ESD has a higher perforation rate than EMR, the reported rate of ESD complication-related surgery is low at <1% as the majority of complications may be treated endoscopically [30]. Prediction models have been developed to stratify the risk of perforation that may be potentially useful in clinical decision-making [40, 41].

The risk of perforation is minimised by ensuring an adequate submucosal cushion with repeated injection during dissection. The incorporation of a contrast dye (e.g. indigo carmine), which stains the submucosa but not the muscularis propria, guides the plane of dissection and allows for identification of exposed muscle during dissection. The use of pure cutting or coagulation current is also avoided to minimise the risk of bleeding and delayed perforation, respectively [14]. Biopsies of the lesion before ESD should be avoided as the resultant fibrosis may predispose to perforation during ESD.

Prompt identification of perforation during ESD enables immediate treatment that reduces mortality and the need for surgery [42]. Upon identification of a perforation, the patient's hemodynamic status should be promptly reviewed to identify a tension pneumoperitoneum. A tension pneumoperitoneum is an emergency characterised by the presence of hypotension and gaseous distension of the abdomen and is treated by immediate needle decompression.

Perforations that are recognised during ESD are amenable to primary endoscopic clip closure. A spectrum of endoscopically recognisable injuries to the muscularis propria that encompasses perforation has been described [43]. The presence of a hole with or without observed contamination, a specimen target sign or a mirror target sign would mandate prompt clip closure of the defect to avoid peritoneal contamination [44].

Successful endoscopic clip closure may be achieved by bearing in mind the following principles. Prior to clip closure, it may be advisable to reduce luminal gas insufflation to reduce the tension on the defect and clean the field by suctioning the fluid pool and repositioning the patient. It may be necessary to continue with dissection of the tissue adjacent to the defect to enable clip deployment without compromising subsequent completion of the dissection. During clip closure, the mucosa is suctioned into the opened clip, gentle pressure from the clip is applied and with further suction the lumen is deflated and the clip is closed. The lumen is re-insufflated to ensure adequate apposition of the defect edges before the clip is deployed [45].

In addition to clips, perforations have also been successfully closed with other devices such as the over-the-scope clips and suturing devices [46, 47].

However, the need for scope withdrawal and reinsertion may potentially compromise outcomes.

Delayed Perforation

Delayed perforation occurs in 0.1–0.4% of cases and results from thermal injury [32, 34]. Patients may present more than one or two days after the ESD. CT is performed to confirm the diagnosis and assess the degree of peritoneal contamination. The presence of peritoneal contamination resulting from egress of luminal contents usually precludes endoscopic closure, and surgery is usually required.

Electrocoagulation Syndrome

Electrocoagulation syndrome is a consequence of transmural thermal injury to the colon resulting in localised peritonitis. It is characterised by clinical features of inflammation (i.e. fever, raised inflammatory markers) and peritoneal signs in the absence of radiological evidence of perforation [48, 49]. Patients usually present within hours to days of the ESD. The incidence of electrocoagulation syndrome following ESD is 8.6–9.5% [50, 51]. It is more common following ESD compared to EMR. Lesion size (>30 mm) and colonic location increase the risk of electrocoagulation syndrome [52]. The vast majority of patients may be treated conservatively with bowel rest, intravenous fluids and antibiotics. Most patients improve within 24 hours without any sequelae and any worsening should prompt re-evaluation.

Strictures

Strictures following ESD are rare and have been reported in a very specific instance – following ESD of near circumferential colorectal lesions. In patients requiring more than 75% circumferential ESD, strictures have been reported in 3.8–19.7% of patients [53, 54]. These strictures may be treated with one or two times endoscopic dilatations.

Histological Assessment of ESD Specimen

Dissected specimens should be retrieved and handled with care to prevent fragmentation. If the resected specimen is large, a rectal overtube may be used to aid removal of the specimen without fragmentation [55]. Once the specimen is retrieved, it is stretched and fixed on the board. It is useful to determine the spatial orientation and cutting direction of the resected specimen.

Resections with clear vertical and horizontal margins, tumour budding grade I, submucosal invasion up to 1 mm, no lymphovascular invasion and no poorly differentiated or mucinous component are considered curative. A positive vertical margin implies deep invasion and is an indication for surgery.

ESD Outcomes

A recent meta-analysis reported a pooled R0 resection rate of 92.9% and *en bloc* resection rates of 91%. However, there was substantial variation in the rates reported in individual studies with significantly lower rates in non-Asian countries compared to Asian countries. The hybrid resection technique was associated with lower rates of R0 resection and *en bloc* resection than the conventional method [29]. The risk of recurrence following ESD is low but higher in Western compared to Asian countries (5.2% vs 1.1%) [29]. Recurrences are more likely with piecemeal resection, with incomplete resections with positive margins on histology, and in cases of non-curative resection [56]. Compared to EMR, ESD achieves higher rates of *en bloc* resection and curative resection. This is, however, at the expense of higher rates of perforation [34].

Conclusions

ESD has emerged as an effective treatment for superficial colorectal neoplasia but still remains a challenging procedure as demonstrated by the wide variation in clinical outcomes. While ESD enables surgery to be avoided in patients with superficial invasion, patients with clear morphological evidence of deep submucosal invasion should be sent for surgery instead. Optimal outcomes may be achieved by careful patient selection, the use of appropriate endoscopic instruments, training in techniques and the management of complications.

References

1. Gotoda T, Kondo H, Ono H, Saito Y, Yamaguchi H, Saito D, et al. A new endoscopic mucosal resection procedure using an insulation-tipped electrosurgical knife for rectal flat lesions: report of two cases. Gastrointest Endosc. 1999;50(4):560–3. PubMed PMID: 10502182.
2. Beaton C, Twine CP, Williams GL, Radcliffe AG. Systematic review and meta-analysis of histopathological factors influencing the risk of lymph node metastasis in early colorectal cancer. Colorectal Dis. 2013;15(7):788–97. PubMed PMID: 23331927.
3. Kitajima K, Fujimori T, Fujii S, Takeda J, Ohkura Y, Kawamata H, et al. Correlations between lymph node metastasis and depth of submucosal invasion in submucosal invasive colorectal carcinoma: a Japanese collaborative study. J Gastroenterol. 2004;39(6):534–43. PubMed PMID: 15235870.
4. Repici A, Pellicano R, Strangio G, Danese S, Fagoonee S, Malesci A. Endoscopic mucosal resection for early colorectal neoplasia: pathologic basis, procedures, and outcomes. Dis Colon Rectum. 2009;52(8):1502–15. PubMed PMID: 19617768.
5. Cao Y, Liao C, Tan A, Gao Y, Mo Z, Gao F. Meta-analysis of endoscopic submucosal dissection versus endoscopic mucosal resection for tumors of the gastrointestinal tract. Endoscopy. 2009;41(9):751–7. PubMed PMID: 19693750.
6. Moss A, Bourke MJ, Williams SJ, Hourigan LF, Brown G, Tam W, et al. Endoscopic mucosal resection outcomes and prediction of submucosal cancer from advanced colonic mucosal neoplasia. Gastroenterology. 2011;140(7):1909–18. PubMed PMID: 21392504.
7. Sano Y, Tanaka S, Kudo SE, Saito S, Matsuda T, Wada Y, et al. Narrow-band imaging (NBI) magnifying endoscopic classification of colorectal tumors proposed by the Japan NBI Expert Team. Dig Endosc. 2016;28(5):526–33. PubMed PMID: 26927367.
8. Kikuchi T, Fu KI, Saito Y, Uraoka T, Fukuzawa M, Fukunaga S, et al. Transcutaneous monitoring of partial pressure of carbon dioxide during endoscopic submucosal dissection of early colorectal neoplasia with carbon dioxide insufflation: a prospective study.

Surg Endosc. 2010;24(9):2231–5. PubMed PMID: 20177925.

9. Wu J, Hu B. The role of carbon dioxide insufflation in colonoscopy: a systematic review and meta-analysis. Endoscopy. 2012;44(2):128–36. PubMed PMID: 22271023.

10. Li X, Dong H, Zhang Y, Zhang G. CO2 insufflation versus air insufflation for endoscopic submucosal dissection: A meta-analysis of randomized controlled trials. PLoS One. 2017;12(5):e0177909. PubMed PMID: 28542645. Pubmed Central PMCID: 5443502.

11. Takano A, Kobayashi M, Takeuchi M, Hashimoto S, Mizuno K, Narisawa R, et al. Capnographic monitoring during endoscopic submucosal dissection with patients under deep sedation: a prospective, crossover trial of air and carbon dioxide insufflations. Digestion. 2011;84(3):193–8. PubMed PMID: 21757910.

12. Saito Y, Uraoka T, Matsuda T, Emura F, Ikehara H, Mashimo Y, et al. A pilot study to assess the safety and efficacy of carbon dioxide insufflation during colorectal endoscopic submucosal dissection with the patient under conscious sedation. Gastrointest Endosc. 2007;65(3):537–42. PubMed PMID: 17321264.

13. Takada J, Araki H, Onogi F, Nakanishi T, Kubota M, Ibuka T, et al. Safety of carbon dioxide insufflation during gastric endoscopic submucosal dissection in patients with pulmonary dysfunction under conscious sedation. Surg Endosc. 2015;29(7):1963–9. PubMed PMID: 25318364.

14. Chino A, Karasawa T, Uragami N, Endo Y, Takahashi H, Fujita R. A comparison of depth of tissue injury caused by different modes of electrosurgical current in a pig colon model. Gastrointest Endosc. 2004;59(3):374–9. PubMed PMID: 14997134.

15. Committee AT, Tokar JL, Barth BA, Banerjee S, Chauhan SS, Gottlieb KT, et al. Electrosurgical generators. Gastrointest Endosc. 2013;78(2):197–208. PubMed PMID: 23867369.

16. Gotoda T, Ho KY, Soetikno R, Kaltenbach T, Draganov P. Gastric ESD: current status and future directions of devices and training. Gastrointest Endosc Clin N Am. 2014;24(2):213–33. PubMed PMID: 24679233.

17. Suzuki S, Gotoda T, Kobayashi Y, Kono S, Iwatsuka K, Yagi-Kuwata N, et al. Usefulness of a traction method using dental floss and a hemoclip for gastric endoscopic submucosal dissection: a propensity score matching analysis (with videos). Gastrointest Endosc. 2016;83(2):337–46. PubMed PMID: 26320698.

18. Yamasaki Y, Takeuchi Y, Uedo N, Kato M, Hamada K, Aoi K, et al. Traction-assisted colonic endoscopic submucosal dissection using clip and line: a feasibility study. Endosc Int Open. 2016;4(1):E51–5. PubMed PMID: 26793785. Pubmed Central PMCID: 4713171.

19. Oyama T. Counter traction makes endoscopic submucosal dissection easier. Clin Endosc. 2012;45(4):375–8. PubMed PMID: 23251884. Pubmed Central PMCID: 3521938.

20. Thompson CC, Ryou M, Soper NJ, Hungess ES, Rothstein RI, Swanstrom LL. Evaluation of a manually driven, multitasking platform for complex endoluminal and natural orifice transluminal endoscopic surgery applications (with video). Gastrointest Endosc. 2009;70(1):121–5. PubMed PMID: 19394008.

21. ASGE, SAGES. ASGE/SAGES Working Group on Natural Orifice Translumenal Endoscopic Surgery White Paper October 2005. Gastrointest Endosc. 2006;63(2):199–203. PubMed PMID: 16427920.

22. Hayashi Y, Sunada K, Takahashi H, Shinhata H, Lefor AT, Tanaka A, et al. Pocket-creation method of endoscopic submucosal dissection to achieve en bloc resection of giant colorectal subpedunculated neoplastic lesions. Endoscopy. 2014;46(Suppl 1 UCTN):E421–2. PubMed PMID: 25314173.

23. Hayashi Y, Miura Y, Yamamoto H. Pocket-creation method for the safe, reliable, and efficient endoscopic submucosal dissection of colorectal lateral spreading tumors. Dig Endosc. 2015;27(4):534–5. PubMed PMID: 25708068.

24. Imai K, Hotta K, Yamaguchi Y, Kakushima N, Tanaka M, Takizawa K, et al. Preoperative indicators of failure of en bloc resection or perforation in colorectal endoscopic submucosal dissection: implications for lesion stratification by technical difficulties during stepwise training. Gastrointest Endosc. 2016;83(5):954–62. PubMed PMID: 26297870.

25. Sakamoto H, Hayashi Y, Miura Y, Shinozaki S, Takahashi H, Fukuda H, et al. Pocket-creation method facilitates endoscopic submucosal dissection of colorectal laterally spreading tumors, non-granular type. Endosc Int Open. 2017;5(2):E123–E9. PubMed PMID: 28337483. Pubmed Central PMCID: 5361878.

26. Toyonaga T, Man IM, Morita Y, Azuma T. Endoscopic submucosal dissection (ESD) versus simplified/hybrid ESD. Gastrointest Endosc Clin N Am. 2014;24(2):191–9. PubMed PMID: 24679231.

27. Tanaka S, Kashida H, Saito Y, Yahagi N, Yamano H, Saito S, et al. JGES guidelines for colorectal endoscopic submucosal dissection/endoscopic mucosal resection. Dig Endosc. 2015;27(4):417–34. PubMed PMID: 25652022.

28. Okamoto K, Muguruma N, Kagemoto K, Mitsui Y, Fujimoto D, Kitamura S, et al. Efficacy of hybrid endoscopic submucosal dissection (ESD) as a rescue treatment in difficult colorectal ESD cases. Dig Endosc. 2017;29(Suppl 2):45–52. PubMed PMID: 28425649.

29. Fuccio L, Hassan C, Ponchon T, Mandolesi D, Farioli A, Cucchetti A, et al. Clinical outcomes after endoscopic submucosal dissection for colorectal neoplasia: a systematic review and meta-analysis. Gastrointest Endosc. 2017;86(1):74–86 e17. PubMed PMID: 28254526.

30. Repici A, Hassan C, De Paula Pessoa D, Pagano N, Arezzo A, Zullo A, et al. Efficacy and safety of endoscopic submucosal dissection for colorectal neoplasia: a systematic review. Endoscopy. 2012;44(2):137–50. PubMed PMID: 22271024.

31. Terasaki M, Tanaka S, Shigita K, Asayama N, Nishiyama S, Hayashi N, et al. Risk factors for

delayed bleeding after endoscopic submucosal dissection for colorectal neoplasms. Int J Colorectal Dis. 2014;29(7):877–82. PubMed PMID: 24825723.

32. Saito Y, Uraoka T, Yamaguchi Y, Hotta K, Sakamoto N, Ikematsu H, et al. A prospective, multicenter study of 1111 colorectal endoscopic submucosal dissections (with video). Gastrointest Endosc. 2010;72(6):1217–25. PubMed PMID: 21030017.

33. Oka S, Tanaka S, Kanao H, Ishikawa H, Watanabe T, Igarashi M, et al. Current status in the occurrence of postoperative bleeding, perforation and residual/local recurrence during colonoscopic treatment in Japan. Dig Endosc. 2010;22(4):376–80. PubMed PMID: 21175503.

34. Fujiya M, Tanaka K, Dokoshi T, Tominaga M, Ueno N, Inaba Y, et al. Efficacy and adverse events of EMR and endoscopic submucosal dissection for the treatment of colon neoplasms: a meta-analysis of studies comparing EMR and endoscopic submucosal dissection. Gastrointest Endosc. 2015;81(3):583–95. PubMed PMID: 25592748.

35. Saito Y, Yamada M, So E, Abe S, Sakamoto T, Nakajima T, et al. Colorectal endoscopic submucosal dissection: Technical advantages compared to endoscopic mucosal resection and minimally invasive surgery. Dig Endosc. 2014;26(Suppl 1):52–61. PubMed PMID: 24191896.

36. Pimentel-Nunes P, Dinis-Ribeiro M, Ponchon T, Repici A, Vieth M, De Ceglie A, et al. Endoscopic submucosal dissection: European Society of Gastrointestinal Endoscopy (ESGE) Guideline. Endoscopy. 2015;47(9):829–4. PubMed PMID: 26317585.

37. Kim ES, Cho KB, Park KS, Lee KI, Jang BK, Chung WJ, et al. Factors predictive of perforation during endoscopic submucosal dissection for the treatment of colorectal tumors. Endoscopy. 2011;43(7):573–8. PubMed PMID: 21448852.

38. Mizushima T, Kato M, Iwanaga I, Sato F, Kubo K, Ehira N, et al. Technical difficulty according to location, and risk factors for perforation, in endoscopic submucosal dissection of colorectal tumors. Surg Endosc. 2015;29(1):133–9. PubMed PMID: 24993172.

39. Yoshida N, Wakabayashi N, Kanemasa K, Sumida Y, Hasegawa D, Inoue K, et al. Endoscopic submucosal dissection for colorectal tumors: technical difficulties and rate of perforation. Endoscopy. 2009;41(9):758–61. PubMed PMID: 19746316.

40. Hong SN, Byeon JS, Lee BI, Yang DH, Kim J, Cho KB, et al. Prediction model and risk score for perforation in patients undergoing colorectal endoscopic submucosal dissection. Gastrointest Endosc. 2016;84(1):98–108. PubMed PMID: 26708921.

41. Kantsevoy SV. A new tool to estimate the risk of perforations during colorectal endoscopic submucosal dissection. Gastrointest Endosc. 2016;84(1):109–14. PubMed PMID: 27315737.

42. Iqbal CW, Cullinane DC, Schiller HJ, Sawyer MD, Zietlow SP, Farley DR. Surgical management and out-comes of 165 colonoscopic perforations from a single institution. Arch Surg. 2008;143(7):701–6; discussion 6–7. PubMed PMID: 18645114.

43. Burgess NG, Bassan MS, McLeod D, Williams SJ, Byth K, Bourke MJ. Deep mural injury and perforation after colonic endoscopic mucosal resection: a new classification and analysis of risk factors. Gut. 2017;66(10):1779–89. PubMed PMID: 27464708.

44. Swan MP, Bourke MJ, Moss A, Williams SJ, Hopper A, Metz A. The target sign: an endoscopic marker for the resection of the muscularis propria and potential perforation during colonic endoscopic mucosal resection. Gastrointest Endosc. 2011;73(1):79–85. PubMed PMID: 21184872.

45. Ma MX, Bourke MJ. Complications of endoscopic polypectomy, endoscopic mucosal resection and endoscopic submucosal dissection in the colon. Best Pract Res Clin Gastroenterol. 2016;30(5):749–67. PubMed PMID: 27931634.

46. Kantsevoy SV, Bitner M, Hajiyeva G, Mirovski PM, Cox ME, Swope T, et al. Endoscopic management of colonic perforations: clips versus suturing closure (with videos). Gastrointest Endosc. 2016;84(3):487–93. PubMed PMID: 26364965.

47. Raithel M, Albrecht H, Scheppach W, Farnbacher M, Haupt W, Hagel AF, et al. Outcome, comorbidity, hospitalization and 30-day mortality after closure of acute perforations and postoperative anastomotic leaks by the over-the-scope clip (OTSC) in an unselected cohort of patients. Surg Endosc. 2017;31(6):2411–25. PubMed PMID: 27633439.

48. Cha JM, Lim KS, Lee SH, Joo YE, Hong SP, Kim TI, et al. Clinical outcomes and risk factors of post-polypectomy coagulation syndrome: a multi-center, retrospective, case-control study. Endoscopy. 2013;45(3):202–7. PubMed PMID: 23381948.

49. Hirasawa K, Sato C, Makazu M, Kaneko H, Kobayashi R, Kokawa A, et al. Coagulation syndrome: delayed perforation after colorectal endoscopic treatments. World J Gastrointest Endosc. 2015;7(12):1055–61. PubMed PMID: 26380051. Pubmed Central PMCID: 4564832.

50. Hong MJ, Kim JH, Lee SY, Sung IK, Park HS, Shim CS. Prevalence and clinical features of coagulation syndrome after endoscopic submucosal dissection for colorectal neoplasms. Dig Dis Sci. 2015;60(1):211–6. PubMed PMID: 25502119.

51. Yamashina T, Takeuchi Y, Uedo N, Hamada K, Aoi K, Yamasaki Y, et al. Features of electrocoagulation syndrome after endoscopic submucosal dissection for colorectal neoplasm. J Gastroenterol Hepatol. 2016;31(3):615–20. PubMed PMID: 26202127.

52. Jung D, Youn YH, Jahng J, Kim JH, Park H. Risk of electrocoagulation syndrome after endoscopic submucosal dissection in the colon and rectum. Endoscopy. 2013;45(9):714–7. PubMed PMID: 23990482.

53. Abe S, Sakamoto T, Takamaru H, Yamada M, Nakajima T, Matsuda T, et al. Stenosis rates after endoscopic submucosal dissection of large rectal tumors involving greater than three quarters of the luminal

circumference. Surg Endosc. 2016;30(12):5459–64. PubMed PMID: 27126623.

54. Ohara Y, Toyonaga T, Tanaka S, Ishida T, Hoshi N, Yoshizaki T, et al. Risk of stricture after endoscopic submucosal dissection for large rectal neoplasms. Endoscopy. 2016;48(1):62–70. PubMed PMID: 26220284.

55. Ikehara H, Saito Y, Uraoka T, Matsuda T, Miwa H. Specimen retrieval method using a sliding overtube for large colorectal neoplasm following endoscopic submucosal dissection. Endoscopy. 2015;47(Suppl 1 UCTN):E168–9. PubMed PMID: 25926185.

56. Watanabe T, Itabashi M, Shimada Y, Tanaka S, Ito Y, Ajioka Y, et al. Japanese Society for Cancer of the Colon and Rectum (JSCCR) Guidelines 2014 for treatment of colorectal cancer. Int J Clin Oncol. 2015;20(2):207–39. PubMed PMID: 25782566. Pubmed Central PMCID: 4653248.

Endoscopic Full-Thickness Resection (EFTR) and Submucosal Tunneling Endoscopic Resection (STER)

Mingyan Cai, Marie Ooi, and Pinghong Zhou

Introduction

Gastrointestinal subepithelial tumors (SETs) are rare and majority of patients are asymptomatic [1]. With the widespread use of cross-sectional imaging and endoscopy in clinical practice, the incidence of SETs is on the rise and more SETs are being detected incidentally on both screening modalities [1]. However, some may experience symptoms such as nonspecific abdominal pain, overt or occult gastrointestinal (GI) hemorrhage, duodenal obstruction, and intussusception [2–4]. SETs with central ulceration are more susceptible to present with overt GI hemorrhage secondary to tumor rupture [3, 4]. Tumors involving the major papilla are more likely to result in jaundice and pancreatitis secondary to biliary or pancreatic duct obstruction, respectively [2].

There has always been a grand vision to develop a minimally invasive, incisionless

Electronic Supplementary Material The online version of this chapter (https://doi.org/10.1007/978-3-030-21695-5_9) contains supplementary material, which is available to authorized users.

M. Cai · P. Zhou (✉)
Endoscopy Center, Zhongshan Hospital of Fudan University, Shanghai, China
e-mail: zhou.pinghong@zs-hospital.sh.cn

M. Ooi
Department of Gastroenterology, Royal Adelaide Hospital, Adelaide, SA, Australia

resection of SETs by accessing a natural orifice using flexible endoscopes. Since the demise of traditional NOTES, the "new NOTES" procedures have been entering an exponential phase of growth with emergence of a large number of new endoscopic techniques and rapid development of new endoscopic devices. The new NOTES evolution has fueled development of new endoscopic techniques, and subepithelial tumors are increasingly amenable to endoscopic curative resection in specialized centers. Endoscopic submucosal dissection (ESD) has been used to resect superficial lesions arising from the mucosal and submucosal layers [5–15]. However, certain SET such as gastrointestinal stromal tumor (GIST) may arise from muscularis propria and have extraluminal or serosal extension. As a result, ESD may not be sufficient to fully resect the tumor that may lead to an incomplete resection. Additional new techniques such as endoscopic submucosal excavation (ESE) or endoscopic muscularis dissection (EMD) have been developed in an attempt to overcome the limitation of ESD and to excavate muscularis propria (MP)-originated subepithelial tumors [16–22]. However, the major drawbacks of ESE and EMD are similar to ESD in that these techniques may fail to guarantee a complete resection of the muscularis propria layer [19]. This may result in partial tumor excavation and positive resected margin especially for tumors that have an extraluminal growth pattern or grow in close proximity to the serosa.

M. S. Wagh, S. B. Wani (eds.), *Gastrointestinal Interventional Endoscopy*,
https://doi.org/10.1007/978-3-030-21695-5_9

In addition, procedure-related complications such as wall perforation, bleeding, and infection are major drawbacks of such techniques [19]. Submucosal tunneling endoscopic resection (STER) and endoscopic full-thickness resection (EFTR) of SET may provide a solution to some of the limitations encountered by the techniques described above.

Endoscopic Full-Thickness Resection (EFTR)

Endoscopic full-thickness resection (EFTR) was first described by Suzuki and colleagues in 1998 [23]. Since then, EFTR has been gaining new proponents all over the world and is now a widely accepted endoscopic treatment option for gastric and colorectal subepithelial tumors in Asian coutries [24–30]. The major advantage of EFTR over other current techniques such as endoscopic mucosal dissection (EMD) and endoscopic submucosal dissection (ESD) that are widely used for en bloc resection of superficial mucosal lesions or submucosal lesions includes the ability to achieve a complete en bloc resection with R0 resected margin especially for tumors arising from the muscularis propria with or without an extraluminal extension [24]. As a result, EFTR of SET may reduce the risk of residual tumor, prevent tumor recurrence, and improve the accuracy of histological diagnosis and tumor staging [24].

EFTR also offers several advantages over surgical resection. EFTR permits endoscopic access into the intra-abdominal cavity through a natural orifice without the need of a skin incision [24]. Based on previous study comparing endoscopic and laparoscopic resection of SET, endoscopic resection was associated with less postoperative pain, postoperative complications, a shorter hospital stay, and less cost [28]. In addition, there may be certain anatomical locations that may not be accessible by laparoscopic surgery, particularly tumors located within retroperitoneal space [31]. However, complete closure of the iatrogenic perforation of GI wall after EFTR remains a major consideration and is the main reason for its limited implementation in clinical practice [29].

EFTR Techniques

EFTR can be performed either with or without laparoscopic assistance [23, 24, 30–33]. For small SETs, EFTR with laparoscopic assistance was previously described [23]. This technique involves endoscopic resection of SET followed by laparoscopic suture of the resected wound. EFTR without laparoscopic assistance also known as "pure free-hand EFTR" was first reported in 2011 [24]. "Pure free-hand EFTR" negates the need for laparoscopic-assisted closure of the wall defect and simplifies the EFTR technique. With the advancement in endoscopic technology and availability of new endoscopic suturing or closure devices, the ability to achieve a curative en bloc resection of SETs is becoming a reality. To date, device-assisted EFTR has been reported for SETs [34, 35]. Device-assisted EFTR such as the over-the-scope clip (OTSC) device also known as full-thickness resection device (FTRD, Ovesco Endoscopy, Tubingen, Germany) has the advantage of a one-step clip-and-snare of pre-closure prior to tumor resection [29, 36, 38].

The full-thickness resection device (FTRD) constitutes of a modified 14 mm OSTC system that can be uploaded on a conventional endoscope with diameter of 11.5–13.2 mm. This modification is in terms of a longer transparent cap which is 23 mm in length, compared to the conventional 6 mm one, so that it can anchor more tissue and grasp up to 30 mm size lesions. Also, the FTRD clip has additional lateral teeth to ensure a safe closure of the defect before resection. It has a 13 mm monofilament high-frequency polypectomy snare which is preloaded into the tip of the cap. Meanwhile the handle of the snare runs on the outer surface of the scope under a plastic sheath not in the working channel. A grasping forceps is introduced into the working channel of the scope to pull the lesion into the transparent cap [38].

Steps of FTRD

- Step (1): Endoscope is introduced without the FTRD to inspect the lesion carefully followed by marking of the lateral margins of the lesion with APC probe. Then the scope is withdrawn.

- Step (2): The endoscope is reintroduced with FTRD mounted on it. The grasping forceps is introduced through the working channel to grasp the lateral margins of the lesion into the transparent cap till the markings are visible.
- Step (3): The preloaded clip is then deployed, and the lesion is resected with the snare applied immediately afterward.
- Step (4): The scope is withdrawn with the cap containing the lesion. Then, reintroduction of the scope is done to inspect if the lesion is fully resected [36].

FTRD was first applied in humans by Schmidt et al. [38] when he published the first case series on three patients with non-lifting adenomas. In several retrospective studies followed but were performed on small number of patients that reached maximum of 33 patients, the technical success ranged from 93 to 100%. R0 ranged from 75 to 100% as shown in table (1). The indications among these studies were non-lifting adenomas from either recurrent or primary incomplete resection, difficult locations as adenoma in diverticulum or in the appendix, submucosal tumors as GIST or NET, and early carcinomas [37–42]. The main adverse outcomes included post-polypectomy syndrome secondary to serosa irritation resulting in fever, leukocytosis and abdominal pain, failure of application of FTRD related to hindrance passage of the scope through the stenotic area, perforation, and bleeding [37, 39–42].

The FTRD was Conformite´ Europe'enne (CE) marked and available throughout Europe since September 2015. FDA in the United States has also recently approved the use of FTRD in clinical practice. Compared to the first FTRD, the current device is smaller and easier to use in the entire colon. Recently, Schmidt and colleagues presented their interim results of an ongoing prospective multicenter study known as the "WALL RESECT" study, involving nine centers in Germany [43]. The purpose of the study is to assess the safety and efficacy of the FTRD system in non-lifting colorectal adenoma. In the interim analysis, 106 patients with indication for endo-

scopic colorectal full-thickness resection were included in the study. Technical success (macroscopically complete and en bloc resection) was achieved in 94 patients (88.7%) and R0-resection rate was 79.6%. More than 70% of all FTRD clips spontaneously detach from the colonic wall within 3 months after full-thickness resection. Complications occurred in 4.7% of cases (two minor bleedings, three perforations) [43].

FTRD-associated complication may necessitate removal of OTSC. An experimental study and small case series have reported on a bipolar direct current (DC) grasping device (remove system, Ovesco, Tubingen, Germany) [44–46]. Short direct current impulses are delivered to the two opposing sites of the OTSC in order to fragment and release it from the tissue.

There are several major drawbacks of FTRD including (i) the limited size of tumor that can be resected, (ii) the inability to ensure a negative tumor margin due to the mobility of the GI wall, and (iii) the large 21 mm outer diameter of the device that may hamper scope passage through the cricopharyngeus limiting its use to mainly colorectal lesions [47].

Table 9.1 summarizes studies published to date on clinical outcomes of FTRD.

Indications and Contraindications of EFTR

To date, several major guidelines recommend that subepithelial tumor in particular GIST ≥2 cm or symptomatic tumors should be resected [48–50]. There is currently no consensus of the maximum size of the lesion amenable to EFTR. Sumiyama proposed that EFTR technique can be used to resect large submucosal tumor and laterally spreading tumor (LST) involving the submucosa or muscularis propria [8].

The management of small tumors less than 2 cm is highly debated. Most guidelines recommend periodic endoscopic surveillance [48–50]. However, limitations of endoscopic surveillance include a delayed diagnosis of malignancy, increased patient's anxiety, and patient's lost to follow-up and therefore may not be cost-effective

Table 9.1 Clinical outcomes of FTRD

Study	N	Site	Mean size (mm)	Indication	Success	R_0	Adverse events	Follow-up	Recurrence
Schmidt et al. [36] (2014)	3	Colon	22 mm	Recurrent non-lifting adenoma	100%	100%	No	3–6 m	No
Schmidt et al. [38] (2015)	25	Colon	24 mm	Non-lifting adenoma SET Adenoma in appendix or diverticulum Coagulopathy Hirschsprung's disease	96%	75%	2 Postpolypectomy syndrome (8%) 1 failed due to stenosis (4%)		No
Schmidt et al. [35] (2015)	4	Duodenum	28.3 mm	Non-lifting adenoma	100%	75%	2 Minor bleeding (50%)	2 m	No
Richter-Schrag et al. [39] (2016)	20	Colon	50 mm	Non-lifting adenoma Early adenocarcinoma	80%	80%	4 failed (20%) 1 perforation (5%)	2 m	2 patients (10%)
Andrisani et al. [40] (2017)	20	Colon	26 mm	Non-lifting adenoma Early adenocarcinoma	100%	100%	1 Postpolypectomy syndrome (5%)	3 m	No
Vitali et al. [44] (2018)	13	Colon	17 mm	Non-lifting adenoma Early adenocarcinoma NET	100%	83.3%	2 Postpolypectomy syndrome (15%)	12 m	3 patients (23%)
Aepli et al. [47] (2018)	33	Colon	27 mm	Non-lifting adenoma NET Adenoma in appendix or diverticulum Early adenocarcinoma	93.9%	87.9%	3 bleeding (9%) 1 delayed perforation (3%) 2 failed (6%)	3 m	2 patients needed surgery (6%)

FTRD full-thickness resection device, *N* number of patients, *SET* subepithelial tumor, *NET* neuroendocrine tumor

Indications and contraindications for endoscopic full-thickness resection	
Indications:	1. Submucosal GI tumors arising from the muscularis propria based on EUS and CT imaging with diameter ≤ 5 cm. Particularly SETs at locations that are difficult to approach with laparoscopic techniques such as the gastroesophageal junction 2. Recurrence of mucosal neoplasms in a post EMR/ESD scar or at a surgical resection site.
Contraindications:	1. High surgical risk due to severe comorbid disease including severe cardiopulmonary disease, blood disorders, coagulation disorders, and anticoagulant/antiplatelet treatment that cannot be interrupted or discontinued. 2. Anesthesia related contraindications such as anesthetic drug allergies, pregnancy. 3. Mucosal neoplasms associated with a high risk of lymph node metastasis or periprocedural intraperitoneal dissemination of carcinoma cells 4. SETs with features on preoperative imaging or histology predicting high risk for aggressive behavior.

Fig. 9.1 Indications for EFTR

in the long term. There is currently no consensus on the association between tumor size and the likelihood of lymph node metastasis [50]. There are several reported cases of small subepithelial tumor <2 cm with malignant potential that presented with early lymph node metastasis [51–53].

We propose the following as indications of EFTR (Fig. 9.1):

We recommend that only skilled endoscopists with experience in ESD, ESE, and the management of perforation should perform EFTR procedures.

Pre-procedural Assessment

Pre-procedural assessment is a crucial step prior to EFTR. As in any other endoscopic procedures, informed consent is necessary. Patients should be fully informed about the intraoperative and postoperative risks that may occur including the possibility of emergency surgery in the event of a major complication such as torrential bleeding or perforation that failed endoscopic closure. Detailed medical history is vital to ensure there are no contraindications to EFTR as highlighted above. For patients on antithrombotic or antiplatelet medications, it is recommended to stop taking both drugs for at least 1 week prior to EFTR if there is no contraindication to cease

these medications temporarily and after discussion with their primary physicians.

Tumor characteristics, size, and location and exclusion of tumor metastasis are also vital information that can be obtained from computed tomography (CT) and endoscopic ultrasound (EUS).

EFTR Procedure

EFTR is a complex procedure that requires the collaboration and support of various departments that include the anesthetist, intensive care unit, surgeon, and pathology department. The success of EFTR not only relies on the endoscopist's technical skill but also experienced trained endoscopic nurses. Both endoscopist and nurses must be familiar with all endoscopic devices and suturing techniques to manage any procedure-related complications. All procedures are performed under general anesthesia with airway intubation. It is recommended to give a single dose of prophylactic intravenous antibiotic at least half an hour prior to EFTR. An infusion of a second- or third-generation cephalosporin tends to be the preferred choice of antibiotic prophylaxis for gastrointestinal tract given the broad-spectrum activity against a wide range of gram-positive and gram-negative bacteria. It is crucial to use carbon dioxide insufflation throughout the EFTR procedure.

Instruments

The instruments used for EFTR were similar to those used for ESD that included a standard single-channel forward-viewing gastroscope (180H Olympus Optical Co., Ltd., Japan) with a transparent cap (D-201-11804, Olympus, Tokyo, Japan) attached to the tip of the endoscope to improve endoscopic visualization, to assist in tissue traction, and to facilitate in hemostasis in the event of bleeding. A dual-channel endoscope (GIF-2T240, Olympus Corporation, Tokyo, Japan) is occasionally used for closure of iatrogenic GI wall defect using a purse-string technique. A grasping forceps (FG-8U-1, Olympus) is also used to prevent inadvertent dislodgment of enucleated tumor into the abdominal cavity.

There are a variety of electrosurgical knives that are available and can be used for EFTR. At our center, an insulated-tip (IT) electrosurgical knife (KD-611L, Olympus), a hook knife (KD-620LR, Olympus), or a needle knife (KD-10Q-1, Olympus) are commonly used to resect the wall layers around the tumor. Other crucial equipment includes injection needles (NM-4L-1, Olympus), snares (SD-230U-20, Olympus), basket (MWB-2 × 4, Cook), hot biopsy forceps (FD-410LR, Olympus), hemostatic clips (HX-610-90, HX-600-135, Olympus), endoloop (MAJ-339, Olympus), over-the-scope-clip (OTSC) (also known as Ovesco device (GmbH, Tubingen, Germany)), argon plasma coagulation unit (APC300, ERBE), and high-frequency electrosurgical generator (VIO200, ERBE).

EFTR Steps

EFTR steps are as follows (Video 9.1, Fig. 9.2):

- *Step 1*: For deep lesions or small lesions (<10 mm), several marking dots around the periphery of the SET are made using either the tip of the electrosurgical knife or argon plasma coagulation catheter because the location may become vague after submucosal injection. Otherwise, marking can be omitted.
- *Step 2*: A submucosal injection of a mixture of 100 ml of normal saline and 1 ml of indigo carmine to create a protective submucosal "cushion" to prevent deep thermal injury during tumor resection.
- *Step 3*: A circumferential mucosal incision is made 1–2 mm outside the marked dots or the contour of the SET. Another option is to perform mucosal excision to unroof the SET.
- *Step 4*: Submucosal and subtumoral dissection is performed surrounding the tumor capsule to ensure a complete en bloc resection of the tumor. Meticulous care must be taken to avoid interruption of the tumor capsule. All visible vessels must be coagulated, and prompt hemostasis must be achieved to avoid accumulation of blood in the GI lumen. To avoid inadvertently losing the specimen into the peritoneal cavity, snare can be used for the final cut of the lesion and immediate specimen retrieval after resection. Another method is to use a double-channel endoscope with a grasping forceps inserted into one channel to grasp the lesion while the electrosurgical knife is inserted into the second channel to excise the lesion.
- *Step 5*: Once the tumor is enucleated, the closure of excisional wall defect can be performed using various available methods as described below depending on the size of the GI wall defect. The diameter of the wall defect can be reduced by air suction to assist in closure of the defect.

In the event of an iatrogenic wall perforation, continuous CO_2 insufflation must be avoided to prevent pneumoperitoneum and regular suction of content within the GI lumen is vital to avoid spillage of fluid and blood into the abdominal cavity. Throughout the procedure, care is taken to constantly monitor the patient's positive end expiratory pressure (PEEP) and for clinical signs of raised intra-abdominal pressure. When necessary, a 20-gauge needle is inserted under aseptic technique directly into the abdominal cavity to relieve pneumoperitoneum during and after the procedure. Patients are on kept nil by mouth after surgery and nursed in semi-Fowler's position. A nasogastric tube is routinely placed to deflate the stomach; in addition it also helps detect early post-procedural bleeding.

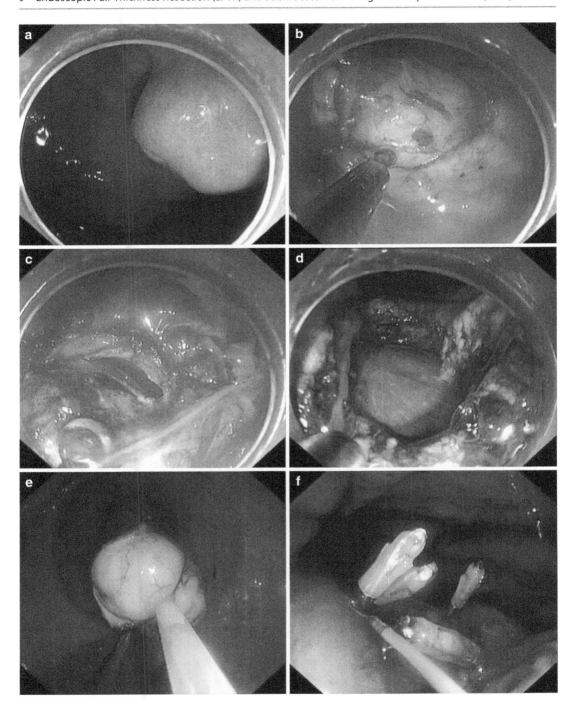

Fig. 9.2 Steps of EFTR for gastric SET originating from muscularis propria. (**a**) Endoscopic view of a gastric SET originating from muscularis propria. (**b**) Circumferential incision was made as deep as muscularis propria around the lesion with IT knife. (**c**) Incision into serosal layer around the lesion was performed with IT knife to create active perforation. (**d**) The full-thickness gastric wall defect after tumor resection. The liver could be seen through the gastric wall defect after EFTR. (**e**) The resected tumor was removed by snare. (**f, g**) The gastric wound was closed with several metallic clips and endoloop by "purse-string" method (double-channel scope). (**h**) The resected specimen

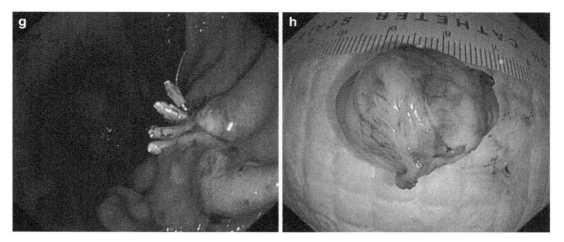

Fig. 9.2 (continued)

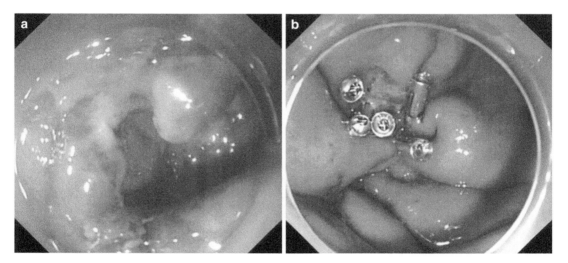

Fig. 9.3 Metallic clips closure. (**a**) The full-thickness gastric wall defect after tumor resection. (**b**) The gastric wound was closed by several metallic clips successfully

Closure of Iatrogenic GI Wall Perforation

There are various endoscopic methods to close the iatrogenic GI wall perforation after EFTR. This step can be very challenging depending on the size of the wall defect and the location of wall defect. An adequate and reliable closure of the GI wall defect is the most important factor to determine the success of the EFTR procedure. We will focus on several closure techniques that include traditional metallic clips, purse-string technique, and other newer closure devices available.

(i) *Metallic clips closure* (Fig. 9.3)

There are a variety of metallic clips available in clinical practice to close GI wall defects. Endoluminal metallic clips have been widely used in clinical practice for closure of GI wall defects, anastomotic fistulas, and small perforations after endoscopic resection and to achieve hemostasis. The successful application of endoscopic metallic clips to close perforation in the stomach was first reported in 1993 by Binmoeller et al. [54] Minami et al. [55] reported a study of 121 patients, in which 117 patient had successful closure of ESD perforation using metallic clips, achieving success rate of 98.3%. At our center, metallic clips are generally used to close elongated wall defects that are less than 2 cm in cross-sectional diameter.

(ii) *Purse-string closure technique (metallic clips combined with endoloop)*

Matsuda first introduced the metallic clips combined with endoloop snare to close EMR defects successfully [56]. This technique can be divided into two ways:

Linear closure: This is applicable for small defects with a single endoloop and two metallic clips anchoring over the proximal and distal edges of the defect to close.

Purse-string closure: This way is suitable for large defects. It uses a single endoloop and about five to six metallic clips gathering mucosa around the defects to the center to close [57] (Video 9.1). This technique has many variations; the commonly used maneuver was performed by a double-channel gastroscope, introducing endoloop through one channel and metallic clips through the other channel. For centers without double-channel gastroscope, single-channel method can be used with a specially designed loop (LeClamp™, LEOMED, Changzhou, China) (Fig. 9.4).

(iii) *Omental patch method*

An omental patch method is not commonly used now; because of the advances in closure devices, most of the defect can be successful closed endoscopically. Hashiba et al. reported successful endoscopic repair of gastric perforation with an omental patch [58]. Dray et al. using animal model reported technical feasibility of omentoplasty for gastrotomy closure [59]. This technique is usually reserved for large wall defects (more than 3 cm in size) that has failed closure using the purse-string technique. This technique utilizes the greater omentum or the lesser omentum as a patch. The omentum is suctioned into the GI lumen through the perforation site to seal the wall defect, and the omentum is anchored to the edge of the wall defect using several metallic clips.

(iv) *Endoscopic suturing device*

Endoscopic suturing device is an indispensable component of any advanced endoscopic resection. There is a recent rapid expansion of endoscopic suturing devices that are currently available, and we are now able to achieve closure of full-thickness resection defects. However, these endoscopic closure devices are generally not widely available, are costly, and are at early stages of development. In addition, there is only very limited preliminary data in regard to its safety and effectiveness. We hereby focus on several endoscopic closure devices that are available and used in clinical practice.

(a) *Over-the-scope clips (OTSC)*

Among all the closure devices available, OTSC has been increasingly used to close various wall defects and bleeding ulcers. The OTSC consists of a nitinol alloy and is installed on an applicator that is mounted onto the tip of the gastroscope. The clip is applied by stretching a wire that is led through the working channel of the endoscope (similar to common endoscopic band ligation systems) [60–62].

In contrast to other mechanical closing devices, the new OTSC clips can grasp much more tissue and offer a strong and long-standing closure of the wound margins in a one-step application technique. The new OTSC system was originally developed and used in humans for hemostasis of ulcer bleeding and for closure of iatrogenic perforations of the GI tract [63–64]. However, one big concern of this device is the device residual in the wound (Fig. 9.5).

(b) *OverStitch™ suturing system*

Apollo OverStitch suturing device has evolved from the previously developed Eagle Claw device. This device was approved in 2011 by the Food and Drug Administration and is used for closure of fistulas and perforations, oversewing ulcers, and bariatric endoscopy in the United States [59]. However, in Asia, the OverStitch is not yet available and many endoscopists used

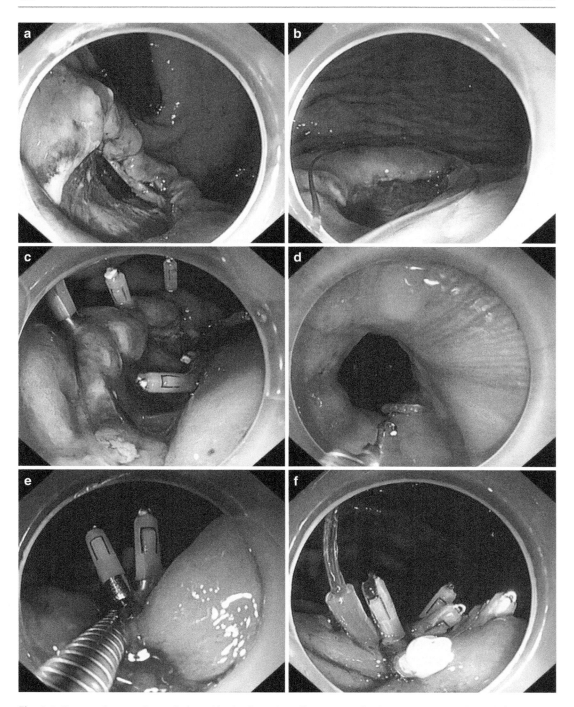

Fig. 9.4 Purse-string suturing technique (single-channel method). (**a**) Endoscopic view of a gastric wall defect after EFTR. (**b**) A loop was placed above the wall defect and detached from the loop hook. (**c**) Several metallic clips were anchoring at the defect edge. (**d–f**) The loop hook was introduced to tighten the loop to achieve complete closure of the full-thickness defect

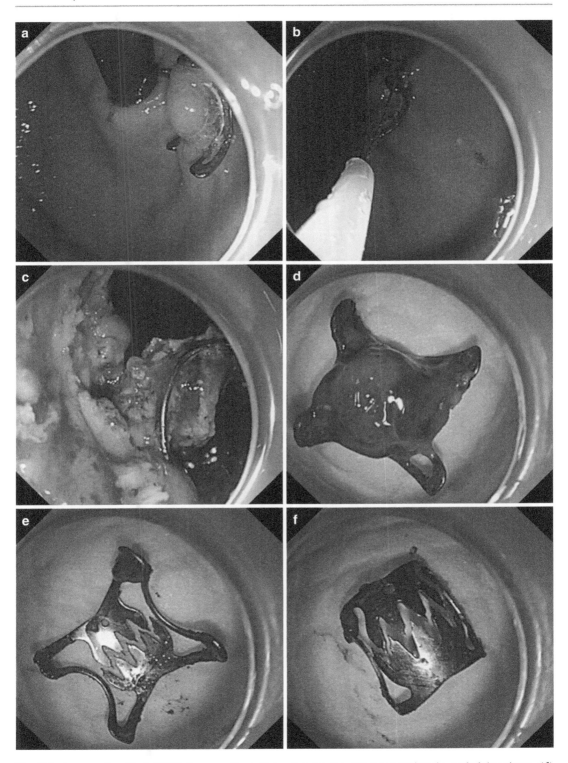

Fig. 9.5 A case of residual OTSC 5 years after initial EFTR. (**a**) Retained OTSC was found on 5-year follow-up endoscopy after initial EFTR. (**b**, **c**) A snare was used to remove the clip by resecting the underlying tissue. (**d**) Removed OTSC with grasped tissue. (**e**, **f**) OTSC

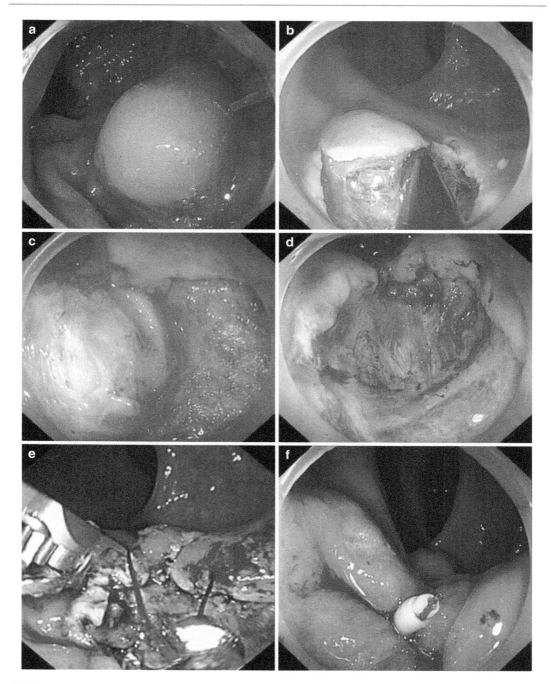

Fig. 9.6 A case of colonic defect after EFTR closed by OverStitch. (**a**) Endoscopic view of a colonic SET. (**b**) Mucosal incision after submucosal injection. (**c**) The SET originated from MP layer. (**d**) The wound after EFTR. (**e, f**) Continuous suture of the wound was achieved successfully by Overstitch suturing device

endoloop and clips to close EFTR defects [65–66]. This device is a single-use device that is mounted onto a double-channel gastroscope. This device enables both inter-rupted and continuous suture application and allows full-thickness suturing as well as tissue approximation or plication in the gastrointestinal tract (Fig. 9.6). This suturing device has been shown to have the ability to attain durable closure of gastric defects ranging from 18 mm to 50 mm in an animal model [66].

Kantsevoy et al. demonstrated in his study that 12 patients who underwent ESD for both gastric and colonic lesions had successful closure of defect using OverStitch device in all patients, and all patients were discharged home on the same day of the procedure [67].

Rajan et al. demonstrated in a porcine study the feasibility of suturing to seal full-thickness gastric defects with an average size of 11 mm without site ulceration [63].

Since then, there are an increased number of studies that demonstrated the effectiveness of OverStitch in closure of wall defect [68, 69].

Pathologic Evaluation

The specimens are fixed, embedded with paraffin, and then sectioned. Hematoxylin and eosin and immunohistochemical staining (CD34, CD117, actin, S-100, desmin, vimentin, Ki-67, etc.) are carried out. Complete resection is defined as en bloc resection, in which the capsule of the tumor is intact and the basal and lateral margins are free of tumor cells.

Post-procedure Management

Post-procedure care is crucial. All patients are kept strictly nil by mouth after EFTR and nursed in a semi-Fowler's position. A nasogastric (NG) tube is recommended to decompress the stomach and to detect early post-procedure bleeding, and vital signs and abdominal signs are monitored closely. At our center, a third-generation cephalosporin is used for the first 3 postoperative days. Oral proton pump inhibitors are prescribed for 2 months and used to protect gastric mucosa in patients with upper GI lesions.

The NG tube is typically removed after 48 hours if there is no sign of bleeding or worsening of abdominal pain. The patients are started on a liquid diet and gradually upgraded to a soft and then finally to a normal diet prior to discharge from hospital.

Clinical Outcomes of EFTR

As shown in Table 9.2, EFTR with closure of the defect has shown promising clinical outcomes, with technical success nearly reaching 100%, with complete en bloc resection in almost all studies. The main indications in these studies were SETs. This may owe to the fact that SETs usually arise from the muscularis propria layer, which requires full-thickness resection. The adverse events are related mainly to the iatrogenic perforation with resultant abdominal pain, distension, fever, and localized peritonitis, all of which had been successfully managed in the mentioned studies. On comparing this to the use of FRTD, inferior results with FTRD as shown in Table 9.1 may be due to the big size of the device that hinders technical success in all cases. FTRD is approved to use only in the colon as it has a wider lumen, and hence most of the studies are on colonic lesions, while EFTR was studied mainly in the stomach and colon. Besides, FTRD is a previously set device with one-step resection technique limiting its use in different locations such as the stomach and in bigger lesions (>3 cm). On the other hand, EFTR, is a free-hand technique, enabling precise full resection of the lesions as well as closure of the defects with variable methods under complete supervision of the endoscopist. Some closure devices such as the suturing device are very expensive and not widely available; however the purse-string technique using the endoloop and metallic clips had offered a convenient substitution. Meanwhile, there are very few studies on the EFTR which are mainly retrospective. So, prospective randomized controlled trials including larger number of patients are required comparing the different closure techniques and comparing FTRD and EFTR to one another.

Post-procedure Complications

(a) *Hemorrhage*

Bleeding can occur during or after EFTR and the severity of bleeding can vary from mild to severe torrential bleeding. Post-procedure bleeding typically occurs within 24 h after EFTR procedure. During EFTR, prophylactic hemostasis of any visible

Table 9.2 Clinical outcomes of EFTR

Study	N	Site	Mean size (mm)	Pathological diagnosis	Closure	Success	R_0	Adverse events	Follow up (m)
Zhou et al. [24] (2011)	26	Gastric	28 mm	GIST (16) Leiomyoma (6) Glomus tumor (1) Schwannoma (1)	Metallic clips	100%	100%	No	8 m
Shi et al. [57] (2013)	20	Gastric	14.7 m	GIST (12) Leiomyoma (4) Schwannoma (2) Granular cell tumor (1) Ectopic pancreas (1)	Purse-string	100%	100%	Abdominal pain and fever (5)	3 m
Feng et al. [27] (2014)	48	Gastric	15.9 mm	GIST (43) Leiomyoma (4) Schwannoma (1)	Metallic clips	100%	100%	Distension (5)	2,6,12& 24 m
Ye et al. [63] (2014)	51	Gastric	24 mm	GIST (30) Leiomyoma (21)	Purse-string	98%	98%	No	22.4 m
Huang et al. [26] (2014)	35	Gastric	28 mm	GIST (25) Leiomyoma (7) Autonomic nerve tumor (2)	Metallic clip ± omental patch	100%	100%	No	6 m
Kantsevoy et al. [67] (2014)	12	Gastric Colon	42.6 mm	Gastric lipoma (2) Ectopic pancreas (1) Intestinal metaplasia (1) Colonic adenoma (6) Intramucosal rectal cancer (2)	Suturing device	100%	100%	No	3 m
Yang et al. [28] (2015)	41	Gastric	16.3 mm	GIST (33) Leiomyoma (4) NET (1) Ectopic pancreas (1) Schwannoma (1) Hyaline degeneration (1)	OTSC or metallic clips	100%	100%	Abdominal pain, fever, dysuria, vomiting (9)	--
Guo et al. [29] (2015)	23	Gastric	12.1 mm	GIST (19) Leiomyoma (4)	OSTC	100%	100%	Localized peritonitis (2) Fever (4)	3 m
Kantsevoy et al. [67] (2016)	16	Colon	5.6 mm	Adenoma	Suturing device	100%	100%	No	3 m

EFTR endoscopic full-thickness resection, *N* number of patients, *GIST* gastrointestinal stromal tumor, *NET* neuroendocrine tumor, *OTSC* over-the-scope clip, *mm* millimeter, *m* months

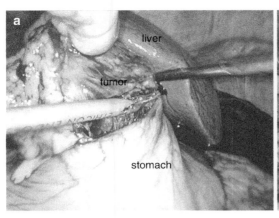
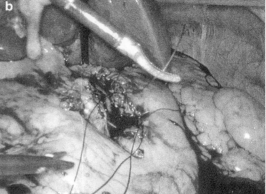

Fig. 9.7 A salvage surgery for uncontrollable bleeding. (**a**) The laparoscopic view of an uncontrollable bleeding of a gastric GIST treated by EFTR. The tumor was lifted by laparoscopic graspers showing the full-thickness defect on gastric wall. (**b**) A salvage surgery was performed laparoscopically to resect the gastric GIST and to suture the full-thickness defect

vessels is recommended to avoid bleeding, and in the event of bleeding, flushing of the bleeding site to identify the bleeding point and prompt hemostasis are crucial to maintain a good endoscopic view. Hemostasis can be achieved by using the tip of the electrosurgical knife or by coagulation grasper. Metallic hemostatic clips can also be used to achieve hemostasis. If there is uncontrollable torrential bleeding, urgent surgical consult should be obtained in preparation for salvage laparoscopic or surgical treatment (Fig. 9.7).

(b) *Pneumoperitoneum*

Pneumoperitoneum during EFTR is unavoidable given iatrogenic wall perforation is necessary to achieve an en bloc resection. During the creation of GI wall perforation, it is important to limit the amount of carbon dioxide insufflation and regular suctioning of any fluid or blood in the lumen to avoid spillage into the abdominal cavity. Endoscopic visibility within the GI lumen can be limited by the expansion of trapped gas within the peritoneal cavity that can collapse the gastric wall inward, and closure of the wall defect can be challenging under this circumstance. A 20-gauge needle is often used to relieve pneumoperitoneum during EFTR and is generally safe.

(c) *Peritonitis and intra-abdominal infections*

As mentioned above, it is vital to avoid fluid or blood escaping into the peritoneal cavity to reduce the risk of post-procedure peritoneal infection that can lead to serious complications such as peritoneal adhesions and intra-abdominal abscess. Occasionally, changing patient's position to shift fluid or blood away from the operative field may be necessary.

Once a wall defect occurs, excessive flushing of fluid should be avoided to prevent transfer of fluid into the peritoneal cavity.

(d) *Adjacent organ injury*

In some animal studies, the reported rate of adjacent organ injury was up to 21.4% [70, 71]. However, in clinical practice, it appears the risk of organ injury is very low.

Submucosal Tunneling Endoscopic Resection (STER)

Since our group first described the STER technique in 2012, there has been evolving experience with this technique throughout the world [73]. This new technique was inspired by the success of peroral endoscopic myotomy (POEM) and was developed as an offshoot of natural orifice transluminal endoscopic surgery (NOTES).

STER is a minimally invasive technique for resection of esophageal or gastric cardia SETs. In contrast to conventional endoscopic procedures, this technique is unique given that it utilizes the submucosal space between the mucosal and muscular layers as a working channel for endoscopic insertion and resection of tumor [74–75].

The key advantage of STER over endoscopic submucosal dissection (ESD) is the ability to maintain mucosal integrity, promote rapid wound healing, and reduce the risk of postoperative GI leaks and cavitary infection compared to ESD. In STER, the mucosal incision is created proximal and away from the tumor site. A submucosal tunnel is created between the mucosal incision site and the tumor to avoid the risk of postoperative GI tract leakage and secondary infection. Therefore, it is crucial to maintain the integrity of the mucosal flap as a protective barrier. Standard ESD technique results in inevitable perforation and direct communication between the GI lumen and the mediastinum. Hence, GI leakage and cavitary infection are much higher [76]. STER permits an en bloc resection even for lesions extending beyond the muscularis propria layer into the extraluminal space where, traditionally, laparoscopic surgery was recommended to remove such tumors [77].

Indications and Contraindications for STER

There is currently no firm consensus on the precise indications for STER; however studies to date demonstrated that STER is indicated for subepithelial lesions (SEL) originating from the muscularis propria layer. For lesions located within the esophagus, the maximum tumor size ranges from 3.5 cm to 5.5 cm confirmed either on EUS or CT scan. For gastric lesions, most studies included tumor size of <3 cm without any high-risk EUS features [78–83].

The majority of resected tumors were leiomyomas or GI stromal tumors (GIST) with the minority including calcifying fibrous tumors, schwannomas, nerve sheath tumors, glomus tumors, intramuscular lipomas, aberrant pancreas, or granular cell tumors [84–89].

STER generally requires a 5 cm tunnel proximal to the location of the tumor [73]. Therefore, lesions located in the proximal (upper) esophagus may be challenging for STER to be performed. For gastric lesions, tumors in the gastric fundus and lesser curvature of the stomach were previously excluded [73].

We propose the following as indications of STER:

Absolute Indications
1. EUS and CT evidence of tumor arising from muscularis propria or extraluminal extension.
2. Diameter ≤ 5 cm. (The reason for limiting the lesion size to 5 cm is due to the narrow space of the submucosal tunnel.)
3. Tumor located in the mid-esophagus, lower esophagus, or cardioesophageal junction.

Absolute Contraindications
1. Severe cardiopulmonary disease (ASA ≥ 3)
2. Coagulation disorders, thrombocytopenic disorders, or on anticoagulant/antiplatelet therapy
3. Pregnancy.
4. Evidence of metastatic disease

We recommend that only skilled endoscopist with experience in ESD, ESE, and the management of perforation should perform STER.

Pre-procedural Assessment

Similar to EFTR, pre-procedural evaluation is crucial to assess the tumor characteristics, size, and location. Routine EUS examinations (high-frequency miniprobe, UM-2R, 12 MHz, UM-3R, 20 MHz; Olympus Optical Co., Ltd., Tokyo, Japan) are often performed: (1) to confirm that

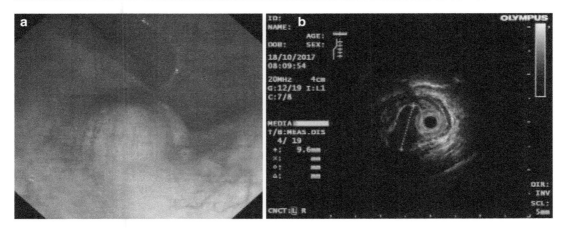

Fig. 9.8 EUS examinations for an esophageal SET. (**a**) An esophageal SET was found in the lower esophagus. (**b**) EUS showed the lesion originated from the MP layer

the tumors originated from the MP layer (Fig. 9.8), (2) to measure the maximum lesion size, (3) to observe the growth pattern of tumor (predominantly intraluminal or extraluminal growth), and (4) to initially distinguish benign from malignant lesions.

Sometimes, EUS-guided FNA is attempted to obtain histological diagnosis. However, the most challenging aspect in the diagnosis of SMTs by needle biopsy is the sampling error, which may show only focal areas of malignant change [85]. CT and/or MRI scan is used not only to assess the origin, size, and growth pattern of tumor but also to provide information of local invasion and distant metastasis.

STER Procedure (Video 9.2, Figs. 9.9 and 9.10)

Most of the equipment used for STER is similar to the tools used for POEM or EFTR as described above. A standard single accessory-channel gastroscope is used during procedure. A transparent cap is attached to the front of the endoscope. The patient is positioned left lateral, and the procedure is carried out under general anesthesia with endotracheal intubation. Prophylactic intravenous antibiotics (third-generation cephalosporin) are given 30 minutes before procedure. Figure 9.10 describes the five major steps in the STER technique [73].

Key Steps in STER Technique (Video 9.2, Fig. 9.10)

- *Step 1: Tumor location.*
  Identifying tumor location can be challenging especially when the tumor is not prominent and located within the deeper layer. Occasionally, prodding using the tip of a biopsy forceps may aid in identifying the surface of the subepithelial tumor.

- *Step 2: Creation of a submucosal tunnel to expose the tumor.*
  Once the subepithelial tumor is identified, submucosal injection using a mixture of saline, indigo carmine, and epinephrine is used to create a submucosal cushion and to expand the submucosal space at 5 cm proximal to the SMT. A 2 cm longitudinal mucosal incision is made using either a hook knife or hybrid knife to enter the third space (submucosal space).

  The submucosal space is used as a working channel. A submucosal longitudinal tunnel is created between the mucosal and muscular layers until the submucosal tumor is identified.

  During the creation of the submucosal tunnel, utmost care is required to avoid injuring the overlying mucosa by dissecting the submucosa closer to the muscularis propria. In addition, care is required to coagulate any

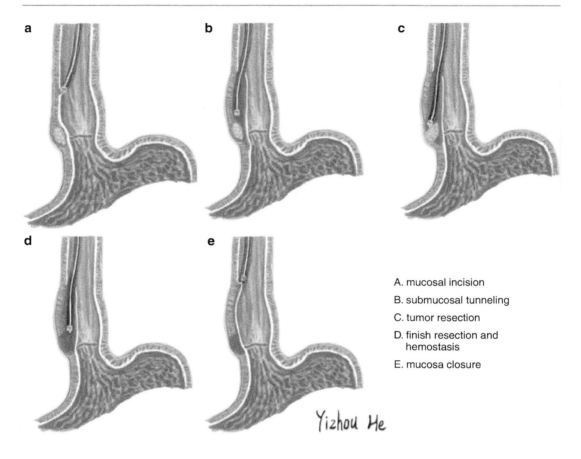

Fig. 9.9 STER technique. (**a**) Mucosal incision: a 2 cm longitudinal mucosal incision is made 5 cm proximal to the tumor. (**b**) Submucosal tunneling: a submucosal tunnel is created 5 cm proximal to and 1–2 cm distal to the tumor. (**c**) Tumor resection: the SMT is resected under direct endoscopic viewing. (**d**) Finished resection and hemostasis: when finishing tumor resection, we perform careful hemostasis of the MP defect and the tunnel. (**e**) Mucosal closure: the mucosal incision site is closed by using four to six hemostatic clips. (Reprinted from Xu et al. [73]. Copyright (2012), with permission from Elsevier)

visible vessel to prevent bleeding within the submucosal tunnel.

- *Step 3: Resection of the SMT under direct endoscopic view.*

  Once the tumor is identified, endoscopic resection of the SET is carried out using either IT knife, hook knife, or hybrid knife. The submucosal tissue is dissected around the tumor capsule. The submucosal tunneling should end at least 1–2 cm distal to the tumor to ensure there is enough working space for tumor resection. Utmost care is needed to avoid interruption of tumor capsule and not to damage the esophageal adventitia or gastric serosa. For extragastrointestinal tumor or tumor located within the deep muscularis propria layer or adjacent to the serosa, full-thickness GI wall dissection is necessary to ensure an en bloc tumor resection. A dual-channel gastroscope is occasionally needed to extract the tumor into submucosal tunnel using a grasping forceps to prevent tumor displacement into the peritoneal cavity. A snare can also be used to retrieve the tumor out of the submucosal tunnel. Care should be taken not to inadvertently resect the tumor during tumor retrieval.

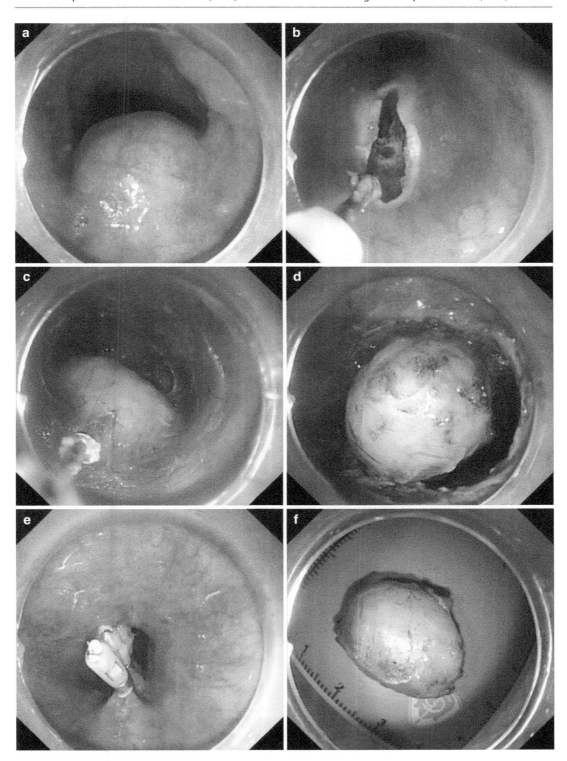

Fig. 9.10 Key major steps in STER technique. (**a**) A SET was found in the esophagus. (**b**, **c**) A submucosal tunnel was created 5 cm above the tumor location. (**d**) The tumor was dissected in the tunnel. (**e**) Several clips were used to seal the mucosal incision site. (**f**) The resected specimen

- *Step 4: Closure of the mucosal incision site.*
  Prior to closure of mucosal incision, close inspection of the submucosal tunnel and adequate hemostasis around the resected site is vital to ensure there is no bleeding into the abdominal cavity. The gastroscope is then withdrawn from the submucosal tunnel and the mucosal incision site is closed using several metallic clips.

Postoperative Care

Postoperative care is similar to that after EFTR. All patients are kept fasting for at least 24 hours and given intravenous proton pump inhibitor and prophylactic intravenous antibiotic. Radiological examinations, such as chest X-ray and CT chest, are routinely performed to assess for pneumothorax and/or hydrothorax after STER. Monitoring for any development of any post-procedure symptoms such as chest pain, dyspnea, abdominal pain, and abdominal distention is important and prompt management of any complications.

If patient remains asymptomatic on day 2, patient is upgraded to liquid diet and subsequently to full diet.

Patient Follow-Up

Patients are followed up with endoscopy and/or EUS at 1, 2, 4, 6, and 12 months after STER and annually thereafter to assess for residual tumor or tumor recurrence. For patients with tumors with malignant potential, a contrast-enhanced CT is performed on an annual basis to rule out distant metastasis.

Clinical Outcomes of STER

STER is becoming a convenient method for the removal of SMTs of the gastrointestinal tract, gaining a lot of attention in the past few years. Many studies came out in the last 6 years of which we included the most important ten studies in Table 9.3. The technical success of the STER reached up to 100% in almost all the studies with the en bloc resection rate around 90 %. The average time taken during the procedure is around 1 hour; meanwhile the size of the lesions included a mean of less than 3 cm [80]. The complications encountered after STER are mainly related to the air leak during tumor resection as pneumoperitoneum, pneumomediastinum, pneumothorax, and very rarely esophageal-pleural fistula [83, 84]. Long-term outcome trials are few, the largest one performed by Chen et al. which included 290 patients with 1 patient needing additional surgery, 2 patients lost for follow-up, and 178 patients who had no recurrence after a mean follow-up period of 36 months [86].

The use of the STER has recently extended for the resection of extraluminal lesions. Cai et al. recently published a study on the use of the STER to excise eight extraluminal lesions whether these lesions originated from the GI wall or just in close proximity to it [90]. The study showed complete resection in all cases with en bloc retrieval for 7 (87.5%.) cases. The complications were unremarkable apart from pneumoperitoneum, which is expected during tumor resection and was managed with decompression needle and a single case of mucosal injury that could be managed endoscopically [90].

Complications

There is a wide variation of reported complications across available studies to date. The complication rates vary from as low as 0% to as high as 42.9% [74, 75, 79–84, 86]. The most common reported complications included subcutaneous emphysema, pneumothorax, pneumomediastinum, pneumoperitoneum, and pleural effusion. There are reported cases of rare complications such as mucosal tunnel perforation, esophageal fistula, and diverticulum. Most of the adverse events can be managed conservatively with good outcomes. A study by Chen and colleagues demonstrated that adverse event rate was 23.4% and only half of these patients (10%) required an intervention to treat the complica-

Table 9.3 Clinical outcomes of STER

Study	N	Mean size (mm)	Site	Pathological diagnosis	Success (%)	En bloc (%)	Adverse events	Mean time (min)	Follow-up (m)
Xu et al. [73] (2012)	15	19 mm (13–30)	Esophagus (9) Cardia (3) Corpus (2) Antrum (1)	Leiomyoma (9) GIST (4) Glomus tumor (1)	100	100	Pneumoperitoneum (1) Pneumothorax (1)	78.7	6
Inoue et al. [87] (2012)	7	18.6	Esophagus (3) Cardia (4)	Leiomyoma (5) GIST (1) Ectopic pancreas (1)	100	100	No	152.4	5.5
Ye et al. [85] (2014)	85	19.2	Esophagus (60) Cardia (16) Corpus (9)	Leiomyoma (65) GIST (19) Calcifying fibrous tumor (1)	100	100	Pneumoperitoneum (4) Pneumothorax (6)	57.2	8
Zhang et al. [74] (2014)	23	15	Esophagus (21) Cardia (2)	Leiomyoma	100	100	Pneumomediastinum (3) Pneumothorax (2) Pleural effusion (1)	40	18
Lu et al. [75] (2014)	18	20.1	Fundus (18)	GIST (13) Leiomyoma (6)	100	100	Pneumoperitoneum (2)	75.1	5
Wang et al. [81] (2015)	80	23.2	Esophagus (67) Cardia (16)	Leiomyoma (68) GIST (15)	100	97.6	Pneumothorax (1) Chest pain (3)	61.2	10.2
Zhou et al. [80] (2015)	21	23	Cardia (21)	Leiomyoma (15) GIST (6)	100	100	Mediastinal emphysema (9)	62.9	12
Li et al. [79] (2015)	32	23	Corpus (18) Fundus (3) Antrum (11)	Leiomyoma (18) GIST (11) Calcifying fibrous tumor (1) Glomus tumor (1) Schwannoma (1)	100	100	Pneumoperitoneum (6) Pneumothorax (3) Bleeding (1)	51.8	28
Chen et al. [86] (2016)	290	21	Esophagus (199) Cardia (68) Stomach (23)	Leiomyoma (226) GIST (53) Calcifying fibrous tumor (23) Schwannoma (3) Glomus tumor (3)	100	89.3	Pneumothorax (22) Major bleeding (5) Mucosal injury (3) Esophageal-pleural fistula (1)	43	36
Cai et al. [90] (2018)	8	28	Extraluminal (8)	GIST (6) Schwannoma (1) Foregut cyst (1)	100	87.5	Pneumoperitoneum (5) Mucosal injury (1)	67	10

STER submucosal tunneling endoscopic resection, *N* number of patients, *mm* millimeters, *min* minutes, *m* months, *GIST* gastrointestinal stromal tumors

tions [72]. On the other hand, Wang and colleagues reported a lower complication rate of 8.8% and none required any intervention to treat the complications [84].

Summary

Over the last few years, an increasing number of patients are being treated with STER and EFTR at our center. In expert hands STER and EFTR appear promising and safe with minimal procedure-related complications. Both techniques are regarded as minimally invasive treatment options for en bloc resection of GI SETs arising from muscularis propria layer. In the future, as we accumulate more experience, we will have more long-term data to establish the long-term outcome of such techniques.

References

1. Sakamoto H, Kitano M, Kudo M. Diagnosis of subepithelial tumors in the upper gastrointestinal tract by endoscopic ultrasonography. World J Radiol. 2010;2:289–97.
2. North JH, Pack MS. Malignant tumors of the small intestine: a review of 144 cases. Am Surg. 2000;66:46–51.
3. Seno K, Itoh M, Endoh K, et al. Schwannoma of the duodenum causing melena. Intern Med. 1994;33:621–3.
4. Cesaretti M, Sulpice L, Farges O. Gastrointestinal bleeding from a submucosal duodenal tumor. Surgery. 2016;159:670–1.
5. Rosch T, Sarbia M, Schumacher B, et al. Attempted endoscopic en bloc resection of mucosal and submucosal tumors using insulated-tip knives: a pilot series. Endoscopy. 2004;36:788–801.
6. Shi Q, Zhong YS, Yao LQ, et al. Endoscopic submucosal dissection for treatment of esophageal submucosal tumors originating from the muscularis propria layer. Gastrointest Endosc. 2011;74:1194–200.
7. Li QL, Yao LQ, Zhou PH, et al. Submucosal tumors of the esophagogastric junction originating from the muscularis propria layer: a large study of endoscopic submucosal dissection (with video). Gastrointest Endosc. 2012;75:1153–8.
8. Sumiyama K, Gostout CJ. Novel techniques and instrumentation for EMR, ESD, and full-thickness endoscopic luminal resection. Gastrointest Endosc Clin N Am. 2007;17:471–85.
9. Bialek A, Wiechowska-Kozlowska A, Huk J. Endoscopic submucosal dissection of large gastric stromal tumor arising from muscularis propria. Clin Gastroenterol Hepatol. 2010;8:119–20.
10. Chun SY, Kim KO, Park DS, et al. Endoscopic submucosal dissection as a treatment for gastric subepithelial tumors that originate from the muscularis propria layer: a preliminary analysis of appropriate indications. Surg Endosc. 2013;27:3271–9.
11. He Z, Sun C, Wang J, et al. Efficacy and safety of endoscopic submucosal dissection in treating gastric subepithelial tumors originating in the muscularis propria layer: a single-center study of 144 cases. Scand J Gastroenterol. 2013;48:1466–73.
12. Lee IL, Lin PY, Tung SY, et al. Endoscopic submucosal dissection for the treatment of intraluminal gastric subepithelial tumors originating from the muscularis propria layer. Endoscopy. 2006;38:1024–8.
13. Li L, Wang F, Wu B, et al. Endoscopic submucosal dissection of gastric fundus subepithelial tumors originating from the muscularis propria. Exp Ther Med. 2013;6:391–5.
14. Meng FS, Zhang ZH, Shan GD, et al. Endoscopic submucosal dissection for the treatment of large gastric submucosal tumors originating from the muscularis propria layer: a single center study. Z Gastroenterol. 2015;53:655–9.
15. Zhang S, Chao GQ, Li M, et al. Endoscopic submucosal dissection for treatment of gastric submucosal tumors originating from the muscularis propria layer. Dig Dis Sci. 2013;58:1710–6.
16. Liu BR, Song JT, Qu B, et al. Endoscopic muscularis dissection for upper gastrointestinal subepithelial tumors originating from the muscularis propria. Surg Endosc. 2012;26:3141–8.
17. Chu YY, Lien JM, Tsai MH, et al. Modified endoscopic submucosal dissection with enucleation for treatment of gastric subepithelial tumors originating from the muscularis propria layer. BMC Gastroenterol. 2012;12:124.
18. Reinehr R. Endoscopic submucosal excavation (ESE) is a safe and useful technique for endoscopic removal of submucosal tumors of the stomach and the esophagus in selected cases. Z Gastroenterol. 2015;53:573–8.
19. Ye LP, Zhu LH, Zhou XB, et al. Endoscopic excavation for the treatment of small esophageal subepithelial tumors originating from the muscularis propria. Hepato-Gastroenterology. 2015;62:65–8.
20. Huang Q, Zhu LH, et al. Endoscopic excavation for gastric heterotopic pancreas: an analysis of 42 cases from a tertiary center. Wien Klin Wochenschr. 2014;126:509–14.
21. Zhang Y, Ye LP, Zhou XB, et al. Safety and efficacy of endoscopic excavation for gastric subepithelial tumors originating from the muscularis propria layer: results from a large study in China. J Clin Gastroenterol. 2013;47:689–94.
22. Zhang Y, Ye LP, Zhu LH, et al. Endoscopic muscularis excavation for subepithelial tumors of the esophago-

gastric junction originating from the muscularis propria layer. Dig Dis Sci. 2013;58:1335–40.

23. Suzuki H, Okuwaki S, Ikeda K, et al. Endoscopic full-thickness resection (EFTR) and waterproof defect closure (ENDC) for improvement of curability and safety in endoscopic treatment of early gastrointestinal malignancies. Prog Dig Endosc. 1998;52:49–53.

24. Zhou PH, Yao LQ, Qin XY, et al. Endoscopic full-thickness resection without laparoscopic assistance for gastric submucosal tumors originated from the muscularis propria. Surg Endosc. 2011;25:2926–31.

25. Xu M, Wang XY, Zhou PH, et al. Endoscopic full-thickness resection of colonic submucosal tumors originating from the muscularis propria: an evolving therapeutic strategy. Endoscopy. 2013;45:770–3.

26. Huang LY, Cui J, Lin SJ, et al. Endoscopic full-thickness resection for gastric submucosal tumors arising from the muscularis propria layer. World J Gastroenterol. 2014;20:13981–6.

27. Feng Y, Yu L, Yang S, et al. Endolumenal endoscopic full-thickness resection of muscularis propria-originating gastric submucosal tumors. J Laparoendosc Adv Surg Tech A. 2014;24(3):171–6.

28. Yang F, Wang S, Sun S, et al. Factors associated with endoscopic full-thickness resection of gastric submucosal tumors. Surg Endosc. 2015;29:3588–93.

29. Guo J, Liu Z, Sun S, et al. Endoscopic full-thickness resection with defect closure using an over-the-scope clip for gastric subepithelial tumors originating from the muscularis propria. Surg Endosc. 2015;29:3356.

30. Wang L, Ren W, Fan CQ, et al. Full-thickness endoscopic resection of nonintracavitary gastric stromal tumors: a novel approach. Surg Endosc. 2011;25:641–7.

31. Walz MK, Alesina PF, Wenger FA, et al. Laparoscopic and retroperitoneoscopic treatment of pheochromocytomas and retroperitoneal paragangliomas: results of 161 tumors in 126 patients. World J Surg. 2006;30:899–908.

32. Schmidt A, Meier B, Caca K. Endoscopic full-thickness resection: current status. World J Gastroenterol. 2015;21:9273–85.

33. Zhou PH, Yao LQ, Qin XYE. Endoscopic full-thickness resection (EFTR). In: Atlas of digestive endoscopic resection. Netherlands: Springer; 2014. p. 218–39.

34. Abe N, Takeuchi H, Shibuya M, et al. Successful treatment of duodenal carcinoid tumor by laparoscopy-assisted endoscopic full-thickness resection with lymphadenectomy. Asian J Endosc Surg. 2012;5:81–5.

35. Schmidt A, Meier B, Cahyadi O, et al. Duodenal endoscopic full- thickness resection (with video). Gastrointest Endosc. 2015;82:728–33.

36. Schmidt A, Damm M, Caca K. Endoscopic full-thickness resection using a novel over-the-scope device. Gastroenterology. 2014;147:740–2.

37. Fahndrich M, Sandmann M. Endoscopic full-thickness resection for gastrointestinal lesions using the over-the-scope clip system: a case series. Endoscopy. 2015;47:76–9.

38. Schmidt A, Bauerfeind P, Gubler C, et al. Endoscopic full-thickness resection in the colorectum with a novel over-the-scope device: first experience. Endoscopy. 2015;47:719–25.

39. Richter-Schrag HJ, Walker C, Thimme R, et al. Full thickness resection device (FTRD). Experience and outcome for benign neoplasms of the rectum and colon. Chirurg. 2016;87:316–25.

40. Andrisani G, Pizzicannella M, Martino M, et al. Endoscopic full-thickness resection of superficial colorectal neoplasms using a new over- scope clip system: a single-centre study. Dig Liver Dis. 2017;49:1009–13.

41. Al-Bawardy B, Rajan E, Wong Kee Song LM. Over-the-scope clip-assisted endoscopic full-thickness resection of epithelial and subepithelial GI lesions. Gastrointest Endosc. 2017;85:1087–92.

42. Dinelli M, Omazzi B, Andreozzi P, et al. First clinical experiences with a novel endoscopic over-the-scope clip system. Endosc Int Open. 2017;5:151–6.

43. Schmidt AR, Meining A, Birk M, et al. Abstract no. 54: endoscopic full-thickness resection in the colorectum using an over-the-scope device—interim results of a prospective multicenter study. Gastrointest Endosc. 2016;83.(Suppl:AB119.

44. Vitali F, Naegel A, Siebler J, Neurath MF, Rath T. Endoscopic full-thickness resection with an over-the-scope clip device (FTRD) in the colorectum: results from a university tertiary referral center. Endosc Int Open. 2018;6(1):98–103.

45. Schostek S, Ho CN, Melbert M, et al. DC current pulses for OTSC clip fragmentation: technology and experimental study. Surg Endosc. 2015;29:2418–22.

46. Schmidt A, Riecken B, Damm M, et al. Endoscopic removal of over-the-scope clips using a novel cutting device: a retrospective case series. Endoscopy. 2014;46:762–6.

47. Aepli P, Criblez D, Baumeler S, et al. Endoscopic full thickness resection (EFTR) of colorectal neoplasms with the full thickness resection device (FTRD): clinical experience from two tertiary referral centers in Switzerland. United Euro Gastro J. 2018;6(3):463–70.

48. Joensuu H. Risk stratification of patients diagnosed with gastrointestinal stromal tumor. Hum Pathol. 2008;39:1411–9.

49. Casali PG, Jost L, Reichardt P, et al. Gastrointestinal stromal tumours: ESMO clinical recommendations for diagnosis, treatment and follow-up. Ann Oncol. 2009;20:64–7.

50. Blackstein ME, Blay JY, Corless C, et al. Gastrointestinal stromal tumours: consensus statement on diagnosis and treatment. Can J Gastroenterol. 2006;20:157–63.

51. Fukami Y, Kurumiya Y, Mizuno K, et al. A 12-mm carcinoid tumor of the minor duodenal papilla with lymph node metastases. Jpn J Clin Oncol. 2013;43:74–7.

52. Demetri GD, Benjamin RS, Blanke CD, et al. NCCN task force report: optimal management of patients with gastrointestinal stromal tumor (GIST)—update of NCCN clinical practice guidelines. J Natl Compr Cancer Netw. 2007:1–26.

53. Soga J. Endocrinocarcinomas (carcinoids and their variants) of the duodenum. An evaluation of 927 cases. J Exp Clin Cancer Res. 2003;22:349–63.

54. Binmoeller KF, Grimm H, Soehendra N. Endoscopic closure of a perforation using metallic clips after snare excision of a gastric leiomyoma. Gastrointest Endosc. 1993;39(2):172–4.

55. Minami S, Gotoda T, Ono H, Oda I, Hamanaka H. Complete endoscopic closure of gastric perforation induced by endoscopic resection of early gastric cancer using endoclips can prevent surgery (with video). Gastrointest Endosc. 2006;63(4):596–601.

56. Matsuda T, Fujii T, Emura F, Kozu T, Saito Y, Ikematsu H, et al. Complete closure of a large defect after EMR of a lateral spreading colorectal tumor when using a two-channel colonoscope. Gastrointest Endosc. 2004;60(5):836–8.

57. Shi Q, Chen T, Zhong YS, Zhou PH, Ren Z, Xu MD, et al. Complete closure of large gastric defects after endoscopic full-thickness resection, using endoloop and metallic clip interrupted suture. Endoscopy. 2013;45(5):329–34.

58. Hashiba K, Carvalho AM, Diniz G Jr, Barbosa de Aridrade N, Guedes CA, Siqueira Filho L, et al. Experimental endoscopic repair of gastric perforations with an omental patch and clips. Gastrointest Endosc. 2001;54(4):500–4.

59. Dray X, Giday SA, Buscaglia JM, Gabrielson KL, Kantsevoy SV, Magno P, et al. Omentoplasty for gastrotomy closure after natural orifice transluminal endoscopic surgery procedures (with video). Gastrointest Endosc. 2009;70(1):131–40.

60. Kratt T, Kuper M, Traub F, Ho CN, Schurr MO, Konigsrainer A, et al. Feasibility study for secure closure of natural orifice transluminal endoscopic surgery gastrotomies by using over-the-scope clips. Gastrointest Endosc. 2008;68(5):993–6.

61. Kirschniak A, Kratt T, Stuker D, Braun A, Schurr MO, Konigsrainer A. A new endoscopic over-the-scope clip system for treatment of lesions and bleeding in the GI tract: first clinical experiences. Gastrointest Endosc. 2007;66(1):162–7.

62. Ozawa S, Yoshida M, Kumai K, Kitajima M. New endoscopic treatments for gastroesophageal reflux disease. Ann Thorac Cardiovasc Surg. 2005;11:146–53.

63. Ye LP, Yu Z, Mao XL, Zhu LH, Zhou XB. Endoscopic full-thickness resection with defect closure using clips and an endoloop for gastric subepithelial tumors arising from the muscularis propria. Surg Endosc. 2014;28:1978–83.

64. Zhang Y, Wang X, Xiong G, Qian Y, Wang H, Liu L, Miao L, Fan Z. Complete defect closure of gastric submucosal tumors with purse-string sutures. Surg Endosc. 2014;28:1844–51.

65. Moran EA, Gostout CJ, Bingener J. Preliminary performance of a flexible cap and catheter-based endoscopic suturing system. Gastrointest Endosc. 2009;69:1375–83.

66. Chiu PW, Phee SJ, Wang Z, Sun Z, Poon CC, Yamamoto T, Penny I, Wong JY, Lau JY, Ho KY. Feasibility of full-thickness gastric resection using master and slave transluminal endoscopic robot and closure by Overstitch: a preclinical study. Surg Endosc. 2014;28:319–24.

67. Kantsevoy SV, Bitner M, Mitrakov AA, Thuluvath PJ. Endoscopic suturing closure of large mucosal defects after endoscopic submucosal dissection is technically feasible, fast, and eliminates the need for hospitalization (with videos). Gastrointest Endosc. 2014;79:503–7.

68. Rajan E, Gostout CJ, Bonin EA, Moran EA, Locke RG, Szarka LA, Talley NJ, Deters JL, Miller CA, Knipschield MA, Lurken MS, Stotlz GJ, Bernard CE, Grover M, Farrugia G. Endoscopic full-thickness biopsy of the gastric wall with defect closure by using an endoscopic suturing device: survival porcine study. Gastrointest Endosc. 2012;76:1014–9.

69. Schmidt A, Bauder M, Riecken B, Caca K. Endoscopic resection of subepithelial tumors. World J Gastrointest Endosc. 2014;6:592–9.

70. Mahmood Z, Ang YS. EndoCinch treatment for gastro-oesophageal reflux disease. Digestion. 2007;76:241–7.

71. Mori H, Kobara H, Fujihara S, Nishiyama N, Rafiq K, Oryu M, Fujiwara M, Suzuki Y, Masaki T. Feasibility of pure EFTR using an innovative new endoscopic suturing device: the double-arm-bar suturing system (with video). Surg Endosc. 2014;28:683–90.

72. Sumiyama K, Gostout CJ, Rajan E, Bakken TA, Deters JL, Knipschield MA. Endoscopic full-thickness closure of large gastric perforations by use of tissue anchors. Gastrointest Endosc. 2007;65(1):134–9.

73. Xu MD, Cai MY, Zhou PH, et al. Submucosal tunneling endoscopic resection: a new technique for treating upper GI submucosal tumors originating from the muscularis propria layer (with videos). Gastrointest Endosc. 2012;75:195–9.

74. Zhang C, Hu JW, Chen T, et al. Submucosal tunnelling endoscopic resection for upper gastrointestinal multiple submucosal tumors originating from the muscular propria layer. A feasibility study. Indian J Cancer. 2014;51:52–5.

75. Lu J, Jiao T, Zheng M, et al. Endoscopic resection of submucosal tumors in muscularis propria: the choice between direct excavation and tunneling resection. Surg Endosc. 2014;28:3401–7.

76. Tao C, Zhou PH, Chu Y, et al. Long-term outcomes of submucosal tunneling endoscopic resection for upper gastrointestinal submucosal tumors. Ann Surg. 2017;265:363–9.

77. Jeong ES, Hong SJ, Han JP, Kwak JJ. Submucosal tunneling endoscopic resection of a leiomyoma originating from the muscularis propria of the gastric car-

dia (with video). Korean J Gastroenterol. 2015;66: 340–4.

78. Lu J, Zheng M, Jiao T, Wang Y, Lu X. Transcardiac tunneling technique for endoscopic submucosal dissection of gastric fundus tumors arising from the muscularis propria. Endoscopy. 2014;46:888–92.

79. Li QL, Chen WF, Zhang C, et al. Clinical impact of submucosal tunneling endoscopic resection for the treatment of gastric submucosal tumors originating from the muscularis propria layer (with video). Surg Endosc. 2015;29:3640–6.

80. Zhou DJ, Dai ZB, Wells MM, Yu DL, Zhang J, Zhang L. Submucosal tunneling and endoscopic resection of submucosal tumors at the esophagogastric junction. World J Gastroenterol. 2015;21:578–83.

81. Wang XY, Xu MD, Yao LQ, et al. Submucosal tunneling endoscopic resection for submucosal tumors of the esophagogastric junction originating from the muscularis propria layer: a feasibility study (with videos). Surg Endosc. 2014;28:1971–7.

82. Tan Y, Lv L, Duan T, et al. Comparison between submucosal tunneling endoscopic resection and video-assisted thoracoscopic surgery for large esophageal leiomyoma originating from the muscularis propria layer. Surg Endosc. 2016;30:3121–7.

83. Liu H, Wei LL, Zhang YZ, et al. Submucosal tunnelling endoscopic resection (STER) for the treatment of a case of huge esophageal tumor arising in the muscularis propria: a case report and review of literature. Int J Clin Exp Med. 2015;8:15846–51.

84. Wang H, Tan Y, Zhou Y, et al. Submucosal tunneling endoscopic resection for upper gastrointestinal submucosal tumors originating from the muscularis propria layer. Eur J Gastroenterol Hepatol. 2015;27:776–80.

85. Ye LP, Zhang Y, Mao XL, Zhu LH, Zhou X, Chen JY. Submucosal tunneling endoscopic resection for small upper gastrointestinal subepithelial tumors originating from the muscularis propria layer. Surg Endosc. 2014;28:524–30.

86. Chen T, Zhang C, Yao LQ, et al. Management of the complications of submucosal tunneling endoscopic resection for upper gastrointestinal submucosal tumors. Endoscopy. 2016;48:149–55.

87. Inoue H, Ikeda H, Hosoya T, et al. Submucosal endoscopic tumor resection for subepithelial tumors in the esophagus and cardia. Endoscopy. 2012;44:225–30.

88. Costache M-I, Iordache S, Karstensen JG, Săftoiu A, Vilmann P. Endoscopic ultrasound-guided fine needle aspiration: from the past to the future. Endosc Ultrasound. 2013;2(2):77–85.

89. Chen H, Xu Z, Huo J, Liu D. Submucosal tunneling endoscopic resection for simultaneous esophageal and cardia submucosal tumors originating from the muscularis propria layer (with video). Dig Endosc. 2015;27:155–8.

90. Cai MY, Zhu BQ, Qin WZ, et al. Submucosal tunnel endoscopic resection for extraluminal tumors: a novel endoscopic method for en bloc resection of predominant extraluminal growing subepithelial tumors or extra-gastrointestinal tumors (with videos). Gastrointest Endosc. 2018;2:160. https://doi.org/10.1016/j.gie.2018.02.032.

Fayez Sarkis, Vijay Kanakadandi,
Mojtaba S. Olyaee, and Amit Rastogi

Colon Polyps

Large colon adenomas, generally defined as those ≥20 mm in size, are associated with a high risk of progression to invasive cancer [1]. These lesions are commonly referred to as lateral spreading tumor (LST) in the literature. With rapid advancements in our endoscopic armamentarium and refinements in endoscopic resection techniques, there has been a shift in the management of LST over the last couple of decades. Endoscopic resection of these lesions is now considered the standard practice as opposed to surgery. It is associated with a lower cost, morbidity, and length of hospitalization compared to surgical resection [2]. Additionally, using validated scores, it has been predicted that surgical removal of large polyps would carry a 3% mortality rate compared to no mortality observed with endoscopic resection [3]. Furthermore, in a population-based study using the SEER database, endoscopic treatment and surgery showed comparable mid- and long-term cancer-free survival rates in patients with malignant colorectal polyps without invasive cancer [4].

Endoscopic mucosal resection (EMR) and endoscopic submucosal dissection (ESD) are the two techniques for removal of LST. EMR is defined as an endoscopic technique for the removal of sessile and flat neoplasms confined to the superficial layers of the GI tract. EMR uses a snare for the removal of LST either en bloc or in a piecemeal fashion. It may involve submucosal injection of fluidlike saline to separate the mucosal lesion from the muscularis propria. ESD, on the other hand, involves removal of the lesion en bloc. After submucosal injection of fluid, meticulous dissection is performed in the deep submucosal plane using a variety of different kinds of knives. This en bloc and potential R0 resection (microscopically margin negative) ensures lower residual/recurrence rates on follow-up and facilitates a more reliable and accurate evaluation of the histopathology specimen, especially if there is invasive cancer. As a result ESD may afford a potential cure for even LST with early invasive cancer. These have been the main arguments set forth by the proponents of ESD. Fragmentation of the lesion associated with piecemeal EMR may lead to suboptimal histologic assessment when invasive cancer is present with respect to the depth of invasion and also whether the lateral and deep margins are clear [5].

Although, with these inherent advantages, it may seem that ESD should be the preferred strategy compared to EMR for removing LST, there are several other aspects that merit discussion in

F. Sarkis · V. Kanakadandi · M. S. Olyaee
A. Rastogi (✉)
Department of Gastroenterology and Hepatology, The University of Kansas Hospital, Kansas City, KS, USA
e-mail: fsarkis@kumc.edu; vkanakadandi@kumc.edu; Molyaee@kumc.edu; arastogi@kumc.edu

© Springer Nature Switzerland AG 2020
M. S. Wagh, S. B. Wani (eds.), *Gastrointestinal Interventional Endoscopy*,
https://doi.org/10.1007/978-3-030-21695-5_10

this debate. Herein, we review the pros and cons of these two procedures for removal of LST with respect to different factors like resection rate, recurrence, adverse events, costs, and procedural complexity.

Resection Rates and Recurrence

A meta-analysis of studies comparing ESD and EMR determined that the rate of en bloc resection of sessile or flat colorectal lesions >20 mm was 90% for ESD compared to 35% for EMR [relative risk (RR) = 1.93; $p < 0.001$] [6]. The same study reported that the rate of R0 resection or curative resection was 79.6% in the ESD group and 36.2% in the EMR group (RR 2.01; $p < 0.001$). The recurrence rate after ESD (0.7%) was significantly lower than after EMR (12.7%), with an overall RR of 0.06 (95% CI 0.03–0.11; $p < 0.001$). Similar results were reported by another meta-analysis [7]. The rate of en bloc resection for ESD was 91.7% compared to 46.7% with EMR, with an odds ratio (OR) of 6.84 (95% CI 3.3–14.18). The rates of curative resection were 80.3% with ESD and 42.3% with EMR, odds ratio of 4.26 (95% CI 3.77–6.57). Rates of recurrence were 0.9% for ESD and 12.2% for EMR (OR 0.08, 95% CI 0.04–0.17). These data would support the use of ESD for these lesions. However, patients undergoing endoscopic resection are typically followed up with a repeat colonoscopy in 3–6 months followed by another one 12 months later. The residual/recurrent adenomas after EMR are usually small and diminutive and can be easily removed on follow-up colonoscopy in majority of the cases. This was shown in a large prospective study evaluating the long-term adenoma recurrence after wide-field EMR. Out of 1000 successful EMRs of lesions ≥20 mm, 799 patients underwent follow-up surveillance colonoscopy at 4 months. Residual/recurrent adenoma was detected in 16% (128) and was diminutive in 72% of these cases. Furthermore, of the 670 patients with normal exam at 4 months, 426 patients underwent second follow-up colonoscopy at 16 months. Late recurrence of adenoma was seen in 17 (4%) patients. Of the total

145 (128 + 17) patients with residual/recurrent adenomas on follow-up, endoscopic treatment was successful in 135 cases (93.1%). Therefore, after initial successful EMR, 98.1% of the patients were adenoma- free and were able to avoid surgery at 16 months [8]. It is important to note that none of the recurrences had cancer. So although EMR may have initial higher rates of residual/recurrent adenoma, but with follow-up colonoscopies, high rates of complete resection can be achieved that are comparable to ESD. One could also argue that patients who would not or may not return for a follow-up colonoscopy after EMR may benefit from ESD of the lesion at the outset, given the lower rates of residual/recurrence.

LST with Submucosal Invasive Cancer

Another central argument favoring the use of ESD over EMR is the possibility of achieving curative or R0 resection in adenomas with invasive cancer limited to the submucosa (T1 disease). This is primarily because pathologists cannot reliably confirm adequacy of resection in terms of negative lateral and deep margins when the lesion is removed and submitted in multiple pieces that are not oriented, as is the case with piecemeal EMR. Resection in one piece by ESD therefore provides superior histologic assessment for the adequacy of resection as well as the precise depth of invasion by cancer. However, even for LST with cancer invading the submucosa, ESD can be considered curative for only a subset. In a meta-analysis of patients diagnosed with T1 adenocarcinoma, the incidence of lymph node metastasis was determined to be 11.4%, the risk being higher among those with lymphovascular invasion, tumor budding, and submucosal invasion of greater than 1000 μm [9]. As the lesions with these poor prognostic features have a significant risk for lymph node metastasis, they would warrant a surgical resection for removal of locoregional nodes, even if the lesion itself was removed successfully by ESD. Therefore, ESD can essentially be deemed curative for lesions with cancer limited to the submucosa and without any of the abovementioned high-risk features [10].

In order to appropriately triage lesions to EMR, ESD, or surgery, endoscopists have to assess for presence of submucosal invasive cancer which can be either evident or covert. A prospective, single-center, cohort study identified endoscopic features associated with the presence of submucosal invasive cancer in LST [11]. These include the presence of Kudo pit pattern V, a depressed component (Paris 0–IIc), rectosigmoid location, 0–Is or 0–IIa + Is Paris classification, non-granular surface morphology, and increasing size. Of these the two strongest predictors of submucosal invasive cancer were Kudo pit pattern V and depressed lesion (Paris 0–IIc). After excluding lesions that had obvious submucosal invasive cancer on endoscopic evaluation, i.e., those with Kudo pit pattern V and depressed component, factors found to be associated with covert submucosal invasive cancer were rectosigmoid location, 0–Is or combined Paris classification, non-granular surface morphology, and increasing size (> 5 cm). It is these select lesions with increased risk of covert malignancy where en bloc resection with ESD may have diagnostic and therapeutic superiority over EMR. Furthermore, it is not clear if there are any strong predictors to differentiate between lesion with superficial and deep invasive submucosal cancer. Therefore if these lesions are removed by ESD and then found to have deep invasive cancer on histopathology, then surgery would still be required to resect the locoregional nodes to decrease the risk of metastatic spread. Risk stratification of lesions based on these features is not perfect, but provides a practical guide in decision-making regarding optimal treatment strategy. While lesions with overt features of invasive cancer should be referred for surgical resection, LST without endoscopic features of overt or covert invasive cancer can be effectively removed by piecemeal EMR as the pathologist is not hampered by the presented multiple disoriented pieces, in the absence of cancer.

With that being said, the crucial question that arises is – how common are these lesions with early submucosal cancer and without the poor prognostic features? The prevalence of these was 3% among lesions ≥20 mm in one study [12]. A recent meta-analysis compiled all colorectal ESD series reporting the histology of dissected lesions. Data on 11,260 colorectal lesions from 51 studies were included [13]. Submucosal cancer was seen in 15.7% lesions, but only 8% had invasion depth of ≤1000 μm. Therefore, the number needed to treat (NNT) by ESD to avoid one surgery would be 12.5. Furthermore, the authors estimated that if the oncologic curative rate was 75% for malignant lesions, the rate of curative resection lowered to 6% with the NNT rising to 16.7. These data highlight that only a select group of lesions benefit from being removed by ESD, i.e., those with invasive cancer and without poor prognostic features. This remains the main counter-argument for proponents of EMR, questioning the indiscriminate use of ESD for all large colonic LST. A selective ESD approach appears to be more justifiable.

Adverse Events

The overall risk of perforation is significantly higher for ESD, estimated to be 4.9%–5.7% compared to 0.9–1.4% with EMR [6, 7]. There is no significant difference in the overall rate of bleeding, ranging from 1.9% to 2% for ESD and 2.9% to 3.5% for EMR [6, 7]. The risk of surgery due to procedural complications, such as perforation, was reported to be significantly higher in the ESD group compared to patients undergoing EMR (3% vs. 0.4%; $p < 0.001$) [6].

Cost

Per procedure, ESD is more expensive than EMR. It is associated with a greater use of endoscopy time, equipment, and anesthesia resources and usually requires inpatient hospital stay. A cost-effectiveness analysis was performed taking into account individual procedural cost, need for follow-up endoscopy, and cost associated with surgery either due to recurrent adenoma or procedural complications [12]. Assuming a 100%

R0 resection with ESD, it was estimated that, per 1000 lesions, the cost of ESD was US $ 6.9 million compared to US $ 4.3 million for EMR. The most cost effective strategy was selective use of ESD for high-risk lesions and use of EMR for the rest. This strategy was estimated to cost US$ 4.2 million. Sensitivity analysis was performed to evaluate the impact of various scenarios on the cost. Even after assuming a higher rate of recurrence after EMR, the cost rose only to US$ 4.7 million. The inclusion of nonmedical costs increased the cost of EMR and ESD per 1000 procedures to US$ 5.3 and US$ 8.3 million, respectively. It was noted that across all the scenarios, the selective utilization of ESD remained the most cost-effective strategy. With the current trends in rising healthcare costs and depleting healthcare resources, endoscopists must be mindful of delivering the most cost-effective care. With that aim, ESD can be justified only in a minority of colorectal LST and will be a superfluous enterprise in the majority.

Procedural Complexity and Other Challenges for the Adoption of ESD in the West

ESD is a complex and time-consuming procedure that originated in Japan and is routinely performed in other Asian countries in both the upper and lower gastrointestinal tract [14]. It is technically more challenging and tedious compared to EMR, and this is reflected in the duration of these respective procedures. A meta-analysis determined that the mean procedure duration for an EMR was 29–30 minutes, while that for ESD ranged from 66 to 108 minutes [7]. Of all the regions in the GI tract, the stomach is probably the safest to learn ESD. As early gastric cancer is more common in Japan, it affords the Japanese endoscopist the opportunity to learn and master the technical aspects of ESD that can then be extended to other regions like the colon. Proficiency can be achieved during fellowship under expert mentors. On the other hand, early gastric lesions are much less common in the West, and therefore the Western endoscopists are limited in the opportunities to learn ESD and hone their skills. They are also handicapped by the lack of experts in ESD in the west. Those wishing to learn ESD have to start with the basics on animal models, attend hands on workshops, or travel to expert centers in Asia. Given the steep learning curve of ESD, these issues continue to be a challenge for the Western endoscopists who have significantly lower rates of en bloc (81.2% versus 93%) and R0 (71.3% versus 85.6%) resections compared to their Asian colleagues [13]. Studies have demonstrated a significant learning curve associated with this ESD before acceptable rates of R0 resection, complications, and procedure duration can be achieved [15, 16]. Although the number of procedures required for achieving proficiency will vary between endoscopists, data from Japan indicate that at least 40 procedures are required for gastric ESD and 80 for colonic ESD [17]. It is recommended to start training in animal models followed by its application in gastric lesions that are more forgiving due to the thick muscularis layer [10, 18].

EMR, on the other hand, is more routinely performed in the West and requires less additional training with a less steep learning curve. It is an outpatient procedure that does not require hospital stay as opposed to ESD where hospitalization is routinely recommended. Compounding these issues is the fact that adverse event rates are higher with ESD compared to EMR as outlined above. This is of relevance given the medicolegal climate in the USA. Furthermore, there is no specific CPT (Common Procedural Terminology) code for ESD in the USA, denying any financial incentive for the endoscopist. Given the higher risk and technical complexity, lower financial gain, and increased expense associated with ESD procedures in the USA, their uptake by even expert endoscopists has been and will continue to be a challenge [19]. EMR will continue to be the preferred option for the vast majority of LST. Hybrid technique that involves a circumferential incision around the lesion as in ESD followed by en bloc EMR, other methods to shorten the ESD learning curves, and tools to make ESD faster and easier may encourage more Western endoscopists to adopt this procedure in the future [19].

Summary

In conclusion, both EMR and ESD are effective procedures for endoscopic resection of LST in the colon and avoid surgery. EMR is technically easier and faster to perform and is associated with lower risk of complications and lower costs compared to ESD. While ESD is a more complex procedure that requires more extensive training, its main advantage over EMR is for colorectal lesions that have invasive cancer limited to <1000 μm of the submucosa and without lymphovascular invasion or tumor budding. For this select subset of lesions, en bloc resection by ESD may be considered curative given the low risk of lymph node metastasis. While piecemeal EMR of these lesions will require referral for surgery, as the pathologist cannot reliably comment on the depth of submucosal invasion or completeness of resection given the fragmented and poorly oriented nature of the piecemeal EMR specimen. Since these lesions represent only a small proportion of large LST, the vast majority can therefore be effectively managed by EMR. The other advantage of ESD is the higher rates of en bloc resection and lower risk of residual/recurrent adenoma on follow-up. This advantage over piecemeal EMR is negated by the easy removal of residual/recurrent lesions on follow-up colonoscopy. Given the higher medicolegal liability and lack of financial incentive for a more time-consuming, complex, and costly procedure, ESD is unlikely to become standard of care for endoscopic resection of large colorectal lesions in the USA. However, with improvements in tools and techniques that can make ESD faster and easier to perform, we may see it being incorporated more into clinical practice in the USA, at tertiary referral centers, tailored for select group of lesions that may benefit from this. In the meantime, EMR will continue to be the more commonly performed procedure for endoscopic resection of large colon polyps.

Esophageal Cancer

Esophageal cancer is the eighth most common cancer worldwide and the sixth leading cause of cancer-related mortality. Squamous cell carcinoma and adenocarcinoma are the two histologic subtypes. While the former is the predominant type in Asia, the latter is seen more commonly in Europe and the USA [20].

Endoscopy is the gold standard for diagnosing precancerous mucosal lesions and early cancers of the esophagus. Subtle mucosal changes in the esophagus can go undetected when evaluated with standard white light. Therefore, dye-based chromoendoscopy and virtual chromoendoscopy, like NBI, are currently being advocated and used to improve detection of early dysplastic lesions [21]. For detecting early neoplastic lesions in the esophagus, endoscopists should be familiar with the associated subtle mucosal changes. A study by Scholvinck et al. showed that 76% of patients with HGD or cancer on random BE biopsies and "no endoscopic abnormalities" reported from community hospitals, in fact, had visible endoscopic lesions when evaluated by expert endoscopists at tertiary centers [22]. Esophagectomy used to be the conventional treatment for high-grade dysplasia and early-stage esophageal cancer in the past. Due to significant associated morbidity, mortality, and poor quality of life post esophagectomy, endoscopic resection has now become the accepted standard of care (Table 10.1).

Table 10.1 Histologic differences of EESC and EEAC and their preferred endoscopic resection technique

	Early esophageal squamous cell cancer	Early esophageal adenocarcinoma
Absolute indication for endoscopic resection	T1 m1–m2	T1 m1–m3
T1 sm1 invasion cutoff for endoscopic resection	200 μm depth into submucosa	500 μm depth into submucosa
Relative indication for endoscopic resection	T1 m3–sm1 without histologic risk factors (good to moderate differentiation, no LV invasion, and radical vertical margin)	T1sm1 without histologic risk factors (good to moderate differentiation, no LV invasion, absence of tumor budding, and radical resection)
Preferred endoscopic resection technique	ESD	EMR

Early Esophageal Adenocarcinoma (EAC) or Barrett's-Related Dysplasia

Barrett's esophagus is the only identifiable premalignant condition for EAC. BE is characterized by the replacement of stratified squamous esophageal mucosa with metaplastic intestinal-type columnar epithelium in distal esophagus. The estimated annual risk of BE progressing to adenocarcinoma is 0.1% to 0.5% and increases to around 5–10% per year if HGD is present. The progression of BE to EAC is believed to be stepwise from intestinal metaplasia to low-grade dysplasia, high-grade dysplasia, intramucosal cancer, and finally invasive EAC [23–25].

Visible lesions on endoscopy are usually classified using the Paris classification (protrude, flat, and excavated). Macroscopic appearance of lesions was shown to correlate with the grade and degree of mucosal/submucosal invasion, in a prospective study by Pech et al. Completely flat lesions (Paris type 0–IIb) had no risk of submucosal involvement. On the contrary, slightly elevated (Paris type 0–IIa) lesions had a 9% risk and protruded lesions (Paris type Is and 0–Ip) had 25–26% risk of submucosal invasion [26]. While there is no risk of nodal involvement in high-grade dysplasia, it is also very low in intramucosal cancer with a reported rate of 0–2%. This makes endoscopic resection the treatment of choice for these early lesions. Although a bit controversial, superficial submucosal cancer (sm1, depth of invasion ≤ 500 μm) with low-risk features (lack of lymphovascular invasion, tumor budding, or poor differentiation) may also be amenable to endoscopic resection [27, 28].

Esophageal Squamous Cell Carcinoma (ESCC)

ESCC is the predominant subtype in the Middle East, Africa, and Asia with abuse of alcohol and tobacco being the most common risk factors [20, 29]. Unlike Barrett's-related neoplasia, early ESCC has a higher rate of nodal metastasis even when confined to the mucosa. The risk of LN invasion in T1 m3–T1sm1 has been reported to be as high as up to 15%, and therefore these lesions are considered relative indications for curative endoscopic resection as long as there are good or moderate differentiation and absence of lymphovascular invasion. Furthermore, the cutoff for depth of invasion for sm1 lesion is 200 μm. Moreover, in ESCC, submucosal glands can harbor epithelial squamous neoplasia that extends from the luminal epithelial layer, and therefore en bloc resection of early ESCC is highly recommended [30, 31].

Endoscopic Resection

This can be accomplished by either EMR or ESD.

Endoscopic Mucosal Resection

En bloc resection is generally possible by EMR for lesions less than 20 mm in diameter. For larger lesions, piecemeal technique is usually required. The two common EMR techniques for resection of esophageal lesions are the cap (lift-suck-cut) technique and the multiband mucosectomy (ligate and cut) technique. In both techniques, the borders of the lesion should ideally be marked with cautery, prior to resection.

The cap technique requires the use of a transparent cap (straight or oblique) attached to the tip of the endoscope. First, the lesion is lifted with submucosal saline injection and then sucked into the cap creating a pseudopolyp. This is then captured by a snare that is pre-positioned along the rim of the cap and resected by electrocautery. These steps can be sequentially repeated for larger lesions that need piecemeal resection.

The multiband mucosectomy technique on the other hand does not require submucosal lifting and uses a modified banding apparatus similar to that used for variceal banding. The identified lesion is sucked into the cap, and a rubber band is released creating a pseudopolyp that is subsequently resected using a hexagonal snare and electrocautery. The banding and resection can be repeated to remove larger lesion in a piecemeal fashion taking precautions not to leave bridges or islands of neoplastic tissues in between the resected areas. Both the cap and band techniques are comparable in effective piecemeal resection and complete eradication of neoplasia, but the former is more time consuming and requires a higher skill level [32, 33].

Endoscopic Submucosal Dissection

En bloc resection of early esophageal cancers by ESD offers the advantage over piecemeal resection due to the superior ability to assess the depth and lateral extent of invasion. ESD can achieve en bloc resection for lesions larger than 20 mm. After marking the margins of the lesion with cautery, submucosal saline injection is performed to lift the lesion. Then a circumferential incision is made using an electrosurgical knife followed by dissection of the submucosa under direct endoscopic visualization until the entire lesion is removed in one piece. As in the colon, ESD is technically more challenging and carries higher rate of complications when compared to EMR in the esophagus [34].

EMR Versus ESD in Early Esophageal Cancer

The goal of using ESD in removing superficial esophageal cancers is to ensure an *en bloc* resection, which is optimal for histopathologic evaluation, with the aim of curative resection. ESD does confer a higher rate of R0 resection when compared to EMR in both subtypes of early esophageal cancer [31, 35]. However, there was no significant difference seen in complete remission of BE-related neoplasia at 3 months in one study. In this randomized control trial from Germany by Terheggen et al. comparing EMR versus ESD in BE, R0 resection was achieved more frequently in the ESD group (58.8%) versus 11.7% in the EMR group. However, there was no difference in complete remission from neoplasia at 3 months or during the follow-up period of the study (23.1 ± 6.4 months). ESD had a higher rate of adverse events, but that was not statistically significant [35]. Therefore, the advantages of ESD do not appear to culminate into clinically impactful difference as any residual BE and related neoplasia after EMR can be treated with adjunctive modalities like radiofrequency ablation. ESD may have an edge over EMR in selective situations like large lesions with higher likelihood of submucosal invasion and those with bulky intraluminal component that may be difficult to capture in a band or cap [36].

On the other hand in early ESCC, ESD is preferred as it offers higher rates of en bloc curative R0 resections and lower rates of local recurrence. A retrospective cohort study from Japan on 300 cases comparing ESD to EMR in early ESCC reported a 100% rate of en bloc resection in the ESD group compared to 53.3% in the EMR group. Subsequently there was lower local recurrence rate in the ESD group versus EMR 0.9% vs. 9.8%, respectively [31].

In the esophagus too, ESD has higher rates of perforation when compared to EMR. A meta-analysis comparing ESD and EMR for resection of superficial esophageal cancers reported a 4% perforation rate in ESD compared to 1.3% for EMR [34]. Many of the perforations can be usually managed endoscopically and do not require surgical intervention. Pneumomediastinum is another complication of ESD, which is not uncommon and seen in up to 30%. This usually resolves within 24 hours as carbon dioxide is used for insufflation [37].

EMR, on the other hand, has a higher risk of esophageal stenosis, up to 26%. The risk of stenosis is higher with longer treated segments and with more circumferential area of resection [38, 39].

As discussed earlier, in the colon section, ESD remains more expensive than EMR, requiring more time and costlier equipment as well being technically more challenging. Furthermore, the complexity of ESD may be more obvious in the esophagus especially in BE-related neoplasia due to the limited endoscopic working space, fibrotic submucosa, angulations in the distal esophagus, and movement due to respiration, motility, and heartbeat [36].

Early Gastric Cancer

Gastric cancer is the fourth most common cancer and the leading cause of cancer-related mortality worldwide. Gastric cancer is more prevalent in the countries of East Asia, Eastern Europe, and South America compared to Europe and North America [40]. Because gastric cancer is more prevalent in those countries, especially Japan, national screening programs have been developed for early detection and endoscopic resection techniques for early gastric cancer have become extremely refined and sophisticated. Endoscopic resection offers a less morbid and less expensive alternative compared to surgery for early gastric cancer.

The Japanese Gastric Cancer Association (JGCA) has recommended criteria for endoscopic resection of EGC. Based on these criteria, to be amenable for endoscopic resection, the tumor had to be differentiated-type adenocarcinoma without ulcerative findings, mucosal based (i.e., invading the lamina propria or muscularis mucosae) with a diameter of 2 cm or less. With the development of ESD in the late 1990s in Japan, allowing for en bloc resection of larger lesions, the JGCA updated their guidelines introducing "expanded indications" for endoscopic resection of EGC [41] (refer to Table 10.2 for JGCA absolute and expanded indication).

Resections Rates and Recurrences

En bloc resections should be the goal of endoscopic therapy of early gastric cancer. This ensures complete pathologic evaluation including vertical and horizontal margins as well as for lymphovascular invasion and also has higher chance of R0 resection and cure. The stomach has a thicker mucosa and muscular layer allowing for more invasive endoscopic techniques, like ESD, to be safer with a relatively low risk of complications. Moreover, the thick gastric mucosa is harder to lift with submucosal injection making EMR technically more challenging with less access to deeper tissue risking positive vertical margin. Therefore ESD has become the preferred technique for endoscopic resection of

Table 10.2 JGCA absolute and relative criteria for endoscopic resection of EGC [41]

Absolute criteria	A differentiated-type adenocarcinoma without ulcerative findings of which the depth of invasion is clinically diagnosed as T1a (invades the lamina propria or muscularis mucosae) and the largest diameter of lesion ≤2 cm
Expanded criteria *(ESD should be employed, not EMR)*	Depth of invasion is clinically diagnosed as T1a (invades the lamina propria or muscularis mucosae) AND (a) Differentiated-type, without ulcerative findings, but >2 cm in diameter (b) Differentiated-type, with ulcerative findings, and ≤3 cm in diameter (c) Undifferentiated-type, without ulcerative findings, and ≤2 cm in diameter

EGC owing to the high rate of curative resections and relatively low risk of complications when compared to other parts of the bowel (esophagus and colon).

A meta-analysis of 10 retrospective case controlled studies and 4328 lesions (8 Japanese, 1 South Korean, and 1 Italian study) showed a significantly higher rate of en bloc and R0 resections in the ESD group compared to EMR, OR 9.7 and 5.7, respectively. This also was reflected in a significant low recurrence rate in ESD group compared to EMR with an OR of 0.09 [42].

Moreover, in the expanded criteria, the JGCA indicates that lesions falling in this category should be resected with ESD and not EMR. This is mainly related to the limitations of EMR with larger EGC owing to the even lower rate of en bloc resections with larger lesions. Expanded criteria were received with a lot of caution especially in Western countries, but studies from Asia are showing comparative outcomes to absolute criteria [43, 44]. A retrospective multicenter Korean study of 1105 patients compared the outcomes of ESD between absolute and expanded criteria based on the EGC lesion characteristics. The study showed similar *en bloc* and curative resection rates on both groups. The rate of disease-free survival at 1 and 3 years was also similar in absolute and expanded criteria groups, 99.3% and 99.6% and 98.1% and 97.1%, respectively [45].

Adverse Events

As previously discussed, the thicker mucosa and muscular layer of stomach are more forgiving than the thinner layers in other parts of the GI tract as it pertains to procedural complications especially perforation. This makes the stomach the organ of choice for those starting to learn ESD. Actually, it is recommended in Japan that an endoscopist should perform 50–100 supervised ESDs in the gastric antrum before moving to other organs to ensure adequate training and competency [46, 47]. However, ESD continues to have a significantly higher risk of perforation in EGC resection compared to EMR albeit lower than the esophagus and colon. The previously referred to meta-analysis reported a higher rate of perforation with ESD compared to EMR, 4.3% versus 0.86%, respectively. There was no significant difference in the rate of bleeding [42]. In a recent case-control study from Italy, 36 cases of ESD of large (>20 mm) EGC were matched and compared to 40 EMR cases. Perforation occurred in two patients in the ESD group, with one requiring emergent surgery for delayed perforation, compared to no perforations in the EMR group, although this difference was not statistically significant [48].

Procedural times are higher in EGC resection with ESD. In the case-control study by Gambitta et al., the mean procedural time in the ESD group was significantly higher than that of the EMR group, 96.7 ± 51.3 versus 24.6 ± 14.6, respectively [48].

In conclusion, ESD is the preferred mode of endoscopic resection of early gastric cancer and should be considered the first line of therapy. As discussed above, ESD has a higher rate of en bloc resections and curative endoscopic resections, as well as lower risk of recurrence when compared to EMR [42, 45]. Unlike other regions of the gastrointestinal tract, the rate of complications of endoscopic resection of EGC does not seem to be significantly different between ESD and EMR [48].

References

1. Stryker SJ, et al. Natural history of untreated colonic polyps. Gastroenterology. 1987;93(5):1009–13.
2. Jayanna M, et al. Cost analysis of endoscopic mucosal resection vs surgery for large laterally spreading colorectal lesions. Clin Gastroenterol Hepatol. 2016;14(2):271–8 e1-2.
3. Ahlenstiel G, et al. Actual endoscopic versus predicted surgical mortality for treatment of advanced mucosal neoplasia of the colon. Gastrointest Endosc. 2014;80(4):668–76.
4. Mounzer R, et al. Endoscopic and surgical treatment of malignant colorectal polyps: a population-based comparative study. Gastrointest Endosc. 2015;81(3):733–740 e2.
5. Hermanek P, Gall FP. Early (microinvasive) colorectal carcinoma. Pathology, diagnosis, surgical treatment. Int J Color Dis. 1986;1(2):79–84.
6. Arezzo A, et al. Systematic review and meta-analysis of endoscopic submucosal dissection vs endoscopic mucosal resection for colorectal lesions. United European Gastroenterol J. 2016;4(1):18–29.
7. Fujiya M, et al. Efficacy and adverse events of EMR and endoscopic submucosal dissection for the treatment of colon neoplasms: a meta-analysis of studies comparing EMR and endoscopic submucosal dissection. Gastrointest Endosc. 2015;81(3):583–95.
8. Moss A, et al. Long-term adenoma recurrence following wide-field endoscopic mucosal resection (WF-EMR) for advanced colonic mucosal neoplasia is infrequent: results and risk factors in 1000 cases from the Australian Colonic EMR (ACE) study. Gut. 2015;64(1):57–65.
9. Bosch SL, et al. Predicting lymph node metastasis in pT1 colorectal cancer: a systematic review of risk factors providing rationale for therapy decisions. Endoscopy. 2013;45(10):827–34.
10. Pimentel-Nunes P, et al. Endoscopic submucosal dissection: European Society of Gastrointestinal Endoscopy (ESGE) guideline. Endoscopy. 2015;47(9):829–54.
11. Burgess NG, et al. Risk stratification for covert invasive cancer among patients referred for colonic endoscopic mucosal resection: a large multicenter cohort. Gastroenterology. 2017;153(3):732–742 e1.
12. Bahin FF, et al. Wide-field endoscopic mucosal resection versus endoscopic submucosal dissection for laterally spreading colorectal lesions: a cost-effectiveness analysis. Gut. 2018;67(11):1965–73.
13. Fuccio L, et al. Clinical outcomes after endoscopic submucosal dissection for colorectal neoplasia: a systematic review and meta-analysis. Gastrointest Endosc. 2017;86(1):74–86 e17.
14. Chung IK, et al. Therapeutic outcomes in 1000 cases of endoscopic submucosal dissection for early gastric neoplasms: Korean ESD Study Group multicenter study. Gastrointest Endosc. 2009;69(7):1228–35.

15. Iacopini F, et al. Stepwise training in rectal and colonic endoscopic submucosal dissection with differentiated learning curves. Gastrointest Endosc. 2012;76(6):1188–96.

16. Probst A, et al. Endoscopic submucosal dissection in large sessile lesions of the rectosigmoid: learning curve in a European center. Endoscopy. 2012;44(7):660–7.

17. Hotta K, et al. A comparison of outcomes of endoscopic submucosal dissection (ESD) for early gastric neoplasms between high-volume and low-volume centers: multi-center retrospective questionnaire study conducted by the Nagano ESD Study Group. Intern Med. 2010;49(4):253–9.

18. Heitman SJ, Bourke MJ. Endoscopic submucosal dissection and EMR for large colorectal polyps: "the perfect is the enemy of good". Gastrointest Endosc. 2017;86(1):87–9.

19. Rex DK, Hassan C, Dewitt JM. Colorectal endoscopic submucosal dissection in the United States: why do we hear so much about it and do so little of it? Gastrointest Endosc. 2017;85(3):554–8.

20. Pennathur A, et al. Oesophageal carcinoma. Lancet. 2013;381(9864):400–12.

21. Lao-Sirieix P, Fitzgerald RC. Screening for oesophageal cancer. Nat Rev Clin Oncol. 2012;9(5):278–87.

22. Scholvinck DW, et al. Detection of lesions in dysplastic Barrett's esophagus by community and expert endoscopists. Endoscopy. 2017;49(2):113–20.

23. Buttar NS, et al. Extent of high-grade dysplasia in Barrett's esophagus correlates with risk of adenocarcinoma. Gastroenterology. 2001;120(7):1630–9.

24. Sharma P. Clinical practice. Barrett's esophagus. N Engl J Med. 2009;361(26):2548–56.

25. Weston AP, et al. Long-term follow-up of Barrett's high-grade dysplasia. Am J Gastroenterol. 2000;95(8):1888–93.

26. Pech O, et al. Prospective evaluation of the macroscopic types and location of early Barrett's neoplasia in 380 lesions. Endoscopy. 2007;39(7):588–93.

27. Alvarez Herrero L, et al. Risk of lymph node metastasis associated with deeper invasion by early adenocarcinoma of the esophagus and cardia: study based on endoscopic resection specimens. Endoscopy. 2010;42(12):1030–6.

28. Manner H, et al. Early Barrett's carcinoma with "low-risk" submucosal invasion: long-term results of endoscopic resection with a curative intent. Am J Gastroenterol. 2008;103(10):2589–97.

29. Wheeler JB, Reed CE. Epidemiology of esophageal cancer. Surg Clin North Am. 2012;92(5):1077–87.

30. Ishihara R, et al. Local recurrence of large squamous-cell carcinoma of the esophagus after endoscopic resection. Gastrointest Endosc. 2008;67(6):799–804.

31. Takahashi H, et al. Endoscopic submucosal dissection is superior to conventional endoscopic resection as a curative treatment for early squamous cell carcinoma of the esophagus (with video). Gastrointest Endosc. 2010;72(2):255–64, 264 e1-2.

32. Alvarez Herrero L, et al. Safety and efficacy of multiband mucosectomy in 1060 resections in Barrett's esophagus. Endoscopy. 2011;43(3):177–83.

33. Pouw RE, et al. Randomized trial on endoscopic resection-cap versus multiband mucosectomy for piecemeal endoscopic resection of early Barrett's neoplasia. Gastrointest Endosc. 2011;74(1):35–43.

34. Guo HM, et al. Endoscopic submucosal dissection vs endoscopic mucosal resection for superficial esophageal cancer. World J Gastroenterol. 2014;20(18):5540–7.

35. Terheggen G, et al. A randomised trial of endoscopic submucosal dissection versus endoscopic mucosal resection for early Barrett's neoplasia. Gut. 2017;66(5):783–93.

36. Bourke MJ, Neuhaus H, Bergman JJ. Endoscopic submucosal dissection: indications and application in Western endoscopy practice. Gastroenterology. 2018;154(7):1887–900.. e5

37. Tamiya Y, et al. Pneumomediastinum is a frequent but minor complication during esophageal endoscopic submucosal dissection. Endoscopy. 2010;42(1):8–14.

38. Peters FP, et al. Stepwise radical endoscopic resection is effective for complete removal of Barrett's esophagus with early neoplasia: a prospective study. Am J Gastroenterol. 2006;101(7):1449–57.

39. Seewald S, et al. Circumferential EMR and complete removal of Barrett's epithelium: a new approach to management of Barrett's esophagus containing high-grade intraepithelial neoplasia and intramucosal carcinoma. Gastrointest Endosc. 2003;57(7):854–9.

40. Ferlay J, et al. Estimates of worldwide burden of cancer in 2008: GLOBOCAN 2008. Int J Cancer. 2010;127(12):2893–917.

41. Japanese Gastric Cancer Association. Japanese gastric cancer treatment guidelines 2014 (ver. 4). Gastric Cancer. 2017;20(1):1–19.

42. Facciorusso A, et al. Endoscopic submucosal dissection vs endoscopic mucosal resection for early gastric cancer: a meta-analysis. World J Gastrointest Endosc. 2014;6(11):555–63.

43. Isomoto H, et al. Endoscopic submucosal dissection for early gastric cancer: a large-scale feasibility study. Gut. 2009;58(3):331–6.

44. Tanabe S, et al. Gastric cancer treated by endoscopic submucosal dissection or endoscopic mucosal resection in Japan from 2004 through 2006: JGCA nationwide registry conducted in 2013. Gastric Cancer. 2017;20(5):834–42.

45. Shin KY, et al. Clinical outcomes of the endoscopic submucosal dissection of early gastric cancer are comparable between absolute and new expanded criteria. Gut Liver. 2015;9(2):181–7.

46. Yamamoto Y, et al. Current status of training for endoscopic submucosal dissection for gastric epithelial neoplasm at Cancer Institute Hospital, Japanese Foundation for Cancer Research, a famous Japanese hospital. Dig Endosc. 2012;24(Suppl 1):148–53.

47. Coman RM, Gotoda T, Draganov PV. Training in endoscopic submucosal dissection. World J Gastrointest Endosc. 2013;5(8):369–78.

48. Gambitta P, et al. Endoscopic submucosal dissection versus endoscopic mucosal resection for type 0-II superficial gastric lesions larger than 20 mm. Ann Gastroenterol. 2018;31(3):338–43.

Training and Competency in Endoscopic Resection

Daniel S. Strand and Andrew Y. Wang

Abbreviations/Acronyms

ACG   American College of Gastroenterology
AET   advanced (therapeutic) endoscopy training
ASGE   American Society for Gastrointestinal Endoscopy
CBE   competency-based education
CRC   colorectal cancer
DOPyS   Direct Observation of Polypectomy Skills
EMR   endoscopic mucosal resection
ESD   endoscopic submucosal dissection
GI   gastrointestinal
NBI   narrow-band imaging
SEER   Surveillance, Epidemiology, and End Results Program
SMI   submucosal invasion
SSAT   Society for Surgery of the Alimentary Tract
STAR   Skills, Training, Assessment, and Reinforcement
USA   United States

D. S. Strand (✉)
Division of Gastroenterology and Hepatology,
University of Virginia Health System,
Charlottesville, VA, USA
e-mail: dss7a@virginia.edu

A. Y. Wang
Section of Interventional Endoscopy, Division of
Gastroenterology and Hepatology, University of
Virginia Health System, Charlottesville, VA, USA
e-mail: ayw7d@virginia.edu

Introduction

The accurate identification and consistent endoscopic removal of intraepithelial neoplasia within the luminal gastrointestinal (GI) tract are a crucial responsibility of the modern endoscopist. When considered alone, colorectal cancer (CRC) represents the fourth most common neoplasm and is the third leading-cause of cancer-related mortality in the United States (USA), according to the National Cancer Institute Surveillance, Epidemiology, and End Results Program (SEER) database [1]. The predictable development of most CRCs from adenomatous or serrated precursor lesions provides the conceptual basis for modern endoscopy-based screening guidelines [2] and likely explains the consistent evidence that CRC incidence and mortality decline following the adoption of such screening [3–5]. Screening on its own does not prevent or cure cancer. Rather, the linchpin of colorectal cancer prevention through colonoscopy is the effective and complete removal of precursor lesions via endoscopic resection [6, 7]. Despite lesser prevalence among Western populations, successful endoscopic management of superficial neoplastic lesions within the esophagus [8], stomach [9], and small intestine [10, 11] is of equivalent value when it comes to providing high-quality care for individual patients.

Broadly, techniques employed in endoscopic resection can be subdivided into traditional polypectomy, endoscopic mucosal resection (EMR), and endoscopic submucosal dissection (ESD). Regardless of the technique chosen by an endoscopist, the complete and durable resection of neoplastic or precursor tissue is critical to a desirable outcome. Failure to achieve complete polypectomy or curative resection can have dire consequences, such as the development of cancer between surveillance intervals [12–14].

Despite these stakes, and the near-ubiquitous practice of colonoscopy among gastroenterologists [15], there is often wide quality variation in the effectiveness of polypectomy among practitioners. In a landmark study done at Dartmouth University and the nearby Veterans' Administration Hospital, Pohl et al. [12] demonstrated that marginal residual neoplastic tissue was routinely left behind (10.1% of the time) during polypectomy, despite the appearance of a macroscopically "complete" excision. More significant, however, was the incredible observed heterogeneity among individual proceduralists for this outcome. In this unblinded study, rates of incomplete resection ranged from 6.5% to nearly 23%, dependent solely upon the endoscopist performing the polypectomy.

This staggering level of variability in colonoscopy quality is not confined to polypectomy alone, but rather includes other metrics of endoscopist performance as well [7]. In an era where the successful removal of superficial mucosal neoplasia increasingly falls to the endoscopist rather than the surgeon, assuring the delivery of consistent, high-quality mucosal resection is of paramount importance to society. These complex procedures require significant training, valuable experience, and meticulous attention to detail in clinical practice. In this chapter, we will review paradigms for institutional training in mucosal resection, the challenges associated with measuring competency, and the importance of feedback and discuss some considerations inherent to training "nontraditional" endoscopic students.

Experiential Learning in Endoscopic Resection

The goal of training in endoscopic resection, be it polypectomy, EMR, or ESD, is the acquisition of a new skill by the learner, along with subsequent

refinement, to the level of consistently demonstrated competence. The process of skill acquisition through experiential learning has been extensively described, modeled, and observed to occur in definable phases [16–19]. The stages of competence model [18], introduced by Noel Burch in the 1970s, subdivides learners into four sequential categories: *unconscious incompetence, conscious incompetence, conscious competence,* and *unconscious competence.* In its purest form, this model implies that all learners arrive as novices within the first category and proceed sequentially to the fourth category in linear fashion. At the *unconscious incompetence* stage, a learner does not understand how to perform a given task but also does not recognize that he or she has a skill deficit. With experience and instruction, the learner first recognizes the deficit in skill (*conscious incompetence*) and then becomes able to perform the task with effort and concentration (*conscious competence*). Finally, with practice dependent upon task difficulty and aptitude, the learner refines and automates the skill so that it no longer requires conscious cognitive involvement to perform (*unconscious competence*).

This progressive model of learning can be applied to a myriad of activities, including the practice of endoscopy. This model does have several limitations: learners may not universally arrive at phase one, not all subjects progress through each of the four phases, and skill regression is entirely possible without maintenance [20]. For example, it is possible for technical skills to be acquired by observation and persistent repetition alone, without conscious understanding by the subject of the precise movements needed to achieve success.

In addition, the achievement of competence in endoscopic resection typically involves ensuring gains in a number of parallel domains, which are supportive of the psychomotor skills required to actually perform the task. Complementary nontechnical domains include both cognitive and less tangible integrative skills [21]. In the context of mucosal resection, cognitive skills include a thorough understanding of the steps involved in EMR or ESD, indications for each procedure, contraindications, selection of equipment, as well as the ability to readily recognize both success and adverse events. Integrative skills are less discrete and prevail at the intersection of cognitive skills, physical skills, and communication. Such ability often requires leadership, team interaction, judgment, adaptability, and situational awareness. It can be successfully argued that the importance of these nontechnical skills is paramount, as a failure to develop them alongside psychomotor prowess can result in significant adverse events regardless of technical expertise [22].

The Apprenticeship Model

Historically, training in EMR in Western countries has followed a traditional mentor-apprentice model, commonplace in both surgical and endoscopic pedagogy. The stage at which trainees are typically first exposed to mucosal resection is variable and may occur either during the course of a structured 3-year gastroenterology fellowship program or as a component of additional, dedicated advanced endoscopy training (AET) [23]. The decision to include learners of different educational levels is center specific and is typically determined by local faculty with expertise in mucosal resection. Frequently, this decision may be the result of long-standing, top-down curriculum design rather than the needs or interests of the individual learner. In addition, exposure of trainees to appropriate cases and overall volume can be unpredictable, often reflective of clinical assignments and the particulars of cases that are scheduled on a given day [24].

Traditional training under the apprenticeship model generally incorporates the learner in a progression of graduated responsibility, beginning with observation of endoscopic resection performed by an expert mentor. Over the course of training, often defined by the term of enrollment, learners are expected to progress to the level of independent practice under direct supervision by their proctor. Put simply, the paradigm of most EMR training programs is "see *one*, do *one*, teach *one*" where *one* is replaced by an integer determined mostly by the instructor. Importantly, the acquisition of competence under this model is frequently defined in nebulous fashion: gestalt on the part of the instructor or the completion of a time-based curriculum. Rarely, if ever, is competence in EMR currently measured among trainees with the use of a validated objectives, observational tools, or other reproducible outcomes [21].

The most frequent objective measure used in order to obtain professional certification in most endoscopic procedures is often caseload. Under the traditional model, this can be defined as a "critical mass" or minimal threshold of procedural volume above which competence can be reliably expected. Such a threshold is frequently variable, and therefore potentially dubious, even for basic procedures such as routine colonoscopy. As an example, the American Board of Surgery recommends that trainees perform a total of 50 colonoscopies during a surgical residency program to obtain basic competence [25]. The UK Joint Advisory Group recommends that learners perform of at least 200 cases [26]. These numbers are widely discordant, and, if both standards are acceptable for certification, such inconsistency raises questions about the concept of using an arbitrary minimum threshold as the sole measure of success [26]. Even so, there exists no well-established algorithm or even an identifiable minimal case volume necessary to confirm competence in EMR under a traditional instructional approach [27].

Western training in ESD is even more problematic than EMR when considered under a traditional model. In Japan, where the practice of ESD is well-established, most training programs fall into the category of a traditional mentor-apprenticeship. These training opportunities are physically located at institutions which possess a discernible history of performing submucosal dissection [28]. In Europe and the United States, no such mature infrastructure of programmatic experience exists, and there are comparatively few endoscopists with sufficient ESD experience to proctor any form of widespread training [23]. Those experts who do possess experience have frequently received their instruction via markedly nontraditional means, usually after extensive experience as a therapeutic endoscopist. This model is disparate from other forms of Western endoscopy training, which are typically incorporated as a part of graduate medical education or structured AET [29]. Further compounding the problem of dissemination, there is a significant paucity of gastric dysplasia and superficial carcinoma in Western populations, which has long been considered by Japanese experts to be the preferred target upon which to begin one's training in ESD [30]. This combined scarcity, of both mentors and disease-state, serves to dramatically inhibit any training model, thereby making experiential learning extremely difficult.

Competency-Based Education

Over the past two decades, there has been a paradigm shift throughout graduate medical education away from traditional structured or time-driven curricula toward competency-based education (CBE). In contrast to traditional approaches, CBE may be distinguished by several features: (1) a focus on outcomes, (2) emphasis on ability, (3) reduced emphasis on time-based learning, and (4) the promotion of learner-centeredness [31]. This model promotes the incorporation of predetermined competencies and the measurement of definable outcomes, rather than assuming that learning has occurred due to time spent in training. Defined competencies should be targeted to reflect the needs of stakeholders (in the case of endoscopic resection, patient outcomes such as residual neoplasia would be logical), and feedback during learning is provided through formal means. This feedback takes the form of assessments and per-competency measures to highlight deficiencies and improve learner performance [31]. When well designed, CBE curricula support the development of learning, target the strengths and weaknesses of individual trainees, and provide both attainable and applicable goals. Such a design could offer significant advantages over traditional training methods for many procedural skills, including mucosal resection.

Even though a CBE model is based upon sound educational principles, there are numerous barriers to the adoption of this format with respect to training in EMR and ESD. First and foremost, there must be clearly defined and validated criteria for identifying competency among learners ("outcomes"). At the present time, no established metrics for measuring competence in mucosal resection training exist. Despite the conspicuous

lack of concrete procedure-based learning objectives, professional societies such as the American Society for Gastrointestinal Endoscopy (ASGE) do provide suggestions for the development of a competency-based mucosal resection training program [27].

The "Core curriculum in EMR and ablative techniques," published in 2012 by the ASGE Training Committee [27], outlines potential goals of training in EMR and sets basic facilities and faculty requirements for an aspiring program. The ASGE also defines expected prerequisites for an incoming trainee (i.e., completion of a 2–3-year GI fellowship program with basic competency in upper and lower diagnostic endoscopy, submucosal injection, and management of complications) and describes the training process. They also present an overall strategy for assessment—as the ASGE adopts the core competency model employed in general by the ACGME for graduate medical education. The ASGE suggests that programs evaluate learners within the established GME competencies of patient care, medical knowledge, interpersonal and communication skills, professionalism, practice-based learning, and systems-based practice [32]. For each competency, the ASGE presents expectations and goals for trainees which, essentially, focus on the important cognitive and integrative funds necessary to successfully perform EMR.

Despite the usefulness of the proposed core curriculum, what is conspicuously lacking are directly observable benchmarks for the technical portion of learning and performing EMR. No formal criteria are presented or discussed in order to delineate a trainee's success in terms of the critical steps of mucosal resection. Rather, instructors are advised to "determine… (the number of procedures necessary)… based upon the trainee's individual performance," to expect competence, and that "objective criteria for competence should be developed and met [27]." In this way, the ASGE Core Curriculum falls short of transitioning entirely away from the traditional apprenticeship model, but does offer an inroad toward the subsequent goal of a CBE curriculum.

Directly Observable Skills as Potential Metrics of Competence in Mucosal Resection

The ASGE has defined competence in endoscopy as "... the minimum level of skill, knowledge, and/or expertise, derived through training and experience, required to safely and proficiently perform a task or procedure." [32] Mucosal resection is considered an advanced technique [23], and, as previously discussed, the metrics by which this specialized procedure should be measured are at best unclear. Although raw procedure numbers have been used in the past, reliance on this metric may be subject to inconsistency. Other metrics of outcome have been proposed including the rate of en bloc resection, the rate of residual or recurrent neoplasia, total procedure time, and adverse events. Unfortunately, none of these metrics have been validated independently as measures of competency in EMR [33]. Also, there are nuances to each of these potential competency measures. For example, the rate of en bloc resection for EMR generally applies only to smaller lesions which do not require piecemeal resection. Residual neoplasia, an important EMR outcome, may be predicted by lesional characteristics that are separate from an endoscopist's capability at performing the procedure [34]. In the following section, we will discuss a few of the various procedural steps involved in mucosal resection and review where and how the inclusion of direct observational assessments could be employed in progressing toward competency-based learning for the technical component of mucosal resection training.

Lesion Identification and Characterization

Regardless of the technique employed, performing high-quality resection of intraepithelial neoplasia begins with a comprehensive and accurate assessment of the lesion to be removed. A variety of inspection and classification schema have been extensively described for lesion morphology, topography, and pit or vascular pattern(s).

Perhaps the most straightforward and widely adopted means of describing lesion morphology is the "Paris classification of superficial neoplastic lesions [35]." In principle, first-stage accurate morphological diagnosis can assist a learner in determining which lesions are most suitable for traditional polypectomy vs. those that require EMR or ESD vs. those that should be referred for laparoscopic surgery. For example, Paris Classification 0-Ip lesions are pedunculated and may be removed without a lift or advanced intervention. Paris 0-IIa + IIc lesions are both superficially elevated and depressed (Fig. 11.1), and such lesions might require more complex intervention and harbor an increased risk of neoplasia associated with submucosal invasion (SMI). Despite its widespread use, there are no reports available that succinctly define the learning curve, inter-rater reliability, or intra-rater reliability of the Paris classification for lesion morphology, particularly among trainees. If such data were available, and there were consensus regarding acceptable proficiency levels, morphologic characterization of lesions would represent a useful and directly observable skill that could be included in CBE for EMR.

The acquisition of other skills in lesion assessment has been evaluated, though these are frequently more complicated. Togashi et al. [36] have described the learning curve and accuracy of optical diagnosis of neoplastic and nonneoplastic polyps using the Kudo pit pattern [37]. In this study, sequential observation of lesions under chromo- and magnification endoscopy demonstrated an improvement to over 90% sensitivity for correctly identifying neoplastic lesions after at least 200 sequential assessments. While this does suggest a threshold for competence, assuming the benchmark of 90% is appropriate, implementation outside of Japan may be challenging. Many endoscopic platforms which are routinely available in the West do not offer a true optical magnification capability. Use of chromoendoscopy for optical diagnosis of the mucosal pit pattern using a high-definition endoscope that lacks optical magnification may introduce issues with fine-detail image resolution and therefore might not be sufficient to perform this task consistently [38].

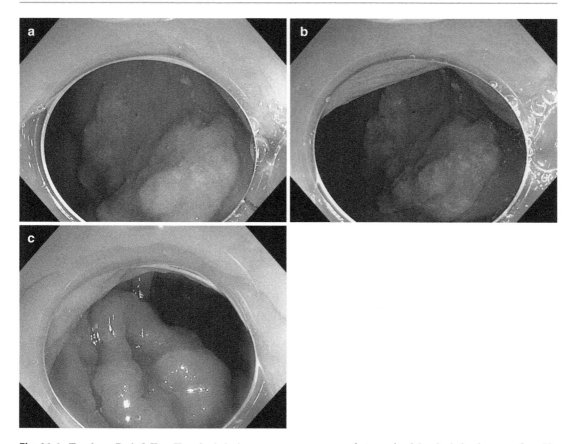

Fig. 11.1 Two large Paris 0-IIa + IIc colonic lesions were found in the same person. High-definition white-light (**a**) and NBI (**b**) images are shown of the lesion in the cecum. White-light images of the second large polyp (**c**) with a mucous cap that remained despite irrigation were found in the ascending colon. Both polyps were removed by underwater EMR and found to be serrated sessile polyps without dysplasia

More applicable to Western training programs, the learning curve for assessment of lesions using narrow-band imaging (NBI) and the meshed capillary pattern [38, 39] has been described [40] (Fig. 11.2). In this study [40], four experienced endoscopists with no NBI experience underwent a 4-hour training course in both NBI principles and the capillary pattern classification system. After as few as 30 cases, the subjects were able to distinguish between lesions appropriate for endoscopic resection (adenomas and superficial neoplasms) and those which required only biopsy (hyperplastic lesions and those with overt deep cancer). The subjects were highly discriminatory, with over 95% diagnostic accuracy. When combining the advantages of a short learning curve, excellent threshold for accurate diagnosis (>95%), and the widespread availability of NBI-capable equipment, assessment of vascular capillary patterns represents an ideal target as a directly observable skill and potential metric that can be included in a mucosal resection training program.

Mucosal Resection Technique

Following lesion identification and characterization, the endoscopist then prepares to tackle the fundamental act of removing the superficial neoplastic lesion. As the practice of mucosal resection has matured, understanding of the technical aspects of both EMR and ESD has become increasingly developed [41, 42]. For

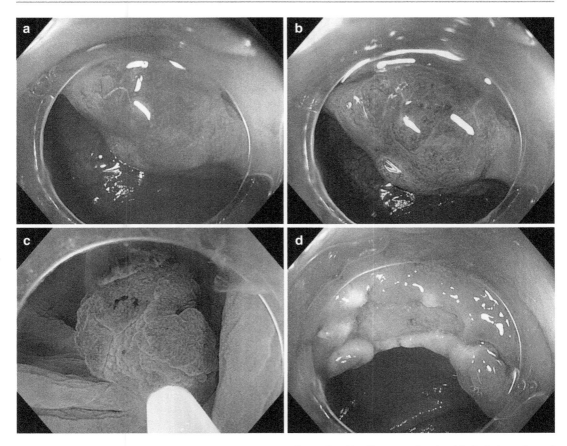

Fig. 11.2 A 1.5-cm sessile polyp (Paris 0-Is) was found in the splenic flexure and high-definition white-light images (**a**) do not show the surface pattern well. NBI (**b**) better demonstrated the meshed capillary pattern, which in this case showed disordered vessels with some areas of avascularity. While there was concern for early invasive cancer (Sano type IIIB), given the relatively small size and lack of other surface features that might suggest deeper invasion (tenting, bridging folds, etc.), en bloc underwater EMR was performed (**c**) with complete resec-tion and no bleeding or perforation (**d**). Pathology showed a well-differentiated adenocarcinoma with invasion into the superficial submucosa but negative margins (>1-mm negative deep margin). In this case, the risk of lymph node metastasis is likely around 5%, and the patient was directed to meet a colorectal surgeon to discuss the risks and benefits of further laparoscopic surgical resection, with the alternative being close endoscopic surveillance and yearly CT scans

each technique that could be employed, there are fundamental steps associated with performance of an optimal resection. These may vary based upon lesion location, characteristics, technique, or equipment utilized. An extensive discussion of *how to perform* these procedures is beyond the scope of this chapter and is discussed elsewhere in the textbook.

In the case of traditional mucosal resection, simply the process of creating a submucosal lift has numerous technical considerations: choosing the proper submucosal injectate solution, injecting the lesion appropriately to facilitate a lift without obscuring visualization, assessing for an adequate or inadequate lift, and interpreting if the presence of poor lifting represents tumor invasion or benign submucosal fibrosis [43]. Snare resection is no less complex with regard to optimal technique and has several facets: lesion and scope orientation to facilitate technical success, incorporating a normal mucosal border within the snare (i.e., a 2–3-mm rim of normal tissue), maintaining a submucosal plane in piecemeal resection using the snare edge, and the application of cautery by using a modern electrosurgical generator. Each and any of these technical steps could be observed and evaluated as a measure of competence, were there a consistent methodology available to do so. Additionally, there are a number of other higher-level decisions made by endoscopists during EMR: attempting en bloc resection whenever possible, removing large or dysplastic appearing nodules in a single piece (given an increased risk of focal malignancy), and minimizing the number of overall fragments when en bloc resection is not possible [43, 44].

Learning Curves and Direct Observation of Polypectomy Skills (DOPyS)

Although no societal recommendation for a threshold number of EMR cases in training has been established, there does exist limited data regarding skill acquisition and the learning curves for EMR among practicing academic interventional endoscopists. In a retrospective series by Bhurwal et al. [34], a total of 578 consecutive colonic EMR procedures, performed by 3 endoscopists over a 9-year period, were tabulated and analyzed. Three relatively narrow outcomes were included: residual neoplasia upon interval surveillance, immediate assessment that an EMR was incomplete, and the occurrence of immediate bleeding as an adverse event. For each of three physicians, the occurrence of residual neoplasia (grossly and by surveillance biopsies) fell below 20% and plateaued by procedure number 100. Immediate bleeding was generally rare throughout the study and was acceptably below 5% by case 100 for all of the endoscopists. Although there were several limitations inherent in this series that may have prolonged the learning curve (referral bias to a tertiary care center, self-teaching environment, retrospective series, etc.), the observed number of cases required to establish a plateau of residual neoplasia was higher than expected. To date, this study represents the only published learning curve data with respect to EMR of large laterally spreading lesions in the colon.

Published data evaluating the rate of acquiring skills necessary to perform ESD in Japan exist and are more robust. In 2005, Gotoda et al. [45] reported that early proficiency in gastric ESD could be seen after 30 cases during intensive training. In 2012, Yamamoto et al. [28] provided observational evidence that by 40 gastric ESDs, trainees may have sufficient skill to reliably remove superficial mucosal lesions, without ulceration, that were less than 2 cm in size. With continued instruction and experience through 80 cases, trainees routinely demonstrated outcomes that approximated their expert instructors. In 2010, Hotta et al. [46] described the first learning curve for colonic ESD in a single endoscopist from Saku Central Hospital in Japan. They demonstrated that 40 ESD procedures were required to avoid an unacceptable rate of perforation (rate dropped from 12.5% to 5%) and that a total of 80 procedures were required to establish an acceptable rate of en bloc, R0 resection (rate increased from 85% to 92.5%). Translation of gastric ESD experience to colonic lesions appears more straightforward. In 2011, Sakamoto et al. [47] reported that trainees with experience in gastric ESD could successfully perform supervised colorectal ESD safely after approximately 30 procedures.

The Western experience with ESD skill acquisition has been more challenging, as the methods used thus far to disseminate ESD skill in Europe and the United States have been fractured and inconsistent. While reports of learning curves for Western endoscopists exist [29, 48, 49], these experiences draw upon training that has been universally disparate. Each published experience is similar only in that the individual pathways to competence have been distinctly different than others. As such, these data likely have only limited translational value to typical Western graduate (fellowship level) or postgraduate endoscopy training concerning ESD.

While learning curves may provide insight into the degree of experience necessary to attain competency in mucosal resection, they may not be reliable measures at the level of an individual trainee. This problem, and how it pertains to routine colonoscopy with polypectomy, has been widely recognized [21]. Out of concerns for inadequate training in routine polypectomy, an expert working group within the United Kingdom deconstructed the process of polypectomy into a 33-item checklist entitled the Direct Observation of Polypectomy Skills (DOPyS) tool [50, 51]. Skills were divided into several sections including (1) optimizing the view of/access to the polyp, (2) stalked polyps, (3) small sessile lesions, and (4) post-polypectomy. Endoscopic nontechnical skills were also included at the end of the assessment form. For each item on the checklist, a 4-point score is given which was intended to evaluate the subject by maneuver: 1 (standards not met), 2 (some uncorrected errors), 3 (competent and safe), and 4 (highly skilled). This methodology was developed, validated, and shown to be reliable in two sequential publications by Gupta et al. [50, 51] These studies demonstrated that assessors who had been formally trained in DOPyS could successfully and consistently delineate between procedures performed by expert endoscopists and those performed by trainees, so long as the assessor was able to observe at least five separate polypectomies performed by each individual.

Despite its promising value, the DOPyS has not been validated for use in more advanced mucosal resection. Polypectomies performed during the DOPyS validation studies were uniformly less than 18 mm in size, which is smaller than lesions typically considered for EMR or ESD (usually >20 mm in size). Further, the tool as written is not applicable to techniques apart from conventional injection-lift EMR. Nonetheless, a similar instrument could be of great value in establishing uniform competency-based mucosal resection training. If validated appropriately, such a method could be applied throughout a graduate or postgraduate training program, and used at intervals guided by data extracted from published learning curves, in order to establish an individual trainee's progression to competence.

The Importance of Feedback

Well-developed CBE is based upon the principle of self-regulated learning. Perhaps the most critical aspect of this process is the capacity of an individual to assess the results of learning (e.g., trainee's performance) and make adjustments, prospectively [52]. Feedback is central to this process of assessment and adaptability, as it allows the trainee to identify areas of weakness that are in need of additional attention. Feedback may be internal (self-assessment) or external, with the latter frequently delivered by one's instructor, mentor, or program-director. Internal feedback is important, but sometimes can be unreliable, and is, in any case, outside the control of an institutional training program. External feedback is more likely to be accurate [53] and, when delivered by a subject matter expert, can include guidance for incremental improvement.

Despite its extremely high value, external feedback typically suffers from poor delivery and inadequate, poorly-timed, or generalized content. Fundamentally, external feedback is difficult because it takes place as an exchange within interpersonal relationships of varying resiliency. A strong relationship, with trust and credibility by both partners, allows for valuable insight and communication. A weak relationship may be harmed by the delivery of criticism or corrective feedback, making this either less effective or less likely to be delivered in the first place. While not explicitly stated, one of the major conceptual advantages of a traditional apprenticeship is this relationship. In the classical sense, a mentor and apprentice are *expected* to have both a close and invested working relationship built on trust and common interest. Such a relationship should allow for the provision of regular and honest formative feedback, which may even be bilateral (How can you/I learn better? How can you/I teach better?).

One potential drawback to an educational model with explicitly defined competencies and learner-directed focus is this need to provide frequent and accurate feedback. Evaluating procedural skills seems particularly susceptible to failures, especially at the outset of mucosal resection training, when trainees are expected to be at the first stage of learning (*unconsciously incompetent*). During this time they may possess only limited insight in order to make self-assessments, and the relationship with a mentor may be nascent or underdeveloped. Great care should be taken at all times to ensure that feedback is given effectively, frequently, and within a nonjudgmental and constructive environment.

Training Considerations for "Nontraditional Students" and Continuing Medical Education (CME)

Much of what has been discussed previously is based upon the assumption that training in mucosal resection occurs in the milieu of a traditional graduate GI fellowship or postgraduate educational program in advanced endoscopy (formal advanced endoscopy fellowship training). While this may be the standard setting in which such skills are developed for new learners, most practicing endoscopists who perform EMR did not develop this technique under such formal circumstances. Regardless of how experience in mucosal resection is acquired, societal and professional expectations would suggest that the practicing endoscopist should demonstrate competency that is on par with graduates of established training programs (and vice versa). This remains inherently problematic, as there are no societally endorsed criteria for judging competency, no validated observational assessment tools, and limited data on learning curves even to suggest a minimum threshold volume of procedures necessary to use as a surrogate for competence.

The previous example of Western experts who perform ESD is perhaps the most striking conglomeration of skill acquisition by nontraditional means [29, 49, 54] and may be beneficial in devising a methodology for practicing endoscopists to acquire EMR skills at the CME level (during active clinical practice and after completion of all endoscopic training). Draganov et al.[29] specifically highlight the impact that observation of live cases can have on acquiring new skills for an already experienced endoscopist. In his pub-

lished experience, Dr. Draganov's ESD learning curve was divided into three phases: (1) *pre-observation*, during which ESD was performed on animal models prior to observation; (2) *observation*, during which Dr. Draganov visited Japan and observed live ESD cases at experienced centers over a 5-week period; and (3) *post-observation*, where additional ex vivo animal models were again used to garner additional experience. Following the observation period, resections were completed on models with significant gains in efficiency (shorter time) and observable trends toward reduced incomplete resection rates and adverse events. This was notable, especially considering that ESD requires significant technical expertise distinctly disparate from traditional polypectomy, while traditional EMR is more akin to an extension or refinement of traditional polypectomy skills [23, 27].

Observation can be accomplished by practicing endoscopists under a number of different circumstances. There are various national and international endoscopy conferences at which practicing endoscopists may attend didactic lectures, breakout sessions, and live demonstrations which showcase EMR or ESD techniques [55, 56]. In keeping with the prior example, these courses may provide a valuable adjunctive experience to solidify skills among practicing physicians who already have extensive polypectomy experience and wish to gain skill in EMR or become exposed to ESD. These courses have several limitations, as many provide short-duration hands-on training limited to a few hours and utilize ex vivo animal models that cannot simulate intraprocedural hemorrhage or clinical instability in the setting of perforation. While these courses offer an important and convenient method for endoscopists to be taught by experts, they may be best digested by the endoscopic *journeyman* rather than the *apprentice*.

Professional societies, including the ASGE, American College of Gastroenterology (ACG), and Society for Surgery of the Alimentary Tract (SSAT), offer several opportunities for hands-on training in mucosal resection which vary in scope, duration, and intensity. These range from introductory 3-hour workshops in EMR and ESD at annual meetings [57] to the formalized ASGE Skills, Training, Assessment, and Reinforcement (STAR) Certificate Programs in Lower GI and

Upper GI EMR [58] and the joint ASGE-Japan Gastrointestinal Endoscopy Society Masters Course in ESD. The STAR EMR courses are multifaceted and are intended to be completed over the course of 3–6 months by enrollees. Enrollment is usually limited to practicing gastroenterologists with at least 2 years of experience, greater than 500 independent colonoscopies, and "proficiency in basic polypectomy, hemostasis, and injection techniques." Each course initially includes a self-directed online curriculum which includes a baseline knowledge assessment (pretest), reading materials, online videos, and a summative assess-

ment upon completion (posttest). The live portion of the course includes 10 hours of EMR-specific didactic and hands-on training, proctored by expert instructors using ex vivo animal models. On the subsequent day, a 4-hour hands-on summative assessment is performed and candidates who pass successfully are awarded a certificate of completion by the ASGE. While the STAR Certification is not a guarantee competency in EMR, it is constructed based upon competency-based educational principles, and the program offers a valuable opportunity for established endoscopists to learn this endoscopic technique (Fig. 11.3).

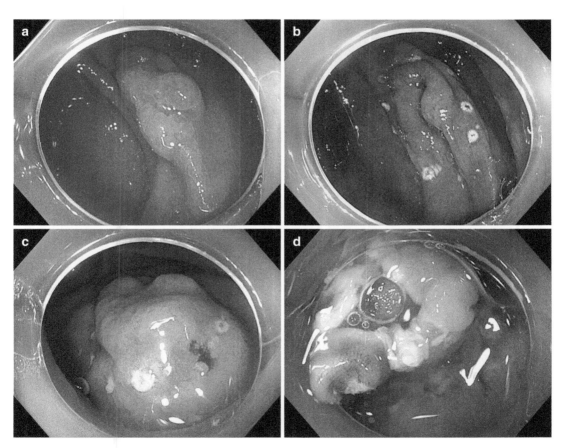

Fig. 11.3 A third-year fellow was being taught to perform conventional EMR. A 15-mm cecal polyp was found and its morphology described using white-light endoscopy as Paris 0-IIa + Is (**a**). The lesion borders were hard to define, and NBI was used to delineate the borders of the polyp, which were then marked by using APC (**b**). No features of invasive cancer were found on high-definition white-light or NBI endoscopy. The lesion was submucosally lifted using a commercially available lifting solution tinted with methylene blue (**c**). En bloc resection using a 15-mm stiff, braided, oval-shaped snare was performed.

The underside of the resected specimen showed no target sign (**d**) nor did the remaining portion of the resected colonic wall. However, a significant amount of mucosa intended for resection remained, as delineated by the marking dots (**e**). This mucosa was removed for completeness sake (**f**). After ablation of the edges using APC, the lesion was closed using two endoclips (**g**). Pathology showed a serrated sessile polyp. This example highlights many of the key steps necessary to teach, learn, and perform EMR, and this is also the standardized approach that is taught in the ASGE STAR EMR course

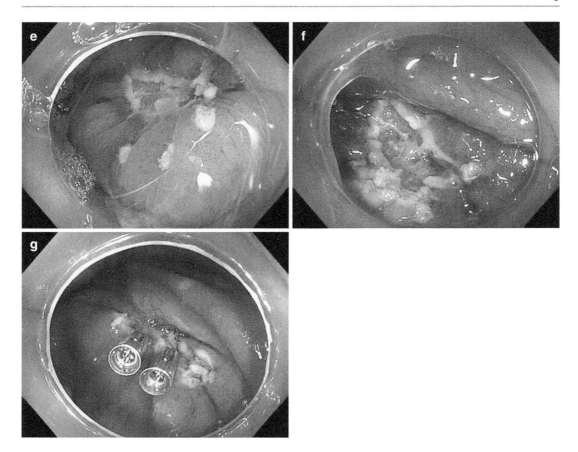

Fig. 11.3 (continued)

Competency Thresholds by Volume and Outcome

As mentioned earlier, there is no established clear-cut methodology to teach trainees EMR, let alone ESD—particularly in countries where the prevalence of gastric cancer is low and where prevalence-based models are adopted where ESD experience (and also often EMR) typically begins in the colorectum [59]. It has been suggested that at least 250–300 procedures are required before competency can be assessed for conventional polypectomy [60]. Similarly, 100 procedures may be required for EMR, 200 procedures for chromoendoscopy, and 30 procedures for NBI prior to assessing or achieving competency [60]. After rigorous theoretical and experimental preparation, a skilled interventional endoscopist can achieve competence after 20–30 untutored ESD proce-

dures, but outcomes data from twice that caseload are often required to support ongoing competence [59]. Importantly, volume thresholds do not necessarily equate to competency [27]. Furthermore, it is understood that to maintain competency a skill should be performed regularly, potentially weekly, or at least 1–2 times each month.

Irrespective of the training methodology, it is critical to remember that high-quality clinical outcomes are paramount. Those seeking to acquire skills in endoscopic resection must remember that these superficial neoplastic lesions are found in patients who present, not to provide a model for gaining experience or for research, but rather to attain a result equivalent to and less risky than surgical resection.

We suggest certain achievable competency thresholds, which can be applied to newly graduated trainees or to experienced endoscopists who have acquired new skills in endoscopic resection. For EMR, the rate of residual neoplasia should be no greater than 20%–25% [61] when only lesions ≥15–20 mm are considered (i.e., for lesions necessitating piecemeal resection). For endoscopically curable lesions (generally those without invasive cancer or risk of lymph node metastasis that do not require surgery, which can vary by organ type), curative resection should be achieved in 90%–95% of cases by the third follow-up procedure [62–64]. For example, if residual neoplasia is found on biopsies during the first follow-up endoscopy, a second endoscopic procedure for eradication of residual neoplasia would be indicated (alternatively, if treatment of suspected macroscopically visible residual neoplasia was carried out at the first follow-up procedure, then a second surveillance procedure would be necessary 3–6 months later). It should be kept in mind that variations in recurrence rates may exist, as the odds of residual or recurrent neoplasia increase with larger lesions that are removed in a greater number of pieces [65]. Thus, a 20% rate of residual/recurrent neoplasia for an endoscopist who only removes lesions up to 2 cm in size might be considered high, whereas the same 20% recurrence rate for an endoscopists who mainly removes very large lesions (>4 cm in size) necessitating piecemeal EMR might be very reasonable.

For ESD, particularly in the West, the focus should probably be on rates of en bloc resection and adverse events such as perforation. Less focus should be applied to other outcomes (e.g., rates of R0 or curative resection), as Western endoscopists who perform ESD are often put in a difficult predicament by referring surgeons and oncologists and asked to resect lesions that fall outside of traditional guidelines. Competency in ESD should be demonstrated by en bloc resection rates of ≥80% with perforation rates of ≤10%; expertise in ESD is associated with en bloc resection rates of ≥90% with perforation rates of ≤5% [59, 66].

Incumbent with use of outcome metrics, patients should be followed closely, and it is recommended not to rely solely on endoscopic visual assessment to rule out recurrent/residual lesions but to also take biopsies from the center and periphery of the resection scar and of any nodularity that might be found.

Conclusion

EMR and by extension ESD have revolutionized the approach treating non-pedunculated, superficial intraepithelial neoplasia at various sites along the GI tract over the past two to three decades. Together, these mucosal resection techniques represent a collection of advanced endoscopic procedures that require significant technical skill, experience, and cognitive training to master. Although there is a long history of producing capable and even expert endoscopists through traditional training pathways, significant variation among practicing physicians suggests the need to establish a mature, competency-based educational process to ensure that both technical and nontechnical skill development has been successful prior to independent practice.

There are several barriers to implementation of such standards and curricula at the present time, which include paucity in information regarding the learning curve to perform EMR, the lack of accepted measures of intraprocedural competency, and the absence of an applicable direct observational tool such as the DOPyS for advanced mucosal resection. Despite these challenges, training in mucosal resection appears to be set on an inexorable tack toward competency-based education, in lockstep with the remainder of undergraduate and graduate medical education. Given the adoption of ACGME principles by professional GI societies, it is likely that a formalized CBE curriculum for mucosal resection could be developed and adopted.

References

1. Siegel RL, Miller KD, Jemal A. Cancer statistics, 2016. CA Cancer J Clin. 2016;66:7–30.
2. Provenzale D, Jasperson K, Ahnen DJ, et al. Colorectal cancer screening, version 1.2015. J Natl Compr Cancer Netw. 2015;13:959–68; quiz 968.

3. Baxter NN, Goldwasser MA, Paszat LF, et al. Association of colonoscopy and death from colorectal cancer. Ann Intern Med. 2009;150:1–8.

4. Nishihara R, Wu K, Lochhead P, et al. Long-term colorectal-cancer incidence and mortality after lower endoscopy. N Engl J Med. 2013;369:1095–105.

5. Doubeni CA, Corley DA, Quinn VP, et al. Effectiveness of screening colonoscopy in reducing the risk of death from right and left colon cancer: a large community-based study. Gut. 2018;67(2):291–8.

6. Winawer SJ, Zauber AG, Ho MN, et al. Prevention of colorectal cancer by colonoscopic polypectomy. The National Polyp Study Workgroup. N Engl J Med. 1993;329:1977–81.

7. Corley DA, Jensen CD, Marks AR, et al. Adenoma detection rate and risk of colorectal cancer and death. N Engl J Med. 2014;370:1298–306.

8. Pimentel-Nunes P, Dinis-Ribeiro M, Ponchon T, et al. Endoscopic submucosal dissection: European Society of Gastrointestinal Endoscopy (ESGE) guideline. Endoscopy. 2015;47:829–54.

9. Gotoda T, Jung HY. Endoscopic resection (endoscopic mucosal resection/endoscopic submucosal dissection) for early gastric cancer. Dig Endosc. 2013;25(Suppl 1):55–63.

10. Gaspar JP, Stelow EB, Wang AY. Approach to the endoscopic resection of duodenal lesions. World J Gastroenterol. 2016;22:600–17.

11. Klein A, Nayyar D, Bahin FF, et al. Endoscopic mucosal resection of large and giant lateral spreading lesions of the duodenum: success, adverse events, and long-term outcomes. Gastrointest Endosc. 2016;84:688–96.

12. Pohl H, Srivastava A, Bensen SP, et al. Incomplete polyp resection during colonoscopy-results of the complete adenoma resection (CARE) study. Gastroenterology. 2013;144:74–80 e1.

13. Farrar WD, Sawhney MS, Nelson DB, et al. Colorectal cancers found after a complete colonoscopy. Clin Gastroenterol Hepatol. 2006;4:1259–64.

14. Rex DK, Schoenfeld PS, Cohen J, et al. Quality indicators for colonoscopy. Gastrointest Endosc. 2015;81:31–53.

15. Joseph DA, Meester RG, Zauber AG, et al. Colorectal cancer screening: estimated future colonoscopy need and current volume and capacity. Cancer. 2016;122:2479–86.

16. Mohamed R, Raman M, Anderson J, et al. Validation of the National Aeronautics and Space Administration Task Load Index as a tool to evaluate the learning curve for endoscopy training. Can J Gastroenterol Hepatol. 2014;28:155–9.

17. Peel JL, Nolan RJ. You can't start a central line? Supervising residents at different stages of the learning cycle. J Grad Med Educ. 2015;7:536–8.

18. Adams L. Gordon Training International. Learning a new skill is easier said than done. Available at: http://www.gordontraining.com/free-workplace-articles/learning-a-new-skill-is-easier-said-than-done.

19. Hershey P. Leadership-Central.com. Hersey-Blanchard situational leadership theory. Available at: http://www.leadership-central.com/situational-leadership-theory.html#axzz3OpFIn2L3.

20. Waschke KA, Anderson J, Macintosh D, et al. Training the gastrointestinal endoscopy trainer. Best Pract Res Clin Gastroenterol. 2016;30:409–19.

21. Dube C, Rostom A. Acquiring and maintaining competency in gastrointestinal endoscopy. Best Pract Res Clin Gastroenterol. 2016;30:339–47.

22. Yule S, Flin R, Paterson-Brown S, et al. Non-technical skills for surgeons in the operating room: a review of the literature. Surgery. 2006;139:140–9.

23. Feurer ME, Draganov PV. Training for advanced endoscopic procedures. Best Pract Res Clin Gastroenterol. 2016;30:397–408.

24. Xiong X, Barkun AN, Waschke K, et al. Current status of core and advanced adult gastrointestinal endoscopy training in Canada: survey of existing accredited programs. Can J Gastroenterol. 2013;27:267–72.

25. Johna S, Klaristenfeld D. Surgery resident training in endoscopy: the saga continues. Arch Surg. 2011;146:899–900.

26. Ward ST, Mohammed MA, Walt R, et al. An analysis of the learning curve to achieve competency at colonoscopy using the JETS database. Gut. 2014;63:1746–54.

27. Training C, Hunt GC, Coyle WJ, et al. Core curriculum for EMR and ablative techniques. Gastrointest Endosc. 2012;76:725–9.

28. Yamamoto Y, Fujisaki J, Ishiyama A, et al. Current status of training for endoscopic submucosal dissection for gastric epithelial neoplasm at Cancer Institute Hospital, Japanese Foundation for Cancer Research, a famous Japanese hospital. Dig Endosc. 2012;24(Suppl 1):148–53.

29. Draganov PV, Chang M, Coman RM, et al. Role of observation of live cases done by Japanese experts in the acquisition of ESD skills by a western endoscopist. World J Gastroenterol. 2014;20:4675–80.

30. Goda K, Fujishiro M, Hirasawa K, et al. How to teach and learn endoscopic submucosal dissection for upper gastrointestinal neoplasm in Japan. Dig Endosc. 2012;24(Suppl 1):136–42.

31. Gruppen LD, Burkhardt JC, Fitzgerald JT, et al. Competency-based education: programme design and challenges to implementation. Med Educ. 2016;50:532–9.

32. Position statement. Maintaining competency in endoscopic skills. American Society for Gastrointestinal Endoscopy. Gastrointest Endosc. 1995;42:620–1.

33. James PD, Antonova L, Martel M, et al. Measures of trainee performance in advanced endoscopy: a systematic review. Best Pract Res Clin Gastroenterol. 2016;30:421–52.

34. Bhurwal A, Bartel MJ, Heckman MG, et al. Endoscopic mucosal resection: learning curve for large nonpolypoid colorectal neoplasia. Gastrointest Endosc. 2016;84:959–968 e7.

35. Endoscopic Classification Review Group. Update on the Paris classification of superficial neoplastic lesions in the digestive tract. Endoscopy. 2005;37:570–8.
36. Togashi K, Konishi F, Ishizuka T, et al. Efficacy of magnifying endoscopy in the differential diagnosis of neoplastic and non-neoplastic polyps of the large bowel. Dis Colon Rectum. 1999;42:1602–8.
37. Kudo S, Hirota S, Nakajima T, et al. Colorectal tumours and pit pattern. J Clin Pathol. 1994;47:880–5.
38. Henry ZH, Yeaton P, Shami VM, et al. Meshed capillary vessels found on narrow-band imaging without optical magnification effectively identifies colorectal neoplasia: a North American validation of the Japanese experience. Gastrointest Endosc. 2010;72:118–26.
39. Sano Y, Ikematsu H, Fu KI, et al. Meshed capillary vessels by use of narrow-band imaging for differential diagnosis of small colorectal polyps. Gastrointest Endosc. 2009;69:278–83.
40. Dai J, Shen YF, Sano Y, et al. Evaluation of narrow-band imaging in the diagnosis of colorectal lesions: is a learning curve involved? Dig Endosc. 2013;25:180–8.
41. Holt BA, Bourke MJ. Wide field endoscopic resection for advanced colonic mucosal neoplasia: current status and future directions. Clin Gastroenterol Hepatol. 2012;10:969–79.
42. ASGE Technology Committee, Hwang JH, Konda V, et al. Endoscopic mucosal resection. Gastrointest Endosc. 2015;82:215–26.
43. Klein A, Bourke MJ. Advanced polypectomy and resection techniques. Gastrointest Endosc Clin N Am. 2015;25:303–33.
44. Klein A, Bourke MJ. How to perform high-quality endoscopic mucosal resection during colonoscopy. Gastroenterology. 2017;152:466–71.
45. Gotoda T, Friedland S, Hamanaka H, et al. A learning curve for advanced endoscopic resection. Gastrointest Endosc. 2005;62:866–7.
46. Hotta K, Oyama T, Shinohara T, et al. Learning curve for endoscopic submucosal dissection of large colorectal tumors. Dig Endosc. 2010;22:302–6.
47. Sakamoto T, Saito Y, Fukunaga S, et al. Learning curve associated with colorectal endoscopic submucosal dissection for endoscopists experienced in gastric endoscopic submucosal dissection. Dis Colon Rectum. 2011;54:1307–12.
48. Berr F, Ponchon T, Neureiter D, et al. Experimental endoscopic submucosal dissection training in a porcine model: learning experience of skilled Western endoscopists. Dig Endosc. 2011;23:281–9.
49. Iacopini F, Bella A, Costamagna G, et al. Stepwise training in rectal and colonic endoscopic submucosal dissection with differentiated learning curves. Gastrointest Endosc. 2012;76:1188–96.
50. Gupta S, Anderson J, Bhandari P, et al. Development and validation of a novel method for assessing competency in polypectomy: direct observation of polypectomy skills. Gastrointest Endosc. 2011;73:1232–9 e2.
51. Gupta S, Bassett P, Man R, et al. Validation of a novel method for assessing competency in polypectomy. Gastrointest Endosc. 2012;75:568–75.
52. Gruppen LD. Competency-based education, feedback, and humility. Gastroenterology. 2015;148:4–7.
53. Kruger J, Dunning D. Unskilled and unaware of it: how difficulties in recognizing one's own incompetence lead to inflated self-assessments. J Pers Soc Psychol. 1999;77:1121–34.
54. Wang AY, Emura F, Oda I, et al. Endoscopic submucosal dissection with electrosurgical knives in a patient on aspirin therapy (with video). Gastrointest Endosc. 2010;72:1066–71.
55. Colorado Uo. Rocky mountain interventional endoscopy course. Available at: https://www.rmiecourse.com/program-overview.
56. Creative. Sydney international endoscopy symposium. Available at: http://www.sies.org.au/symposium/topics.
57. ASGE. DDW hands-on workshops: EMR. Available at: https://www.asge.org/home/education-meetings/advanced-education-training/ddw-digestive-disease-week.
58. ASGE. ASGE STAR certificate programs. Available at: https://www.asge.org/home/education-meetings/advanced-education-training/star-certificate-programs.
59. Oyama T, Yahagi N, Ponchon T, et al. How to establish endoscopic submucosal dissection in Western countries. World J Gastroenterol. 2015;21:11209–20.
60. Lee RF, Heitman SJ, Bourke MJ. Training and competency in endoscopic mucosal resection. Tech Gastrointest Endosc. 2017;19:125–36.
61. Belderbos TD, Leenders M, Moons LM, et al. Local recurrence after endoscopic mucosal resection of non-pedunculated colorectal lesions: systematic review and meta-analysis. Endoscopy. 2014;46:388–402.
62. Wang AY, Ahmad NA, Zaidman JS, et al. Endoluminal resection for sessile neoplasia in the GI tract is associated with a low recurrence rate and a high 5-year survival rate. Gastrointest Endosc. 2008;68:160–9.
63. Ahmad NA, Kochman ML, Long WB, et al. Efficacy, safety, and clinical outcomes of endoscopic mucosal resection: a study of 101 cases. Gastrointest Endosc. 2002;55:390–6.
64. Schenck RJ, Jahann DA, Patrie JT, et al. Underwater endoscopic mucosal resection is associated with fewer recurrences and earlier curative resections compared to conventional endoscopic mucosal resection for large colorectal polyps. Surg Endosc. 2017;31:4174.
65. Sakamoto T, Matsuda T, Otake Y, et al. Predictive factors of local recurrence after endoscopic piecemeal mucosal resection. J Gastroenterol. 2012;47:635–40.
66. Wang AY, Draganov PV. Training in endoscopic submucosal dissection from a Western perspective. Tech Gastrointest Endosc. 2017;19:159–69.

Intragastric Balloons and Aspiration Therapy

Chetan Mittal and Shelby Sullivan

Introduction

The prevalence of obesity and its associated comorbidities including diabetes, hypertension, and hyperlipidemia is exponentially increasing, across all age groups [1]. Lifestyle intervention is considered the first line of therapy with pharmacotherapy and bariatric surgery used for patients meeting BMI criteria in addition to failure to achieve weight loss with lifestyle intervention alone [2]. Lifestyle interventions including dietary change, exercise, and behavior modification have limited effectiveness in providing sustained long-term weight loss [3]. Bariatric surgery is the most effective modality for weight loss [4–6]. Bariatric surgery is associated with procedural morbidity and potential long-term complications but in general is considered safe procedure with acceptable adverse event rates [4–6]. Despite this, rates of bariatric surgery among patients who would qualify for surgery remain low, with only 1.068% of eligible patients undergoing bariatric surgery in 2015 [7]. There are likely multiple reasons why patients avoid bariatric surgery including but not limited to risks associated with surgery, cost, access to care, physician referral, and

recovery time. Endoscopic bariatric therapies (EBTs) may overcome some of these barriers to bariatric surgical treatments. EBTs are less invasive, reversible procedures and can be performed at lower BMIs than bariatric surgery. These characteristics are extremely attractive to patients seeking effective weight loss without the potential complications associated with bariatric surgery.

The EBTs currently approved by the FDA including three intragastric balloons and aspiration therapy with the AspireAssist primarily reduce calorie intake leading to weight loss through different mechanisms, but they are all considered gastric EBTs. In general, gastric EBT's improvement on metabolic function is weight loss dependent. This is in contrast to small bowel EBTs which may have both weight loss-dependent and weight loss-independent effects on metabolism, in particular glucose control. This chapter will focus on the currently approved EBTs for primary obesity treatment, which include the ReShape Dual Balloon, the Orbera Balloon, the Obalon Balloon System, and the AspireAssist System for aspiration therapy as well as two IGBs which are currently being studied in multicenter randomized controlled trials in the United States.

Intragastric Balloons

IGBs are space-occupying devices that promote weight loss by reducing food intake. The Garren-Edwards gastric bubble (American Edwards

C. Mittal
Division of Gastroenterology, University of Colorado-Denver, Aurora, CO, USA

S. Sullivan (✉)
University of Colorado School of Medicine, Aurora, CO, USA
e-mail: shelby.sullivan@ucdenver.edu

© Springer Nature Switzerland AG 2020
M. S. Wagh, S. B. Wani (eds.), *Gastrointestinal Interventional Endoscopy*,
https://doi.org/10.1007/978-3-030-21695-5_12

Laboratories, USA) was the first commercially available air-filled polyurethane balloon. It was approved by the US Food and Drug Administration in 1985 but was later removed due to risk of serious adverse events including gastric ulceration, gastric perforation, and bowel obstruction. Also, the size of these balloons was not large enough to promote effective weight loss [8]. Data suggests that at least 400 ml of volume is needed to for a space-occupying device to result in weight loss [9]. The currently approved IGBs have introduced design changes in addition to the volume of space occupation in the stomach to mitigate the adverse events seen with the Garren-Edwards gastric bubble including spherical or ellipse shape, soft pliable materials for balloon construction, and elimination of sharp edges. In addition, the fluid-filled IGBs have been shown to delay gastric emptying, which, in turn, reduces the frequency of food intake. A secondary analysis conducted on a subset of 29 patients in the Orbera pivotal trial evaluated baseline 1- and 2-hour gastric retention values between IGB and control groups [10]. Gastric retention more than doubled during the duration of IGB placement (8 and 16 weeks) and returned to normal within 3 weeks of IGB removal. Also, greater increase in gastric retention was significantly associated with higher total body weight loss at 24 and 52 weeks. Fluid-filled IGBs have also been shown to reduce the fasting and postprandial serum concentration of cholecystokinin and pancre-

atic peptide hormones, which lead to delayed gastric emptying [11]. Mion et al. showed that plasma ghrelin concentrations were reduced with IGB placement and correlated with degree of weight loss [12]. This is in contrast to the effect of weight loss with lifestyle therapy alone on ghrelin concentrations, which increase with weight loss and correlate with visual analogue scores for hunger and desire to eat [13]. These changes may contribute to the effect of IGBs on weight loss maintenance. The weight loss achieved with IGB appears to be maintained for a longer period of time as compared to lifestyle modifications and weight loss medications. In one study reporting 5-year outcomes after IGB removal, the proportion of patients maintaining >20% total body weight loss was 53%, 27%, and 23% at 1-, 2-, and 5-year follow-up, respectively [14]. Moreover, weight loss maintenance of 70–90% has been seen in the US pivotal trials of IGBs [15, 16].

Currently, there are three IGBs – Orbera, ReShape and Obalon, FDA approved for treatment of obesity in patients with a BMI of 30–40 kg/m². Two other IGBs are in the process of obtaining FDA approval – Spatz balloon and Elipse balloon.

Orbera Balloon

The Orbera balloon (Apollo Endosurgery, Austin, Texas, USA, Table 12.1) was previously

Table 12.1 FDA-approved intragastric balloons

Device	Device image	Characteristics	FDA status
Reshape Dual Balloon System ReShape Medical, San Clemente, CA		Two medical-grade silicone spheres joined by a flexible shaft Each balloon filled with 375–450 ml of saline dyed with methylene blue Endoscopically placed and removed after 6 months	Approved July 28, 2015 BMI 30–40kg/m² with one obesity-related comorbidity
Orbera Intragastric Balloon, Apollo Endosurgery, Austin, TX		Medical-grade silicone sphere, filled with 400-700 ml of saline Endoscoically placed and removed	Approved August 5, 2015 BMI 30–40kg/m²
Obalon Balloon System, Obalon Therapeutics, Carlsbad, CA		Thin polymer ellipse shape Filled with 250 ml of a nitrogen mix gas Three balloons administered over 8 to 12-week period Swallowed and endoscopically removed 6 months after first balloon administration	Approved September 8, 2016 BMI 30–40kg/m²

known as the BioEnterics Intragastric Balloon (BIB, BioEnterics Corporation, Allergan, Irvine, CA), which has been commercially available since 1991 outside of the United States. It is made of a silicone elastomer, filled with 400 to 700 mL of saline. The saline can be mixed with methylene blue to aid in detection of leaks, but this is not approved in the United States. It required endoscopic placement and endoscopic removal for a maximum duration of 6 months [17]. The initial use of BIB was in patients with BMI > 40 kg/m² as a bridge to bariatric surgery or in patients with BMI 30–40 kg/m² with associated comorbidities. The largest case series evaluating the safety and outcomes data on BIB reported a 33.8% ± 18.7% EWL at 6 months of follow-up [18]. The study reported improvement or resolution of diabetes and hypertension in 86.9% and 93.7% of patients, with an acceptable adverse event rate of 2.8%. Gastric perforations were reported in five patients, four of whom had previous gastric surgery. Gastric outlet obstruction, balloon rupture, esophagitis, and gastric ulcer were other complications, managed either with endoscopic removal of balloon or with conservative treatment.

In the US pivotal multicenter non-blinded randomized controlled trial, 273 patients with a BMI of 30–40 kg/m² were randomized into one of two groups: Orbera balloon plus behavioral modification program (n = 125, BMI 35.2 ± 3.2 kg/m²) or behavioral modification alone (n = 130, BMI 35.4 ± 2.7 kg/m²) [15]. At 26 and 52 weeks after balloon placement, 71.8% and 45.9% patients in the Orbera balloon group achieved ≥25% EWL compared to 31.9% and 32.6% of patients in behavioral modification alone group. The mean %TBWL at 26 and 52 weeks in the completed analysis was 10.5% and 7.7% in patients who received the balloon compared to 4.7% and 3.9% in patients on behavioral modification alone, respectively [19].

A recent meta-analysis by American Society for Gastrointestinal Endoscopy (ASGE) Bariatric Endoscopy Task Force reported that Orbera meets Preservation and Incorporation of Valuable Endoscopic Innovations (PIVI) thresholds for both primary and non-primary bridge therapy for obesity [20]. The PIVI thresholds were published in 2011 from a joint ASGE/American Society for Metabolic and Bariatric Surgery (ASMBS) Task Force which recommended that 25% excess weight loss (EWL) at 12 months and difference between active and control subjects in a randomized controlled trial should be at least 15% EWL for primary therapies [21]. Although there are issues with this white paper, namely, the differential effects of sham-controlled study design and intensity of lifestyle therapy on overall weight loss, the recommendations in this white paper were used to evaluate Orbera. This analysis included 17 studies and 1683 patients for weight loss outcomes with %EWL using random effect model at 12 months at 25.4%. The pooled percent total body weight loss (%TBWL) at 3, 6, and 12 months after Orbera balloon placement was 12.3%, 13.2% and 11.3%.

A few studies have evaluated the utility of sequential or repeated IGB placements. Dumonceau et al. reported outcomes on 19 patients who had repeat IGB therapy (using BIB) per their own request, either immediately (n = 8) or after device-free period (n = 11). Overall, the %EWL at 6 months and 1 year was higher for patients with repeat IGB placement (49.3% vs 30.7% and 40.9% vs 20.8%, respectively), but the difference was not significant at 3 years [22]. Another study reported outcomes on endoscopic BIB placement (600–700 mL saline with 10 mL methylene blue) in 714 consecutive patients. Mean %EWL at 6 months was 41.6 ± 21.8.

Hundred twelve patients underwent second BIB placement, and mean %EWL at second balloon removal was 31.5 ± 23.2 [23]. Genco et al. compared dietary therapy vs second balloon placement after removal of first IGB in 100 patients with obesity (BMI 40 to 44.9 kg/m²). At the end of study period, mean excess BMI loss was significantly higher in patients with a second balloon placement as compared to dietary therapy alone (51.9 ± 24.6% and 25.1 ± 26.2%, respectively) [24].

In addition to weight loss, IGBs have been shown to be associated with improvement in metabolic syndrome and obesity-associated comorbidities. In a multicenter European study including 261 patients, the %EWL was 29.1% at 3 years [25]. The rate of hypertension decreased from 29% to 16% at 3 years, diabetes decreased from 15% to 10%, hypercholesterolemia decreased from 32% to 21%, and osteoarthritis decreased from 25% to 13%.

Orbera IGB is generally well tolerated in clinical practice with a low rate of serious adverse events. In the above meta-analysis, pain and nausea were reported in about one third of the patients [20]. Migration and gastric perforation were seen in 1.4% and 0.1%, respectively. The most common nonserious adverse events in the Orbera US pivotal trial include vomiting, nausea, and abdominal pain which occurred in 86.8%, 75.6%, and 57.5% of subjects, respectively. Of note, 30% of subjects either developed or had worsening gastroesophageal reflux disease, which may be a consideration when helping patients choose an IGB. The rate of serious adverse events in the Orbera US pivotal trial was 10%, half of which were device intolerance followed by dehydration (two cases), gastric outlet obstruction (one case), gastric perforation (one case), aspiration pneumonia (one case), and infected balloon (one case), all of which resolved without permanent sequelae [15]. As with any new device or therapy, the rates of adverse events were significantly lower in clinical practice than in original clinical trials, likely related to lack of experience and heightened awareness in the clinical trial phase. Data from a US registry demonstrated a serious adverse event rate requiring hospitalization of 1.7% [26].

The FDA recently issued warning statements regarding hyperinsufflation, pancreatitis, and death, which were not previously identified in the US pivotal trials [27]. Pancreatitis likely results from compression of pancreatic body from the IGB, which resolves with balloon aspiration, but likely affects <0.01% of patients treated with IGB [28]. Moreover, a death rate of 0.08% was previously reported in the ASGE meta-analysis listed above [20], and based on recent publications from Apollo Endosurgery, the current rate is likely <0.01%, which may be related to improved patient selection and adverse event prevention [29].

ReShape Balloon

The ReShape Integrated Dual Balloon System (ReShape Medical, San Clemente, CA,

Table 12.1) is unique in design, consisting of two medical grade silicone spheres connected by a flexible shaft. Each balloon is filled with 375–450 mL of saline mixed with methylene blue depending on the height of the patient [30]. Both placement and removal after 6 months of implantation are performed under direct endoscopic visualization. The dual balloon system is designed to provide higher gastric volume occupation and lower chances of migration into the small bowel. The REDUCE pivotal trial was a multicenter double-blind randomized sham-controlled trial comparing ReShape Dual Balloon System plus diet and exercise ($n = 187$, BMI 35.3 ± 2.8 kg/m^2) with sham endoscopy plus diet and exercise ($n = 139$, BMI 35.4 ± 2.6 kg/m^2) [31]. Patients in the balloon group had a significantly higher %EWL at 24 weeks (25.1%) compared with diet and exercise alone group (11.3%) in an intention-to-treat analysis. For completed cases, balloon group had a 7.6%TBWL as compared to 3.6% TBWL for diet and exercise group. For patients that completed a 48-week follow-up, the mean %EWL was 18.8%. Hemoglobin A1c, serum triglyceride concentrations, low-density lipoprotein cholesterol (LDL-C), systolic blood pressure, and diastolic blood pressure significantly decreased in the ReShape Dual Balloon group compared with baseline, with continued improvement compared with baseline in all parameters except for serum triglyceride concentration. Improvement in quality-of-life score and obesity-related quality-of-life scores, as measured by physical function, public distress, self-esteem, sexual life, and work productivity, were significantly higher in the balloon group. Balloon retrieval was required in 9.1% [24] cases due to early intolerance and in 6% due to symptoms associated with ulceration. No gastric perforations, balloon migration, or bowel obstruction was reported. Nausea, vomiting, and abdominal pain were experienced by 54.5%–86.7% of subjects, some of which required emergency room visits (21 cases). The serious adverse event rate was 10.6%; however, the majority of serious adverse events were due to hospitalization or ER visit for intravenous treatment of post-placement accommodative symptoms (nausea, vomiting, abdominal pain). Non-accommodative serious adverse events were uncommon and included esophageal mucosal tear during retrieval (one case), GE junction ulcer (one case), contained cervical esophageal perforation (one case), and pneumonitis post retrieval (one case), all of which were managed conservatively. Gastric ulceration, mostly near incisura, occurred in 39% of patients in the initial trial phase, which was reduced to 10% after subtle changes in balloon distal tip design. However, it is to be noted that gastric ulceration rates were highest with ReShape balloon as compared to Orbera or Obalon balloon, which may be a factor in choosing the right balloon for patients at high risk for gastric ulcers.

Similar to Orbera balloon, weight loss in clinical practice is higher with ReShape balloon as compared to the above reported clinical trial. Lopez-Nava et al. reported outcomes in 60 patients who underwent ReShape dual intragastric balloon system placement, filled with a total of 900 cc fluid, for 6 months. The study reported 15.4% TBWL and 47.1% EWL, compared to 7.6% TBWL and 25.1% EWL in the REDUCE trial. Only one early removal for patient intolerance, one early deflation without migration, and one gastric perforation were reported [32].

The overall weight loss in REDUCE trial was lower as compared to the Orbera balloon trial. This is likely the result of difference in trial design as the Orbera trial was not sham controlled, and subject knowledge of intervention may be associated with higher weight loss. A recent retrospective cohort study compared 14 Orbera and 26 ReShape balloon cases [33] and showed similar weight loss results despite higher baseline BMI in Orbera group (10.5% ±1.8% TBWL in ReShape and 10.2 ± 1.9% TBWL in Orbera group). The overall adverse events requiring intervention (defined as early IGB removal due to intolerance, IGB deflation requiring replacement, and upper gastrointestinal symptoms requiring emergency room visit or inpatient admission) were significantly more common in Orbera patients (43% vs 12%, $P = 0.04$) [33]. Another recent study compared tolerability of Orbera and ReShape IGBs in a retrospective study of 100 patients. The overall rate and severity of accommodative symptoms (nausea, vomiting, and abdominal pain) were similar between the two groups, but duration of nausea and vomiting was longer in Orbera balloon group. Overall weight loss was similar for both groups though early retrieval rate due to intolerance was higher in Orbera group (15.7%) as compared to ReShape group (7.8%) [34]. These data suggest that the weight loss seen with ReShape Dual Balloon is the same as the Orbera balloon in clinical practice and that the ReShape Dual Balloon may be slightly better tolerated by patients; however more data is necessary to understand these differences.

Obalon Balloon

The Obalon Balloon System (Obalon Therapeutics, Carlsbad, CA, Table 12.1) is the most recent FDA-approved IGB. The Obalon Balloon System consists of a thin polymer Elipse balloon filled with 250 cc of a proprietary nitrogen gas mixture. The Obalon balloon is enclosed inside a 6-gram dissolvable capsule, attached to a thin catheter. The balloon is swallowed in the capsule form, and placement in stomach is confirmed using fluoroscopy and pressure monitor readings using a manometer connected to the catheter. As the capsule dissolves, the pressure reading on manometer drops under 7 KPa. After confirming on fluoroscopy, balloon can be inflated (9–13 KPa) and catheter is removed. Three balloons are administered over an 8- to 12-week period, followed by endoscopic removal of all balloons at 6 months from the first balloon placement [16].

The pivotal US multicenter double-blind randomized sham controlled trial (SMART trial) compared Obalon IGB plus lifestyle counseling ($n = 198$, BMI 35.1 ± 2.7 kg/m^2) to a sham control group of non-balloon capsules and lifestyle counseling ($n = 189$, BMI 35.4 ± 2.7 kg/m^2). For the per protocol analysis, %TBWL at 24 weeks was 6.86% ± 5.1% in the Obalon IGB plus lifestyle counseling group as compared to 3.59 ± 5% in the control group. For the modified intention-to-treat analysis (including patients who swallowed at least 1 capsule), %TBWL at 24 weeks was 6.6 ± 5.1% in the treatment group and 3.4 ± 5% in the control group ($p = 0.0354$). For the completer analysis (including patients who completed study testing through week 24), %TBWL at 24 weeks was 7.1 ± 5.0% in the Obalon IGB plus lifestyle counseling group as compared to 3.6 ± 5.1% in the control group, $p = 0.0085$) In addition to weight loss, significant improvement was noticed in systolic blood pressure, fasting glucose, LDL cholesterol and triglyceride levels in the intervention group [35].

The most common nonserious adverse events in the SMART trial included abdominal pain, nausea, and vomiting occurring in 72.6%, 56.0%, and 17.3% of subjects respectively, with 99.6% of all nonserious adverse events reported as mild or moderate. Only one serious adverse event of a bleeding gastric ulcer was reported in a patient taking high dose NSAIDs which was prohibited per protocol [36].

Obalon balloon has been used off-label in the pediatric and adolescent population. De Peppo et al. reported outcomes of a small study including 17 children with obesity (BMI > 30 kg/m^2) and a mean age of 13.6 years (Range 9.9 to 17.1). The overall %EWL was 20.1 ± 9.8 (range 2.3–35.1) with significant reductions in mean BMI (35.27 ± 5.89 to 32.25 ± 7.1), mean excess weight (36.2 ± 15.9 to 29.4 ± 18.3 kg) and waist circumference (109 ± 12.3 cm to 99 ± 10.5 cm) [37]. No studies comparing the Obalon Balloon System to the ReShape or Orbera balloons have been published to date.

Spatz Balloon

The Spatz balloon system (Spatz FGIA, Great Neck, NY, Table 12.2) is a spherical silicone saline-filled balloon with an attached inflation catheter. The balloon requires endoscopic placement and the volume of the balloon can be adjusted endoscopically. The second generation of the Spatz Balloon (Spatz3) balloon is currently under FDA approval but has been studied for use up to 12 months after placement outside of the United States. The main advantage of Spatz balloon is the volume adjustability, which allows for increase in size when more weight gain is desired or reduction in size to improve tolerability.

The first-generation Spatz balloon was studied in 18 patients and showed a 26.4% EWL at 24 weeks and 48.8% EWL at 52 weeks. Adjustments were successfully performed for additional weight loss in ten cases. However, seven balloons had to be removed prematurely due to valve malfunction, gastritis, Mallory-Weiss tear, NSAID-related perforation ulcer, and balloon deflation [38].

A UK study including 73 patients with 1-year Spatz balloon placement (mean volume 417 mL) showed 45.7% EWL (excluding 21

Table 12.2 Investigational intragastric balloons in the United States

Device	Device Image	Characteristics	FDA Status
Spatz III Adjustable Balloon System Spatz FGIA, Inc., Great Neck, NY		Spherical silicone balloon around a curved catheter which extends outside the balloon to adjust fill volume after implantation Filled with saline dyed with methylene blue 300-900 ml	Pivotal trial
Elipse Intragastric Balloon Allurion Technologies, Wellesley, MA)		Spherical balloon made of a polymer film Filled with 550 ml of saline Swallowed Self-deflates and passes through GI tract at 4 months	Pivotal trial

early removals). Balloon volume adjustment was considered in 51 patients for plateaued weight loss, but adjustment failed in 6 cases and did not lead to additional weight loss in 7 cases. Catheter impaction requiring surgical removal (4.1%) and failure of volume adjustment (5.5%) were the main concerns in post-marketing phase [39].

A recent study reported outcomes in 206 patients from three centers, implanted with the second-generation Spatz3 adjustable IGB. The overall %EWL was 55.6%, and %TBWL was 15.2% on balloon removal at 12 months. Downward adjustment of balloon volume by 100–150 mL successfully allowed continuation of IGB in 80% (12/15) cases. Increase in balloon volume for weight loss plateau leads to additional mean weight loss of 9.3 kg (range 3–24 kg). No serious adverse events were noted [40].

Elipse Balloon

The Elipse balloon system (Allurion Technologies, Wellesley, MA, Table 12.2) consists of a single spherical balloon made of polymer filled with 550 mL of saline. The balloon contained in a capsule is swallowed, and gastric placement is confirmed using fluoroscopy. The main design advantage of Elipse balloon is the presence of an internal release valve that spontaneously deflates at 4 months, and the deflated balloon passes through the GI tract, saving the need for endoscopic removal.

The first European trial included 34 patients with a mean BMI of 34.4 kg/m^2 and reported a 9.5% TBWL and 37.2% EWL at 4 months. All patients safely excreted the balloon [41]. A recent prospective Italian study included 38 patients with a mean BMI of 38.6 kg/m^2 and reported 26% EWL and 11.6% TBWL at 16 weeks. The study also reported significant improvement in metabolic syndrome parameters including blood pressure, waist circumference, blood glucose, and triglyceride levels. No serious adverse events were noted [42].

Another single-center prospective pilot study from Kuwait including 51 patients reported 10.4% TBWL, 40.84% EWL, and 3.42 kg/m^2 change in BMI at 4 months. Five balloon removals were reported due to intolerance, including one case vomiting the balloon [43]. A recent multicenter prospective study including 135 patients reports safety and efficacy outcomes. At 4 months, mean BMI reduction was 4.9 units and mean %TWL was 15.1%. Two patients vomited the balloon, three patients required early removal due to intolerance, three patients had early deflation, and one patient suffered small bowel obstruction that required balloon removal via laparoscopic enterotomy [44].

Aspiration Therapy

The Aspire Assist System (AspireAssist; Aspire Bariatrics, King of Prussia, PA) functions on the principle of removing a portion of ingested food via a percutaneous endoscopic gastrostomy (PEG) tube, to reduce the amount of food available for absorption. In addition, the device also results in a decrease in food consumed at a meal [45]. The device is FDA approved for use in patients 21 years or older with BMI 35–55 kg/m^2. The device consists of components that are implanted and components that are only used during aspiration (Figs. 12.1 and 12.2).

The A-Tube is placed endoscopically with a standard pull technique similar to a PEG tube. General anesthesia is not required for A-Tube

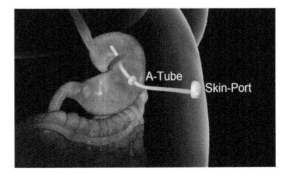

Fig. 12.1 Implanted A-Tube with attached Skin-Port

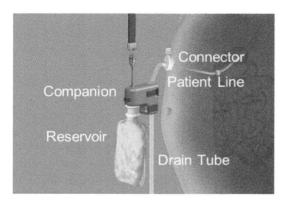

Fig. 12.2 Assembled AspireAssist System with implanted A-Tube and components only used during aspiration

placement, which makes it an attractive option for patients with BMI > 50 kg/m² and who have significant perioperative mortality associated with bariatric surgery. One to two weeks after placement, the skin port is attached to the external cut end of tube and aspiration sessions can begin. The patients remove about 30% of the ingested meal 20 min after eating, and the process takes about 5–15 min. In addition to aspiration of a portion of caloric intake, patients also notice a change in behavior leading to reduced food intake. In order to avoid clogging of the A-Tube, food particles must be <5 mm in diameter on average, which requires patients to chew food significantly longer than before initiation of aspiration therapy and to drink sufficient water with meals. These mealtime behaviors likely contribute to the reduced intake of food at mealtimes reported by patients [46].

In the pivotal multicenter US trial, 171 subjects with BMI 35–55 kg/m² were randomly assigned in a 2:1 fashion and included in the modified intention-to-treat analysis to AspireAssist plus lifestyle counseling ($n = 111$, mean BMI 42.2 ± 5.1 kg/m²) or lifestyle counseling alone ($n = 70$, mean BMI 40.9 ± 3.9 kg/m²). The A-Tube was successfully placed in 97% of patients with a mean procedure time of 15 min. Three failed cases were due to inability to transilluminate, presence of gastric varices, and Roux-en-Y anatomy diagnosed during endoscopy. The

mean %EWL and %TBWL at 52 weeks were significantly higher in AspireAssist group as compared to lifestyle counseling alone group in the modified intention-to-treat analysis (31.5 ± 26.7% vs 9.8 ± 15.5% and 12.1 ± 9.6% vs 3.5 ± 6.0% respectively), with 58.6% of patients in the AspireAssist group achieving at least 25% EWL and 59% of subjects with at least 10% TBWL. Also, metabolic syndrome parameters improved significantly in the AspireAssist group, including HbA1c, triglyceride, and HDL cholesterol levels, though the difference in metabolic parameters between the two groups was statistically significant only for HbA1c. It is important to note that most patients had normal glucose control, lipid concentrations, and blood pressure at baseline and would not be expected to have significant changes with weight loss. A total of five severe adverse events were reported including one case of mild peritonitis after A-Tube placement, two hospitalizations related to abdominal pain after tube placement, one prepyloric ulcer at 53 weeks causing abdominal pain, and one case of product malfunction requiring replacement of A-Tube, all of which resolved without long-term sequelae [46].

A European study including 11 patients with a mean BMI of 66.5 kg/m² reported outcomes of aspiration therapy. Overall, the %TBWL and %EWL were 14.5% and 28.5% at 6 months, 21.4% and 33.9% at 1 year, and 25.5% and 38.8% at 2 years. No serious adverse events were reported and procedure was successful in all cases [47].

A recent European registry study including 201 patients with mean BMI of 43.6 ± 7.2 kg/m² reported 1- to 4-year safety and effectiveness outcomes. Mean %TBWL at 1, 2, 3, and 4 years was 18.2% ± 9.4% ($n/N = 155/173$), 19.8% ± 11.3% ($n/N = 82/114$), 21.3% ± 9.6% ($n/N = 24/43$), and 19.2% ± 13.1% ($n/N = 12/30$). The mean %EWL at 1, 2, 3, and 4 years was 46.3% ± 26.3%, 48.2% ± 28.2%, 50.3% ± 26.2%, and 47.9% ± 36.2%. There was significant reduction in HbA1c (−0.39% ± 0.44%), systolic blood pressure (−12.1 ± 19.3 mm Hg), diastolic blood pressure (−6.0 ± 14.0 mm Hg), and triglyceride levels (−25.5 ± 49.1 mg/dL) including a significant

HbA1c reduction in diabetics ($-1.0\% \pm 0.5\%$) at 1 year. A few serious complications were reported including seven cases of buried bumpers and one case of peritonitis, which resolved with 2-day course of antibiotics [48].

There are no studies comparing AspireAssist device directly to IGBs. However, aspiration therapy has been studied in comparison with bariatric surgery [49]. A total of 103 patients were sequentially enrolled to either the aspiration therapy group ($n = 54$, BMI 42.0 ± 5.1 kg/m^2, 120.2 ± 23.6 kg) or Roux-en-Y gastric bypass surgery $n = 49$, BMI 41.1 ± 5.0 kg/m^2, 115.3 ± 17.8 kg). At 1 year, patients in the aspiration therapy group achieved $21 \pm 11\%$TBWL compared with $32 \pm 9\%$ TBWL in the Roux-en-Y gastric bypass surgery group. Although weight loss was higher in the Roux-en-Y gastric bypass surgery group, five serious adverse events requiring a total of five additional surgeries and seven additional endoscopies occurred in the Roux-en-Y gastric bypass surgery group compared with three serious adverse events that required a total of six endoscopies and no surgeries in the aspiration therapy group.

Conclusion

EBTs represent a new category of treatment options for obesity. There are a variety of available EBTs, with different routes of placement, weight loss outcomes, metabolic benefits, and safety profiles. The three FDA-approved intragastric balloons and the AspireAssist for aspiration therapy are gastric EBTs and are able to be placed with minimal additional training for most endoscopists. Two additional intragastric balloons are currently under evaluation in the United States. Although not discussed in this chapter, a comprehensive weight loss program involving endoscopists, nutritionists, counselors, and bariatric surgeons is essential for maximizing weight loss and metabolic goals for patients with obesity undergoing EBT. As all EBTs are increasingly used, safety profiles will continue to improve with experience.

References

1. Ward ZJ, Long MW, Resch SC, Gortmaker SL, Cradock AL, Giles C, et al. Redrawing the US obesity landscape: bias-corrected estimates of state-specific adult obesity prevalence. PLoS One. 2016;11(3):e0150735.
2. Jensen MD, Ryan DH, Apovian CM, Ard JD, Comuzzie AG, Donato KA, et al. 2013 AHA/ACC/TOS guideline for the management of overweight and obesity in adults: a report of the American College of Cardiology/American Heart Association Task Force on Practice Guidelines and The Obesity Society. Circulation. 2014;129(25 Suppl 2):S102–38.
3. Turk MW, Yang K, Hravnak M, Sereika SM, Ewing LJ, Burke LE. Randomized clinical trials of weight loss maintenance: a review. J Cardiovasc Nurs. 2009;24(1):58–80.
4. Schauer PR, Kashyap SR, Wolski K, Brethauer SA, Kirwan JP, Pothier CE, et al. Bariatric surgery versus intensive medical therapy in obese patients with diabetes. N Engl J Med. 2012;366(17):1567–76.
5. Buchwald H, Oien DM. Metabolic/bariatric surgery worldwide 2011. Obes Surg. 2013;23(4):427–36.
6. Chang SH, Stoll CR, Song J, Varela JE, Eagon CJ, Colditz GA. The effectiveness and risks of bariatric surgery: an updated systematic review and meta-analysis, 2003-2012. JAMA Surg. 2014;149(3):275–87.
7. Ponce J, DeMaria EJ, Nguyen NT, Hutter M, Sudan R, Morton JM. American Society for Metabolic and Bariatric Surgery estimation of bariatric surgery procedures in 2015 and surgeon workforce in the United States. Surg Obes Relat Dis. 2016;12(9):1637–9.
8. Kirby DF, Wade JB, Mills PR, Sugerman HJ, Kellum JM, Zfass AM, et al. A prospective assessment of the Garren-Edwards gastric bubble and bariatric surgery in the treatment of morbid obesity. Am Surg. 1990;56(10):575–80.
9. Geliebter A, Westreich S, Gage D. Gastric distention by balloon and test-meal intake in obese and lean subjects. Am J Clin Nutr. 1988;48(3):592–4.
10. Gómez V, Woodman G, Abu Dayyeh BK. Delayed gastric emptying as a proposed mechanism of action during intragastric balloon therapy: results of a prospective study. Obesity. 2016;24(9):1849–53.
11. Mathus-Vliegen EM, de Groot GH. Fasting and meal-induced CCK and PP secretion following intragastric balloon treatment for obesity. Obes Surg. 2013;23(5):622–33.
12. Mion F, Napoleon B, Roman S, Malvoisin E, Trepo F, Pujol B, et al. Effects of intragastric balloon on gastric emptying and plasma ghrelin levels in non-morbid obese patients. Obes Surg. 2005;15(4):510–6.
13. Sumithran P, Prendergast LA, Delbridge E, Purcell K, Shulkes A, Kriketos A, et al. Long-term persistence of hormonal adaptations to weight loss. N Engl J Med. 2011;365(17):1597–604.

14. Kotzampassi K, Grosomanidis V, Papakostas P, Penna S, Eleftheriadis E. 500 Intragastric balloons: what happens 5 years thereafter? Obes Surg. 2012;22(6):896–903.

15. Courcoulas A, Abu Dayyeh BK, Eaton L, Robinson J, Woodman G, Fusco M, et al. Intragastric balloon as an adjunct to lifestyle intervention: a randomized controlled trial. Int J Obes. 2017;41(3):427–33.

16. FDA. Summary of safety and effectiveness data (SSED) Obalon balloon system. In: FDA, editor. 2016. p. 1–46. https://fda.report/PMA/P160001/16/P160001B.pdf.

17. FDA. Summary of safety and effectiveness data (SSED) ORBERA intragastric balloon system. In: FDA, editor. 2015. p. 1–32. https://www.accessdata.fda.gov/cdrh_docs/pdf14/P140008b.pdf.

18. Genco A, Bruni T, Doldi SB, Forestieri P, Marino M, Busetto L, et al. BioEnterics Intragastric balloon: the Italian experience with 2,515 patients. Obes Surg. 2005;15(8):1161–4.

19. Abu Dayyeh BK, Eaton LL, Woodman G, Fusco M, Shayani V, Billy HT, et al. 444 A randomized, multicenter study to evaluate the safety and effectiveness of an intragastric balloon as an adjunct to a behavioral modification program, in comparison with a behavioral modification program alone in the weight management of obese subjects. Gastrointest Endosc. 2015;81(5 Suppl):AB147.

20. Abu Dayyeh BK, Kumar N, Edmundowicz SA, Jonnalagadda S, Larsen M, Sullivan S, et al. ASGE Bariatric Endoscopy Task Force systematic review and meta-analysis assessing the ASGE PIVI thresholds for adopting endoscopic bariatric therapies. Gastrointest Endosc. 2015;82(3):425–38 e5.

21. Ginsberg GG, Chand B, Cote GA, Dallal RM, Edmundowicz SA, Nguyen NT, et al. A pathway to endoscopic bariatric therapies. Gastrointest Endosc. 2011;74(5):943–53.

22. Dumonceau JM, Francois E, Hittelet A, Mehdi AI, Barea M, Deviere J. Single vs repeated treatment with the intragastric balloon: a 5-year weight loss study. Obes Surg. 2010;20(6):692–7.

23. Lopez-Nava G, Rubio MA, Prados S, Pastor G, Cruz MR, Companioni E, et al. BioEnterics(R) intragastric balloon (BIB(R)). Single ambulatory center Spanish experience with 714 consecutive patients treated with one or two consecutive balloons. Obes Surg. 2011;21(1):5–9.

24. Genco A, Cipriano M, Bacci V, Maselli R, Paone E, Lorenzo M, et al. Intragastric balloon followed by diet vs intragastric balloon followed by another balloon: a prospective study on 100 patients. Obes Surg. 2010;20(11):1496–500.

25. Genco A, Lopez-Nava G, Wahlen C, Maselli R, Cipriano M, Sanchez MM, et al. Multi-centre European experience with intragastric balloon in overweight populations: 13 years of experience. Obes Surg. 2013;23(4):515–21.

26. Vargas EJ, Kadouh HC, Bazerbachi F, Acosta Cardenas AJ, Lorentz PA, Pesta CM, et al. 547 Single fluid-filled intragastric balloon for weight loss: us post-regulatory approval multicenter clinical experience in 245 patients. Gastrointest Endosc. 2017;85(5):AB82.

27. https://www.fda.gov/MedicalDevices/Safety/LetterstoHealthCareProviders/ucm570707.htm.

28. Aljiffry M, Habib R, Kotbi E, Ageel A, Hassanain M, Dahlan Y. Acute pancreatitis: a complication of intragastric balloon. Surg Laparosc Endosc Percutan Tech. 2017;27(6):456–9.

29. http://ir.apolloendo.com/press-release/company/apollo-endosurgery-provides-update-and-clarity-fda-letter-health-care.

30. FDA. Summary of safety and effectiveness data (SSED) ReShape integrated dual balloon system; 2015. p. 1–43. https://www.accessdata.fda.gov/cdrh_docs/pdf14/p140012b.pdf.

31. Ponce J, Woodman G, Swain J, Wilson E, English W, Ikramuddin S, et al. The REDUCE pivotal trial: a prospective, randomized controlled pivotal trial of a dual intragastric balloon for the treatment of obesity. Surg Obes Relat Dis. 2015;11(4):874–81.

32. Lopez-Nava G, Bautista-Castaño I, Jimenez-Baños A, Fernandez-Corbelle JP. Dual intragastric balloon: single ambulatory center Spanish experience with 60 patients in endoscopic weight loss management. Obes Surg. 2015;25(12):2263–7.

33. Bennett MC, Early DS, Sullivan SA, Maday RE, Bell SM, Mullady D, et al. Sa2020 Comparison of two intragastric balloon systems for weight loss in a clinical setting. Gastrointest Endosc. 2017;85(5):AB280.

34. Curry T, Pitt T. Sa2016 Intragastric balloon intolerance: a retrospective review of 100 patients treated with two different devices. Gastrointest Endosc. 2017;85(5):AB277–AB8.

35. Sullivan S, Woodman G, Edmundowicz S, Hassanein T, Shayani V, Fang JC, Noar M, Eid G, English WJ, Tariq N, Larsen M, Jonnalagadda SS, Riff DS, Ponce J, Early D, Volkmann E, Ibele AR, Spann MD, Krishnan K, Bucobo JC, Pryor A. Randomized sham-controlled trial of the 6-month swallowable gas-filled intragastric balloon system for weight loss. Surg Obes Relat Dis. 2018;14(12):1876–89.

36. Sullivan S, Swain JM, Woodman G, Edmundowicz S, Hassanein TI, Shayani V, et al. 812d The Obalon Swallowable 6-month balloon system is more effective than moderate intensity lifestyle therapy alone: results from a 6- month randomized sham controlled trial. Gastroenterology. 2016;150(4):S1267.

37. De Peppo F, Caccamo R, Adorisio O, Ceriati E, Marchetti P, Contursi A, et al. The Obalon swallowable intragastric balloon in pediatric and adolescent morbid obesity. Endosc Int Open. 2017;5(1):E59–63.

38. Machytka E, Klvana P, Kornbluth A, Peikin S, Mathus-Vliegen LEM, Gostout C, et al. Adjustable intragastric balloons: a 12-month pilot trial in endoscopic weight loss management. Obes Surg. 2011;21(10):1499–507.

39. Brooks J, Srivastava ED, Mathus-Vliegen EM. One-year adjustable intragastric balloons: results in

73 consecutive patients in the UK. Obes Surg. 2014;24(5):813–9.

40. Machytka E, Divi VP, Saenger F, Sorio R, Brooks J. Mo1296a adjustable balloons for weight loss: a higher yield of responders compared with non-adjustable balloons. Gastrointest Endosc. 2017;85(5):AB495.

41. Chuttani R, Machytka E, Raftopoulos I, Bojkova M, Kupka T, Buzga M, et al. 102 The first procedureless gastric balloon for weight loss: final results from a multi-center, prospective study evaluating safety, efficacy, metabolic parameters, quality of life, and 6-month follow-up. Gastroenterology. 2016;150(4):S26.

42. Genco A, Ernesti I, Ienca R, Casella G, Mariani S, Francomano D, et al. Safety and efficacy of a new swallowable intragastric balloon not needing endoscopy: early Italian experience. Obes Surg. 2018;28(2):405–9.

43. Al-Subaie S, Khalifa S, Buhaimed W, Al-Rashidi S. A prospective pilot study of the efficacy and safety of Elipse intragastric balloon: a single-center, single-surgeon experience. Int J Surg (London, England). 2017;48:16–22.

44. Alsabah S, Al Haddad E, Ekrouf S, Almulla A, Al-Subaie S, Al Kendari M. The safety and efficacy of the procedureless intragastric balloon. Surg Obes Relat Dis. 2018;14(3):311–7.

45. Sullivan S, Stein R, Jonnalagadda S, Mullady D, Edmundowicz S. Aspiration therapy leads to weight loss in obese subjects: a pilot study. Gastroenterology. 2013;145(6):1245–52.e5.

46. Thompson CC, Abu Dayyeh BK, Kushner R, Sullivan S, Schorr AB, Amaro A, et al. Percutaneous gastrostomy device for the treatment of class II and class III obesity: results of a randomized controlled trial. Am J Gastroenterol. 2017;112(3):447–57.

47. Machytka E, Turro R, Huberty V, Buzga M, Bojkova M, Espinos JC, et al. Mo1944 Aspiration therapy in super obese patients – pilot trial. Gastroenterology. 2016;150(4):S822–S3.

48. Nyström M, Machytka E, Norén E, Testoni PA, Janssen I, Turró Homedes J, et al. Aspiration therapy as a tool to treat obesity: 1- to 4-year results in a 201-patient multi-center post-market European Registry Study. Obes Surg. 2018;28:1860.

49. Wilson E, Noren E, Axelsson L, Nystrom M, Gruvaes J, Paradis C, et al. A comparative 100-participant 5-year study of aspiration therapy versus roux-en-Y gastric bypass: first year results. Surg Obes Relat Dis. 2107;13(10):S25–S6.

Endoscopic Sleeve Gastroplasty (ESG)

13

Gontrand Lopez-Nava
and Inmaculada Bautista-Castaño

Introduction

The goal of endoscopic sleeve gastroplasty (ESG) is to reduce the gastric lumen into a tubular configuration, with the greater curvature modified by a line of sutured plications [1]. Lopez-Nava et al. have published clinical experiences with ESG, showing that the use of ESG for the treatment of obesity is safe and feasible, and resulted in both significant weight loss and altered patient eating behaviors [2–5].

Standard Scheme for Pre-, Peri-, and Postoperative Treatment of ESG Patients

ESG Indication Criteria

Specific indications for the procedure are based on obesity parameters (body mass index [BMI] 30–49 kg/m^2) with previous failed attempts at weight loss with conventional treatment of obe-

G. Lopez-Nava (✉)
Bariatric Endoscopy Unit, Madrid Sanchinarro University Hospital, Madrid, Spain

I. Bautista-Castaño
Bariatric Endoscopy Unit, Madrid Sanchinarro University Hospital, Madrid, Spain

Ciber of Obesity and Nutrition Pathophysiology (CIBEROBN), Instituto de Salud Carlos III, Madrid, Spain

sity and the willingness and ability of patients to be treated by a multidisciplinary team for at least 1 year. Table 13.1 shows the pre- ESG evaluation.

Peri-ESG Management

- *Pre-procedure*
  A liquid diet is initiated 1 day before the procedure. Pre-procedure antibiotics are given (cefotaxime 2 gm IV).
- *Procedure*
  The goal of the procedure is to reduce the gastric cavity to resemble a tubular lumen with the greater curvature modified by a line of cinched plications. An esophageal overtube (US Endoscopy, Mentor, OH, USA) is used to facilitate both atraumatic passage of the endoscope with the suturing device and repeated intubation with a second endoscope when needed. Carbon dioxide gas insufflation is used to distend the gastric lumen. The gastroplasty uses an endoscopic suture device (OverStitch; Apollo Endosurgery Inc., Austin, Texas, USA) fitted to a dual-channel endoscope (GIF-2 T160; Olympus Medical Systems Corp., Tokyo, Japan).

The technique uses endoscopic transmural suturing throughout the gastric wall to provide a gastric sleeve similar but not identical to sleeve

© Springer Nature Switzerland AG 2020
M. S. Wagh, S. B. Wani (eds.), *Gastrointestinal Interventional Endoscopy*,
https://doi.org/10.1007/978-3-030-21695-5_13

Table 13.1 Pre-ESG evaluation

Complete history and physical examination, nutrition evaluation Routine labs Special labs	Causes and obesity-related comorbidities, weight, BMI, weight loss history, commitment. Complete blood count, coagulation profile. Fasting blood glucose, lipid panel, kidney functions, liver panel	*Exclusions*: Related to clinical risk: previous gastric surgery, gastric ulceration, hiatal hernia ≥5 cm, or pregnancy anticoagulation or coagulopathy
Psychological evaluation	Psychosocial-behavioral assessment	*Exclusions*: Psychiatric disorders and abnormal psychologist interview
Endocrine evaluation	HbA$_{1c}$ with suspected or diagnosed prediabetes or diabetes TSH with symptoms or increased risk of thyroid disease	Goal: Optimize abnormal results
Anesthesiology evaluation	ECG, CXR, echocardiography if cardiac disease or pulmonary hypertension suspected	Goal: Assessment of anesthetic risk
Personal interview with results	Check/improved analytical parameters	Goal: Sign informed consent

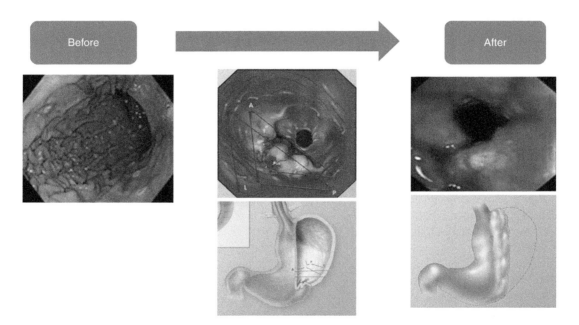

Fig. 13.1 Endoscopic sleeve gastroplasty

gastrectomy in shape. To perform the gastroplasty, we deploy interrupted sutures from distal to proximal body. Each suture consists of six bites along the anterior/greater curvature/posterior gastric wall before it is cinched. Because this is not a continuous staple line, but, rather, an invagination of the greater curvature of the stomach, intraluminal gaps exist along the plication line. These gaps are of no clinical consequences as far as trapping food and are analogous to gaps seen with surgical plications of the greater curvature for weight loss. Reinforcing stitches are usu-

ally placed in the upper body of the stomach. The suture pattern has evolved from a very few cases addressing the fundus to the majority in which we leave the fundus open, so the patient can have a pouch and some accommodation ability.

The technique is performed under general anesthesia with the patient in the left lateral position and using endotracheal intubation. After procedure completion a second endoscopy is carried out to ensure the final tubular configuration, to examine any defects requiring supplemental closure, and to rule out potential bleeding [3] (Fig. 13.1).

Early Post-ESG

The immediate postoperative period includes inpatient surveillance for 24 hours. Medication during hospitalization includes omeprazole 20 mg/12 hours IV (optional: analgesia (metamizole IV) and antiemetic (ondansetron IV)). Lopez-Nava et al. [4] showed that the procedure does produce discomfort for patients in the immediate post-procedure period, with 50% experiencing moderate abdominal pain and 20% experiencing nausea, both of which can be controlled pharmacologically.

At 8 hours after the procedure, liquid tolerance is tested. Blood tests are performed at 6 and 24 hours after the procedure to rule out bleeding [3]. An oral contrast study is performed the day after the procedure (Fig. 13.2). Discharge is planned within 24 hours.

Activity restrictions are not specifically recommended after the procedure (lifting weights, return to work, travel, flight, etc.), beyond the feeling of weakness that the patient could have due to the low caloric intake.

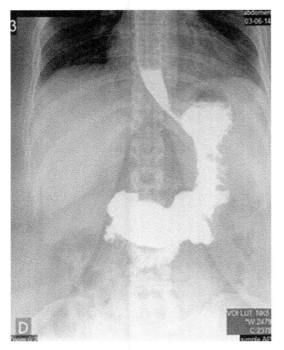

Fig. 13.2 Post-procedure (next day) barium radiographs (Lopez-Nava et al. 2015)

Follow-Up of Patients

Post-procedure care with a nutritionist and a psychologist weekly or biweekly is maintained. Patient communication includes personal interviews (face-to-face), telephone interviews, e-mails, and text messages.

Nutritional intervention changes during the course of treatment. Initially, the focus is on a transitional diet post-intervention. A liquid diet is initiated on the day before the procedure and is continued for at least 2 weeks after. The patient then progresses from hypocaloric liquids to small semisolid meals over 4 weeks.

After patients are started on solid food, the focus is on following the prescribed hypocaloric diet and discussing healthy food choices and alternatives. Once the first phase is completed, nutritional support is shifted to providing patients with a workable diet program that they could follow over the long term, which is personalized to their individual needs. The psychologist coaches patients to follow the recommended lifestyle modification program necessary to maintain their weight loss over the long term. Furthermore, patients were coached on how to interact with food cues and obesogenic environmental stimuli. Finally, they are taught how to recognize emotional eating cues and deal with them. Gastric cavity restriction facilitates caloric limitation. Dietitians and psychologist are in continuous contact to resolve problems and to design the best strategy for treatment of each individual patient.

Exercise is recommended, taking into account each patient's limitations and as prescribed by an exercise physiologist. An exercise plan that avoids increase in intra-abdominal pressure is recommended during the first month. Initially, walking is encouraged, with a progressive increase in the intensity of exercise as the diet progresses.

The team verifies weight loss results at different times post-procedure.

Results

Fogel in 2008 [6] and Brethauer in 2010 [7] showed the feasibility of endoscopic gastric volume reduction for management of obesity using a

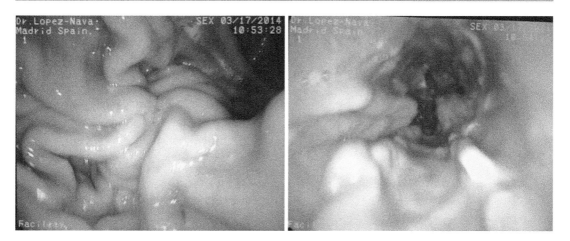

Fig. 13.3 Endoscopic findings after endoscopic sleeve gastroplasty

Table 13.2 Comparison of %TWL between the three centers in the study at 6 and 24 months (Multicenter Study)[a]

N Total	N Lost to follow-up	%TWL Madrid	%TWL Rochester	%TWL New York	%TWL All	P-value
6 months						
248	33	15.8 (0.62) [14.6–17]	14 (1.2) [11.5–16.3]	14.2 (1.0) [12.2–16.25]	15.17 (0.45) [14.2–16.25]	0.25
24 months (18–24)						
92	35	19.3 (2.1) [15.1–23.5]	16.8 (2.6) [11.5–22.1]	19.5 (3) [13.5–25.6]	18.6 (1.43) [15.7–21.5]	0.7

[a]Both standard deviation and 95% confidence intervals shown

superficial endoscopic suturing device that mimicked vertical banded gastroplasty surgical anatomy. Subsequent to a pilot feasibility study in 2013 [1], that demonstrated the feasibility of the ESG multiple groups have further demonstrated the technical feasibility, safety, and short-term efficacy in a variety of clinical settings [2–5, 8–10]. A recent study also demonstrated statistically significant physiologic changes associated with ESG including early satiety, delayed gastric emptying, and a trend toward increased insulin sensitivity [11]. Lopez-Nava et al. showed that at 1 year after the procedure, the number of nutritional and psychological interaction was predictive of success (Fig. 13.3). Sartoretto et al. [12] showed that male sex, greater baseline body weight, and lack of prior endoscopic bariatric therapy were predictors of greater weight loss at 6 months.

In our experience with a sample of 25 patients, a high percentage of patients improved nutritional habits, level of physical activity, and sleep quality. Initially, the worst habits were "not eating 5 meals a day" (94.1%) and "not eating slowly" (93.3%). One year after the procedure, the most notable changes were "not eating 5 meals a day" (from 94.1% to 29.4%) and binge eating (from 68.8% to 12.5%). Among the initially sedentary patients, 55.6% began physical activity (walking or doing cardiovascular exercises in the gym), and 75% of those who were initially not sedentary improved their level of physical activity (e.g., increasing walking time or doing other activities in the gym) [4].

We have recently reported the effectiveness, safety, weight evolution, and 2-year outcome data from a Multicenter Study of 248 Patients [5]. At 6 and 24 months, percentage of initial body weight loss (%TBWL) was 15.2 [95%CI 14.2–16.3] and 18.6 [15.7–21.5], respectively. Weight loss was similar between centers at both follow-up intervals (Table 13.2). At 24 months, the percentage of patients achieving ≥10% TBWL was 84.2 and 53% with per-protocol and intention-to-treat analyses, respectively. On multivariable linear regression analysis, only %TBWL at 6 months strongly predicted %TBWL at 24 months.

Five (2%) serious adverse events occurred: two perigastric inflammatory fluid collections (adjacent to the fundus) that resolved with percutaneous drainage and antibiotics, one self-limited hemorrhage from splenic laceration, one pulmonary embolism 72 hours after the procedure, and one pneumoperitoneum and pneumothorax requiring chest tube placement. All five patients recovered fully.

Conclusions

Most individuals who opt for weight loss procedures have usually struggled for many years with their weight. Endoscopic bariatric techniques, like the ESG procedure, provide an opportunity to lose weight and help change lifestyle habits necessary to perpetuate long-term success. A team of healthcare professionals must be available to provide patients with ongoing education and support.

The durability of the endoscopic sleeve gastroplasty at 2-year, along with the weight loss results, suggests that this endolumenal technique remains effective and helpful. It should be noted that no irreversible anatomical alteration occurs in the gastric cavity and the technique is reproducible and repeatable, thus allowing reintervention in the future to achieve lasting results.

References

1. Abu Dayyeh BK, Rajan E, Gostout CJ. Endoscopic sleeve gastroplasty: a potential endoscopic alternative to surgical sleeve gastrectomy for treatment of obesity. Gastrointest Endosc. 2013;78:530–5.

2. Lopez-Nava G, Galvão MP, da Bautista-Castaño I, et al. Endoscopic sleeve gastroplasty for the treatment of obesity. Endoscopy. 2015;47:449–52.

3. Lopez-Nava G, Galvão MP, Bautista-Castaño I, Jimenez-Baños A, Fernandez-Corbelle JP. Endoscopic sleeve gastroplasty: how I do it? Obes Surg. 2015;25:1534.

4. Lopez-Nava G, Galvão MP, Bautista-Castaño I, et al. Endoscopic sleeve gastroplasty with 1 year follow-up: predictive factors of success. Endosc Int Open. 2016;4(2):E222–7.

5. Lopez-Nava G, Sharaiha RZ, Vargas EJ, Bazerbachi F, Manoel GN, Bautista-Castaño I, Acosta A, Topazian MD, Mundi MS, Kumta N, Kahaleh M, Herr AM, Shukla A, Aronne L, Gostout CJ, Abu Dayyeh BK. Endoscopic sleeve gastroplasty for obesity: a multicenter study of 248 patients with 24 months follow-up. Obes Surg. 2017;27:2649.

6. Fogel R, De Fogel J, Bonilla Y, et al. Clinical experience of transoral suturing for an endoluminal vertical gastroplasty: 1-year follow-up in 64 patients. Gastrointest Endosc. 2008;68:51–8.

7. Brethauer SA, Chand B, Schauer PR, et al. Transoral gastric volume reduction for weight management: technique and feasibility in 18 patients. Surg Obes Relat Dis. 2010;6:689–94.

8. Sharaiha RZ, Kedia P, Kumta N, et al. Initial experience with endoscopic sleeve gastroplasty: technical success and reproducibility in the bariatric population. Endoscopy. 2015;47(2):164–6.

9. Galvao-Neto MD, Grecco E, Souza TF, et al. Endoscopic sleeve gastroplasty—minimally invasive therapy for primary obesity treatment. Arq Bras Cir Dig. 2016;29(Suppl 1):95–7.

10. Kumar N, Lopez-Nava G, Sahdala HNP, et al. Endoscopic sleeve gastroplasty: multicenter weight loss results. Gastroenterology. 2015;148(4):S179.

11. Abu Dayyeh BK, Acosta A, Camilleri M, et al. Endoscopic sleeve gastroplasty alters gastric physiology and induces loss of body weight in obese individuals. Clin Gastroenterol Hepatol. 2017;15(1):37–43.e1.

12. Sartoretto A, Sui Z, Hill C, Dunlap M, Rivera AR, Khashab MA, Kalloo AN, Fayad L, Cheskin LJ, Marinos G, Wilson E, Kumbhari V. Endoscopic Sleeve Gastroplasty (ESG) is a reproducible and effective endoscopic bariatric therapy suitable for widespread clinical adoption: a large, international multicenter study. Obes Surg. 2018;28(7):1812–21. https://doi.org/10.1007/s11695-018-3135-x. PubMed PMID:29450845.

Emerging Endoscopic Therapies for Weight Loss

Thomas J. Wang and Marvin Ryou

Introduction

The prevalence of obesity (defined as BMI $\geq$ 30) in the US adult population was 36.5% between 2011 and 2014 [1]. Estimates of obesity-associated healthcare costs ranged from $ 146 to 190 billion between 2005 and 2006 [2–3] and are most likely even higher over the past few years due to inflation and rising healthcare costs. Lifestyle modifications are frequently attempted by both clinicians and the general public, but they are often inadequate in maintaining weight loss and suppressing metabolic disease. Surgical interventions have been shown to be effective for weight loss but do require morbid obesity (defined as BMI $\geq$ 40 or BMI $\geq$ 35 with an obesity-associated comorbidity) and can put patients at risk for significant postsurgical com-

plications, though the safety profiles of these procedures have increased over the years [4]. Bariatric endoscopic interventions are often seen as the middle ground between lifestyle modifications, which harbor the lowest risk, and surgical procedures; over the past decade, these interventions have become increasingly appealing given their lower cost and invasiveness.

As of 2018, there exist four endoscopic devices that have gained FDA approval as therapeutic interventions for weight loss, including three intra-gastric balloons and one aspiration device [5]. These devices are discussed in detail in a prior chapter. Many more interventions exist but have not received or have only very recently received FDA approval. Many are undergoing various stages of development, ranging from pre-clinical concepts to devices that have seen multiple iterations through randomized controlled trials. These devices, however, all still require alterations or additional, larger studies to demonstrate their safety profile and efficacy.

Within this chapter, we will discuss each intervention one by one in detail, along with a table at the end of the chapter that summarizes the highlights of what we know about these devices: their therapeutic benefits, mechanism of action, existing clinical trial results, and plans for the future. We will start our discussion with gastroduodenal implants, which can propagate both mechanical and neurohormonal effects in achieving weight loss, and then proceed to malabsorptive sleeves

Disclosures Thomas J. Wang: None.
Marvin Ryou: Covidien/Medtronic (consultant); GI Windows (co-founder).

T. J. Wang
Massachusetts General Hospital, Department of Medicine, Boston, MA, USA

Harvard Medical School, Boston, MA, USA

M. Ryou (✉)
Harvard Medical School, Boston, MA, USA

Brigham and Women's Hospital, Division of Gastroenterology, Hepatology, and Endoscopy, Boston, MA, USA
e-mail: mryou@bwh.harvard.edu

© Springer Nature Switzerland AG 2020
M. S. Wagh, S. B. Wani (eds.), *Gastrointestinal Interventional Endoscopy*,
https://doi.org/10.1007/978-3-030-21695-5_14

and interventions that impact gastric motility. We will then end the chapter by discussing therapeutic options aimed toward alterations of the small intestine and colon, which have been shown to not only help achieve weight loss but also other aspects of metabolic syndrome, such as glycemic control and fatty liver disease.

Gastroduodenal Implants

BAROnova Transpyloric Shuttle

The TransPyloric Shuttle (BAROnova, Inc., San Carlos, California, USA, Fig. 14.1) is a silicone device composed of two bulbs connected by a flexible tether that sits at the pylorus to enable to weight loss by delaying gastric emptying and promoting early and extended satiety. The device is deployed into the stomach endoscopically and migrates toward the pylorus via natural peristalsis, with the smaller bulb stationed in the duodenum. The larger bulb serves as the anchor and prevents migration by sitting at the pylorus. Clinical data for the efficacy of the device is limited, with only one prospective, non-randomized trial consisting of two groups of ten patients showing successful excess weight loss of $25.1 \pm 14.0\%$ (mean ± SD) in the 3 months group and $41.0 \pm 21.1\%$ in the 6 months group [6]. Notably, two patients (10%) from the study required early device removal due to acute-onset epigastric pain. The most significant complication was gastric ulcers larger than 5 mm in the antrum, seen in 50% of patients endoscopically, most of which were asymptomatic and all resolved with medications alone [6]. Since then, the device has been reiterated, and the company has recently presented their results from their multicenter, double-blind, randomized sham-controlled trial (ENDObesity II) of 302 patients in Obesity Week 2018, in which they reported an average weight loss of 9.5% for patients who were treated with the device versus 2.8% for patients with the sham device [7]. The company also reported greater improvement in blood pressure and cardiometabolic factors. Most common adverse events were reported to be stomach pain, nausea, vomiting, and dyspepsia, though notably there were no mention of gastric ulcers for this trial. Detailed results are not published or publicly available. As of April 2019, the device has gained FDA approval for patients with BMI of 30–40 kg/m for up to 12 months of treatment [8].

SatiSphere System

The SatiSphere Duodenal Insert (EndoSphere Inc., Columbus, Ohio, USA, Fig. 14.2) is an endoscopically implanted device designed to delay passage of nutrients through the duodenum. It consists of a nitinol backbone with two pigtails to stabilize the device between the pylorus and duo-

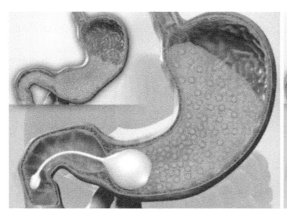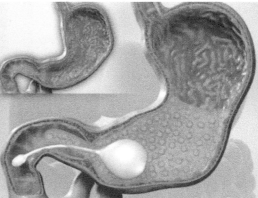

Fig. 14.1 The left image shows a digital model of the device obstructing the pylorus, and the right image shows intermittent migration that allows chyme to pass at a slower rate. (Images taken with permission from video at original site at: https://baronova.com/technology/baronova-products/)

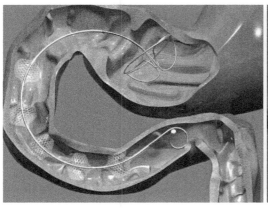 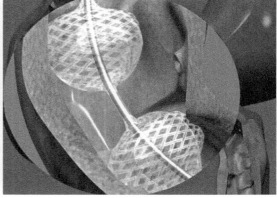

Fig. 14.2 Left image shows a digital model of the SatiSphere system in the duodenum after deployment, with a magnified image on the right. (Original images taken with permission from https://www.e-sciencecentral. org/articles/?scid=SC000010392)

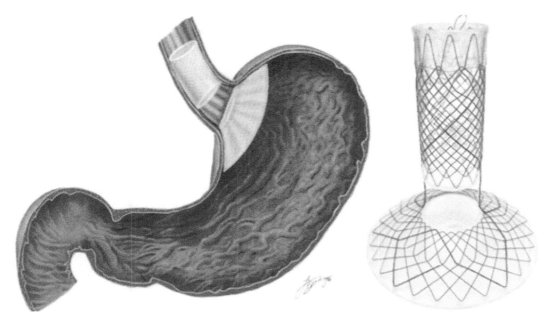

Fig. 14.3 Artwork of the device implanted in the distal esophagus and gastric cardia. (Original image available at: http://www.obesityhelp.com/articles/new-full-sense-device-to-combat-obesity)

denum and a series of polyethylene terephthalate spheres attached to the backbone that slows down the flow of chyme in the duodenum. The theoretical benefits of this device relate to hormonal regulation and are twofold: first, the spheres and increased chyme in the duodenum from slower passage may cause increased mechanical stimulation of duodenal walls, resulting in earlier satiety. Second, delayed passage in the duodenum may also cause prolonged neurohormonal signaling (i.e., CCK and GLP-1) to promote extended appetite suppression. An initial small randomized controlled trial of 31 (2:1 ratio for intervention arm) patients showed a significant excess weight loss of 18.4% at 3 months for those who completed the study ($n = 9$) versus 4.4% in the control group [9]. However, 10 out of the 21 patients who received the device resulted in migrations before the 3-month period, with two requiring surgical removal, and thus the trial was prematurely terminated. Device modifications have since been made to address issues with migration.

Full Sense Device

The Full Sense Device (BFKW LLC., Grand Rapids, Michigan, Fig. 14.3) is a modified esophagogastric stent with the intent to induce satiety. It has two components, a cylindrical stent placed above the gastroesophageal junction that is connected to a disk situated below the junction, placing pressure on the distal esophagus and gastric cardia. Although the exact mechanism is unknown, it is thought theoretically that the mechanical pressure from the device would likely trigger gastric stretch receptors and neurohormonal signaling, which would promote a constant state of fullness and thus appetite suppression. The device is currently undergoing internal clinical trials, most recently reporting having done studies of 100 obese patients in Mexico. However, no peer-reviewed data is available to date.

Malabsorptive Sleeves

EndoBarrier

The EndoBarrier (GI Dynamics, Boston, MA, USA, Fig. 14.4) is a malabsorption bypass filter that prevents mixing of chyme and pancreaticobiliary juice and digestion in the proximal intestinal tract. The device is composed of a 60 cm fluoropolymer liner reversibly anchored to the duodenal bulb and extending to the proximal jejunum. Chyme passes from the stomach and into the EndoBarrier, while pancreatic enzymes and bile flow outside the liner. To date, dozens of multicenter clinical trials and observational studies around the world have been conducted with success in achieving excess weight loss as well as better glycemic control when combined with other diabetic therapies [10–13]. A recent meta-analysis of recent trials showed significant reduction in excess weight loss of 12.6% (95% CI 9.0, 16.2) at 12 weeks when compared to diet changes only. In addition, the meta-analysis showed a decrease in glycated hemoglobin of 0.9% (95% CI −1.8, 0.0) and a reduction of fasting plasma glucose of 3.7 mM (95% CI −8.2, 0.8) [14]. Neither of the glycemic markers on aggregate reached statistical significance, although the results were close. The device so far is not FDA approved due to a 3.3% incidence of hepatic abscesses (7/212 in intervention arm) in the recent US pivotal trial, which is higher than the 2% safety threshold and thus resulted in early termination of the trial [15]. Other complications include abdominal pain and GI bleeding, each noted to occur in 3.8% (8/212) of patients in the interventional arm [14]. Overall, the EndoBarrier appears to be a promising therapeutic option for weight loss and glycemic control. Further trials are planned following device reiteration.

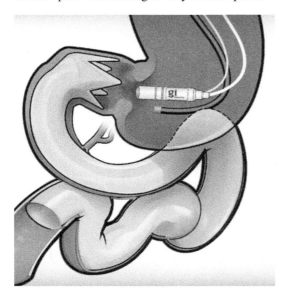

Fig. 14.4 Artwork of the device after full deployment of the EndoBarrier sleeve. (Image is credited to original video available at: http://gidynamics.com/endobarrier/)

ValenTx Sleeve

The ValenTx Sleeve is a fluoropolymer bypass sleeve that aims to mimic the physiological benefits of a Roux-en-Y bypass, promoting early satiety and malabsorption by circumventing the stomach and proximal small bowel. The device extends from the gastroesophageal junction at the Z-line to the proximal jejunum, with a total length of 120 cm. So far, one 12-week pilot study and a follow-up year-long single-center trial have been published. The pilot study of 17 patients reported an excess weight loss of 39.7% after 12 weeks. In addition, patients taking antihyperglycemic or antihypertensive medications prior to the trial no longer required the medications at the end of the 12-week trial due to improvements in glucose control and blood pressure. Five out of the original 22 patients could not complete the trial due to early postoperative dysphagia [16]. The follow-up trial followed ten patients for a year after device placement and reported a mean excess weight loss of 36%. Four out of ten patients had a partial cuff detachment. When those patients were excluded, the excess weight loss on average was higher at 54%. The device was otherwise well tolerated [17]. A larger follow-up study of 40 patients is set to be complete by October 2018 [18].

Gastric Motility Therapies

Botulinum Toxin A Injection

Botulinum toxin injections are commonly used for patients with GI smooth muscle disorders, including achalasia, diffuse esophageal spasms, gastroparesis, and sphincter of Oddi dysfunction [19]. Over the past decade, botulinum injections have also been considered as a possible option in treating morbid obesity. Injected onto the gastric antrum, botulinum has been thought to delay gastric emptying by inhibiting peristalsis, thus helping achieve earlier satiety. There currently exist three randomized control trials that have so far explored this option, with mixed results [20]. One double-blind, randomized control trial with 24 patients showed significant weight loss (11.0 vs. 5.7 kg, $p < 0.001$), higher satiety, reduction in gastric capacity, and delayed emptying 8 weeks after 200 IU of botulinum injection when compared to the placebo group [21]. However, the two other studies showed no significant weight loss after 5 and 16 weeks postinjection, respectively, even at higher doses of 500 IU botulinum [22, 23]. It is unclear the reason behind these mixed results, though possibly due to the studies' small cohort

size. Due to these mixed results, botulinum injections are currently not medically indicated or FDA approved for weight loss therapy. Currently, one longer clinical trial of a cohort of 20 patients is underway to determine the benefit of repeated botulinum injections with follow-up over the span of 5 years [24]. The current study is set to be completed in 2022.

Endoscopically Placed Gastric Stimulator

Although the exact mechanism is currently unclear, implantable gastric stimulators are hypothesized to impair physiological electrical activity in the gastric system, causing delayed gastric emptying and increased satiety. Currently, multiple devices are actively undergoing clinical trials, with all studies achieving some level of statistically significant weight loss in the first 12 months [25]. At the moment, larger and longer studies are actively being pursued. However, these gastric stimulators currently require laparoscopic implantation due to the size of the device. Versions of these devices that can be endoscopically placed do exist, although they are still in the preclinical stage (Fig. 14.5) [26]. Further modifications and clinical trials of these devices will need to be conducted in the future before they can be considered as possible therapeutic options for weight loss.

Intestinal Alterations

Revita Duodenal Mucosal Resurfacing

The Revita Duodenal Mucosal Resurfacing (Fractyl Laboratories, Cambridge, MA) procedure aims to improve glycemic control in diabetic patients via duodenal hydrothermal ablation. The technique for the ablation first entails a mucosal lift via submucosal saline injection to protect the deep muscularis, followed by circumferential thermal ablation (at a

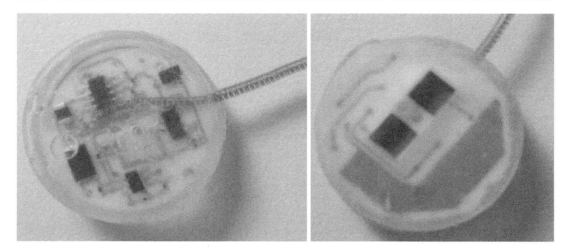

Fig. 14.5 Front and back images of a preclinical version of the device. (Original images available from Springer article Lonys et al. [26])

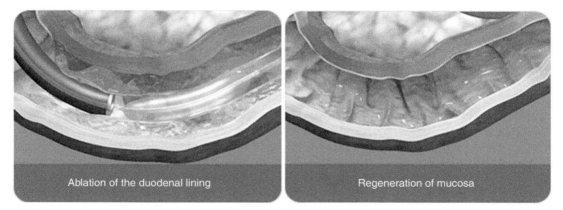

Ablation of the duodenal lining

Regeneration of mucosa

Fig. 14.6 Left image shows a digital model of the ablated duodenal lining immediately after the procedure, and the right image shows regeneration of the mucosa multiple weeks after. (Original images available at: http://www.fractyl.com/medical-professionals/#revita-dmr-procedure)

temperature of 90 °C) of the duodenal walls by a balloon catheter. The mucosa walls then naturally regenerate, which is hypothesized to modify enteroendocrine cell signaling and thus glycemic control and insulin resistance (Fig. 14.6). An initial trial of 39 patients was conducted, with 28 receiving long-segment (average 9.3 cm) and 11 receiving short-segment (average 3.4 cm) ablations between the ampulla of Vater and ligament of Treitz [27]. Three months post-procedure, those who received the long segment ablation saw a larger reduction in hemoglobin A1c (2.5%, from an average baseline of 9.5%) than those who received a short-segment ablation (1.2%). No significant difference was noted at 6 months, with 1.4% reduction in hemoglobin A1c for long-segment ablation and 0.7% reduction for short segment [28]. Patients also saw a reduction in their hepatic transaminases (AST 32 ± 17 from baseline to 22 ± 6 at 6 months; ALT 40 ± 23 from baseline to 27 ± 12 at 6 months), thus invoking possible benefit for fatty liver disease as well. Effects on weight loss were minimal, with a mild decrease in total weight from 86 ± 11 kg at baseline to 82 ± 11 kg

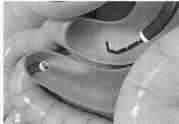
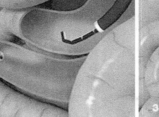
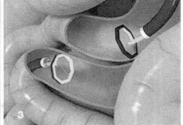

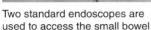

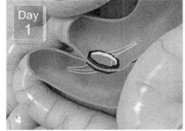
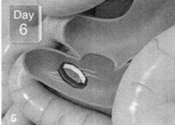
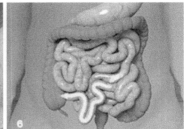

Two standard endoscopes are used to access the small bowel

Self-forming magnets are deployed from the working channel of each endoscope

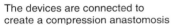

The devices are connected to create a compression anastomosis

When the anastomosis is fully formed, the devices are passed

A treatment path is created, by-passing a portion of the small

Fig. 14.7 Six panels visually demonstrating how the magnetic anastomosis system is deployed and the results of the procedure 6 days after. (Original images taken with permission from GI Windows and available at: http://giwindows.com/main-pages/product)

at 1 month post-procedure that subsequently reverted to near baseline at 6 months [1]. Although not aimed specifically at weight loss, the procedure has shown metabolic benefits to sequelae linked with obesity and metabolic syndrome. The company is currently actively recruiting patients for a larger clinical trial with a longer follow-up of 48 weeks to further evaluate the procedure as a possible therapeutic option for type 2 diabetes and nonalcoholic fatty liver disease (NAFLD) [29].

Partial Jejunal Diversion Procedure Using Incisionless Magnetic Anastomosis System

The Partial Jejunal Diversion procedure is an endoscopic therapy designed to treat type 2 diabetes and obesity, performed using the Incisionless Magnetic Anastomosis System (IMAS; GI Windows, Boston, MA, USA). The procedure uses simultaneous enteroscopy and colonoscopy to place two self-assembling octagonal magnets in the jejunum and ileum, respectively. The procedure concludes with the coupling of these two magnets under endoscopic and fluoroscopic visualization. Within 1 week, a large-caliber, side-to-side anastomosis forms between the jejunum and ileum, creating a partial diversion for chyme while preserving the native pathway to mitigate against complications of malabsorption [30]. The coupled magnets are naturally expelled in the stool (Fig. 14.7). Early clinical results indicate significant durable glycemic control from changes in neurohormonal control in addition to sustained weight loss. GIW has completed their first pilot study of ten patients with reported post-procedure results up to 12 months [32]. All anastomoses formed within 1 week and continued to be patent. Mean weight loss at 6 and 12 months was 28.3% and 40.2% EWL, respectively. Seven out of ten patients were diabetic or prediabetic, and all patients received significant reduction in HbA1c (1.9% for diabetic and 1.0% for prediabetic at 12 months) and fasting blood glucose. No serious complications were noted [31, 32]. Post-procedure nausea and diarrhea were reported in some patients, with most symptoms resolving within 2 weeks and all cases resolving with diet modifications or standard medical therapy. Larger prospective trials are planned to be conducted in the future.

Fecal Microbiota Transplant (FMT)

Fecal microbiota transplantation (FMT) is an accepted treatment for refractory *Clostridium difficile* infection and is currently being studied as a treatment option for inflammatory bowel disease, irritable bowel disease, and pouchitis [33]. Given its impressive results in *C. difficile* colitis, FMT is also in clinical studies for treatment of metabolic syndrome. At the moment, there is one clinical trial published in the literature. In that trial, 29 patients received FMT from lean donors and after 6 weeks were found to have significantly increased peripheral insulin sensitivity [34]. With continued advances in this field, FMT represents an experi-

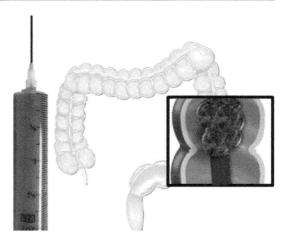

Fig. 14.8 Image showing a syringe filled with fecal microbiota and an illustration of the fecal microbiota deployed endoscopically

mental, but certainly thought-provoking treatment option for obesity and diabetes (Fig. 14.8). Multiple small clinical trials to evaluate FMT's efficacy in this domain are currently actively recruiting patients [35–38], and therefore we should see results for this possible therapeutic option for weight loss within the next few years.

Summary Table 14.1

Table 14.1 Summary of emerging endoscopic therapies for weight loss

Name	Anatomic location	Weight loss	Glycemic control	Putative mechanism	Existing published trials	Summary of key results	Reported adverse events	Future plans
Gastroduodenal implants								
BAROnova Transpyloric shuttle	Pylorus and duodenum	X		Delay gastric emptying from mechanical obstruction, earlier satiety	2 prospective trials, first with 20 patients and the second 302 patients (data presented, but not published)	1st trial: 25% EWL and 41% EWL at 3 and 6 months, respectively. 2nd trial: 9.5% (device) versus 2.8% (control) weight loss at 12 months	1st trial: Epigastric pain in 2/20 of patients, requiring early device removal	Device is now FDA approved.
SatiSphere system	Duodenum	X		Earlier and prolonged appetite suppression from both mechanical and neurohormonal effects	1 randomized control trial of 31 patients	18% EWL at 3 months vs. 4% EWL for control	Device migration in 10/21 patients, resulting in early termination of trial	Unknown, require device modification
Full sense device	GE junction and gastric cardia	X[a]		Earlier satiety from mechanical pressure	None (internal trials only)	Unknown	Unknown	Unknown
Malabsorptive sleeves								
EndoBarrier	Duodenum to proximal jejunum	X	X	Delayed absorption and mixing of chyme and pancreatobiliary juice	Dozens of known trials	Meta-analysis: 13% higher EWL at 3 months vs. diet only. Decrease of HbA1c by 0.9%	Hepatic abscess (3.3%, 7/212 patients), early termination of US trial	Further trials after device reiteration
ValenTx sleeve	GE junction to proximal jejunum	X	X	Malabsorption similar to roux-en-Y bypass, early satiety	1 pilot study of 17 patients with 1-year follow-up	40% EWL after 12 weeks with device (n = 17). 36% EWL at 1-year follow-up (n = 10)	5/22 patients could not complete trial due to post-op dysphagia	Larger follow-up study to be complete in late 2018

(continued)

Table 14.1 (continued)

Name	Anatomic location	Weight loss	Glycemic control	Putative mechanism	Existing published trials	Summary of key results	Reported adverse events	Future plans
Gastric motility therapies								
Botulinum toxin A injection	Gastric antrum	Unclear		Delayed gastric emptying from inhibition of peristalsis, earlier satiety	3 randomized, double-blind, controlled trials with numerous observational studies	Overall mixed. Only 1 out of 3 studies was significant for weight loss of 11.0 kg vs. 5.7 kg (placebo) at 8 weeks		One longer follow-up study on benefit of repeated botulinum injections
Endoscopically placed gastric stimulator	Stomach	X		Delayed gastric emptying from disruption of physiological electrical activity	None (preclinical stage)	None		Unknown
Intestinal alterations								
Revita duodenal mucosal resurfacing	Duodenum		X	Alteration in neuroendocrine signaling in regenerated duodenal mucosa	1 clinical trial of 39 patients	Reduction in HbA1c of 1.4% for long-segment ablation at 6 months. Minimal benefit for weight loss		Larger clinical trial with 48-week follow-up; actively recruiting
Partial jejunal diversion with magnetic anastomosis	Jejunum and ileum	X	X	Partial diversion of chyme via anastomosis, resulting in changes in neurohormonal signaling and some malabsorption	1 pilot study of 10 patients	28% and 40% EWL at 6-month and 1-year follow-up. Reduction of 1.9% in HbA1c for diabetic patients		Randomized controlled trial in Argentina 2018
Fecal microbiota transplant	Colon	Unclear	X	Changes in gut flora. Exact mechanism unknown	1 trial of 29 patients for studying of metabolic syndrome	Significant increase in peripheral insulin sensitivity		Multiple follow-up studies for weight loss and diabetes

Abbreviations: *EWL* estimated weight loss, *GE* gastroesophageal, *HbA1c* glycated hemoglobin, *FPG* fasting plasma glucose, *NASH* nonalcoholic steatohepatitis, *IBD* inflammatory bowel disease, *IBS* irritable bowel syndrome

[a]Results not published

Conclusion

New endoscopic bariatric therapies continue to emerge. Some are geared for weight loss, some focus on metabolic outcomes including glycemic control, and some target both endpoints. Since bariatric surgery reaches only 2% of the eligible population, it is important to have a robust pipeline of future, minimally invasive therapeutic options. While all of these emerging interventions still require further studies to demonstrate their safety, benefits, and cost-effectiveness, many of them appear promising and some may have an impact in the field of bariatric management in the near future.

References

1. National Center for Health Statistics. National Health and Nutrition Examination Survey. 2014. URL: http://www.cdc.gov/nchs/nhanes.htm [accessed 2014-09-08][WebCite Cache]. 2014.
2. Finkelstein EA, Trogdon JG, Cohen JW, Dietz W. Annual medical spending attributable to obesity: payer-and service-specific estimates. Health Aff. 2009;28(5):w822–31.
3. Cawley J, Meyerhoefer C. The medical care costs of obesity: an instrumental variables approach. J Health Econ. 2012;31(1):219–30.
4. Ma IT, Madura JA. Gastrointestinal complications after bariatric surgery. Gastroenterol Hepatol. 2015;11(8):526.
5. Ryou M, McQuaid KR, Thompson CC, Edmundowicz S, Mergener K, Force AE. ASGE EndoVators Summit: defining the role and value of endoscopic therapies in obesity management. Obesity surgery. 2018;28(1):3–14.
6. Marinos G, Eliades C, Muthusamy VR, Greenway F. Weight loss and improved quality of life with a nonsurgical endoscopic treatment for obesity: clinical results from a 3-and 6-month study. Surg Obes Relat Dis. 2014;10(5):929–34.
7. Densford F. BaroNova touts TransPyloric Shuttle pivotal study data. In: MassDevice Medical Network. 2018. https://www.massdevice.com/baronova-touts-transpyloric-shuttle-pivotal-study-data/. Accessed 21 July 2019.
8. Densford F. BaroNova wins FDA nod for TransPyloric Shuttle weight loss device. In: MassDevice Medical Network. 2019. https://www.massdevice.com/baronova-wins-fda-nod-for-transpyloric-shuttle-weight-loss-device/. Accessed 21 July 2019.
9. Sauer N, Rösch T, Pezold J, Reining F, Anders M, Groth S, Schachschal G, Mann O, Aberle J. A new endoscopically implantable device (SatiSphere) for treatment of obesity—efficacy, safety, and metabolic effects on glucose, insulin, and GLP-1 levels. Obes Surg. 2013;23(11):1727–33.
10. Gersin KS, Rothstein RI, Rosenthal RJ, Stefanidis D, Deal SE, Kuwada TS, Laycock W, Adrales G, Vassiliou M, Szomstein S, Heller S. Open-label, sham-controlled trial of an endoscopic duodenojejunal bypass liner for preoperative weight loss in bariatric surgery candidates. Gastrointest Endosc. 2010;71(6):976–82.
11. Koehestanie P, de Jonge C, Berends FJ, Janssen IM, Bouvy ND, Greve JW. The effect of the endoscopic duodenal-jejunal bypass liner on obesity and type 2 diabetes mellitus, a multicenter randomized controlled trial. Ann Surg. 2014;260(6):984–92.
12. Cohen RV, et al. A pilot study of the duodenal-jejunal bypass liner in low body mass index type 2 diabetes. J Clin Endocrinol Metab. 2013;98:E279–82.
13. Sen Gupta P, Drummond RS, Lugg ST, McGowan BM, Amiel SA, Ryder RE. One year efficacy, safety and tolerability outcomes of endoscopic duodenal exclusion using EndoBarrier as an adjunct to glucagon-like peptide-1 (GLP-1) therapy in suboptimally controlled type 2 diabetes: a randomised controlled trial. In Novel treatment for diabetes-focusing on GLP-1 and SGLT2. Endocrine Society; 2016. p. PP15–PP11. https://onlinelibrary.wiley.com/page/journal/14631326/homepage/editorialboard.html.
14. Rohde U, Hedbäck N, Gluud LL, Vilsbøll T, Knop FK. Effect of the EndoBarrier gastrointestinal liner on obesity and type 2 diabetes: a systematic review and meta-analysis. Diabetes Obes Metab. 2016;18(3):300–5.
15. Safety and efficacy of EndoBarrier in subjects with type 2 diabetes who are obese. In: ClinicalTrials.gov. 2016. https://clinicaltrials.gov/ct2/show/study/NCT01728116. Accessed 22 Oct 2017.
16. Sandler BJ, Rumbaut R, Swain CP, Torres G, Morales L, Gonzales L, Schultz S, Talamini M, Horgan S. Human experience with an endoluminal, endoscopic, gastrojejunal bypass sleeve. Surg Endosc. 2011;25(9):3028–33.
17. Sandler BJ, Rumbaut R, Swain CP, Torres G, Morales L, Gonzales L, Schultz S, Talamini MA, Jacobsen GR, Horgan S. One-year human experience with a novel endoluminal, endoscopic gastric bypass sleeve for morbid obesity. Surg Endosc. 2015;29(11):3298–303.
18. The ValenTx endo bypass system in obese subjects. In: ClinicalTrials.gov. 2016. https://clinicaltrials.gov/ct2/show/NCT02954003. Accessed 22 Oct 2017.
19. Lacy BE, Weiser K, Kennedy A. Botulinum toxin and gastrointestinal tract disorders: panacea, placebo, or pathway to the future? Gastroenterol Hepatol. 2008;4(4):283.
20. Pero R, Coretti L, Lembo F. Botulinum toxin a for controlling obesity. Toxins. 2016;8(10):281.

21. Foschi D, Corsi F, Lazzaroni M, Sangaletti O, Riva P, La Tartara G, Bevilacqua M, Osio M, Alciati A, Bianchi Porro G, Trabucchi E. Treatment of morbid obesity by intraparietogastric administration of botulinum toxin: a randomized, double-blind, controlled study. Int J Obes. 2007;31(4):707.

22. Gui D, Mingrone G, Valenza V, Spada PL, Mutignani M, Runfola M, Scarfone A, Mugno M, Panunzi S. Effect of botulinum toxin antral injection on gastric emptying and weight reduction in obese patients: a pilot study. Aliment Pharmacol Ther. 2006;23(5):675–80.

23. Topazian M, Camilleri M, Enders FT, Clain JE, Gleeson FC, Levy MJ, Rajan E, Nehra V, Dierkhising RA, Collazo-Clavell ML, et al. Gastric antral injections of botulinum toxin delay gastric emptying but do not reduce body weight. Clin Gastroenterol Hepatol. 2013;11:45–50.

24. Intragastric injections of Botox for the treatment of obesity. In: ClinicalTrials.gov. 2017. https://clinicaltrials.gov/ct2/show/NCT02035397. Accessed 22 Oct 2017.

25. Cha R, Marescaux J, Diana M. Updates on gastric electrical stimulation to treat obesity: systematic review and future perspectives. World J Gastrointest Endosc. 2014;6(9):419–31.

26. Lonys L, Vanhoestenberghe A, Julémont N, Godet S, Delplancke MP, Mathys P, Nonclercq A. Silicone rubber encapsulation for an endoscopically implantable gastrostimulator. Med Biol Eng Comput. 2015;53(4):319–29.

27. Neto MG, Rajagopalan H, Becerra P, Rodriguez P, Vignolo P, Caplan J, Rodriguez L. 829 Endoscopic duodenal mucosal resurfacing improves glycemic and hepatic parameters in patients with type 2 diabetes: data from a first-in-human study. Gastroenterology. 2016;150(4):S174.

28. Rajagopalan H, Cherrington AD, Thompson CC, Kaplan LM, Rubino F, Mingrone G, Becerra P, Rodriguez P, Vignolo P, Caplan J, Rodriguez L. Endoscopic duodenal mucosal resurfacing for the treatment of type 2 diabetes: 6-month interim analysis from the first-in-human proof-of-concept study. Diabetes Care. 2016;39(12):2254–61.

29. Effect of DMR using the Revita system in the treatment of type 2 diabetes (T2D). In: ClinicalTrials.gov. 2017.

https://clinicaltrials.gov/ct2/show/NCT02879383. Accessed 30 Oct 2017.

30. Machytka E, Buzga M, Ryou M, Lautz DB, Thompson CC. 1139 Endoscopic dual-path enteral anastomosis using self-assembling magnets: first-in-human clinical feasibility. Gastroenterology. 2016;150(4):S232.

31. Machytka E, Buzga M, Lautz DB, Ryou M, Simonson D, Thompson CC. 103 A dual-path enteral bypass procedure created by a novel incisionless anastomosis system (IAS): 6-month clinical results. Gastroenterology. 2016;150(4):S26.

32. Machytka E, Bužga M, Zonca P, Lautz DB, Ryou M, Simonson DC, Thompson CC. Partial jejunal diversion using an incisionless magnetic anastomosis system: 1-year interim results in subjects with obesity and diabetes. Gastrointest Endosc. 2017;86:904.

33. Rossen NG, MacDonald JK, de Vries EM, D'Haens GR, de Vos WM, Zoetendal EG, Ponsioen CY. Fecal microbiota transplantation as novel therapy in gastroenterology: a systematic review. World J Gastroenterol: WJG. 2015;21(17):5359.

34. Vrieze A, Van Nood E, Holleman F, Salojärvi J, Kootte RS, Bartelsman JF, Dallinga-Thie GM, Ackermans MT, Serlie MJ, Oozeer R, Derrien M. Transfer of intestinal microbiota from lean donors increases insulin sensitivity in individuals with metabolic syndrome. Gastroenterology. 2012;143(4):913–6.

35. Transplantation of microbes for treatment of metabolic syndrome & NAFLD. In: ClinicalTrials.gov. 2016. https://clinicaltrials.gov/ct2/show/results/NCT02496390. Accessed 22 Oct 2017.

36. Fecal microbiota transplantation for diabetes mellitus type II in obese patients. In: ClinicalTrials.gov. 2016. https://clinicaltrials.gov/ct2/show/NCT02346669. Accessed 22 Oct 2017.

37. Fecal microbiota transplantation for the treatment of obesity (FMT obesity). In: ClinicalTrials.gov. 2017. https://clinicaltrials.gov/ct2/show/NCT02741518. Accessed 22 Oct 2017.

38. Fecal microbiota transplant for obesity and metabolism. In: ClinicalTrials.gov. 2017. https://clinicaltrials.gov/ct2/show/study/NCT02530385. Accessed 22 Oct 2017.

Endoscopic Therapy of Post-Bariatric Surgery Strictures, Leaks, and Fistulas

Filippo Filicori and Lee L. Swanström

Introduction

Over two-third of US adults are classified as overweight and obese, and one-third are classified as morbidly obese [1]. The rising prevalence of obesity is coupled with the rising number of bariatric procedures performed each year in this country. Surgical treatment of obesity offers the most substantial and durable weight loss in this population [2, 3]. The safety profile of these procedures has also improved dramatically. However, despite such improvement, up to 5% of patients undergoing Roux-en-Y gastric bypass (RYGB) or sleeve gastrectomy (SG) will experience a postoperative leak [4] which has a mortality rate of 0.1–0.5% [5, 6], and between 3 and 27% will experience strictures of varying severity [7–9]. Historically, complications of bariatric surgery have required operative therapy. The role of endoscopy, however, is emerging as a more common option to manage many of these complications with a minimally invasive approach.

F. Filicori
Lenox Hill Hospital-Hofstra Northwell School of Medcine, New York, NY, USA

L. L. Swanström (✉)
Division of Gastrointestinal and Minimally Invasive Surgery, The Oregon Clinic, Portland, OR, USA
e-mail: lswanstrom@orclinic.com

Strictures

Bariatric procedures are unique because they partly function by limiting the size of the conduits, and thus, some degree of stricture serves a beneficial purpose. The pathogenesis of strictures is not completely understood but is likely related to technical factors such as choice of stapler or suture, inflammatory response, ulceration caused by acid-producing parietal cells remaining in the stomach, ischemia, nonsteroidal anti-inflammatory drug (NSAID) therapy, or alcohol consumption [10, 11].

Strictures in RYGB at the gastrojejunostomy and in SG patients can cause dysphagia, vomiting, and unwanted, accelerated weight loss and occur in 3–27% of patients [7–9]. Typically a diagnosis of anastomotic stricture is suggested at fluoroscopic evaluation and confirmed by narrowing of the lumen or the lack of passage of the gastroscope at endoscopic evaluation. Several techniques have been used to treat strictures, although endoscopic balloon dilations are often the first-line treatment. Occasionally, serial dilations every couple of weeks over a period of time are necessary to achieve lasting results usually starting with a 10 mm balloon and progressing to a 15–18 mm balloon. This approach can achieve sustained long-term results in >80% of patients [7, 8, 12] with a low risk of perforation. More chronic or difficult anastomotic strictures may require more

© Springer Nature Switzerland AG 2020
M. S. Wagh, S. B. Wani (eds.), *Gastrointestinal Interventional Endoscopy*,
https://doi.org/10.1007/978-3-030-21695-5_15

aggressive endoscopic therapy such as steroid injections or even a needle-knife strictureplasty [13, 14]. When endoscopic management of strictures fails, operative revision of the anastomosis or surgical strictureplasty is appropriate. The enteroenterostomy, when strictured, is more difficult to manage endoscopically due to its location. Such distal strictures often require surgical revision. Strictures in SG appear to be associated to a smaller bougie size, misapplied staple lines, or efforts to make a tighter sleeve [15]. Strictures close to the incisura appear to be more refractory to balloon dilation then proximal strictures and might require repeated dilations, stenting, or surgical revision. More aggressive dilation with larger balloons (30–35 mm) have been advocated in the specific instance of mid-sleeve strictures, although data to support this approach is lacking and many surgeons resort to conversion to a RYGB in this instance [15–18].

Leaks

Anastomotic or staple line leaks after bariatric surgery are uncommon but usually morbid and potentially lethal. Their incidence is 2%–5% of cases [4, 12]. Postoperative leaks carry a high morbidity and a mortality of 0.5%–10% in most series [4, 19]. However, as many as 50% of patients may be asymptomatic, with leaks detected only on X-ray studies [19]. A slow leak or chronic manifestation of an acute, self-limited leak is termed a fistula, which occurs in 1.5%–12.5% cases after RYGB.

Endoscopic treatment strategies may attempt to exclude a leak (stenting) and/or occlusion of the orifice (clips, plugs, glues, or sutures) [14, 20–23]. However as the time interval between leak formation and attempted closure increases, the more difficult it becomes to deploy clips because of the inflammatory changes in the surrounding tissues. When the orifice caliber is too large for clip deployment or additional endoluminal drainage is needed, a pigtail catheter or an EndoVAC can be used to obtain additional source

control [24, 25]. These complications require a thoughtful, multidisciplinary, and often long-term approach to management. Control of abdominal contamination, systemic antimicrobials, and nutritional support are essential components of treatment in these cases but are outside the scope of this chapter.

Etiologies

Postoperative leaks occurring in the first 4 days are most commonly attributed to a technical flaw. A leak presenting 4 or more days after surgery may be due to ischemia at the staple line or anastomosis, poor nutrition, tension, or other host factors. With gastric bypass, most leaks occur at the gastrojejunostomy [19, 26, 27]. After a sleeve gastrectomy, high pressure in the gastric conduit can result in a leak which most commonly occurs at the former angle of His, where the staple line meets the esophagogastric junction [28, 29]. After ligation of the short gastric arteries, this area may be particularly susceptible to ischemic perforation. These leaks are especially prone to becoming chronic fistulas that resist attempts at closure. Timing of the leak can offer valuable information regarding its etiology. Despite sound surgical principles, gastric ischemia or technical failure may occur unpredictably resulting in such complication.

Diagnosis and Classification

An early postoperative leak after bariatric surgery can be challenging to diagnose. The abdominal exam is often not reflective of the severity of intra-abdominal spillage and usually misleading in the obese patient. One of the most sensitive indicators of a leak is isolated tachycardia. Although normally patients are feeling well and ambulating on the night of surgery, someone who complains of severe pain, is not ambulating, or is deviating from the standard postoperative course should prompt suspicion of a leak. Computed tomography performed with oral, water-soluble contrast provides the most information and has a near 100% sensitivity [30]. Contrast esophagograms or upper gastrointestinal (GI) series are often employed but have a sensitivity that as been reported as low as 33% [31].

Acute self-limited leaks, small, intermediate leaks or failed closure attempts may present late as chronic fistulas. These can present insidiously, months to years after surgery, with nonspecific abdominal complaints such as pain or malaise. Additionally, fistulas between the gastric pouch and gastric remnant can occur after RYGB and may present with weight regain and/or nausea, pain, or new-onset GERD. With appropriate clinical suspicion, upper endoscopy or contrast upper GI radiographs will usually make the diagnosis. Careful endoscopic examination of the gastric pouch or sleeve will demonstrate a granulated fistula tract, often too small to permit passage of the gastroscope. Cross-sectional imaging may exclude other diagnoses or reveal occult abscesses but is unlikely to show a fistula directly. Without specific symptoms or apparent findings on clinical exam, these diagnoses rely on clinical intuition and interpretation of the imaging.

The literature suggests a classification of leaks into (a) early leaks, occurring <3 days after surgery; (b) intermediate leaks, occurring between 4 and 7 days after surgery; and (c) late leaks/fistulas, occurring 8 or more days after surgery [15, 18]. In early leaks, the local inflammatory and the systemic responses to peritoneal contamination can be dramatic but are often limited. With intermediate leaks, inflammatory responses are likely at their height, with friable tissue and substantial contamination. Traditional surgical remedies have high failure rates in these scenarios [18]. For late leaks, local inflammation may have subsided, but the chronic healing of a fistulous tract may hamper spontaneous closure. Fistulas resulting from such leaks remain a complex process requiring synchronous application of multiple techniques. Fistulas may form to the gastric remnant after RYGB, resulting in a gastrogastric fistula, often presenting as a loss of the benefits of bariatric surgery. They can also form between

hollow viscous organs with variable effects or the skin along a drain tract. Though less common, bronchogastric fistulas have been reported [32].

Management

Patients with a systemic response to the leak, particularly if hemodynamically unstable, should be aggressively resuscitated prior to interventions for source control; nevertheless, it is crucial not to delay their care. Nonoperative and endoscopic therapies should be attempted only in hemodynamically stable patients. Broad-spectrum antimicrobials and close monitoring are essential adjuncts. These are the treatment modalities commonly available for endoscopic therapy:

Stents

The use of fully covered self-expandable metallic stents (SEMS, Fig. 15.1) is a minimally invasive and relatively safe and effective treatment approach for leaks after bariatric surgery. SEMS placement can be considered in patients who are hemodynamically stable, have favorable anatomy to allow for stent deployment and retention and adequate source control [33].

It is important to point out that stent deployment requires suitable anatomy and sometimes it can be challenging to securely place a stent through a gastrojejunostomy leak. Sleeve leaks which occur most often at the angle of His might require a "nested" SEMS deployment to prevent stent migration and to "depressurize the conduit, which can result in significant pain and discomfort for the patient.

Endoscopic stenting diverts enteric contents past the leak while maintaining GI continuity allowing for immediate reintroduction of PO intake; this allows for a significant decrease of patient discomfort. In studies employing routine stenting for early leaks, healing was complete for >80% of patients at the predetermined time of stent removal: usually 6 weeks [22, 33–35]. Despite being an attractive therapeutic option, stent migration is a commonly reported complication in about 16% of cases [33] which can

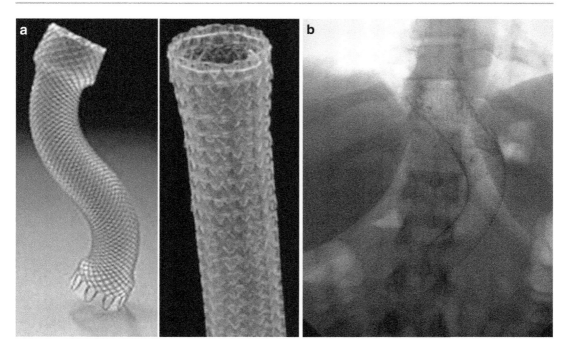

Fig. 15.1 Self-expanding metallic stents (SEMS). (**a**) Commercially available stents. (**b**) Radiographic image of deployed stents

require stent revision or discontinuation. For this reason one or multiple clips or an over-the-scope clip (OTSC) can be deployed between the mucosa and the proximal side of the stent to decrease its likelihood to migrate [36, 37]. More secure fixation is possible with endoscopic suturing, though this does adds cost to the procedure [38]. Less commonly, stents have resulted in migration beyond endoscopic reach, clinically significant bleeding, and GI erosion requiring surgery [22, 39]. Other potential therapies such as endoscopic clips, OTSC, fibrin sealants, plugs, or endoscopic suturing (Figs. 15.2 and 15.3) exist and can be coupled with stenting.

Internal Drainage

Internal drainage has been reported as a quite effective, inexpensive, and safe means to drain an enteric leak in bariatric patients. The pigtail can be introduced through the operative channel over a guide wire with the help of a pigtail pusher.

When the degree of contamination is high as testified by purulent material exiting the cavity and source control is incomplete, pigtail drain placement (Fig. 15.4) with one lumen communicating with the cavity and one in the enteric side appears to be a safe option allowing for resolution in the majority of cases. In a retrospective study, examining 100 patients with leaks after sleeve gastrectomies internal drainage was successful in 86% of cases [40] despite a median resolution time of 6 months. An extramural cavity diameter > 5 cm was associated with failure of internal drainage.

Fibrin Glues

Good quality data about the use of fibrin sealants in the early treatment of leaks following bariatric surgery is lacking. One study examined 3 patients which underwent fibrin injections and found that 2/3 had resolution at mean time of 33 days [41]. The efficacy of fibrin glue injections appeared even lower in patients with late leaks [42]. This treatment modality will require more extensive investigation before implementation on a large scale.

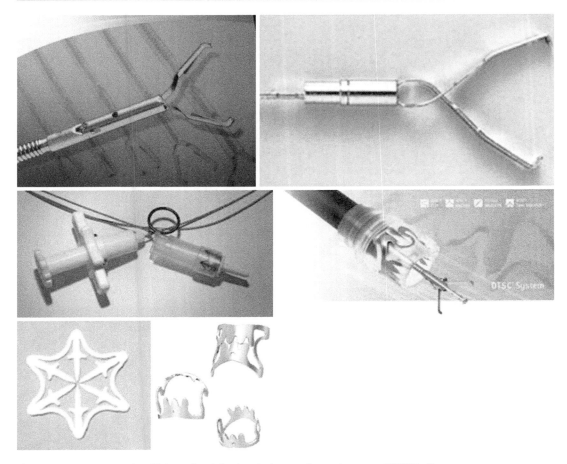

Fig. 15.2   Endoscopic clips, fibrin sealant injection devices, and over-the-scope (OTSC) clips

Fig. 15.3   Endoscopic
suturing device

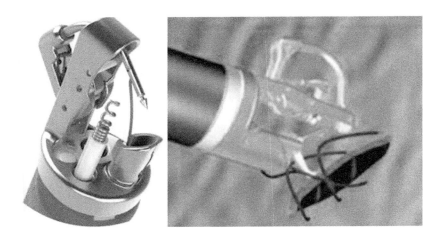

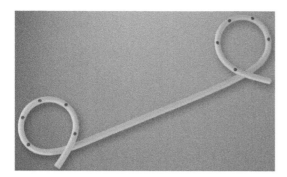

Fig. 15.4 Pigtail internal drainage catheter (double J stent)

Clips

Traditional hemostatic clips are usually not effective when used alone for the closure of fistulas. The larger over-the-scope clips, such as the Ovesco OTSC (Ovesco Endoscopy, Germany) or Padlock Clip (US Endoscopy, OH), on the other hand, create a full-thickness closure like a "bear trap" which is more suitable for this application. Specialized grasping forceps are also available for pulling tissue up into the cap prior to deployment. Occasionally multiple clips can be deployed next to each other to seal linear defects >2 cm. Feasibility of any endoscopic closure with over-the-scope clips needs to take into the account the narrow working space of a tubular gastroesophageal junction, the size and orientation of the defect, the surrounding tissue quality, and the difficulty in removing the clips once fired.

While OTSC have been described in a variety of intestinal leaks, the experience in bariatric patients is limited. Surace et al. have described a series of 19 patients, 11 with gastric fistulas following sleeve gastrectomy and a successful closure rate of 91% [43]. Another study by Winder et al. with a patient population composed of 55% bariatric patients demonstrated a similar pattern in success rates, with long-term closure achieved in 77.3 and 100% of fistulas and leak cases, respectively [44]. Both studies emphasize the necessity of multiple interventions and attempts to close the leaks. Deployment of a stent over these clips has been advocated in some previous studies [45] to further aid in closure.

Chronic fistulae are difficult to treat endoscopically for multiple reasons; fibrosis and inflammation which cause friability of the tissues tend to increase the technical difficulty of endoscopic closure. In cases where the tissue is fibrotic and difficult to draw into the firing cap with suction, two devices are available to help assist with this which are the OTSC Twin Grasper and the OTSC Anchor (Ovesco Endoscopy, Germany). Both devices are used to grasp the fibrotic edges of more chronic fistulae to help draw the entire opening into the cap prior to firing. Although these devices can effectively grasp tissue and may assist in fistula closure, the reported long-term failure rate exceeds 80% in chronic fistulae [44].

EndoVAC

Endoluminal vacuum (E-Vac) (Fig. 15.5) therapy has emerged as an alternative in management of large leaks resulting from bariatric surgery. It uses the same treatment principles seen with vacuum-assisted closure therapy of external

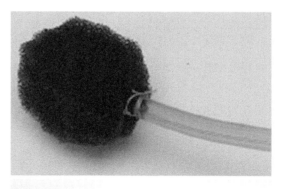

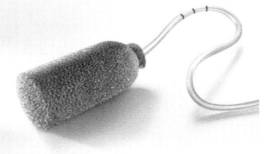

Fig. 15.5 Self-assembled and commercially available E-Vac devices. (Endo-SPONGE, Braun, Germany)

wounds. Both improve and accelerate healing by removing infected secretions, reducing edema, increasing local perfusion, and promoting granulation tissue formation [46, 47].

Most reported studies from European institutions show an average closure rate approximating 90% and mortality rates of around 10% [46, 48–53]. A commercially assembled system (Endo-SPONGE, B. Braun Medical, Germany) is available in Europe, but this system is only FDA approved for treatment of colorectal leaks in the United States. Therefore, it is necessary to self-assemble the available devices in the United States for implementation of this therapy.

The E-Vac insertion is performed under general anesthesia for airway protection. A 16-Fr Silastic nasogastric tube (NGT) is passed through one of the nostrils and pulled out of the mouth through the bite block. At this point, the E-Vac is created and attached to the end of the NGT. The E-Vac is adapted from the small granulofoam package from KCI (San Antonio, Texas) negative pressure system. The size of the actual E-Vac is limited by the necessity to pass it through the esophageal lumen, so 3–4 cm width and 6–8 cm length is the maximum size that can be safely passed through the esophagus. Once the E-Vac is cut to the appropriate size, a tunnel is created through its center to the tip without exiting the sponge. The NGT is then placed into this tunnel to encompass the extent of the foam making sure that all fenestrations on the NGT are within the sponge. The tube may need to be trimmed at the tip to accommodate this. Once in place, a 2–0 permanent suture is used to fix the E-Vac to the proximal portion of the NGT. A U-stitch is used to wrap the suture around the circumference of the E-Vac. Another suture is used at the tip of the NGT, through the E-Vac, and an air knot is created. This knot is used is to grasp the E-Vac with rat tooth forceps and facilitate carrying it into place. The scope should be driven into the cavity to get the tip of the NGT and E-Vac extraluminally. The E-Vac can be pushed, from its proximal portion into the fistula cavity with the rat tooth forceps, and then should be left in place. The NGT then should be adapted to connect to the KCI negative pressure machine

(San Antonio, TX), and settings should be set to 175 mmHg, high, and continuous. The sponge should be changed every 3 days. This procedure should be repeated as the fistula cavity closes and eventually seals.

Early/Intermediate Leaks

When diagnosed promptly, early and intermediate leaks have the best prognosis for the patient. Early leaks can be approached through multiple therapeutic options although there is little comparative data available in the literature. In the appropriate setting and in most contained leaks, a regimen of drainage, antimicrobials, nil per os, and nutritional support (parenteral or jejunal) result in closure within 5 weeks in 90% of patients [19, 26, 54, 55]. Despite high resolution rates, a traditional percutaneous approach comes at the cost of significant distress for the patient that needs to be placed nil per os in case of high output leaks for several weeks and places him at risk for the complications derived from parenteral nutrition and/or additional procedures to gain enteric access which might be difficult to obtain in a bariatric patient. On the other end, surgical exploration and repair with drainage show similar efficacy in early but not intermediate/late leaks. Primary surgical repair performed after 2–3 days or in the face of significant peritoneal contamination is unlikely to succeed [18]. In both early and intermediate leaks, endoscopic therapies offer important alternatives to classical therapy. Further management should take into account the diameter of the opening, the time since inception, and size and degree of contamination of the cavity. Generally speaking all the previously described techniques used alone or in combination provide successful means to achieve resolution of the leaks.

Late Leaks and Fistulas

When presenting or diagnosed late, leaks will be associated with significant and persistent soiling. Similarly, leaks that have failed previous management may have inflammation or granulation complicating treatment. In series with late leaks, nonoperative strategies had success rates between 40% and 80% [27, 29]. Failure requiring alternative treatments was higher in patients with late leaks and fistulas compared with those with early leaks. However, in most of these series, failures of nonoperative and operative therapies responded to stenting. Fully covered esophageal stents can improve healing by minimizing soiling and inflammation of the wound. Several small case series involving late leaks diagnosed after postoperative day 8 reported 100% success rates when stents were left in situ for 2–4 months, demonstrating complete healing on contrast esophagogram when removed [28, 34, 56]. Other series of stenting on the other end were less successful and demonstrated 50%–80% healing rates of delayed fistulas with stents alone [32, 57].

Other treatment options are available for late leaks not amenable to stenting. Fibrin sealants, fistula plugs, and endoscopic suturing are only a few of the other modalities attempted for closure of fistulas. Though most series are small, results are promising. Injection of fibrin glue, biologic and degradable, into the leak orifice was uniformly successful in 11 selected patients coming from 4 series with no adverse events [23, 25]. Similarly, fistula plugs can provide a scaffolding for healing a chronic fistula and were particularly useful for fistulas 1.5 cm or wider, resulting in healing in ~80% of patients in small series [58, 59]. Endoscopic plication of the mucosa adjacent to the fistula over the orifice has also been described [60, 61]. Increasingly complex fistulas may require several technologies simultaneously. A few series examined outcomes of multimodality therapy for complex fistulas after bariatric procedures. Employing a combination of transluminal debridement, OTSC, fibrin sealants, and stenting was shown to achieve 100% success in a series of 27 patients with complex late fistulas larger than 10 mm at a mean of 86 days and a median of 4.4 endoscopies per patient [45].

Fistulization between the gastric pouch and gastric remnant can occur after gastric bypass and demands a separate discussion. This was more common due to staple line failure when the pouch was created with a nondividing stapler, which has fallen out of favor. Other causes include incomplete division of the fundus during gastric bypass, pouch staple line leak with abscess formation and decompression into the remnant, and marginal ulcer that erodes into the gastric remnant [62]. These fistulas can present with symptoms similar to marginal ulcer, or with weight regain and lack of satiety. Upper gastrointestinal series and endoscopy are the initial diagnostic modalities of choice. For small fistulas of a less than 5 mm in size, endoscopic closure with over-the-scope clip is a useful technique to achieve closure [20]. Surgical treatment including total gastrectomy with esophagojejunostomy, conversion of SG to RYGB, should be reserved only to patients with chronic leaks that have failed initial endoscopic management [17, 63, 64].

Conclusion

Historically, complications of bariatric surgery required operative therapy. This was morbid and sometimes even deadly for patients. Over the last decade, the role of endoscopy has emerged as an effective and less invasive approach to manage many of these complications.

There are several endoscopic approaches that have been found to achieve success in these difficult scenarios. Over-the-scope type of clips appears to be particularly suited for small early leaks <1 cm. Internal drainage with a pigtail stent seems to achieve comparable resolution rates and is useful for more chronic leaks with contained extramural fluid collections. E-Vac application is useful in leaks which have failed other therapeutic means and where high degree of contamination is present. Fully covered SEMS are successful in early as well as late leaks and fistulas, as a stand-alone treatment or as adjunct modality when the anatomy of the patient favors their placement.

References

1. Zipf G, Chiappa M, Porter KS, Ostchega Y, Lewis BG, Dostal J. National health and nutrition examination survey: plan and operations, 1999–2010. Vital Health Stat 1. 2013;(56):1–37.
2. Adams TD, Davidson LE, Litwin SE, Kim J, Kolotkin RL, Nanjee MN, Gutierrez JM, Frogley SJ, Ibele AR, Brinton EA, Hopkins PN, McKinlay R, Simper SC, Hunt SC. Weight and metabolic outcomes 12 years after gastric bypass. N Engl J Med. 2017;12377(21):1143–55. https://doi.org/10.1056/NEJMoa1700459.
3. Buchwald H, Avidor Y, Braunwald E, et al. Bariatric surgery. JAMA. 2004;292(14):1724. https://doi.org/10.1001/jama.292.14.1724.
4. Kim J, Azagury D, Eisenberg D, Demaria E, Campos GM. ASMBS position statement on prevention, detection, and treatment of gastrointestinal leak after gastric bypass and sleeve gastrectomy, including the roles of imaging, surgical exploration, and nonoperative management. Surg Obes Relat Dis. 2015;11(4):739–48. https://doi.org/10.1016/j.soard.2015.05.001.
5. Buchwald H, Estok R, Fahrbach K, et al. Weight and type 2 diabetes after bariatric surgery: systematic review and meta-analysis. Am J Med. 2009;122(3):248–256.e5. https://doi.org/10.1016/j.amjmed.2008.09.041.
6. Rosenthal R, Szomstein S, Kennedy C, Soto F, Zundel N. Laparoscopic surgery for morbid obesity: 1,001 consecutive bariatric operations performed at the Bariatric Institute, Cleveland Clinic Florida. Obes Surg. 2006;16(2):119–24. https://doi.org/10.1381/096089206775565230.
7. Ukleja A, Afonso BB, Pimentel R, Szomstein S, Rosenthal R. Outcome of endoscopic balloon dilation of strictures after laparoscopic gastric bypass. Surg Endosc Other Interv Tech. 2008;22(8):1746–50. https://doi.org/10.1007/s00464-008-9788-0.
8. Caro L, Sánchez C, Rodríguez P, Bosch J. Endoscopic balloon dilation of anastomotic strictures occurring after laparoscopic gastric bypass for morbid obesity. Dig Dis. 2009;26(4):314–7. https://doi.org/10.1159/000177015.
9. Puig CA, Waked TM, Baron TH, Wong Kee Song LM, Gutierrez J, Sarr MG. The role of endoscopic stents in the management of chronic anastomotic and staple line leaks and chronic strictures after bariatric surgery. Surg Obes Relat Dis. 2014;10(4):613–7. https://doi.org/10.1016/j.soard.2013.12.018.
10. Gonzalez R, Lin E, Venkatesh KR, Bowers SP, Smith CD. Gastrojejunostomy during laparoscopic gastric bypass: analysis of 3 techniques. Arch Surg. 2003;138:181–4. https://doi.org/10.1001/archsurg.138.2.181.
11. Kataoka M, Masaoka A, Hayashi S, et al. Problems associated with the EEA stapling technique for esophagojejunostomy after total gastrectomy. Ann Surg. 1989;209(1):99–104.
12. Updated position statement on sleeve gastrectomy as a bariatric procedure. Surg Obes Relat Dis. 2010;6(1):1–5. https://doi.org/10.1016/j.soard.2009.11.004.
13. Neto MG, Silva LB, Campos JM. International perspective on the endoscopic treatment of bariatric surgery complications. In: Bariatric surgery complications. Cham: Springer International Publishing; 2017. p. 77–84. https://doi.org/10.1007/978-3-319-43968-6_7.
14. Shada AL, Beard KW, Reavis KM. Role of endoscopy, stenting, and other nonoperative interventions in the management of bariatric complications: a US perspective. In: Bariatric surgery complications. Cham: Springer International Publishing; 2017. p. 85–92. https://doi.org/10.1007/978-3-319-43968-6_8.
15. Rosenthal RJ, International Sleeve Gastrectomy Expert Panel, Diaz AA, et al. International sleeve gastrectomy expert panel consensus statement: best practice guidelines based on experience of >12,000 cases. Surg Obes Relat Dis. 2012;8(1):8–19. doi:https://doi.org/10.1016/j.soard.2011.10.019.
16. Vilallonga R, Himpens J, Van De Vrande S. Laparoscopic management of persistent strictures after laparoscopic sleeve gastrectomy. Obes Surg. 2013;23(10):1655–61. https://doi.org/10.1007/s11695-013-0993-0.
17. Mahmoud M, Maasher A, Al Hadad M, Salim E, Nimeri AA. Laparoscopic roux En Y Esophago-Jejunostomy for chronic leak/fistula after laparoscopic sleeve gastrectomy. Obes Surg. 2016;26(3):679–82. https://doi.org/10.1007/s11695-015-2018-7.
18. Deitel M, Gagner M, Erickson AL, Crosby RD. Third international summit: current status of sleeve gastrectomy. Surg Obes Relat Dis. 2011;7(6):749–59. https://doi.org/10.1016/j.soard.2011.07.017.
19. Ballesta C, Berindoague R, Cabrera M, Palau M, Gonzales M. Management of anastomotic leaks after laparoscopic roux-en-Y gastric bypass. Obes Surg. 2008;18(6):623–30. https://doi.org/10.1007/s11695-007-9297-6.
20. Fernandez-Esparrach G, Lautz DB, Thompson CC. Endoscopic repair of gastrogastric fistula after roux-en-Y gastric bypass: a less-invasive approach. Surg Obes Relat Dis. 2010;6(3):282–8. https://doi.org/10.1016/j.soard.2010.02.036.
21. Quezada N, Maiz C, Daroch D, et al. Effect of early use of covered self-expandable endoscopic stent on the treatment of postoperative stapler line leaks. Obes Surg. 2015;25(10):1816–21. https://doi.org/10.1007/s11695-015-1622-x.
22. Iqbal A, Miedema B, Ramaswamy A, et al. Long-term outcome after endoscopic stent therapy for complications after bariatric surgery. Surg Endosc Other Interv Tech. 2011;25(2):515–20. https://doi.org/10.1007/s00464-010-1203-y.
23. Kowalski C, Kastuar S, Mehta V, Brolin RE. Endoscopic injection of fibrin sealant in repair of gastrojejunostomy leak after laparoscopic Roux-en-Y gastric bypass. Surg Obes Relat Dis. 2007;3(4):438–42. https://doi.org/10.1016/j.soard.2007.02.012.

24. Smallwood NR, Fleshman JW, Leeds SG, Burdick JS. The use of endoluminal vacuum (E-Vac) therapy in the management of upper gastrointestinal leaks and perforations. Surg Endosc Other Interv Tech. 2016;30(6):2473–80. https://doi.org/10.1007/s00464-015-4501-6.

25. Papavramidis ST, Eleftheriadis EE, Papavramidis TS, Kotzampassi KE, Gamvros OG. Endoscopic management of gastrocutaneous fistula after bariatric surgery by using a fibrin sealant. Gastrointest Endosc. 2004;59(2):296–300. https://doi.org/10.1016/S0016-5107(03)02545-8.

26. Gonzalez R, Sarr MG, Smith CD, et al. Diagnosis and contemporary management of anastomotic leaks after gastric bypass for obesity. J Am Coll Surg. 2007;204(1):47–55. https://doi.org/10.1016/j.jamcollsurg.2006.09.023.

27. Spyropoulos C, Argentou MI, Petsas T, Thomopoulos K, Kehagias I, Kalfarentzos F. Management of gastrointestinal leaks after surgery for clinically severe obesity. Surg Obes Relat Dis. 2012;8(5):609–15. https://doi.org/10.1016/j.soard.2011.04.222.

28. Casella G, Soricelli E, Rizzello M, et al. Nonsurgical treatment of staple line leaks after laparoscopic sleeve gastrectomy. Obes Surg. 2009;19(7):821–6. https://doi.org/10.1007/s11695-009-9840-8.

29. De Aretxabala X, Leon J, Wiedmaier G, et al. Gastric leak after sleeve gastrectomy: analysis of its management. Obes Surg. 2011;21(8):1232–7. https://doi.org/10.1007/s11695-011-0382-5.

30. Lyass S, Khalili TM, Cunneen S, et al. Radiological studies after laparoscopic Roux-en-Y gastric bypass: routine or selective? Am Surg. 2004;70:918–21.

31. Doraiswamy A, Rasmussen JJ, Pierce J, Fuller W, Ali MR. The utility of routine postoperative upper GI series following laparoscopic gastric bypass. Surg Endosc Other Interv Tech. 2007;21(12):2159–62. https://doi.org/10.1007/s00464-007-9314-9.

32. Serra C, Baltasar A, Andreo L, et al. Treatment of gastric leaks with coated self-expanding stents after sleeve gastrectomy. Obes Surg. 2007;17(7):866–72. https://doi.org/10.1007/s11695-007-9161-8.

33. Puli SR, Spofford IS, Thompson CC. Use of self-expandable stents in the treatment of bariatric surgery leaks: a systematic review and meta-analysis. Gastrointest Endosc. 2012;75(2):287–93. https://doi.org/10.1016/j.gie.2011.09.010.

34. Blackmon SH, Santora R, Schwarz P, Barroso A, Dunkin BJ. Utility of removable esophageal covered self-expanding metal stents for leak and fistula management. Ann Thorac Surg. 2010;89(3):931–7. https://doi.org/10.1016/j.athoracsur.2009.10.061.

35. Chang J, Sharma G, Boules M, Brethauer S, Rodriguez J, Kroh MD. Endoscopic stents in the management of anastomotic complications after foregut surgery: new applications and techniques. Surg Obes Relat Dis. 2016;12(7):1373–81. https://doi: 10.1016/j.soard.2016.02.041.

36. Speer E, Dunst CM, Shada A, Reavis KM, Swanström LL. Covered stents in cervical anastomoses following esophagectomy. Surg Endosc. 2016;30(8):3297–303. https://doi.org/10.1007/s00464-015-4661-4.

37. Diana M, Swanström LL, Halvax P, et al. Esophageal covered stent fixation using an endoscopic over-the-scope clip. Mechanical proof of the concept and first clinical experience. Surg Endosc. 2015;29(11):3367–72. https://doi.org/10.1007/s00464-015-4078-0.

38. Rieder E, Dunst C, Martinec D, Cassera M, Swanstrom L. Endoscopic suture fixation of gastrointestinal stents: proof of biomechanical principles and early clinical experience. Endoscopy. 2012;44(12):1121–6. https://doi.org/10.1055/s-0032-1325730.

39. Tan JT, Kariyawasam S, Wijeratne T, Chandraratna HS. Diagnosis and management of gastric leaks after laparoscopic sleeve gastrectomy for morbid obesity. Obes Surg. 2010;20(4):403–9. https://doi.org/10.1007/s11695-009-0020-7.

40. Lorenzo D, Guilbaud T, Gonzalez JM, et al. Endoscopic treatment of fistulas after sleeve gastrectomy: a comparison of internal drainage versus closure. Gastrointest Endosc. 2017;87:429. https://doi.org/10.1016/j.gie.2017.07.032.

41. Brolin RE, Lin JM. Treatment of gastric leaks after roux-en-Y gastric bypass: a paradigm shift. Surg Obes Relat Dis. 2013;9(2):229–33. https://doi.org/10.1016/j.soard.2012.01.006.

42. Gumbs AA, Duffy AJ, Bell RL. Management of gastrogastric fistula after laparoscopic Roux-en-Y gastric bypass. Surg Obes Relat Dis. 2006;2(2):117–21. https://doi.org/10.1016/j.soard.2005.12.002.

43. Surace M, Mercky P, Demarquay JF, et al. Endoscopic management of GI fistulae with the over-the-scope clip system (with video). Gastrointest Endosc. 2011;74(6):1416–9. https://doi.org/10.1016/j.gie.2011.08.011.

44. Winder JS, Kulaylat AN, Schubart JR, Hal HM, Pauli EM. Management of non-acute gastrointestinal defects using the over-the-scope clips (OTSCs): a retrospective single-institution experience. Surg Endosc Other Interv Tech. 2016;30(6):2251–8. https://doi.org/10.1007/s00464-015-4500-7.

45. Bège T, Emungania O, Vitton V, et al. An endoscopic strategy for management of anastomotic complications from bariatric surgery: a prospective study. Gastrointest Endosc. 2011;73(2):238–44. https://doi.org/10.1016/j.gie.2010.10.010.

46. Weidenhagen R, Hartl WH, Gruetzner KU, Eichhorn ME, Spelsberg F, Jauch KW. Anastomotic leakage after esophageal resection: new treatment options by endoluminal vacuum therapy. Ann Thorac Surg. 2010;90(5):1674–81. https://doi.org/10.1016/j.athoracsur.2010.07.007.

47. Wedemeyer J, Brangewitz M, Kubicka S, et al. Management of major postsurgical gastroesophageal intrathoracic leaks with an endoscopic vacuum-assisted closure system. Gastrointest Endosc. 2010;71(2):382–6. https://doi.org/10.1016/j.gie.2009.07.011.

48. Ahrens M, Schulte T, Egberts J, et al. Drainage of esophageal leakage using endoscopic vacuum therapy:

a prospective pilot study. Endoscopy. 2010;42(9):693–8. https://doi.org/10.1055/s-0030-1255688.

49. Brangewitz M, Voigtländer T, Helfritz FA, et al. Endoscopic closure of esophageal intrathoracic leaks: stent versus endoscopic vacuum-assisted closure, a retrospective analysis. Endoscopy. 2013;45(6):433–8. https://doi.org/10.1055/s-0032-1326435.

50. Schniewind B, Schafmayer C, Voehrs G, et al. Endoscopic endoluminal vacuum therapy is superior to other regimens in managing anastomotic leakage after esophagectomy: a comparative retrospective study. Surg Endosc Other Interv Tech. 2013;27(10):3883–90. https://doi.org/10.1007/s00464-013-2998-0.

51. Schorsch T, Müller C, Loske G. Endoscopic vacuum therapy of perforations and anastomotic insufficiency of the esophagus. Chirurg. 2014;85(12):1081–93. https://doi.org/10.1007/s00104-014-2764-4.

52. Bludau M, Hölscher AH, Herbold T, et al. Management of upper intestinal leaks using an endoscopic vacuum-assisted closure system (E-VAC). Surg Endosc Other Interv Tech. 2014;28(3):896–901. https://doi.org/10.1007/s00464-013-3244-5.

53. Heits N, Stapel L, Reichert B, et al. Endoscopic endoluminal vacuum therapy in esophageal perforation. Ann Thorac Surg. 2014;97(3):1029–35. https://doi.org/10.1016/j.athoracsur.2013.11.014.

54. Csendes A, Braghetto I, León P, Burgos AM. Management of leaks after laparoscopic sleeve gastrectomy in patients with obesity. J Gastrointest Surg. 2010;14(9):1343–8. https://doi.org/10.1007/s11605-010-1249-0.

55. Thodiyil PA, Yenumula P, Rogula T, et al. Selective nonoperative management of leaks after gastric bypass: lessons learned from 2675 consecutive patients. Ann Surg. 2008;248(5):782–92. https://doi.org/10.1097/SLA.0b013e31818584aa.

56. Salinas A, Baptista A, Santiago E, Antor M, Salinas H. Self-expandable metal stents to treat gastric leaks. Surg Obes Relat Dis. 2006;2(5):570–2. https://doi.org/10.1016/j.soard.2006.08.007.

57. Eubanks S, Edwards CA, Fearing NM, et al. Use of endoscopic stents to treat anastomotic complications after bariatric surgery. J Am Coll Surg. 2008;206(5):935–8. https://doi.org/10.1016/j.jamcollsurg.2008.02.016.

58. Maluf-Filho F, Hondo F, Halwan B, De Lima MS, Giordano-Nappi J, Sakai P. Endoscopic treatment of Roux-en-Y gastric bypass-related gastrocutaneous fistulas using a novel biomaterial. Surg Endosc Other Interv Tech. 2009;23(7):1541–5. https://doi.org/10.1007/s00464-009-0440-4.

59. Kim Z, Kim YJ, Kim YJ, Goo DE, Cho JY. Successful management of staple line leak after laparoscopic sleeve gastrectomy with vascular plug and covered stent. Surg Laparosc Endosc Percutan Tech. 2011;21(4):e206–8. https://doi.org/10.1097/SLE.0b013e3182258bf5.

60. Schweitzer M, Steele K, Mitchell M, Okolo P. Transoral endoscopic closure of gastric fistula. Surg Obes Relat Dis. 2009;5(2):283–4. https://doi.org/10.1016/j.soard.2008.11.014.

61. Overcash WT. Natural orifice surgery (NOS) using StomaphyX for repair of gastric leaks after bariatric revisions. Obes Surg. 2008;18(7):882–5. https://doi.org/10.1007/s11695-008-9452-8.

62. Pauli EM, Beshir H, Mathew A. Gastrogastric fistulae following gastric bypass surgery—clinical recognition and treatment. Curr Gastroenterol Rep. 2014;16(9):405. https://doi.org/10.1007/s11894-014-0405-1.

63. Vilallonga R, Himpens J, van de Vrande S. Laparoscopic roux limb placement for the management of chronic proximal fistulas after sleeve gastrectomy: technical aspects. Surg Endosc. 2015;29(2):414–6. https://doi.org/10.1007/s00464-014-3684-6.

64. Ramos AC, Ramos MG, Campos JM, Galvão Neto MDP, Bastos ELDS. Laparoscopic total gastrectomy as an alternative treatment to postsleeve chronic fistula. Surg Obes Relat Dis. 2015;11(3):552–6. https://doi.org/10.1016/j.soard.2014.10.021.

Endoscopic Management of Weight Regain

Eric J. Vargas, Andrew C. Storm, Fateh Bazerbachi, and Barham K. Abu Dayyeh

Introduction

Obesity has reached epidemic proportions with almost 40% of Americans considered to have obesity [1–3]. The evidence is clear that bariatric surgery induces the most durable weight loss as compared to other modalities and also results in improvement of obesity-related comorbidities [4–7]. However, despite this success, all bariatric surgeries are associated with a degree of weight recidivism [8–10]. After Roux-en-Y gastric bypass (RYGB), over a third of patients will regain more than 5% of their nadir weight, with some groups reporting rates of weight regain over 50%, depending on the criteria used to define weight regain. While a consensus on the definition of weight regain has not been reached, *greater than or equal to* 15% weight regain has been associated with decreased quality of life and recrudescence of obesity-related comorbidities [11]. The etiology of weight regain is multifactorial [12, 13], including anatomical and nonanatomical factors such as a dilated gastrojejunal anastomosis (GJA), an enlarged surgical pouch,

E. J. Vargas · A. C. Storm · F. Bazerbachi
Department of Gastroenterology and Hepatology,
Mayo Clinic, Rochester, MN, USA
e-mail: Vargas.Eric@mayo.edu; Storm.Andrew@mayo.edu

B. K. Abu Dayyeh (✉)
Mayo Clinic, Rochester, MN, USA
e-mail: abudayyeh.barham@mayo.edu

presence of a gastrogastric fistula (GGF), nutritional nonadherence, mental health disorders, and poor post-bariatric clinical follow-up [10, 11, 14–17]. Indeed, GJA dilation (>20 mm) is one of the most frequently identified and implicated abnormalities associated with weight regain, and revisional surgeries were increasingly being performed for this indication [14, 15, 17]. However, due to the increased risk of major complications, including mortality, associated with surgical revision procedures [18], endoscopic approaches were developed aimed at reducing GJA diameter in a minimally invasive and safe approach. These procedures include GJA sclerotherapy, GJA argon plasma coagulation (APC) therapy, and the endoscopic transoral outlet reduction (TORe) procedures.

Sclerotherapy, APC, and Plication/Suturing Platforms

Sclerotherapy was the first popularized endoscopic approach to reducing the size of the GJA using 5% sodium morrhuate. This sclerosing agent is typically injected around the anastomosis site over several endoscopic sessions (2+) aiming for a final GJA diameter of 10–12 mm with an average reported weight loss of 6.8–19.9 kg [19]. While some studies revealed durable weight loss outcomes at 6–12 months, the decreasing commercial availability of the toxic

© Springer Nature Switzerland AG 2020
M. S. Wagh, S. B. Wani (eds.), *Gastrointestinal Interventional Endoscopy*,
https://doi.org/10.1007/978-3-030-21695-5_16

sclerosing agent has limited its growth and use [19, 20]. The widespread availability of argon plasma coagulation (APC) and familiarity with its use led to its utilization to "resurface" the GJA using electrocautery for outlet revision [21]. In the most popular technique, the APC probe is intentionally placed against the mucosa in order to allow deeper submucosal extension of electrocautery energy, presumably inducing fibrosis that over several endoscopic treatments has been shown to reduce the aperture size (typically 10–12 mm). A pulsed APC with settings of flow 0.8 L/s, effect 2, and 55 W has been preferred, though expert centers have begun using higher energy settings (flow 1.0 L/s, effect 2, 100 W) without allowing the probe to touch the mucosa. One non-randomized study demonstrated an average 15.5 kg weight loss of the 19 kg regained post-bariatric surgery was observed after three sessions performed every 8 weeks [22]. APC is performed alone in or conjunction with full-thickness suturing approaches like TORe for improved efficacy [23].

With the advent of endoscopic suturing and plication devices came procedural innovation in the approach to endoscopic revision of dilated GJA for weight regain after RYGB. The StomaphyX was one of the earliest endoscopic suturing devices (EndoGastric Solutions) used for TORe and pouch reduction. Using vacuum assistance, plications were placed in the pouch and outlet to reduce their aperture. Unfortunately, the randomized sham-controlled clinical trial was terminated early due to preliminary results indicating failure to achieve the primary endpoint [24]. The revision obesity surgery endolumenal (ROSE) is another endoscopic approach using the Incisionless Operating Platform (IOP; USGI Medical, San Clemente, CA, USA). The device uses tissue anchors to create full-thickness plications reducing the size of the gastric pouch and GJA resulting in a mean 6.5 ± 6.5 kg weight loss at 6 months [25]. However to date, the only randomized clinical trial showing device efficacy over sham or placebo has been the Bard EndoCinch suturing system (C.R. BARD, Inc., Murray Hill, NJ, USA), a superficial thickness suturing device initially used for GERD, which was used to reduce the

size of the GJA diameter. The randomized multicenter sham-controlled clinical trial (RESTORe) using this device established level 1 evidence that the TORe procedure was effective in the management of weight regain after RYGB, with a mean % weight loss treatment difference of 3.2% compared to the sham group (3.5% vs. 0.4%; $p = 0.21$). Following the randomized trial, a study compared full-thickness suturing using the OverStitch platform (Fig. 16.1) (Apollo Endosurgery, Austin TX, USA) with superficial thickness suturing with the EndoCinch for TORe, revealing superior 12 month outcomes with full thickness over superficial thickness (8.6 ± 2.5 kg vs 2.9 ± 1.0 kg; $P < .01$), leading to the international adoption of full-thickness suturing using the OverStitch platform for TORe [26].

Transoral Outlet Reduction (TORe) Using the OverStitch Device

TORe using the OverStitch full-thickness suturing platform has been shown effective at inducing clinically significant long-term weight loss in patients who experienced weight regain after RYGB [27–29]. Mean weight loss experienced 12 months after the procedure ranges from 5.7 to 10.6 kg, with % excess weight loss ranging from 11.3% to over 25%. Improved outcomes are consistently seen when APC is combined with full-thickness TORe [23].

Procedures are typically performed under general anesthesia with endotracheal intubation. A routine upper endoscopy is first completed to evaluate the diameter and health of the anastomosis along with the size of the gastric pouch. Pouch diameter and length can be used to estimate gastric volume (diameter x length). The OverStitch platform is then mounted on the distal tip double-channel endoscope (GIF-2T160 or 180 Olympus America, Central Valley, Pennsylvania, USA) which allows the use of the Helix device for tissue acquisition for deep suture placement and the catheter-based actuating needle for driving and reloading sutures.

Prior to performing the TORe procedure, the authors prefer to use APC along the gastric side

Fig. 16.1 The Apollo OverStitch device (Apollo EndoSurgery)

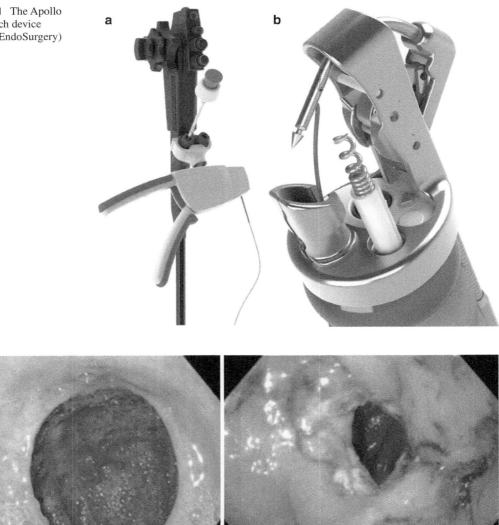

Fig. 16.2 GJA pre- and post-TORe

of the anastomosis to prepare the tissue for suturing and to minimize bleeding. An esophageal overtube may be placed prior to passing the suturing system through the esophagus in order to protect the esophagus from repeated intubations with the suturing device but is not employed across all expert centers.

Multiple suturing patterns have been used and studied for TORe including simple interrupted, figure of eight, and purse string. The end goal is to reduce the aperture to 8–10 mm (Fig. 16.2), as

smaller diameters are associated with increased nausea and vomiting that result in higher stitch loss and poorer weight loss outcomes. Endoscopists can expect to use anywhere from 1 to 12 sutures depending on the size of the GJA and suturing technique employed. The patient is maintained NPO for 24 hours after the procedure. The authors occasionally prescribe a 5-day course of antibiotics and at least 2 weeks of proton pump inhibitor therapy along with a liquid diet for at least 2 weeks after the procedure, with gradual progression to solid food over the next 2 weeks. Nausea and abdominal pain are the most common symptoms after the procedure, but with intraoperative dexamethasone or aprepitant injection, these are reduced significantly. A small proportion (<2%) can experience stenosis after revision, necessitating endoscopy to perform balloon dilation of the stenosed GJA.

Simple Interrupted

The simple interrupted technique is illustrated in Fig. 16.3. After the OverStitch device is mounted on the endoscope and APC has been performed around the mucosa, stitches are placed through the gastric mucosa with aid of the tissue helix from the lower left to the upper right. The revised GJA may be edematous afterward, but a standard endoscope should transverse the aperture in order to ensure patency. Figure of eight suturing pattern is employed in a similar fashion, and at times a combination of simple interrupted and figure of eight sutures is used due to the GJA anatomy.

Purse-String Technique

The second most common suturing technique used for TORe is the purse-string technique. This technique involves using a single suture (or in some cases two running sutures) placed around the margin of the GJA in a continuous ring. APC is used to ablate the gastric side of the GJA prior to suture placement. After the running suture has made at least one full circle around the GJA, a balloon is then passed through the second endoscope channel and inflated inside the anastomosis to 6–8 mm. The suture is then tightened around the balloon and cinched (Fig. 16.4). The advantages of the purse-string technique include the low number of sutures used, control over the final aperture by using the balloon to tighten the suture, and superior weight loss outcomes compared to simple interrupted techniques [28, 29].

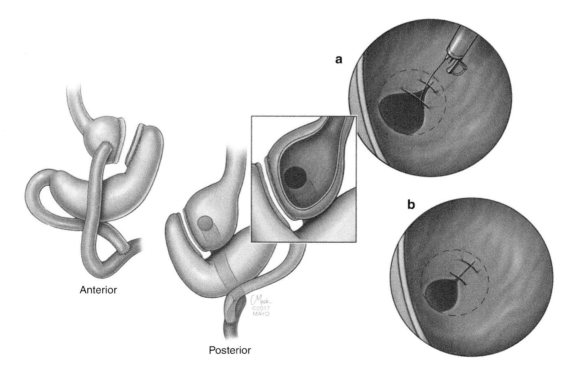

Anterior

Posterior

Fig. 16.3 TORe using simple interrupted suture technique. The GJA is reduced to approximately 8–10 mm

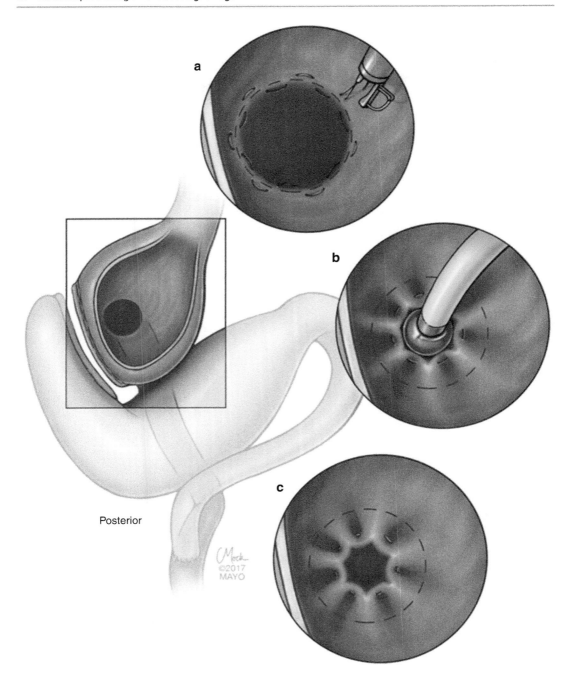

Fig. 16.4 TORe using a purse-string technique. The suture is tightened and cinched over a through-the-scope balloon to size the final aperture

Tubular Reinforced TORe

A novel approach to TORe involves the creation of a reinforced tubular sleeve proximal to the revised GJA anastomosis. The reinforced proximal tubular sleeve uses the same triangular suturing pattern as the endoscopic sleeve gastroplasty, reducing the size of the pouch. The GJA is reduced first using a combination of interrupted and figure of eight sutures, and the proximal sleeve gastroplasty is then created (Fig. 16.5). The technique was developed for those with an eccentric GJA location, making it difficult to perform the purse-string technique with a concomitantly enlarged gastric pouch. Unpublished data suggests superior weight loss outcomes at 3 months compared to simple interrupted suturing.

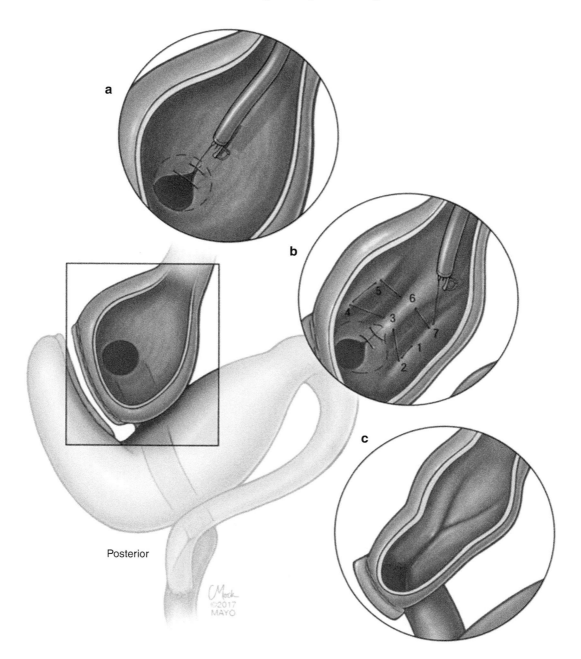

Fig. 16.5 Reinforced "tubular" TORe. A reinforced tubular gastroplasty exit proximal to the revised GJA is performed

Pouch Revision

A variety of novel endoscopic techniques have more recently been employed to reduce the size of the gastric pouch. One study described the use of radiofrequency ablation (Barrx™, Medtronic, Minneapolis, MN) across the entire pouch and GJA in 25 patients. The authors repeated the procedure at 4 and 8 months if the patients had not met target weights. At 12 months, the median %EWL was 18.4% [IQR 10.8–33.7] with an absolute weight loss of 14 kg. The majority of patients (>80%) required three RFA treatments over the course of the study [30]. Further comparative trials are needed.

Sleeve Gastrectomy Revision

While the bariatric endoscopists have traditionally focused on RYGB, a few case series have reported successful revision of the sleeve gastrectomy using the full-thickness suturing platform as an alternative to conversion to RYGB, or "resleeving" with endoscopic suture gastroplasty for the treatment of weight regain or primary failure. A pilot series of five patients reported 12-month mean % EWL of 33% with %weight loss ranging from 6.7% to 17.2% [31]. Further retrospective studies are forthcoming.

Conclusion

Advances in endoluminal techniques have allowed endoscopists to manage a variety of complications after bariatric surgery in a safe and effective fashion. With the rising prevalence of obesity and number of bariatric surgeries being performed, endoscopists are poised to play an instrumental role in the advanced management of bariatric patients who experience leaks, fistulas, and weight regain. Endoscopic revisions of the anatomical factors associated with weight regain are effective at inducing weight loss and weight stabilization. TORe with full-thickness suturing techniques is effective in the revision of dilated

GJAs and should be offered to patients as part of a comprehensive treatment approach with level 1 data supporting its use. Concomitant pouch revision is regaining popularity, with innovative treatments such as RFA and pouch gastroplasty representing the newest endoscopic approaches.

References

1. Releases CN. Cancers associated with overweight and obesity make up 40 percent of cancers diagnosed in the United States 2017 [11/11/2017]. Available from: https://www.cdc.gov/media/releases/2017/p1003-vs-cancer-obesity.html.
2. Organization WH. Global Health Observatory (GHO) data: overweight and obesity 2016 [11/11/2017]. Available from: http://www.who.int/gho/ncd/risk_factors/overweight_text/en/(2016).
3. Flegal KM, Carroll MD, Ogden CL, Curtin LR. Prevalence and trends in obesity among US adults, 1999–2008. JAMA. 2010;303(3):235–41. Epub 2010/01/15. PubMed PMID: 20071471. https://doi.org/10.1001/jama.2009.2014.
4. Diabetes Prevention Program Research G. The diabetes prevention program (DPP): description of lifestyle intervention. Diabetes Care. 2002;25(12):2165–71. Epub 2002/11/28. PubMed PMID: 12453955; PubMed Central PMCID: PMCPMC1282458
5. The Look ARG. Eight-year weight losses with an intensive lifestyle intervention: the look AHEAD study. Obesity (Silver Spring). 2014;22(1):5–13. https://doi.org/10.1002/oby.20662. PubMed PMID: PMC3904491
6. Adams TD, Davidson LE, Litwin SE, Kim J, Kolotkin RL, Nanjee MN, et al. Weight and metabolic outcomes 12 years after gastric bypass. N Engl J Med. 2017;377(12):1143–55. https://doi.org/10.1056/NEJMoa1700459. Epub 2017/09/21. PubMed PMID: 28930514; PubMed Central PMCID: PMCPMC5737957
7. Colquitt JL, Pickett K, Loveman E, Frampton GK. Surgery for weight loss in adults. Cochrane Database Syst Rev. 2014;8:CD003641. Epub 2014/08/12. PubMed PMID: 25105982. https://doi.org/10.1002/14651858.CD003641.pub4.
8. Cooper TC, Simmons EB, Webb K, Burns JL, Kushner RF. Trends in weight regain following Roux-en-Y gastric bypass (RYGB) bariatric surgery. Obes Surg. 2015;25(8):1474–81. Epub 2015/01/18. PubMed PMID: 25595383. https://doi.org/10.1007/s11695-014-1560-z.
9. Maciejewski ML, Arterburn DE, Van Scoyoc L, Smith VA, Yancy WS Jr, Weidenbacher HJ, et al. Bariatric surgery and long-term durability of weight

loss. JAMA Surg. 2016;151(11):1046–55. https://doi.org/10.1001/jamasurg.2016.2317. Epub 2016/09/01. PubMed PMID: 27579793; PubMed Central PMCID: PMCPMC5112115

10. Karmali S, Brar B, Shi X, Sharma AM, de Gara C, Birch DW. Weight recidivism post-bariatric surgery: a systematic review. Obes Surg. 2013;23(11):1922–33. https://doi.org/10.1007/s11695-013-1070-4.

11. Jirapinyo P, Abu Dayyeh BK, Thompson CC. Weight regain after Roux-en-Y gastric bypass has a large negative impact on the bariatric quality of life index. BMJ Open Gastroenterol. 2017;4(1):e000153. https://doi.org/10.1136/bmjgast-2017-000153. Epub 2017/09/26. PubMed PMID: 28944069; PubMed Central PMCID: PMCPMC5596836

12. Mechanick JI, Kushner RF, Sugerman HJ, Gonzalez-Campoy JM, Collazo-Clavell ML, Guven S, et al. American Association of Clinical Endocrinologists, The Obesity Society, and American Society for Metabolic & Bariatric Surgery medical guidelines for clinical practice for the perioperative nutritional, metabolic, and nonsurgical support of the bariatric surgery patient. Surg Obes Relat Dis. 2008;4(5, Suppl):S109–S84. https://doi.org/10.1016/j.soard.2008.08.009.

13. Magro DO, Geloneze B, Delfini R, Pareja BC, Callejas F, Pareja JC. Long-term weight regain after gastric bypass: a 5-year prospective study. Obes Surg. 2008;18(6):648–51. Epub 2008/04/09. PubMed PMID: 18392907. https://doi.org/10.1007/s11695-007-9265-1.

14. Catalano MF, Rudic G, Anderson AJ, Chua TY. Weight gain after bariatric surgery as a result of a large gastric stoma: endotherapy with sodium morrhuate may prevent the need for surgical revision. Gastrointest Endosc. 2007;66(2):240–5. Epub 2007/03/03. PubMed PMID: 17331511. https://doi.org/10.1016/j.gie.2006.06.061.

15. Abu Dayyeh BK, Lautz DB, Thompson CC. Gastrojejunal stoma diameter predicts weight regain after Roux-en-Y gastric bypass. Clin Gastroenterol Hepatol. 2011;9(3):228–33. https://doi.org/10.1016/j.cgh.2010.11.004. Epub 2010/11/26. PubMed PMID: 21092760; PubMed Central PMCID: PMCPMC3043151

16. Heneghan HM, Yimcharoen P, Brethauer SA, Kroh M, Chand B. Influence of pouch and stoma size on weight loss after gastric bypass. Surg Obes Relat Dis. 2012;8(4):408–15. Epub 2011/11/08. PubMed PMID: 22055390. https://doi.org/10.1016/j.soard.2011.09.010.

17. Yimcharoen P, Heneghan HM, Singh M, Brethauer S, Schauer P, Rogula T, et al. Endoscopic findings and outcomes of revisional procedures for patients with weight recidivism after gastric bypass. Surg Endosc. 2011;25(10):3345–52. Epub 2011/05/03. PubMed PMID: 21533520. https://doi.org/10.1007/s00464-011-1723-0.

18. Spyropoulos C, Kehagias I, Panagiotopoulos S, Mead N, Kalfarentzos F. Revisional bariatric surgery: 13-year experience from a tertiary institution. Arch Surg. 2010;145(2):173–7. Epub 2010/02/17. PubMed PMID: 20157086. https://doi.org/10.1001/archsurg.2009.260.

19. Giurgius M, Fearing N, Weir A, Micheas L, Ramaswamy A. Long-term follow-up evaluation of endoscopic sclerotherapy for dilated gastrojejunostomy after gastric bypass. Surg Endosc. 2014;28(5):1454–9. Epub 2014/01/31. PubMed PMID: 24477936. https://doi.org/10.1007/s00464-013-3376-7.

20. Abu Dayyeh BK, Jirapinyo P, Weitzner Z, Barker C, Flicker MS, Lautz DB, et al. Endoscopic sclerotherapy for the treatment of weight regain after Roux-en-Y gastric bypass: outcomes, complications, and predictors of response in 575 procedures. Gastrointest Endosc. 2012;76(2):275–82. https://doi.org/10.1016/j.gie.2012.03.1407. Epub 2012/07/24. PubMed PMID: 22817783; PubMed Central PMCID: PMCPMC4428559

21. Aly A. Argon plasma coagulation and gastric bypass—a novel solution to stomal dilation. Obes Surg. 2008;19(6):788. https://doi.org/10.1007/s11695-008-9763-9.

22. Baretta GA, Alhinho HC, Matias JE, Marchesini JB, de Lima JH, Empinotti C, et al. Argon plasma coagulation of gastrojejunal anastomosis for weight regain after gastric bypass. Obes Surg. 2015;25(1):72–9. Epub 2014/07/10. PubMed PMID: 25005812. https://doi.org/10.1007/s11695-014-1363-2.

23. Brunaldi VO, Jirapinyo P, de Moura DTH, Okazaki O, Bernardo WM, Galvão Neto M, et al. Endoscopic treatment of weight regain following Roux-en-Y gastric bypass: a systematic review and meta-analysis. Obes Surg. 2018;28(1):266–76. https://doi.org/10.1007/s11695-017-2986-x.

24. Eid GM, McCloskey CA, Eagleton JK, Lee LB, Courcoulas AP. StomaphyX vs a sham procedure for revisional surgery to reduce regained weight in Roux-en-Y gastric bypass patients: a randomized clinical trial. JAMA Surg. 2014;149(4):372–9. Epub 2014/02/21. PubMed PMID: 24554030. https://doi.org/10.1001/jamasurg.2013.4051.

25. Horgan S, Jacobsen G, Weiss GD, Oldham JS Jr, Denk PM, Borao F, et al. Incisionless revision of post-Roux-en-Y bypass stomal and pouch dilation: multicenter registry results. Surg Obes Relat Dis. 2010;6(3):290–5. Epub 2010/06/01. PubMed PMID: 20510293. https://doi.org/10.1016/j.soard.2009.12.011.

26. Kumar N, Thompson CC. Comparison of a superficial suturing device with a full-thickness suturing device for transoral outlet reduction (with videos). Gastrointest Endosc. 2014;79(6):984–9. Epub 2014/04/12. PubMed PMID: 24721521; PubMed Central PMCID: PMCPMC5038592. https://doi.org/10.1016/j.gie.2014.02.006.

27. Vargas EJ, Bazerbachi F, Rizk M, Rustagi T, Acosta A, Wilson EB, et al. Transoral outlet reduction with full thickness endoscopic suturing for weight regain after gastric bypass: a large multicenter international

experience and meta-analysis. Surg Endosc. 2017. Epub 2017/07/01. PubMed PMID: 28664438; https://doi.org/10.1007/s00464-017-5671-1.

28. Schulman AR, Kumar N, Thompson CC. Transoral outlet reduction: a comparison of purse-string with interrupted stitch technique. Gastrointest Endosc. 2017. Epub 2017/11/08. PubMed PMID: 29108984; https://doi.org/10.1016/j.gie.2017.10.034.

29. Jirapinyo P, Kroner PT, Thompson CC. Purse-string transoral outlet reduction (TORe) is effective at inducing weight loss and improvement in metabolic comorbidities after Roux-en-Y gastric bypass. Endoscopy.

2017. Epub 2017/12/19. PubMed PMID: 29253919; https://doi.org/10.1055/s-0043-122380.

30. Abrams JA, Komanduri S, Shaheen NJ, Wang Z, Rothstein RI. Radiofrequency ablation for the treatment of weight regain after Roux-en-Y gastric bypass surgery. Gastrointest Endosc. 2018;87(1):275–9.e2. https://doi.org/10.1016/j.gie.2017.06.030.

31. Eid G. Sleeve gastrectomy revision by endoluminal sleeve plication gastroplasty: a small pilot case series. Surg Endosc. 2017;31(10):4252–5. Epub 2017/04/02. PubMed PMID: 28364152. https://doi.org/10.1007/s00464-017-5469-1.

POEM: Pre-procedural Work-Up and Indications

17

Joseph Rayfield Triggs and John E. Pandolfino

Introduction

Over the past decade, POEM has developed into one of the three principle treatments for achalasia, along with pneumatic dilation (PD) and laparoscopic Heller myotomy (LHM) [1, 2]. These therapies aim to disrupt the lower esophageal sphincter (LES) with the goal of relieving esophagogastric junction outflow obstruction (EGJOO). POEM was first introduced in 2007, when Pasricha et al. described endoscopic myotomy using a porcine model in which a submucosal tunnel was created using a biliary dilating balloon followed by circular muscle myotomy using a needle knife [3]. Subsequently, Inoue et al. performed the first endoscopic esophageal myotomy in humans in 2008 and published a case series of 17 patients with promising results for the treatment of achalasia [4].

Achalasia is a rare disorder with a mean age of diagnosis of 56 and an incidence rate of 2.3–2.9 per 100,000 [5, 6]. The pathophysiology is incompletely understood, but it is thought to result from an inflammatory process that leads to the loss of ganglions of the myenteric plexus and fibrosis ultimately resulting in aberrant neuromuscular signaling of both the esophageal body and LES [7–9]. This aberrant signaling leads to an absence of peristalsis in the esophageal body and failure of the LES to relax. These are the two quintessential physiologic features of achalasia although current definitive therapies focus on only one component, LES dysfunction.

Coincident with the development of POEM was the widespread adoption of high-resolution manometry and its interpretation using the Chicago Classification (CC) [10]. The CC which was originally proposed in 2008 led to a major reclassification of esophageal motility disorders [11, 12]. It is currently in its third version which was published in 2015 and subdivides motility disorders into minor and major disorders based on the presence or absence of findings in asymptomatic controls, respectively [10]. The CC uses high-resolution manometry (HRM) which was developed in the early 2000s and is measured using a catheter-based system that has intraluminal pressure sensors closely spaced to ensure little data loss between them. HRM is most commonly viewed using esophageal pressure topography (EPT) plots or Clouse plots which were named after the individual who developed them [13–15]. These plots place time on the x-axis and esophageal position on the y-axis with

J. R. Triggs
Section of Gastroenterology and Hepatology in the Department of Medicine, Northwestern Feinberg School of Medicine, Chicago, IL, USA
e-mail: joseph.triggs@northwestern.edu

J. E. Pandolfino (✉)
Division of Gastroenterology, Department of Medicine, Northwestern University's Feinberg School of Medicine, Chicago, IL, USA
e-mail: j-pandolfino@northwestern.edu

© Springer Nature Switzerland AG 2020
M. S. Wagh, S. B. Wani (eds.), *Gastrointestinal Interventional Endoscopy*,
https://doi.org/10.1007/978-3-030-21695-5_17

pressure represented as a color. Diagnoses are made through the analysis of 10 supine or reclined 5 ml saline swallows. HRM replaced traditional line tracing manometry and has led to increased ease of use and uniformity, standardization of objective measures used in the diagnosis of motility disorders, improved processes for interpretation, and finally, improved diagnostic yield from 84% to 97% for achalasia [16–18]. Despite these advances, HRM is a diagnostic tool that requires special expertise and training to reliably preform high-quality studies [19–21]. Healthcare professionals reading these studies must be able to assess for technical adequacy, which includes ensuring proper placement and recognizing common artifacts and equipment failure, in addition to being able to accurately report the measurements used in the CC to allow for an accurate diagnosis. HRM and interpretation using the CC are essential in the work-up and evaluation prior to POEM. Unfortunately, equivocal cases can make the diagnosis and subsequent treatment decisions of motility disorders difficult. For this reason, in addition to HRM and prior to treatment with POEM, patients may often need further testing to ensure an accurate diagnosis. These tests include esophagogastroduodenoscopy (EGD), timed barium esophagram (TBE), and functional luminal imaging probe (FLIP) analysis. Once a global picture is obtained, the physician may then make an informed decision regarding the best treatment options.

The goal of this chapter will be to review the work-up and indications of POEM. The remainder of this section will go into further detail regarding the technical aspects, efficacy, safety, and training.

POEM Work-Up

Patients presenting for work-up and evaluation of POEM most often present with nonobstructive dysphagia, regurgitation, or chest pain [1, 22, 23]. After careful evaluation, a subset of these patients may ultimately benefit from LES myotomy via POEM. Current practice suggests that at a minimum, the work-up requires an upper endoscopy and an appropriate HRM diagnosis in the correct clinical context. Here we will discuss

HRM and upper endoscopy as well as additional diagnostic tools (impedance manometry, TBE, and FLIP) which may aid in identifying the subset of patients who will benefit from POEM.

High-Resolution Manometry

HRM interpreted using the CC v3.0 is the current gold standard in diagnosing esophageal motility disorders. This in combination with EGD is the minimum work-up required prior to POEM [10]. Patients presenting with dysphagia, reflux, regurgitation, or chest pain should start with an EGD to rule out high-grade (Los Angeles classification grade C or D) esophagitis or an anatomic abnormality for their symptoms (e.g., stricture). These findings obviate the need for motility testing, and in addition to a history of prior foregut surgery are exclusions to using the CC for interpretation of HRM.

In the hierarchical model of the CC, the initial assessment is to determine deglutitive LES relaxation [10]. This is done using the integrated relaxation pressure (IRP) which is the median value of 10 supine swallows of the 4 s of maximal deglutitive relaxation (contiguous or noncontiguous) in the 10-s window beginning at UES relaxation referenced to gastric pressure [24] (Fig. 17.1). Of note, although used as the measure of LES relaxation, the IRP is actually measuring EGJ resistance which is the sum of the pressure from the LES, crural diaphragm, and intrabolus pressure [25]. Outflow obstruction is defined as an IRP ≥ upper limit of normal (15 mmHg for Sierra design catheters). The IRP needs to be interpreted with great care as patients may have achalasia with normal IRP values [26]. In fact, patients with type I achalasia can have values below 15 mmHg, and a diagnosis of achalasia should always be considered in patients with absent contractility, pan-esophageal pressurization, or spasm.

Once the IRP is determined, the next step in making a manometric diagnosis is to determine the peristaltic activity of the esophagus. The key parameters used to define the peristaltic activity of the esophagus are distal latency (DL) and distal contractile integral (DCI) (Fig. 17.1). The DL identifies premature contractions (spasms) and is defined as the time from the start of upper esophageal sphincter relaxation to the contractile deceleration point (CDP) which is the inflection point along the 30 mmHg isobaric contour at which the propagation velocity slows [10, 27]. Values of less than 4.5 s are considered prema-

ture. Contractions are also assessed for their adequacy according to the DCI which is defined as the amplitude∗duration∗length (mmHg∗s∗cm) of a contraction distal to the transition zone and above 20 mmHg [10]. Using the combination of these values, the CC can then be applied to define achalasia, EGJOO, distal esophageal spasm (DES), and jackhammer, the diagnoses amenable to POEM. Beyond diagnosis, HRM can also be used to assess for technical success following POEM with multiple studies showing improvement in IRP and lower esophageal basal pressure following treatment [28–31].

A unique capability of POEM is to perform an extended proximal myotomy, typically dictated by HRM metrics, which is recommended for patients with type III achalasia, type I or II with symptoms of chest pain, abdominal contractions on initial inspection, or spastic motility disorders such as DES or jackhammer [32]. These data are consistent with results that suggest that noncardiac chest pain may be associated with sustained esophageal contractions and studies supporting efficacy in extended surgical myotomy in relieving the pain [33, 34]. Figure 17.2 represents such an example in which a patient had complete

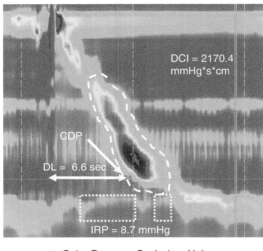

Fig. 17.1 High-resolution manometry parameters. (Courtesy of the Northwestern Esophageal Center)

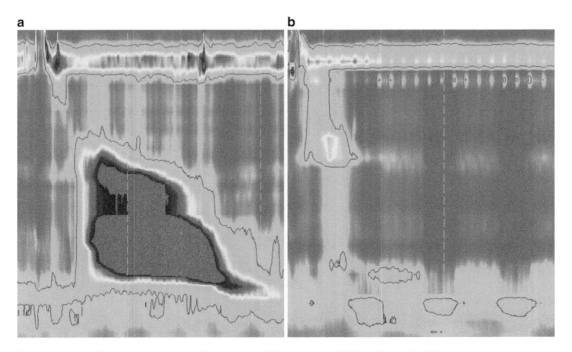

Fig. 17.2 Type III achalasia treated with extended POEM, (**a**) Pre-POEM HRM, (**b**) HRM post 19 cm myotomy. (Courtesy of the Northwestern Esophageal Center)

symptomatic response (Eckardt score (ES) 6 pretreatment to 0 posttreatment) following an extended 19 cm myotomy for type III achalasia. The pre- and post-POEM EPT plots are shown which demonstrate an improved LES pressure and almost complete loss of the premature hypercontractile segment following therapy.

In addition to standard high-resolution manometry, advanced metrics using impedance manometry may also be useful in identifying those patients that may benefit from POEM. Impedance values decrease with bolus/fluid retention. This allows impedance to act as a surrogate for this cardinal feature of EGJ dysfunction. The impedance bolus height which can be measured during manometry with the addition of a 200 ml saline challenge has been shown to correlate with bolus retention on TBE (Fig. 17.3a) [35]. Furthermore, the esophageal impedance integral ratio, defined as the ratio of bolus that *does not* clear the esophagus (Z2) to that of bolus that *does* clear the esophagus (Z1), has also been shown to be aid in the diagnosis of nonobstructive dysphagia and can be used to evaluate treatment outcomes in achalasia (Fig. 17.3b) [36, 37]. Beyond assessing retention, manometry with impedance is also able to measure bolus flow time (BFT) which uses impedance manometry to evaluate EGJ opening and bolus flow using a virtual high-resolution sleeve. This approach relies on a flow-permissive pressure gradient and assesses the nadir impedance as a surrogate of bolus presence within the EGJ [38]. A recent study demonstrated significantly reduced BFTs (median (IQR)) in patients with achalasia compared to healthy controls, 0.45 s (0.0–1.2 s) vs 3.5 s (2.3–3.9 s), respectively. Additionally, BFT was able to identify patients with clinical achalasia and a normal IRP [39].

Fig. 17.3 Impedance manometry, (**a**) impedance bolus height corresponds to barium retention on TBE, (**b**) EII ratio approaches 1 in patient with achalasia (Z2÷Z1), demonstrating significant bolus retention. (Courtesy of the Northwestern Esophageal Center)

a

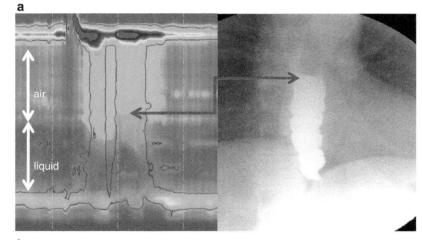

b

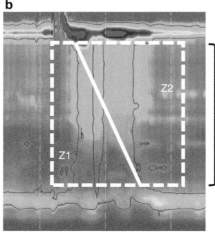

Esophageal Impedance Integral (EII ratio) = the ratio of residual bolus volume (Z2) relative to the intra-esophageal bolus volume following the swallow, but before the peristaltic wave (Z1) (Z2 ÷ Z1)

Esophagogastroduodenoscopy

As described above, EGD is necessary for the evaluation prior to POEM to ensure a patient does not have high-grade esophagitis or an anatomic etiology for their symptoms. EGD can also be useful in assessing for esophageal dilatation, the presence and location of diverticula, and tortuosity which although is not a contraindication to POEM should be recognized prior to treatment to ensure proper procedural planning. There is also debate in the literature regarding the necessity of EGD to rule out fungal infections prior to POEM. Some centers administer empiric fluconazole or nystatin in all patients for 2–3 days before the procedure, due to the high rate of esophageal stasis and candidiasis, while others treat only overt evidence of fungal overgrowth [40–42]. It is our practice to treat only overt disease prior to POEM.

Timed Barium Esophagram

TBE is a modified version of the barium swallow where patients drink 100–200 ml of low-density barium followed by upright radiographs at defined time intervals, typically 1, 2, and 5 min, post-swallow [43]. This test has classically been used to assess esophageal emptying in patients with achalasia and post-LES targeted therapy to assess for response to treatment. Multiple studies have reported that improvements in TBE correlate with improvement in patient-reported outcomes following treatment for achalasia [44–46]. The test has not been rigorously evaluated as a diagnostic tool but can often aid in defining esophageal anatomy and assessing for esophageal retention which is one of the hallmarks of achalasia aiding in its diagnosis (Fig. 17.4). Furthermore, in the subset of patients with absent peristalsis and borderline IRP values, liquid barium retention may suggest that a patient would benefit from LES targeted therapy such as POEM.

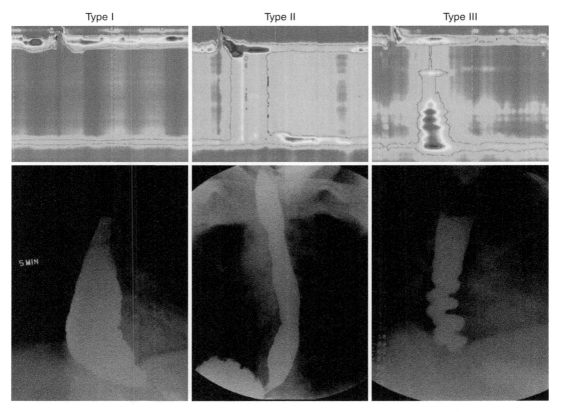

Fig. 17.4 Achalasia subtypes on high-resolution manometry (top panels) and associated timed barium esophagrams (bottom panels). (Courtesy of the Northwestern Esophageal Center)

Endoscopic Ultrasound (EUS) and Computerized Tomography (CT)

These tests are not regularly needed for the assessment of esophageal disease prior to treatment with POEM; however, in specific circumstances, they may help rule out pseudoachalasia due to infiltrative disease or a vascular anomaly

[23, 47–53]. A careful history and endoscopic examination may prompt these tests if there is lymphadenopathy, weight loss, or abnormal anatomy on a thorough endoscopic examination including retroflexion to assess the cardia of the stomach.

This is exemplified in Fig. 17.5 which demonstrates a HRM and an esophagram of a patient

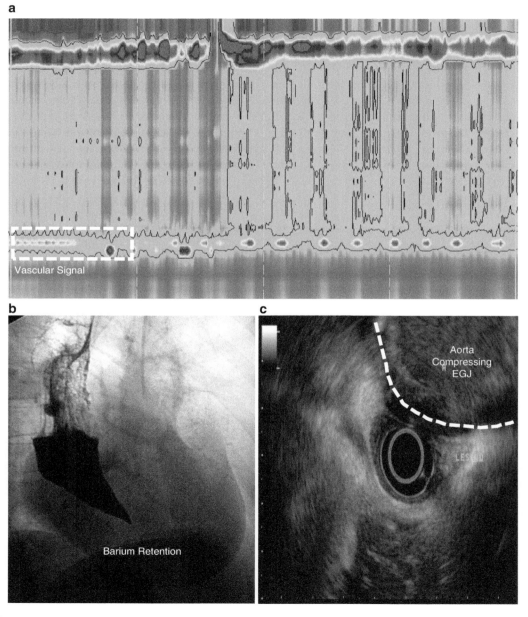

Fig. 17.5 Pseudoachalasia due to vascular obstruction. (**a**) HRM, (**b**) esophagram, (**c**) EUS. (Courtesy of the Northwestern Esophageal Center)

referred to our esophageal center for pneumatic dilatation. The esophagram has the classic bird-beak pattern associated with achalasia, and the HRM met the criteria for type II achalasia; however, the LES pressure appeared to vary with the patient's heart rate prompting an EUS. The EUS revealed a large aortic aneurysm compressing the EGJ leading to an outflow obstruction. Fortunately, the patient underwent vascular surgery in lieu of a potentially life-threatening pneumatic dilation.

Functional Luminal Imaging Probe

The FLIP uses high-resolution impedance planimetry to measure esophageal cross-sectional area and simultaneous pressure (distensibility, $mm^2/mmHg$) during volumetric distention. This technology is unique as it allows for the assessment of esophageal motility during sedated upper endoscopy [54]. Patients with treatment-naïve achalasia have consistently demonstrated esophagogastric junction distensibilities (EGJ-DI) less than 2.8 $mm^2/mmHg$, and patients posttreatment for achalasia with an EGJ-DI that remains below 2.8 $mm^2/mmHg$ have demonstrated worse outcomes [55–58]. At this point, this technology functions as an adjunct to formal HRM motility diagnoses, but more recent work identifying esophageal body contractions has led to a diagnostic algorithm similar to that used in the CC [54]. In combination with the correct clinical context (HRM with absent peristalsis and normal IRP, barium retention on esophagram, or EGD suggestive of achalasia without evidence of obstructive dysphagia), a FLIP distensibility index of <2.8 $mm^2/mmHg$ suggests that these patients may benefit from LES targeted therapy. This has been demonstrated previously in a study of 13 patients with symptoms consistent with achalasia, absent peristalsis but normal IRP on HRM, and distensibility indices consistent with achalasia. These patients were treated with LES targeted therapy (1 Botox, 9 PD, 3 LHM) and subsequently had improvement in EGJ-DI and Eckardt scores [59]. It is our experience that POEM may also be an effective therapy for these

patients. Figure 17.6 demonstrates a patient who presented with dysphagia and had absent peristalsis with a normal IRP on HRM. This patient would not meet the criteria for achalasia according to the CC; however, she had an 11 cm barium column on TBE at 5 min and a FLIP with an EGJ-DI of 1.6 $mm^2/mmHg$. Following POEM, she had complete resolution of her symptoms.

This technology also offers the ability to assess the LES in real time during POEM, and several studies have demonstrated immediate increases in EGJ-DI at the completion of the procedure [60–63]. Furthermore, a recent study reported that a final intraoperative EGJ-DI in the range of 4.5–8.5 $mm^2/mmHg$ was optimal for reducing dysphagia and minimizing gastroesophageal reflux disease at 6 months post-POEM [62].

Indications

POEM was first performed for uncomplicated achalasia, but the technique was quickly adopted for more complex cases including patients with sigmoid anatomy of their esophagus [4]. There is currently no consensus regarding formal indications for POEM, but substantial work has been done to study various treatment applications including achalasia (all three clinical subtypes), non-achalasia motility disorders (DES and jackhammer esophagus), and following failed prior LES targeted therapy for achalasia (Table 17.1).

Achalasia

Achalasia is defined according to the CC as a major motility disorder with an IRP ≥ upper limit of normal (15 mmHg for Sierra design transducers) and 100% failed peristalsis or spasm. Achalasia is subtyped into type I, no contractility; type II, ≥20% pan-esophageal pressurization (with an isobaric contour line of 30 mmHg); or type III, ≥20% spasm with a distal latency of <4.5 s (Fig. 17.4). These subtypes define distinct clinical entities with varying response to different treatments; however, studies suggest that POEM

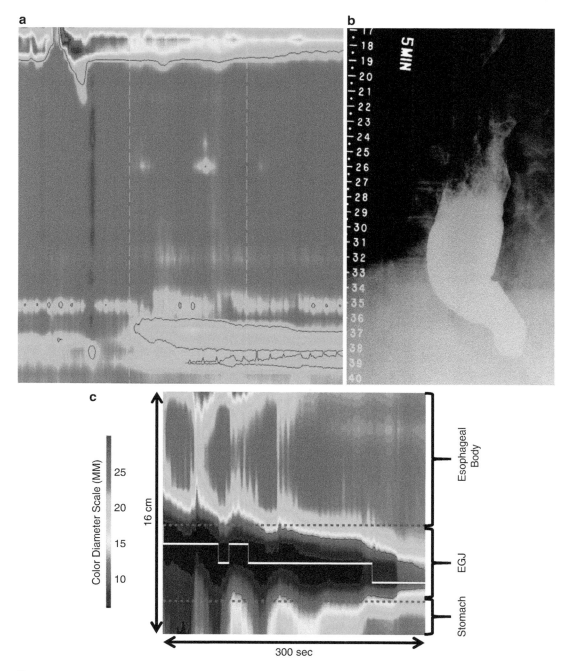

Fig. 17.6 Achalasia in the setting of a normal IRP. (**a**) HRM, (**b**) esophagram, (**c**) FLIP topography. (Courtesy of the Northwestern Esophageal Center)

is effective at treating all types of achalasia [64–66]. A prospective multicenter study of POEM demonstrated a 90% clinical success rate [67]. Two meta-analyses of more than 1000 patients each also demonstrated the short-term success of POEM in treating achalasia as measured by reduced ES and LES pressures [68, 69]. Furthermore, POEM appears to be a durable

Table 17.1 Indications for POEM

Indications
Achalasia (all subtypes)
Failed LHM
Failed PD
Failed POEM
Sigmoid anatomy/end stage
Pediatric population
EGJOO
DES
Jackhammer

treatment for achalasia with continued response rates >88% in studies assessing patient outcomes ranging from 2 to 5 years [44, 70, 71]. When comparing POEM to PD and LHM, POEM appears to be at least as effective in treating type I and II achalasia and is likely more effective due to the ability to extend the myotomy length in treating type III achalasia [40, 72–74]. FLIP analysis pre- and posttreatment with POEM compared to LHM shows similar increases in the EGJ-DI [60, 61]. Furthermore, POEM had operative times that were similar or up to 30 min faster, less blood loss, similar or less post-op pain, shorter length of hospital stay, and faster return to normal activity compared to LHM [41, 42, 75, 76].

Non-achalasia Motility Disorders

In the hierarchical scheme put forth in the CC, EGJOO, like achalasia, is defined as an elevated IRP; however, there is sufficient peristalsis in isolated EGJOO to exclude classic or spastic achalasia [10] (Fig. 17.7). Intuitively, POEM would seem an ideal treatment for this disease; however, EGJOO currently functions as a catchall diagnosis for a heterogeneous clinical entity making management decisions difficult. Within EGJOO, there is a subset of diseases which have been shown to benefit from POEM including incomplete achalasia or achalasia in evolution, but this represents only a small proportion of patients [52, 77]. A large proportion of patients with EGJOO (20–40%) improve without therapy, and the majority has etiologies which will not respond to LES targeted therapy (e.g., infiltrative disease or cancer, vascular obstruction, hiatal hernia, eosinophilic esophagitis, stricture, abdominal obesity, or prior foregut surgery) [23, 51, 53, 78, 79]. Although some patients with EGJOO may benefit from POEM, the heterogeneity of this diagnosis dictates further evaluation which may include impedance manometry, endoscopic ultrasound, computed tomography, timed barium esophagram, or FLIP. Figure 17.7a demonstrates representative images of HRM (left panel), FLIP (top right panel), and EUS (bottom right panel) for patients with EGJOO who would likely benefit from POEM. The HRM shows a normal distal latency with an elevated IRP to 19.9 mmHg. FLIP analysis of this patient demonstrated an EGJ-DI of 0.73 mm^2/mmHg which is less than the cut-off of 2.8 mm^2/mmHg and suggests that this patient would benefit from LES targeted therapy. The EUS shown here was also performed on a patient with EGJOO to rule alternative etiologies for the cause of the outlet obstruction. The EUS did not identify an alternative etiology for the outlet obstruction, but it did reveal a thickened muscularis propria to 8 mm suggesting this patient may benefit from POEM.

In 2013, an international survey of 16 expert centers performing POEM demonstrated that 22.5% of patients undergoing POEM at that time were treated for spastic esophageal disorders including DES (≥20% premature contractions, distal latency <4.5 s) and jackhammer esophagus (≥20% of swallows with a distal contractile integral >8000 mmHg/s/cm) [80] (Fig. 17.7b, c). A growing literature and a recent meta-analysis demonstrate the efficacy of this approach with 88% and 72% success in DES and jackhammer, respectively [80–84]. POEM is especially attractive in these diseases as it allows for customization of the myotomy length based on the area of high pressure on HRM, thickening on endoscopic ultrasound, or intraoperative FLIP. Figure 17.7b shows an HRM (left panel), FLIP (top right panel), and esophagram (bottom right panel) of a patient with a manometric diagnosis of DES. The HRM meets the criteria for DES with a normal IRP and a distal latency of less than 4.5 s. The FLIP and esophagram further support the deci-

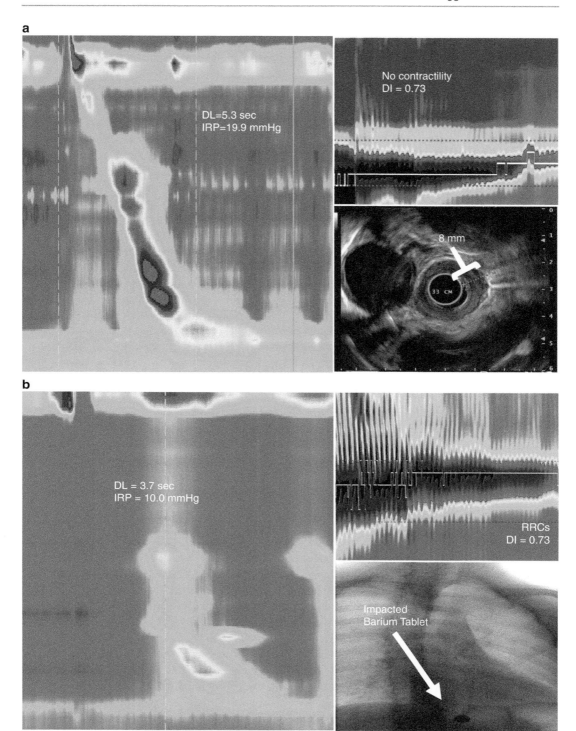

Fig. 17.7 Non-achalasia motility disorders for which POEM is indicated. (**a**) EGJOO on HRM, FLIP topography with low DI and absent contractility, and muscularis propria thickening on EUS. (**b**) DES on HRM, FLIP topography with repetitive retrograde contractions, and an impacted barium tablet on esophagram. (**c**) Jackhammer on HRM with poor bolus clearance and compartmentalization on both impedance manometry 200 ml challenge and an esophagram. (Courtesy of the Northwestern Esophageal Center)

c

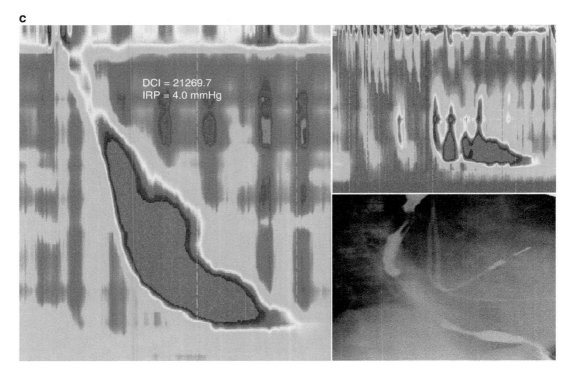

DCI = 21269.7
IRP = 4.0 mmHg

Fig. 17.7 (continued)

sion to proceed with myotomy given the low EGJ-DI on FLIP and impaction of a 12.5 mm barium tablet on the esophagram. Similarly, Fig. 17.7c demonstrates the HRM (left panel), impedance manometry (top right panel), and an esophagram (bottom right panel) for a patient with jackhammer. The DCI on HRM is significantly elevated to >20,000 mmHg∗s∗cm, and both the impedance manometry and the esophagram demonstrate spastic activity with compartmentalization and liquid retention. These findings suggest that this patient would benefit most from an extended myotomy to the top of the hypercontractile segment.

Special Populations

In the treatment of achalasia, special consideration is given to patients who have failed prior LES targeted therapy (PD, LHM, or POEM) or have abnormal anatomy (esophageal dilatation, sigmoid anatomy, diverticula, and hernias) due to the increased complexity of these individuals. Primary treatment with PD, LHM, and POEM shows near 90% clinical success rates; however, there is a subset of patients who will fail treatment or have recurrent symptoms [1]. In either case, whether it is primary treatment failure due to incomplete myotomy focused at the LES or a more proximal myotomy in type III patients or symptom recurrence due to disease progression or scarring and remodeling at the previous myotomy site, POEM appears to be an effective option for retreatment with clinical success rates ranging from 81% to 100% [4, 70, 85–92].

As a chronic disease, achalasia has the propensity to worsen over time resulting in esophageal dilatation which can often lead to the esophagus taking on a sigmoid shape. POEM has been shown to be >95% effective in both end-stage achalasia and in patients with sigmoid deformity; however, these studies are limited by small numbers of patients and short follow-up periods [4, 93–95]. It is our practice to discuss complex cases at an interdisciplinary meeting

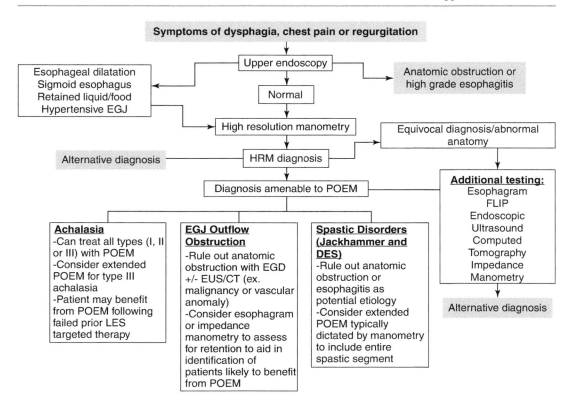

Fig. 17.8 POEM pre-procedural algorithm. (Courtesy of the Northwestern Esophageal Center)

with esophagologists and surgeons to determine the best treatment options for these patients with difficult anatomy.

Although the mean age of diagnosis of achalasia is 56, patients can present at any age. There does not appear to be specific age cutoffs for POEM in the treatment of achalasia with case studies demonstrating clinical success in patients ranging from 3 to >90 years old [70, 96–100].

Summary

POEM was first performed less than a decade ago, and its role in the treatment of esophageal motility disorders continues to evolve. There is evidence to support its use in patients with a diagnosis of achalasia (all clinical subtypes), DES and jackhammer esophagus, and a subset of patients with EGJOO. In current practice, these entities are diagnosed with EGD and HRM at a

minimum. In difficult cases, additional studies including impedance manometry, TBE, CT, EUS, or FLIP can be used to differentiate patients who may benefit from myotomy and those that will not (Fig. 17.8).

References

1. Pandolfino JE, Kahrilas PJ. Presentation, diagnosis, and management of achalasia. Clin Gastroenterol Hepatol. 2013;11(8):887–97.
2. Vaezi MF, Pandolfino JE, Vela MF. ACG clinical guideline: diagnosis and management of achalasia. Am J Gastroenterol. 2013;108(8):1238–49; quiz 50
3. Pasricha PJ, Hawari R, Ahmed I, Chen J, Cotton PB, Hawes RH, et al. Submucosal endoscopic esophageal myotomy: a novel experimental approach for the treatment of achalasia. Endoscopy. 2007;39(9):761–4.
4. Inoue H, Minami H, Kobayashi Y, Sato Y, Kaga M, Suzuki M, et al. Peroral endoscopic myotomy (POEM) for esophageal achalasia. Endoscopy. 2010;42(04):265–71.

5. Samo S, Carlson DA, Gregory DL, Gawel SH, Pandolfino JE, Kahrilas PJ. Incidence and prevalence of achalasia in Central Chicago, 2004–2014, since the widespread use of high-resolution manometry. Clin Gastroenterol Hepatol. 2017;15(3):366–73.

6. Duffield JA, Hamer PW, Heddle R, Holloway RH, Myers JC, Thompson SK. Incidence of achalasia in South Australia based on esophageal manometry findings. Clin Gastroenterol Hepatol. 2017;15(3):360–5.

7. Goldblum JR, Rice TW, Richter JE. Histopathologic features in esophagomyotomy specimens from patients with achalasia. Gastroenterology. 1996;111(3):648–54.

8. Sodikoff JB, Lo AA, Shetuni BB, Kahrilas PJ, Yang GY, Pandolfino JE. Histopathologic patterns among achalasia subtypes. Neurogastroenterol Motil. 2016;28(1):139–45.

9. Kahrilas PJ, Boeckxstaens G. The spectrum of achalasia: lessons from studies of pathophysiology and high-resolution manometry. Gastroenterology. 2013;145(5):954–65.

10. Kahrilas PJ, Bredenoord AJ, Fox M, Gyawali CP, Roman S, Smout AJPM, et al. The Chicago classification of esophageal motility disorders, v3.0. Neurogastroenterol Motil. 2015;27(2):160–74.

11. Bredenoord AJ, Fox M, Kahrilas PJ, Pandolfino JE, Schwizer W, Smout AJ. Chicago classification criteria of esophageal motility disorders defined in high resolution esophageal pressure topography. Neurogastroenterol Motil. 2012;24(Suppl 1):57–65.

12. Kahrilas PJ, Ghosh SK, Pandolfino JE. Esophageal motility disorders in terms of pressure topography: the Chicago classification. J Clin Gastroenterol. 2008;42(5):627–35.

13. Clouse RE, Staiano A. Topography of the esophageal peristaltic pressure wave. Am J Physiol. 1991;261(4 Pt 1):G677–84.

14. Clouse RE, Staiano A, Alrakawi A, Haroian L. Application of topographical methods to clinical esophageal manometry. Am J Gastroenterol. 2000;95(10):2720–30.

15. Gyawali CP. High resolution manometry: the Ray Clouse legacy. Neurogastroenterol Motil. 2012;24(Suppl 1):2–4.

16. Grubel C, Hiscock R, Hebbard G. Value of spatiotemporal representation of manometric data. Clin Gastroenterol Hepatol. 2008;6(5):525–30.

17. Soudagar AS, Sayuk GS, Gyawali CP. Learners favour high resolution oesophageal manometry with better diagnostic accuracy over conventional line tracings. Gut. 2012;61(6):798–803.

18. Roman S, Huot L, Zerbib F, Bruley des Varannes S, Gourcerol G, Coffin B, et al. High-resolution manometry improves the diagnosis of esophageal motility disorders in patients with dysphagia: a randomized multicenter study. Am J Gastroenterol. 2016;111(3):372–80.

19. Carlson DA, Kahrilas PJ. How to effectively use high-resolution esophageal manometry. Gastroenterology. 2016;151(5):789–92.

20. Yadlapati R, Keswani RN, Dunbar KB, Gawron AJ, Gyawali CP, Kahrilas PJ, et al. Benchmarks for the interpretation of esophageal high-resolution manometry. Neurogastroenterol Motil. 2017;29(4).

21. Yadlapati R, Keswani RN, Ciolino JD, Grande DP, Listernick ZI, Carlson DA, et al. A system to assess the competency for interpretation of esophageal manometry identifies variation in learning curves. Clin Gastroenterol Hepatol. 2017;15(11):1708–14.e3.

22. van Hoeij FB, Bredenoord AJ. Clinical application of esophageal high-resolution manometry in the diagnosis of esophageal motility disorders. J Neurogastroenterol Motil. 2016;22(1):6–13.

23. Schupack D, Katzka DA, Geno DM, Ravi K. The clinical significance of esophagogastric junction outflow obstruction and hypercontractile esophagus in high resolution esophageal manometry. Neurogastroenterol Motil. e13105-n/a.

24. Pandolfino JE, Ghosh SK, Zhang Q, Jarosz A, Shah N, Kahrilas PJ. Quantifying EGJ morphology and relaxation with high-resolution manometry: a study of 75 asymptomatic volunteers. Am J Physiol Gastrointest Liver Physiol. 2006;290(5):G1033–40.

25. Kahrilas PJ, Bredenoord AJ, Fox M, Gyawali CP, Roman S, Smout AJPM, et al. Expert consensus document: advances in the management of oesophageal motility disorders in the era of high-resolution manometry: a focus on achalasia syndromes. Nat Rev Gastroenterol Hepatol. 2017;advance online publication.

26. Lin Z, Kahrilas PJ, Roman S, Boris L, Carlson D, Pandolfino JE. Refining the criterion for an abnormal integrated relaxation pressure in esophageal pressure topography based on the pattern of esophageal contractility using a classification and regression tree model. Neurogastroenterol Motil. 2012;24(8):e356–63.

27. Pandolfino JE, Leslie E, Luger D, Mitchell B, Kwiatek MA, Kahrilas PJ. The contractile deceleration point: an important physiologic landmark on oesophageal pressure topography. Neurogastroenterol Motil. 2010;22(4):395–400, e90.

28. Nabi Z, Ramchandani M, Chavan R, Kalapala R, Darisetty S, Rao GV, et al. Per-oral endoscopic myotomy for achalasia cardia: outcomes in over 400 consecutive patients. Endosc Int Open. 2017;5(5):E331–e9.

29. Benedict JJ, Golas AA, Richter JE, Velanovich V. Health-related quality of life and physiological outcomes of peroral endoscopic myotomy for achalasia. J Laparoendosc Adv Surg Tech A. 2017;27(8):778–83.

30. Tang Y, Xie C, Wang M, Jiang L, Shi R, Lin L. Association of high-resolution manometry

metrics with the symptoms of achalasia and the symptomatic outcomes of peroral esophageal myotomy. PLoS One. 2015;10(9):e0139385.

31. Ju H, Ma Y, Liang K, Zhang C, Tian Z. Function of high-resolution manometry in the analysis of peroral endoscopic myotomy for achalasia. Surg Endosc. 2016;30(3):1094–9.

32. Khashab MA, Messallam AA, Onimaru M, Teitelbaum EN, Ujiki MB, Gitelis ME, et al. International multicenter experience with peroral endoscopic myotomy for the treatment of spastic esophageal disorders refractory to medical therapy (with video). Gastrointest Endosc. 2015;81(5):1170–7.

33. Leconte M, Douard R, Gaudric M, Dumontier I, Chaussade S, Dousset B. Functional results after extended myotomy for diffuse oesophageal spasm. Br J Surg. 2007;94(9):1113–8.

34. Balaban DH, Yamamoto Y, Liu J, Pehlivanov N, Wisniewski R, DeSilvey D, et al. Sustained esophageal contraction: a marker of esophageal chest pain identified by intraluminal ultrasonography. Gastroenterology. 1999;116(1):29–37.

35. Cho YK, Lipowska AM, Nicodeme F, Teitelbaum EN, Hungness ES, Johnston ER, et al. Assessing bolus retention in achalasia using high-resolution manometry with impedance: a comparator study with timed barium esophagram. Am J Gastroenterol. 2014;109(6):829–35.

36. Carlson DA, Lin Z, Kahrilas PJ, Sternbach J, Hungness ES, Soper NJ, et al. High-resolution impedance manometry metrics of the esophagogastric junction for the assessment of treatment response in achalasia. Am J Gastroenterol. 2016;111(12):1702–10.

37. Carlson DA, Omari T, Lin Z, Rommel N, Starkey K, Kahrilas PJ, et al. High-resolution impedance manometry parameters enhance the esophageal motility evaluation in non-obstructive dysphagia patients without a major Chicago Classification motility disorder. Neurogastroenterol Motil. 2017;29(3).

38. Lin Z, Imam H, Nicodeme F, Carlson DA, Lin CY, Yim B, et al. Flow time through esophagogastric junction derived during high-resolution impedance-manometry studies: a novel parameter for assessing esophageal bolus transit. Am J Physiol Gastrointest Liver Physiol. 2014;307(2):G158–63.

39. Lin Z, Carlson DA, Dykstra K, Sternbach J, Hungness E, Kahrilas PJ, et al. High-resolution impedance manometry measurement of bolus flow time in achalasia and its correlation with dysphagia. Neurogastroenterol Motil. 2015;27(9):1232–8.

40. Kumbhari V, Tieu AH, Onimaru M, El Zein MH, Teitelbaum EN, Ujiki MB, et al. Peroral endoscopic myotomy (POEM) vs laparoscopic Heller myotomy (LHM) for the treatment of type III achalasia in 75 patients: a multicenter comparative study. Endosc Int Open. 2015;3(3):E195–201.

41. Bhayani NH, Kurian AA, Dunst CM, Sharata AM, Rieder E, Swanstrom LL. A comparative study on comprehensive, objective outcomes of laparoscopic Heller myotomy with per-oral endoscopic myotomy (POEM) for achalasia. Ann Surg. 2014;259(6):1098–103.

42. Chan SM, Wu JC, Teoh AY, Yip HC, Ng EK, Lau JY, et al. Comparison of early outcomes and quality of life after laparoscopic Heller's cardiomyotomy to peroral endoscopic myotomy for treatment of achalasia. Dig Endosc. 2016;28(1):27–32.

43. de Oliveira JM, Birgisson S, Doinoff C, Einstein D, Herts B, Davros W, et al. Timed barium swallow: a simple technique for evaluating esophageal emptying in patients with achalasia. AJR Am J Roentgenol. 1997;169(2):473–9.

44. Teitelbaum EN, Dunst CM, Reavis KM, Sharata AM, Ward MA, DeMeester SR, et al. Clinical outcomes five years after POEM for treatment of primary esophageal motility disorders. Surg Endosc. 2018;32(1):421–7.

45. Vaezi MF, Baker ME, Achkar E, Richter JE. Timed barium oesophagram: better predictor of long term success after pneumatic dilation in achalasia than symptom assessment. Gut. 2002;50(6):765–70.

46. Nicodeme F, de Ruigh A, Xiao Y, Rajeswaran S, Teitelbaum EN, Hungness ES, et al. A comparison of symptom severity and bolus retention with Chicago classification esophageal pressure topography metrics in patients with achalasia. Clin Gastroenterol Hepatol. 2013;11(2):131–7; quiz e15

47. Agrusa A, Romano G, Frazzetta G, De Vita G, Chianetta D, Di Buono G, et al. Achalasia secondary to submucosal invasion by poorly differentiated adenocarcinoma of the cardia, Siewert II: consideration on preoperative workup. Case Rep Surg. 2014;2014:654917.

48. Choi MK, Kim GH, Song GA, Nam HS, Yi YS, Ahn KH, et al. Primary squamous cell carcinoma of the liver initially presenting with pseudoachalasia. Gut Liver. 2012;6(2):275–9.

49. Branchi F, Tenca A, Bareggi C, Mensi C, Mauro A, Conte D, et al. A case of pseudoachalasia hiding a malignant pleural mesothelioma. Tumori. 2016;102(Suppl 2).

50. Carter M, Deckmann RC, Smith RC, Burrell MI, Traube M. Differentiation of achalasia from pseudoachalasia by computed tomography. Am J Gastroenterol. 1997;92(4):624–8.

51. Clayton SB, Patel R, Richter JE. Functional and anatomic esophagogastric junction outflow obstruction: manometry, timed barium esophagram findings, and treatment outcomes. Clin Gastroenterol Hepatol. 2016;14(6):907–11.

52. Ihara E, Muta K, Fukaura K, Nakamura K. Diagnosis and treatment strategy of achalasia subtypes and esophagogastric junction outflow obstruction based on high-resolution manometry. Digestion. 2017;95(1):29–35.

53. Okeke FC, Raja S, Lynch KL, Dhalla S, Nandwani M, Stein EM, et al. What is the clinical significance of esophagogastric junction outflow obstruction? Evaluation of 60 patients at a tertiary referral center. Neurogastroenterol Motil. 2017;29(6):e13061-n/a.

54. Carlson DA, Kahrilas PJ, Lin Z, Hirano I, Gonsalves N, Listernick Z, et al. Evaluation of esophageal motility utilizing the functional lumen imaging probe. Am J Gastroenterol. 2016;111(12):1726–35.

55. Rohof WO, Hirsch DP, Kessing BF, Boeckxstaens GE. Efficacy of treatment for patients with achalasia depends on the distensibility of the esophagogastric junction. Gastroenterology. 2012;143(2):328–35.

56. Rieder E, Swanström LL, Perretta S, Lenglinger J, Riegler M, Dunst CM. Intraoperative assessment of esophagogastric junction distensibility during per oral endoscopic myotomy (POEM) for esophageal motility disorders. Surg Endosc. 2013;27(2):400–5.

57. Carlson DA, Lin Z, Kahrilas PJ, Sternbach J, Donnan EN, Friesen L, et al. The functional lumen imaging probe detects esophageal contractility not observed with manometry in patients with achalasia. Gastroenterology. 2015;149(7):1742–51.

58. Pandolfino JE, de Ruigh A, Nicodeme F, Xiao Y, Boris L, Kahrilas PJ. Distensibility of the esophagogastric junction assessed with the functional lumen imaging probe (FLIP) in achalasia patients. Neurogastroenterol Motil. 2013;25(6):496–501.

59. Ponds FA, Bredenoord AJ, Kessing BF, Smout AJ. Esophagogastric junction distensibility identifies achalasia subgroup with manometrically normal esophagogastric junction relaxation. Neurogastroenterol Motil. 2017;29(1).

60. Teitelbaum EN, Boris L, Arafat FO, Nicodeme F, Lin Z, Kahrilas PJ, et al. Comparison of esophagogastric junction distensibility changes during POEM and Heller myotomy using intraoperative FLIP. Surg Endosc. 2013;27(12):4547–55.

61. Teitelbaum EN, Soper NJ, Pandolfino JE, Kahrilas PJ, Boris L, Nicodème F, et al. An extended proximal esophageal myotomy is necessary to normalize EGJ distensibility during Heller myotomy for achalasia, but not POEM. Surg Endosc. 2014;28(10):2840–7.

62. Teitelbaum EN, Soper NJ, Pandolfino JE, Kahrilas PJ, Hirano I, Boris L, et al. Esophagogastric junction distensibility measurements during Heller myotomy and POEM for achalasia predict postoperative symptomatic outcomes. Surg Endosc. 2015;29(3):522–8.

63. Teitelbaum EN, Sternbach JM, El Khoury R, Soper NJ, Pandolfino JE, Kahrilas PJ, et al. The effect of incremental distal gastric myotomy lengths on EGJ distensibility during POEM for achalasia. Surg Endosc. 2016;30(2):745–50.

64. Kim WH, Cho JY, Ko WJ, Hong SP, Hahm KB, Cho JH, et al. Comparison of the outcomes of peroral endoscopic myotomy for achalasia according to manometric subtype. Gut Liver. 2017;11(5):642–7.

65. Pandolfino JE, Kwiatek MA, Nealis T, Bulsiewicz W, Post J, Kahrilas PJ. Achalasia: a new clinically relevant classification by high-resolution manometry. Gastroenterology. 2008;135(5):1526–33.

66. Rohof WO, Salvador R, Annese V, Bruley des Varannes S, Chaussade S, Costantini M, et al. Outcomes of treatment for achalasia depend on manometric subtype. Gastroenterology. 2013;144(4):718–25; quiz e13-4

67. Von Renteln D, Fuchs KH, Fockens P, Bauerfeind P, Vassiliou MC, Werner YB, et al. Peroral endoscopic myotomy for the treatment of achalasia: an international prospective multicenter study. Gastroenterology. 2013;145(2):309–11.e3.

68. Talukdar R, Inoue H, Reddy DN. Efficacy of peroral endoscopic myotomy (POEM) in the treatment of achalasia: a systematic review and meta-analysis. Surg Endosc. 2015;29(11):3030–46.

69. Patel K, Abbassi-Ghadi N, Markar S, Kumar S, Jethwa P, Zaninotto G. Peroral endoscopic myotomy for the treatment of esophageal achalasia: systematic review and pooled analysis. Dis Esophagus. 2016;29(7):807–19.

70. Inoue H, Sato H, Ikeda H, Onimaru M, Sato C, Minami H, et al. Per-oral endoscopic myotomy: a series of 500 patients. J Am Coll Surg. 2015;221(2):256–64.

71. Ngamruengphong S, Inoue H, Chiu PW-Y, Yip HC, Bapaye A, Ujiki M, et al. Long-term outcomes of per-oral endoscopic myotomy in patients with achalasia with a minimum follow-up of 2 years: an international multicenter study. Gastrointest Endosc. 2017;85(5):927–33.e2.

72. Meng F, Li P, Wang Y, Ji M, Wu Y, Yu L, et al. Peroral endoscopic myotomy compared with pneumatic dilation for newly diagnosed achalasia. Surg Endosc. 2017;31(11):4665–72.

73. Leeds SG, Burdick JS, Ogola GO, Ontiveros E. Comparison of outcomes of laparoscopic Heller myotomy versus per-oral endoscopic myotomy for management of achalasia. Proc (Bayl Univ Med Cent). 2017;30(4):419–23.

74. Schneider AM, Louie BE, Warren HF, Farivar AS, Schembre DB, Aye RW. A matched comparison of per oral endoscopic myotomy to laparoscopic Heller myotomy in the treatment of achalasia. J Gastrointest Surg. 2016;20(11):1789–96.

75. Hungness ES, Teitelbaum EN, Santos BF, Arafat FO, Pandolfino JE, Kahrilas PJ, et al. Comparison of perioperative outcomes between peroral esophageal myotomy (POEM) and laparoscopic Heller myotomy. J Gastrointest Surg. 2013;17(2):228–35.

76. Ujiki MB, Yetasook AK, Zapf M, Linn JG, Carbray JM, Denham W. Peroral endoscopic myotomy: a short-term comparison with the standard laparoscopic approach. Surgery. 2013;154(4):893–7; discussion 7-900

77. Kahrilas PJ, Katzka D, Richter JE. Clinical practice update: the use of per-oral endoscopic myotomy in achalasia: expert review and best practice advice from the American Gastroenterological Association. Gastroenterology. 2017;153(5):1205–11.

78. Scherer JR, Kwiatek MA, Soper NJ, Pandolfino JE, Kahrilas PJ. Functional esophagogastric junction obstruction with intact peristalsis: a heterogeneous syndrome sometimes akin to achalasia. J Gastrointest Surg. 2009;13(12):2219–25.

79. van Hoeij FB, Smout AJPM, Bredenoord AJ. Characterization of idiopathic esophagogastric junction outflow obstruction. Neurogastroenterol Motil. 2015;27(9):1310–6.

80. Stavropoulos SN, Modayil RJ, Friedel D, Savides T. The international per oral endoscopic myotomy survey (IPOEMS): a snapshot of the global POEM experience. Surg Endosc. 2013;27(9):3322–38.

81. Swanstrom LL, Rieder E, Dunst CM. A stepwise approach and early clinical experience in peroral endoscopic myotomy for the treatment of achalasia and esophageal motility disorders. J Am Coll Surg. 2011;213(6):751–6.

82. Shiwaku H, Inoue H, Beppu R, Nakashima R, Minami H, Shiroshita T, et al. Successful treatment of diffuse esophageal spasm by peroral endoscopic myotomy. Gastrointest Endosc. 2013;77(1):149–50.

83. Louis H, Covas A, Coppens E, Deviere J. Distal esophageal spasm treated by peroral endoscopic myotomy. Am J Gastroenterol. 2012;107(12):1926–7.

84. Khashab MA, Saxena P, Kumbhari V, Nandwani M, Roland BC, Stein E, et al. Peroral endoscopic myotomy as a platform for the treatment of spastic esophageal disorders refractory to medical therapy (with video). Gastrointest Endosc. 2014;79(1):136–9.

85. Zhang X, Modayil RJ, Friedel D, Gurram KC, Brathwaite CE, Taylor SI, et al. Per-oral endoscopic myotomy in patients with or without prior Heller myotomy: comparing long-term outcomes in a large U.S. single-center cohort (with videos). Gastrointest Endosc. 2018;87(4):972–85.

86. Ngamruengphong S, Inoue H, Ujiki MB, Patel LY, Bapaye A, Desai PN, et al. Efficacy and safety of peroral endoscopic myotomy for treatment of achalasia after failed heller myotomy. Clin Gastroenterol Hepatol. 2017;15(10):1531–7.e3.

87. Zhou PH, Li QL, Yao LQ, Xu MD, Chen WF, Cai MY, et al. Peroral endoscopic remyotomy for failed Heller myotomy: a prospective single-center study. Endoscopy. 2013;45(03):161–6.

88. Vigneswaran Y, Yetasook AK, Zhao J-C, Denham W, Linn JG, Ujiki MB. Peroral endoscopic myotomy (POEM): feasible as reoperation following heller myotomy. J Gastrointest Surg. 2014;18(6):1071–6.

89. Fumagalli U, Rosati R, De Pascale S, Porta M, Carlani E, Pestalozza A, et al. Repeated surgical or endoscopic myotomy for recurrent dysphagia in patients after previous myotomy for achalasia. J Gastrointest Surg. 2016;20(3):494–9.

90. Ling T, Guo H, Zou X. Effect of peroral endoscopic myotomy in achalasia patients with failure of prior pneumatic dilation: a prospective case-control study. J Gastroenterol Hepatol. 2014;29(8):1609–13.

91. Li QL, Yao LQ, Xu XY, Zhu JY, Xu MD, Zhang YQ, et al. Repeat peroral endoscopic myotomy: a salvage option for persistent/recurrent symptoms. Endoscopy. 2016;48(2):134–40.

92. Tyberg A, Seewald S, Sharaiha RZ, Martinez G, Desai AP, Kumta NA, et al. A multicenter international registry of redo per-oral endoscopic myotomy (POEM) after failed POEM. Gastrointest Endosc. 2017;85(6):1208–11.

93. Duan T, Tan Y, Zhou J, Lv L, Liu D. A retrospective study of peroral endoscopic full-thickness myotomy in patients with severe achalasia. J Laparoendosc Adv Surg Tech A. 2017;27(8):770–6.

94. Hu J-W, Li Q-L, Zhou P-H, Yao L-Q, Xu M-D, Zhang Y-Q, et al. Peroral endoscopic myotomy for advanced achalasia with sigmoid-shaped esophagus: long-term outcomes from a prospective, single-center study. Surg Endosc. 2015;29(9):2841–50.

95. Lv L, Liu J, Tan Y, Liu D. Peroral endoscopic full-thickness myotomy for the treatment of sigmoid-type achalasia: outcomes with a minimum follow-up of 12 months. Eur J Gastroenterol Hepatol. 2016;28(1):30–6.

96. Maselli R, Inoue H, Misawa M, Ikeda H, Hosoya T, Onimaru M, et al. Peroral endoscopic myotomy (POEM) in a 3-year-old girl with severe growth retardation, achalasia, and down syndrome. Endoscopy. 2012;44(Suppl 2 UCTN):E285–7.

97. Chen WF, Li QL, Zhou PH, Yao LQ, Xu MD, Zhang YQ, et al. Long-term outcomes of peroral endoscopic myotomy for achalasia in pediatric patients: a prospective, single-center study. Gastrointest Endosc. 2015;81(1):91–100.

98. Li C, Tan Y, Wang X, Liu D. Peroral endoscopic myotomy for treatment of achalasia in children and adolescents. J Pediatr Surg. 2015;50(1):201–5.

99. Tang X, Gong W, Deng Z, Zhou J, Ren Y, Zhang Q, et al. Usefulness of peroral endoscopic myotomy for treating achalasia in children: experience from a single center. Pediatr Surg Int. 2015;31(7):633–8.

100. Chen Y-I, Inoue H, Ujiki M, Draganov PV, Colavita P, Mion F, et al. An international multicenter study evaluating the clinical efficacy and safety of per-oral endoscopic myotomy in octogenarians. Gastrointest Endosc. 2018;87(4):956–61.

Chetan Mittal and Mihir S. Wagh

Introduction

Peroral endoscopic myotomy (POEM) is a novel natural orifice flexible endoscopic procedure which involves a submucosal tunnel approach accessed through an esophageal mucosal incision, to perform endoscopic myotomy in the esophagus and cardia. The technique was initially developed in Japan by Inoue et al. [1] as a minimally invasive procedure for treatment of achalasia but has evolved significantly as potential primary therapy for many different conditions of the gastrointestinal (GI) tract.

Endoscopic Techniques for POEM

Pre-procedure Preparation

Risks and benefits of the different treatment options, including medical, endoscopic, and

Electronic Supplementary Material The online version of this chapter (https://doi.org/10.1007/978-3-030-21695-5_18) contains supplementary material, which is available to authorized users.

C. Mittal
Division of Gastroenterology, University of Colorado-Denver, Aurora, CO, USA

M. S. Wagh (✉)
Interventional Endoscopy, Division of Gastroenterology, University of Colorado-Denver, Aurora, CO, USA
e-mail: mihir.wagh@cuanschutz.edu

surgical therapies, should be discussed with patients and their families, ideally during a clinic visit before the procedure. A full liquid diet is recommended for 1–2 days before the procedure to allow adequate esophageal clearance for visualization during POEM and to minimize the risk of adverse events. General anesthesia with endotracheal intubation and muscle paralysis is required for POEM to safely perform the precise dissection required during the procedure. In some centers, POEM is performed in the operating room, while others use the GI endoscopy suite for POEM. There are no direct comparative studies in terms of differences in efficacy and safety outcomes between POEM performed by endoscopists in the endoscopy unit and the operating room. POEM can be safely performed in the endoscopy unit [2]; however, appropriate surgical and interventional radiology backup should be available in case of any adverse events.

Since POEM involves dissection into the submucosa and muscle layers of the esophagus and stomach, with a risk of mediastinitis and perforation, periprocedural antibiotics are generally given though there is no definite evidence to suggest for or otherwise. Usually a fluoroquinolone and metronidazole, third-generation cephalosporin, or semisynthetic penicillin with beta-lactamase inhibitor (ampicillin-sulbactam) is preferred as broad-spectrum coverage. We also continue antibiotic coverage for 7 days after POEM.

© Springer Nature Switzerland AG 2020
M. S. Wagh, S. B. Wani (eds.), *Gastrointestinal Interventional Endoscopy*,
https://doi.org/10.1007/978-3-030-21695-5_18

Setup for Endoscopy

Typically, the patient is placed in the supine position for POEM, but the procedure can also be performed with the patient in left lateral position. The main advantage of the supine position is easy identification of anterior and posterior orientations during endoscopy, based on pooling of fluids posteriorly in the esophagus due to gravity. Also, abdominal examination for distention and decompression with a percutaneous needle can be easily performed in the supine patient, if needed.

The use of carbon dioxide is an absolute must for insufflation during endoscopy, and the procedure should not be performed with air insufflation due to risk of major adverse events due to barotrauma. We use a low-flow carbon dioxide insufflator to further reduce the risk of hemodynamic and cardiorespiratory compromise from barotrauma resulting from the inevitable capno/pneumomediastinum and capno/pneumoperitoneum that is associated with submucosal endoscopy and myotomy.

Serial abdominal examination is performed at baseline and every 5–10 min during the procedure by the assisting nurse to assess for abdominal distention. Peak airway pressures are monitored during the procedure by the anesthesia team, and increased peak pressures associated with cardiorespiratory compromise and/or difficulty with ventilation may suggest capno/pneumoperitoneum requiring urgent decompression. In this situation, the stomach is first suctioned to reduce distention, and if hemodynamic instability persists, urgent percutaneous decompression is needed. We therefore recommend having a percutaneous abdominal decompression kit (containing a Veress needle or an angiocath) available in the endoscopy room, if urgent abdominal decompression is needed due to capno/pneumoperitoneum.

A diagnostic upper endoscopy is first performed to assess the esophagus, gastroesophageal junction (GEJ), and stomach. Any residual food and fluid is suctioned to clear the endoscopic field. This also allows inspection of the mucosa for the presence of esophagitis, ulcers, bleeding, and mass lesions, which may preclude POEM. The GEJ is carefully traversed to assess the resistance while crossing the lower esophageal sphincter (LES) and to minimize trauma to the mucosa at the GEJ. Normal esophageal and gastric anatomical landmarks should be appreciated such as pulsations from the left atrium (12–1 o'clock position) and the longitudinal ridgelike prominence of the spine (7–8 o'clock position) posteriorly in the esophagus, as shown in Fig. 18.1a, b.

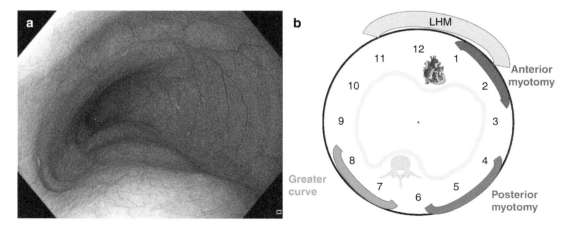

Fig. 18.1 (**a**) Prominence of the spine seen posteriorly in the esophagus. (**b**) Schematic representation of esophageal landmarks and myotomy location. LHM laparoscopic heller myotomy

Technique

POEM has evolved significantly since inception with varying technical approaches based on the indication and per endoscopist preference. To understand the concept of POEM, it is critical to understand the anatomy of the layers of gastrointestinal wall – mucosa, submucosa, muscularis propria (inner circular and outer longitudinal muscle layers), and adventitia/serosa. It is important to note that the esophagus lacks a serosal layer unlike other parts of the GI tract. The beauty of POEM lies in the expansion of the microscopic submucosa to a space large enough to pass a >1 cm diameter upper endoscope with a distal attachment/cap, to perform myotomy under the protective net of the mucosal flap [3]. The technique for esophageal POEM is discussed here (Fig. 18.2a–e and Video 18.1), though the concept remains the same for other sites in the GI tract (the pylorus and rectum described elsewhere in this book).

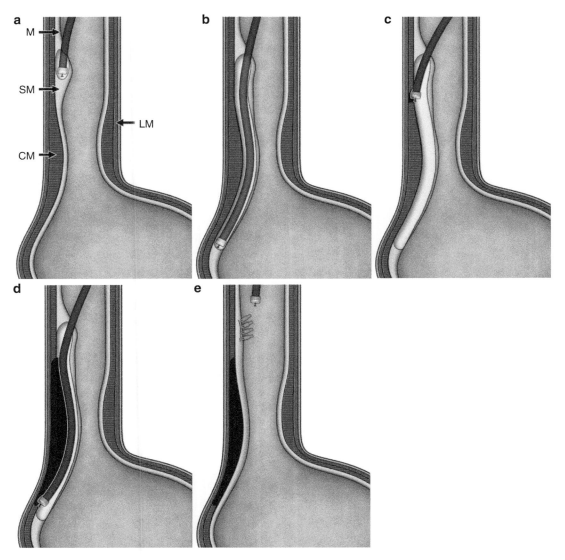

Fig. 18.2 (**a**) Mucosotomy and endoscope entry into the submucosal space. M mucosa, SM submucosa, CM circular muscle, LM longitudinal muscle. (**b**) Submucosal tunnel extended beyond the GE junction and into the cardia. (**c**) Start of myotomy distal to the site of mucosal entry. (**d**) Myotomy extended to the cardia. (**e**) Mucosotomy closure [3]

Mucosal Incision

A distal attachment cap is fitted onto the tip of the endoscope, which helps to improve endoscopic visualization and accuracy of dissection during the procedure, in addition to facilitating entry into the submucosal space. A mucosal site for entry into the submucosal space is first chosen about 10–12 cm from the GEJ or based on the desired length of myotomy, which can vary depending on the indication (e.g., longer myotomy performed for type III achalasia). Any visible mucosal vessels or esophageal tortuosity is avoided when choosing the site for mucosal incision which may make submucosal entry challenging.

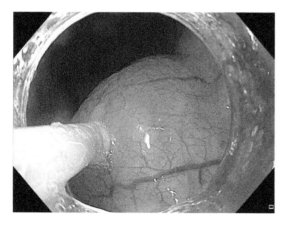

Fig. 18.3 Submucosal injection

An injection needle is used to inject saline-methylene blue mixture (or saline-indigo carmine) at the site of the desired mucosal entry to create a submucosal lift (Fig. 18.3). Some endoscopists also add epinephrine (0.5–1 mg/100 ml of fluid) in the injection solution. After injection, an endoscopic knife is used with blended current (Endocut, ERBE USA, Marietta, GA) to make a 10–20 mm longitudinal mucosal incision. A transverse incision is used by some endoscopists as well, but less commonly since a longitudinal incision is easier to close at the end of the procedure. The mucosal incision is performed in the 1–2 o'clock position for an anterior myotomy or in the 4–5 o'clock position for a posterior myotomy (Fig. 18.4a, b).

We typically use Endocut Q: effect 3, duration 1 and interval 1 for the mucosotomy, but other variations such as Endocut Q: effect 2, duration 1 and interval 6, or effect 3, duration 2 and interval 4, or other settings can be used as well. The procedure can be performed with any endoscopic knife, based on endoscopist preference, usually a triangle tip knife (Olympus America, Center Valley, PA) or a hybrid knife (ERBE USA, Marietta, GA). Tang et al. showed shorter procedure time and less frequent device exchange with hybrid knife as compared to triangular tip knife, despite similar rates of procedure success and adverse events [4].

After mucosal incision, the exposed submucosa is dissected to create space for advance-

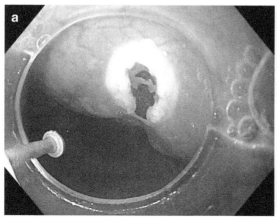

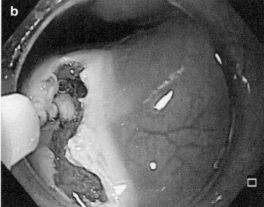

Fig. 18.4 (**a**) Incision for anterior myotomy. (**b**) Incision for posterior myotomy

ment of the endoscope. Special attention needs to be paid to identify the esophageal wall layers at this site and to not accidentally cut the underlying muscle layer since this would result in a full-thickness esophageal perforation at the site of mucosotomy. The endoscope is then carefully inserted into the submucosal space via the mucosotomy.

Submucosal Tunneling

Once the endoscope with the distal cap is in the submucosal space, the region is diligently inspected to confirm orientation of the esophageal wall layers. The loose submucosal tissue (stained blue after injection) has a characteristic blue "cotton candy" appearance (Fig. 18.5), with the mucosa on one side and the white muscle fibers on the other side. A submucosal tunnel is created with frequent injection of saline-methylene blue (or indigo carmine) solution and careful dissection of submucosal tissue using spray coagulation (effect 2, 50 W) or Endocut Q (effect 3, duration 1 and interval 1; or effect 3, duration 2 and interval 4) or forced coagulation (effect 2, 50 W) (ERBE USA, Marietta, GA). During tunneling, submucosal dissection should be performed with the knife closer to the muscle layer rather than toward the mucosal layer to avoid inadvertent mucosal perforation. The submucosal tunnel should extend at least 2–3 cm

into the cardia beyond the GEJ. Extension of the tunnel into the cardia is confirmed by typical landmarks (distance from the incisors, submucosal space narrowing at the level of the lower esophageal sphincter and widening once the stomach is entered, and larger penetrating vessels and spindle veins seen in the stomach) as shown in Fig. 18.6a, b. This is also confirmed by retroflexed examination from the luminal side showing a submucosal blue bleb at the cardia bulging in the stomach (Fig. 18.7). Another strategy for confirming the location of the GEJ during tunneling is to pass a tandem ultrathin endoscope in the esophageal and gastric true lumen and visualizing transillumination from the endoscope in the

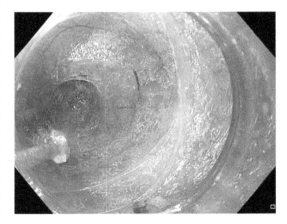

Fig. 18.5 Submucosal tunnel showing the submucosa stained blue

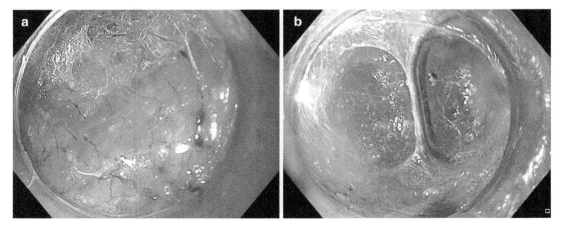

Fig. 18.6 Submucosal tunnel extending to the cardia showing (**a**) spindle veins and (**b**) penetrating vessels

submucosal tunnel [5]. Kumbhari et al. recently described fluoroscopic visualization of an endoscopically placed GEJ clip or fluoroscopy-guided placement of a 19G needle on the skin as marker for GEJ. The authors reported extension of the tunnel by a mean of 1.4 cm in about 20% cases while adding 2–4 min to total procedure time [6].

Intervening submucosal vessels are coagulated with spray or forced coagulation with the dissection knife or with a Coagrasper (Olympus America, Center Valley, PA) with soft coagulation (effect 5, 50 or 80 W, ERBE USA, Marietta, GA).

Gentamicin lavage of the submucosal tunnel can be performed before beginning the myotomy but is not mandatory. Bayer et al. showed no major infectious complications post-procedure

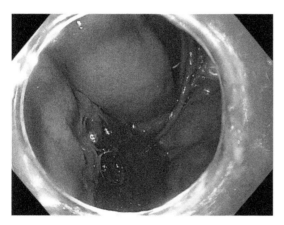

Fig. 18.7 Retroflexed view of gastroesophageal junction showing bluish bleb extending into the cardia

with or without gentamicin lavage, though leukocyte count and CRP levels were lower in the lavage group suggesting a possible reduction in systemic inflammatory response [7].

Myotomy

Tunneling is followed by endoscopic myotomy. Myotomy is started about 2 cm distal to mucosal entry site to avoid esophageal perforation or leak at the mucosotomy site. Just as for submucosal tunneling, the choice of electrosurgical settings during myotomy are variable as well, mainly dependent on endoscopist preference. Spray coagulation (effect 2, 50 W) or Endocut Q (effect 3, duration 1 and interval 1; or effect 3, duration 2 and interval 4; or effect 2, duration 1 and interval 6) or forced coagulation (effect 2, 50 W) (ERBE USA, Marietta, GA) can be used, but these are often modified based on the endoscopist, indication and location for myotomy, and the presence of scarring from prior interventions. The location, type, and direction of myotomy is evolving and being studied extensively.

Anterior Versus Posterior Myotomy
Anterior myotomy (2 o' clock position, lesser curve side of the stomach) was the original location described in early Japanese literature as an extrapolation of the ventral approach during laparoscopic Heller myotomy (LHM) (Fig. 18.8a and Video 18.2) [1]. A posterior myotomy, on the

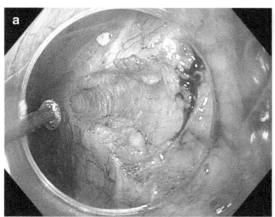
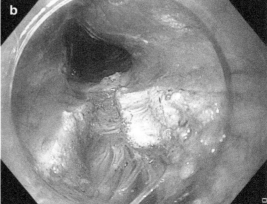

Fig. 18.8 (**a**) Anterior myotomy. (**b**) Posterior myotomy

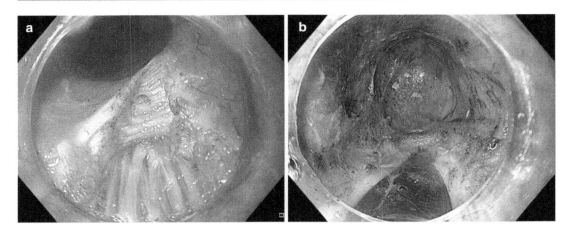

Fig. 18.9 (**a**) Partial-thickness myotomy. The yellowish cut ends of the circular muscle are seen on the sides, and the intact longitudinal muscle layer is seen deep to the circular muscles. (**b**) Full-thickness myotomy

other hand, is performed at the 4–5 o'clock position (Fig. 18.8b and Video 18.1).

Partial-Thickness, Full-Thickness, and Progressive Myotomy

Partial-thickness myotomy involves selective incision of the circular muscles only, preserving the longitudinal muscle layer (Fig. 18.9a and Video 18.1), while a full-thickness myotomy is an incision of both the circular and longitudinal layers (Fig. 18.9b and Video 18.3). A progressive myotomy is a partial-thickness myotomy proximally in the esophagus which then blends into a full-thickness myotomy distally in the esophagus and at the level of the GEJ and cardia. A progressive myotomy toward the GEJ has been shown to reduce procedure time with similar efficacy and adverse events [8].

Antegrade Versus Retrograde Myotomy

An antegrade myotomy is performed in the proximal to distal direction. Another variation includes a retrograde myotomy starting at the GEJ and extending proximally. Ponsky et al. described this technique in five patients with similar technical and clinical success as antegrade myotomy, without significant adverse events [9]. One potential advantage of retrograde myotomy is that the most critical portion of myotomy (myotomy at the level of the LES and cardia) is performed first, in case the procedure has to be aborted due to hemodynamic changes

or adverse events such as uncontrolled bleeding during the procedure. However, there is no data to suggest that isolated myotomy at GEJ is adequate to relieve symptoms.

One of the more common approaches nowadays is an antegrade, progressive posterior myotomy, starting 2 cm distal to the mucosal entry site and extending 2–3 in to gastric cardia. This technique may be easier and may reduce risk of serious adverse events such as intra-procedural bleeding. However, posterior myotomy may be associated with a higher rate of post-procedure acid reflux by disrupting the angle of His. Ominaru et al. reported data on POEM in 21 patients, performed posteriorly due to either prior surgery or other anatomical constraints preventing an anterior myotomy. The study showed a high rate of reflux esophagitis on endoscopy performed post-procedure (52% cases), though <10% patients were symptomatic and easily controlled with proton pump inhibitor (PPI) therapy [10]. Currently, there are multiple prospective comparative studies being performed (clinicaltrials.gov) assessing types of myotomy. Optical coherence tomography (OCT) can be also used to assess the submucosal vascularity and thickness of circular muscle layer, which can determine the location of myotomy. Desai et al. used OCT as a guide in 51 patients who underwent anterior (47%) or posterior (53%) POEM and showed a reduction in procedural bleeding (8% vs 43%) and therefore total procedure time (85.8 min vs 121.7 min) [11].

Use of EndoFLIP during POEM

Endoscopic functional luminal imaging probe (EndoFLIP) is a novel technology that uses impedance planimetry to evaluate esophagogastric junction distensibility and cross-sectional area at GEJ. Familiari et al. showed that GEJ diameter and cross-sectional area as measured by endoFLIP improved significantly after POEM in 23 cases, though there was no correlation between symptom improvement or GERD incidence and GEJ diameter [12]. Another study showed that intraoperative GEJ cross-sectional area correlated with response to POEM and reflux esophagitis after POEM [13]. Therefore, endoFLIP may be an important tool to guide the location and extent of myotomy in POEM.

The myotomy is extended 2–3 cm into the cardia beyond the GEJ during POEM. Grimes et al. described a double endoscope technique (one endoscope in the submucosal tunnel and a second slim endoscope in the esophageal and gastric true lumen) to confirm extension of myotomy into the gastric cardia using transillumination from the first endoscope in the tunnel as a landmark, in a prospective randomized controlled trial ($n = 100$ total). Using a second endoscope added 17 min to procedure time but resulted in significant myotomy extension in 34% cases by an average of 0.6 cm [14].

The extent of gastric myotomy has been an area of debate, as LHM typically extends gastric myotomy to about 3 cm. However, the length of gastric myotomy can be adjusted in POEM, to potentially reduce the chances of postoperative reflux. Ramirez et al. compared outcomes in 35 prospectively enrolled POEM cases and 35 historical LHMs. LHM patients had >3 cm gastric myotomy as compared to <2 cm in POEM. The rates of postoperative reflux were similar in POEM and LHM patients, defined by symptoms (20% vs 17.1%), esophagitis seen on endoscopy (4.7% vs 4.5%), or PPI requirement (22.8% vs 20%) [15].

After completion of the myotomy, the submucosal tunnel is carefully inspected for exposed or bleeding vessels, which are diligently coagulated.

Mucosotomy Closure

The mucosal entry site is closed using multiple hemostatic clips or with endoscopic sutures. During clip closure, the first clip is placed at the distal end of the incision, and then subsequent clips are deployed proximally (Fig. 18.10). Pescarus et al. compared endoscopic suturing versus clip closure in a case-control study design and showed that both techniques were similar in clinical efficacy at preventing post-procedure leaks, but closure time was significantly shorter with endoscopic clips (16 min) as compared to suturing (33 min). Procedure cost was slightly higher with endoscopic suturing but can be used if endoscopic clips fail to approximate the defect [16].

POEM Techniques in Special Situations

(a) *Type 3 achalasia and spastic esophageal disorders* (such as diffuse esophageal spasm [DES] and jackhammer esophagus).

POEM has the advantage that a longer proximal myotomy can be performed, tailored to esophagram and manometric findings, and recent studies have shown high rates of clinical success in type III achalasia [17]. Type III achalasia is traditionally considered most dif-

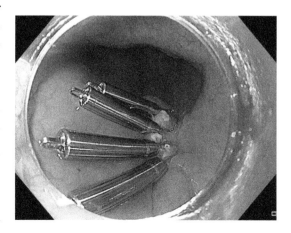

Fig. 18.10 Mucosotomy closure with endoscopic clips

ficult to treat with lower response rates to LHM and PD [18]. However, POEM may be the answer for type III achalasia since a longer myotomy can be performed and the myotomy can be adjusted and even guided by FLIP intra-operatively. Khan et al. performed a recent meta-analysis showing 92.5% clinical success rate in type III achalasia with an average myotomy length of 17.2 cm. The study also showed good clinical outcomes in diffuse esophageal spasm (88%) and jackhammer esophagus (72%) [19].

Kumbhari et al. reported significantly higher clinical response rate of POEM compared to LHM (98% vs 80.8%) and longer myotomy length (16 cm vs 8 cm) in 75 patients with type III achalasia, despite shorter mean procedure time (102 min vs 264 min) [20].

(b) *Advanced   achalasia   with   sigmoid esophagus.*

POEM can be challenging in patients with advanced achalasia and sigmoid esophagus due to difficulty in maintaining orientation during submucosal tunneling and myotomy and due to submucosal fibrosis that limits expansion of the submucosal space. Hence, careful attention must be paid during tunneling to dissect close to the muscle layer, keeping the direction of tunneling perpendicular to the circular muscle. The endoscope can also be intermittently withdrawn and inserted into the true esophageal lumen assessing the progress of the tunnel in the desired orientation. Repeated injections of fluid into the submucosa also help delineate tissue planes separating mucosa from the muscle.

(c) *POEM after prior interventions.*

Multiple prior interventions for achalasia such as botulinum toxin injections, pneumatic dilation, as well as prior surgical (Heller myotomy with fundoplication) or endoscopic (previous failed POEM) myotomy pose a special technical challenge for POEM. These interventions may result in submucosal fibrosis and increased submucosal neovascularization, reduced distensibility of the submucosal space, and also may make identification of tissue planes difficult. Diligent submucosal dissection along the muscle layer along with repeated injections, coagulation of intervening vessels, and carefully maintaining spatial orientation in the tunnel is crucial as described above for patients with sigmoid achalasia. POEM can be performed safely and effectively regardless of these prior interventions as shown in a few retrospective studies. Tang et al. showed similar operative time, improvement in Eckardt score, and manometric outcomes at 1-year follow-up in patients with and without prior endoscopic interventions. The incidence of intraoperative complications and gastroesophageal reflux rates was also similar [21]. Tyberg et al. showed that POEM can be successfully repeated after a failed POEM ($n = 46$) with excellent technical (100%) and clinical success (85%), with an acceptable rate of adverse events, primarily intra-procedural bleeding, which can be managed endoscopically [22]. POEM has been performed after failed LHM in small retrospective series with good outcomes overall and may be preferred over repeating LHM in a previous operative field. Kristensen et al. showed significant improvement in post-POEM Eckardt score in 14 patients with prior LHM, though rates of improvement were lower than patients without prior LHM at 3,12, and 24 months [23].

Louie et al. performed a prospective study comparing three groups of patients undergoing POEM – (1) no intervention ($n = 19$), (2) prior intervention (submucosal injection or dilation) ($n = 11$), and (3) sigmoid esophagus, prior esophageal surgery, and/or balloon dilation >30 mm ($n = 8$). The authors found no difference in clinical improvement between the groups though operative time was significantly longer in the highest complexity group [24]. Another study by van Hoeij et al. showed modest clinical success (63% for POEM, 45%

for LHM, and <20% for PD) with repeat intervention for recurrent symptoms after failed POEM [25].

Conclusion

The technique for POEM is evolving based on patient characteristics, expanding indications, operator experience and preference, and advances in available tools and accessories. POEM in patients with advanced achalasia and complex anatomy is technically challenging, and understanding the anatomy of esophagogastric wall layers is critical. POEM has been a game changer in the practice of gastrointestinal endoscopy, and this technique promises further novel treatments using the submucosal space.

References

1. Inoue H, Minami H, Kobayashi Y, et al. Peroral endoscopic myotomy (POEM) for esophageal achalasia. Endoscopy. 2010;42(4):265–71.
2. Yang D, Pannu D, Zhang Q, White JD, Draganov PV. Evaluation of anesthesia management, feasibility and efficacy of peroral endoscopic myotomy (POEM) for achalasia performed in the endoscopy unit. Endosc Int Open. 2015;3(4):E289–95.
3. Mittal C, Wagh M. Technical advances in per-oral endoscopic myotomy (POEM). Am J Gastroenterol. 2017;112(11):1627–31.
4. Tang X, Gong W, Deng Z, Zhou J, Ren Y, Zhang Q, Chen Z, Jiang B. Comparison of conventional versus hybrid knife peroral endoscopic myotomy methods for esophageal achalasia: a case-control study. Scand J Gastroenterol. 2016;51(4):494–500.
5. Grimes K, Inoue H, Onimaru M, et al. Double-scope per oral endoscopic myotomy (POEM): a prospective randomized controlled trial. Surg Endosc. 2016;30(4):1344–51.
6. Kumbhari V, Besharati S, Abdelgelil A, et al. Intraprocedural fluoroscopy to determine extent of cardiomyotomy during POEM. Gastrointest Endosc. 2015;81(6):1451–6.
7. Bayer J, Vackova Z, Svecova H, et al. Gentamicin sub-mucosal lavage during per-oral endoscopic myotomy (POEM): a retrospective analysis. Surg Endosc. 2018;32(1):300–6.
8. Li C, Gong A, Zhang J, et al. Clinical outcomes and safety of partial full-thickness myotomy versus circular muscle myotomy in peroral endoscopic myotomy for achalasia patients. Gastroenterol Res Pract. 2017:2676513.
9. Ponsky J, Marks J, Orenstein S. Retrograde myotomy: a variation in per-oral endoscopic myotomy technique. Surg Endosc. 2014;28:3257–9.
10. Ominaru M, Inoue H, Ikeda H, et al. Greater curve myotomy is a safe and effective modified technique for per-oral endoscopic myotomy. Gastrointest Endosc. 2015;81(6):1370–7.
11. Desai A, Tyberg A, Kedia P, et al. Optical coherence tomography prior to POEM reduces procedure time and bleeding: a multicenter international collaborative study. Surg Endosc. 2016;30:5126–33.
12. Familiari P, Gigante G, Marchese M, Boskoski I, Bove V, Tringali A, Perri V, Onder G, Costamagna G. EndoFLIP system for the intraoperative evaluation of peroral endoscopic myotomy. United European Gastroenterol J. 2014;2(2):77–83.
13. Ngamruengphong S, von Rahden BH, Filser J, Tyberg A, Desai A, Sharaiha RZ, Lambroza A, Kumbhari V, El Zein M, Abdelgelil A, Besharati S, Clarke JO, Stein EM, Kalloo AN, Kahaleh M, Khashab MA. Intraoperative measurement of esophagogastric junction cross-sectional area by impedance planimetry correlates with clinical outcomes of peroral endoscopic myotomy for achalasia: a multicenter study. Surg Endosc. 2016;30(7):2886–94.
14. Grimes K, Inoue H, Onimaru M, et al. Double scope POEM: a prospective randomized controlled trial. Surg Endosc. 2016;30:1344–51.
15. Ramirez M, Zubieta C, Ciotola F, et al. Per oral endoscopic myotomy vs. laparoscopic Heller myotomy, does gastric extension length matter? Surg Endosc. 2018;32(1):282–8.
16. Pescarus R, Shlomovitz E, Sharata A, et al. Endoscopic suturing versus endoscopic clip closure of the mucosotomy during a per-oral endoscopic myotomy (POEM): a case–control study. Surg Endosc. 2016;30:2132–5.
17. Zhang W, Linghu EQ. Peroral endoscopic myotomy for type III achalasia of Chicago classification: outcomes with a minimum follow-up of 24 months. J Gastrointest Surg. 2017;21:785–91.
18. Rohof WO, Salvador R, Annese V, et al. Outcomes of treatment for achalasia depend on manometric subtype. Gastroenterology. 2013;144:718–25.
19. Khan MA, Kumbhari V, Ngamruengphong S, et al. Is POEM the answer for management of spastic esophageal disorders? A systematic review and meta-analysis. Dig Dis Sci. 2017;62(1):35–44.
20. Kumbhari V, Tieu AH, Onimaru M, et al. Peroral endoscopic myotomy (POEM) vs laparoscopic Heller

myotomy (LHM) for the treatment of type III achalasia in 75 patients: a multicenter comparative study.
Endosc Int Open. 2015;3:E195–201.

21. Tang X, Gong W, Deng Z, et al. Feasibility and safety
of peroral endoscopic myotomy for achalasia after
failed endoscopic interventions. Dis Esophagus.
2017;30(3):1–6.

22. Tyberg A, Seewald S, Sharaiha RZ, et al. A multicenter
international registry of redo per-oral endoscopic
myotomy (POEM) after failed POEM. Gastrointest
Endosc. 2016;83:AB175.

23. Kristensen HO, Kirkegard J, Kjaer DW, et al. Long-
term outcome of peroral endoscopic myotomy for
esophageal achalasia in patients with previous Heller
myotomy. Surg Endosc. 2017;31(6):2596–601.

24. Louie B, Schneider A, Schembre D, et al. Impact of
prior interventions on outcomes during peroral endoscopic myotomy. Surg Endosc. 2017;31(4):1841–8.

25. Van Hoeij F, Ponds F, Werner Y, et al. Management
of recurrent symptoms after per-oral endoscopic
myotomy in achalasia. Gastrointest Endosc.
2018;87(1):95–101.

Juergen Hochberger and Volker Meves

Introduction

Peroral endoscopic myotomy (POEM) is the endoscopic approach of surgical myotomy for patients with spastic esophageal disorders [1]. It uses the concept of natural orifice transluminal endoscopic surgery (NOTES) introduced by the Apollo Group in 2004 [2–4]. Inoue et al. were the first ones to perform POEM in human after initial experimental steps by Pasricha et al. in 2007 [5, 6]. A submucosal esophago-cardial tunnel is created as an operating space, and an endoscopic myotomy is carried out by means of a microknife and the tunnel subsequently closed by clips. Due to its minimally invasive character, it appears to be effective and safe even in old or multimorbid patients, regardless of prior therapy undertaken [7–10]. POEM and balloon dilation have replaced other endoscopic treatment modalities such as intersphincteric botulinum toxin A injection [11, 12]. Multiple studies during the last 5 years have proven the clinical value of POEM [13]. However, the POEM procedure can be a

J. Hochberger (✉)
Gastroenterology, GI Oncology, Interventional Endoscopy, Vivantes Klinikum im Friedrichshain, Berlin, Germany
e-mail: juergen.hochberger@vivantes.de

V. Meves
Gastroenterology, Klinikum Oldenburg AöR, Oldenburg, Germany
e-mail: meves.volker@klinikum-oldenburg.de

challenge for even advanced endoscopists. Serious adverse events can arise, and endoscopists starting with POEM should be well trained to handle these complications endoscopically or minimally invasive and avoid open surgery. These include bleeding, perforation, pneumothorax, pneumomediastinum, pneumoperitoneum, as well as infections such as mediastinitis and abscess formation [14, 15].

Appropriate training and continuous practice are crucial for success of this procedure. With this chapter, we would like to give a short overview on efficacy, safety, training, and competency in POEM.

Efficacy of POEM

POEM Versus Heller Myotomy

POEM has shown to be highly effective in the management of achalasia in several short-term follow-up studies. Its technical success does not seem to differ significantly from that of Heller myotomy (HM) [16]. Table 19.1 shows a summary of different series comparing the efficacy of POEM in comparison to Heller myotomy (HM) in a non-randomized retrospective fashion [17]. We did not find any results of a prospective direct comparison until july 2019. Beside the management of achalasia, preliminary data suggest that POEM is an effective option for the management of spastic

© Springer Nature Switzerland AG 2020
M. S. Wagh, S. B. Wani (eds.), *Gastrointestinal Interventional Endoscopy*,
https://doi.org/10.1007/978-3-030-21695-5_19

Table 19.1 Non-randomized comparisons for laparoscopic Heller myotomy (LHM) versus peroral endoscopic myotomy (POEM)

Study, year	Number of patients	Follow-up in month	Posttreatment reflux, %	Efficacy, %
Peng, 2017 [25]	POEM 13 LHM 18	54.2	No significant difference in GERD	POEM 83.3 LHM 83
Leeds, 2017 [26]	POEM 12 LHM 11	>6	Not reported	POEM 82 LHM 66
Chan, 2016 [27]	POEM 33 LHM 23	>6	POEM 15 LHM 26	POEM 100 LHM 87
Schneider, 2016 [28]	POEM 42 LHM 84	12	Not reported	POEM 91 LHM 84
Sanaka, 2016 [16]	POEM 36 LHM 142	2	Not reported	No significant difference in HREM after 2 months (p >0.05)
Kumbhari, 2015 [29]	POEM 49 LHM 26	9	POEM 39 LHM 46	POEM 98
Bhayani, 2014 [30]	POEM 37 LHM 64	6	POEM 39 LHM 32	POEM 100 LHM 92
Teitelbaum, 2013 [23]	POEM 17 LHM 12	Not reported	POEM 17 LHM 31	POEM 100 LHM 87

From Kahrilas et al. [31]
HREM high-resolution manometry

esophageal disorder. It permits an adapted myotomy according to HR-manometric changes and radiologic findings even in the mid- and proximal esophagus which is usually longer compared to classical achalasia [18–21].

The majority of studies define technical success as a post-procedure Eckardt score of ≤3, decreased lower esophageal sphincter pressure, and improved esophageal emptying [22–24]. Crespin et al. conducted a systematic review including 1299 POEM procedures. Median follow-up was 13 months (range 3–24). Pre- and post-POEM Eckardt scores and lower esophageal sphincter pressures differed significantly with a reported technical and clinical success of 80–100% [13]. The most frequently reported complications were mucosal perforation or mucosotomies (circumscript minimal defects), subcutaneous emphysema, pneumoperitoneum, pneumothorax, pneumomediastinum, pleural effusion, and pneumonia (see Table 19.1).

POEM after Heller Myotomy

Zhang, Stavropoulos and colleagues from Mineola, NY, followed 318 patients for at least 3 months after POEM, performed between

October 2009 and October 2016 [9]. They compared efficacy and safety of POEM in 46 patients with prior Heller myotomy (HM) and the remaining 272 patients without myotomy pretreatment. Patients with prior HM had longer disease history, more advanced disease, more type I and less type II achalasia, and lower before-POEM Eckardt scores. Procedure parameters and follow-up results (clinical success rate, Eckardt score, LES pressure, GERD score, esophagitis, and pH testing) showed no significant difference between the two groups [9].

POEM Long-Term Data

There are only few long-term data exceeding 5-years follow-up at present [9, 10, 32–36]. The group led by P.H. Zhou recently analyzed a collective of 564 patients having undergone a POEM procedure between August 2010 and December 2012 in Shanghai, China [36]. Major perioperative adverse events occurred in 36 patients (6.4%). After a median follow-up of 49 months (range, 3–68), the Eckardt score and lower esophageal sphincter (LES) pressure were significantly decreased (median Eckardt score, 2 vs. 8 [p <0.05]; median LES pressure,

11.9 vs. 29.7 mm Hg [p <0.05]). Fifteen failures occurred within 3 months, 23 between 3 months and 3 years, and 10 after 3 years. The estimated clinical success rates at 1, 2, 3, 4, and 5 years were 94.2%, 92.2%, 91.1%, 88.6%, and 87.1%, respectively. Multivariate Cox regression revealed long disease duration ($\geq$10 years) and history of prior interventions to be risk factors for recurrence. Clinical reflux occurred in 37.3% of patients (155/416). The authors concluded that POEM is a highly safe and effective treatment for esophageal achalasia with favorable long-term outcomes [36]. Teitelbaum and Swanstrom analyzed their long-term data on 36 patients who had undergone a POEM procedure from October 2010 to February 2012 in Portland, Oregon. Current symptom scores were obtained from 29 patients at a median follow-up of 65 months. In the 23 patients with achalasia, Eckardt scores were significantly improved from preoperative baseline (mean preoperative 6.4, mean current 1.7; p <0.001). Nineteen patients (83%) with achalasia had a symptomatic success (Eckardt $\leq$3) and none required re-treatment for symptoms. Eckardt scores were dramatically improved at 6 months and maintained at 2 years. However, there was a small but significant worsening of symptoms between 2 and 5 years. Of the 5 patients with EGJ outflow obstruction, all had current Eckardt scores $\leq$3, but two needed re-intervention for persistent or recurrent symptoms, one with a laparoscopic Heller myotomy and another with an endoscopic cricomyotomy and proximal esophageal myotomy extension. At 6-month follow-up, repeat manometry showed decreased EGJ relaxation pressures, and esophagram demonstrated improved emptying. 24-h pH monitoring showed abnormal distal esophageal acid exposure in 38% of patients. Fifteen patients underwent endoscopy at 5 years, revealing erosive esophagitis in two (13%), new hiatal hernia in two, and new non-dysplastic Barrett's esophagus in one. The authors concluded that POEM resulted in a successful palliation of symptoms in the majority of patients after 5 years, though the results confirmed the importance of a systematic long-term follow-up in all patients.

Adverse Events

As Peter Cotton et al. state: The most feared negative outcome is when something "goes wrong" and the patient experiences a "complication" [37]. This term has unfortunate medicolegal connotations and is perhaps better avoided. Describing these deviations from the plan as "unplanned events" fits nicely with the principles of informed consent, but the term "adverse events" (AEs) is in common parlance [37].

Adverse events with POEM have to be classified in intra- and post-procedural AEs [15]. Pre-interventional AEs such as aspiration pneumonia in achalasia should be excluded prior to the procedure. There is up to now no consensus on a standard classification of AEs associated with the procedure [8, 10, 15, 32, 38–45].

In general, the POEM procedure can be seen as safe procedure in the hands of an expert endoscopist at a specialized referral center [8, 10, 32, 38–45]. Until 2015 only 1 death in about 4000 procedures had been reported [45]. Inoue et al. presented in 2015 a large cohort study of 500 POEM procedures [32]. Adverse events were observed in 3.2% of patients. However, complication rates in small series are not clear yet.

Single Center and Multicenter Analysis of AEs in POEM

Haito-Chavez published in 2017 an international multicenter study on adverse events in association with POEM performed in a total of 1826 patients at 12 tertiary care academic centers between 2009 and 2015 [8]. All authors were expert endoscopists and pioneers in the field of POEM. They found 156 AEs occurring in 137 of 1826 patients (7.5% of patients). Mild, moderate, and severe AEs had a frequency of 116 (6.4%), 31 (1.7%), and 9 (0.5%), respectively. An AE was defined as any symptomatic event related to the POEM procedure itself or to anesthesia, requiring temporary stop of the procedure and/or further action to solve the event and/or to treat the symptoms [8]. Any event that prevented completion and/or resulted in prolongation of hospital stay required another procedure, or subsequent medical consultation was considered as AEs as well. The ASGE lexicon's severity grading system was used to grade the AEs [37]. Incidental findings of capnoperitoneum, capnothorax, or capnomediastinum on post-procedure imaging and subcutaneous emphysema were not considered AEs. The authors included different multivariate analyses to find out predictors for AEs. They analyzed factors related to the patient including age, gender, Charlson comorbidity index, American Society of Anesthesiologists (ASA) class, history of antiplatelet or anticoagulation, immunosuppression drug or steroid use, and previous therapies including botulinum toxin injection, pneumatic dilation, and LHM. There was no significant association between these patient-related predictors and occurrence of AEs.

Multivariate analysis demonstrated that sigmoid-type esophagus (odds ratio (OR) 2.28, $p = 0.05$), endoscopist experience <20 cases (OR 1.98, $p = 0.04$), use of a triangular tip knife (OR 3.22, $p = 0.05$), and use of an electrosurgical current different than spray coagulation (OR 3.09, $p = 0.02$) were significantly associated with the occurrence of AEs [8].

The most common time of presentation of AEs was intraprocedural in 89 patients (57.1%). A total of 64 (41.0%) AEs presented during the first 48 h, and only 3 (1.9%) AEs presented after 48 h. The most common AEs that presented during the first 48 h were esophageal leak ($n = 13$), submucosal hematoma ($n = 10$) (Fig. 19.1a, b), and pneumonia ($n = 8$). A total of 51 (2.8%) inadvertent mucosotomies occurred, mostly closed by clips (Fig. 19.2a, b). Only three AEs occurred after 48 h. There was one case of empyema requiring thoracotomy and chest tube insertion. The two remaining cases were one patient with pneumonia and one patient with delayed bleeding, both of whom were treated conservatively [8].

As discussed most of the AEs were graded as mild in 116 (6.4%), followed by moderate and severe in 31 (1.7%) and 9 (0.5%), respectively.

Among the nine severe AEs, two were esophageal leaks, two bleeding episodes during tunneling (one resulted in conversion to LHM and one resulted in intensive care unit admission), one perforation, one aspiration pneumonia, one empyema, one capnomediastinum, and one severe cardiac arrhythmia. There were two patients with heavy bleeding during tunneling; one patient with secondary bleeding could not be managed endoscopically and required balloon tamponade with a Sengstaken–Blakemore tube. The second patient experienced intraprocedural bleeding with extensive submucosal hematoma that rendered completion of POEM impossible. LHM was performed successfully during the same session [8].

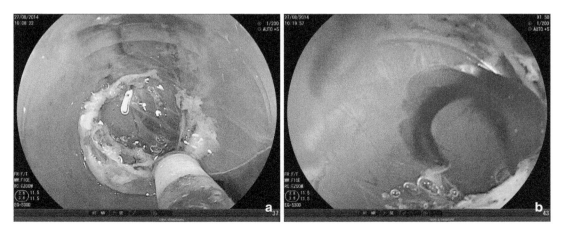

Fig. 19.1 Submucosal vessels at the enterance site appearing after mucosal incision (**a**). Bleeding submucosal vessel after transsection during mucosal incision for tunnel creation (**b**)

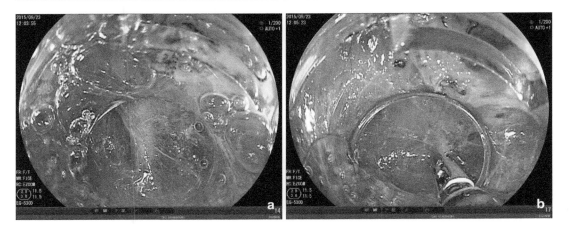

Fig. 19.2 2 mm arterial vessel crossing the submucosal tunnel. Soft or low wattage Forced Coagulation using a coaggrasper over 3-5 mm before transsection of the vessel

Among the 13 patients who presented with esophageal leak, there were two with severe esophageal leaks; one of them required surgery (washout surgery and drainage), while the second patient was treated with endoclipping. However, this latter patient progressed with a pleural effusion requiring insertion of a chest tube and then progressed with empyema requiring thoracotomy and drainage.

Overall inadvertent mucosotomy was the most common intraprocedural AE occurring in 51 patients, followed by insufflation related AEs in 28 patients (22 capnoperitoneum, 4 capnothorax, 1 pneumothorax, and 1 capnomediastinum), and bleeding during tunneling in 6 patients [8].

Other successful treatment of the 13 esophageal leaks included stent placement ($n = 2$) and endoscopically assisted vacuum therapy ($n = 1$). Three patients presented with contained leak into the submucosal tunnel and responded to conservative management.

Zhang and Zhou et al. presented their retrospective single-center analysis on only major perioperative adverse events (mAE) in 1680 patients who underwent POEM between August 2010 and July 2015 at Zhongshan Hospital, Shanghai, China [38]. They identified a total of 55 patients experiencing major adverse events (3.3%): they found delayed mucosal barrier failure ($n = 13$; 0.8%), delayed bleeding ($n = 3$;

0.2%), hydrothorax ($n = 8$; 0.5%), pneumothorax ($n = 25$; 1.5%), and miscellaneous ($n = 6$; 0.4%). Four patients (0.2%) required ICU admission. No surgical conversion occurred, and 30-day mortality was zero. In stepwise multivariate regression, institution experience of <1 year (odds ratio [OR] 3.85; 95%CI 1.49–9.95), air insufflation (OR 3.41; 95%CI 1.37–8.50), and mucosal edema (OR 2.01; 95%CI 1.14–3.53) were identified as related risk factors. After introducing CO_2 insufflation, the major Adverse Event rate declined to 1.9% (95%CI 1.2–2.7%) and seemed to plateau after 3.5 years at ~1%. The authors concluded that POEM appeared to be a safe procedure. Major adverse events were rare and could usually be managed effectively.

CO_2-Associated Problems and Anesthesiologic Considerations

Already in early series, the need for CO_2 insufflation instead of room air during POEM became evident [46, 47]. CO_2 may inadvertently track into surrounding tissues during POEM, causing systemic CO_2 uptake and tension capnoperitoneum. This in turn may affect cardiorespiratory function. Gas-associated AEs include also pneumomediastinum, subcutaneous emphysema, and pneumothorax. In a meta-analysis of Akintoye et al., subcutaneous emphysema was found in 7.5%, pneumothorax in 1.2%, pneumomediastinum in 1.1%, and pneumoperitoneum in 6.8% [48]. Important guiding parameters indicating the need for an intervention were significant abdominal distension, increased end-tidal CO_2 and increased peak airway pressure [40]. In cases of tension pneumoperitoneum, a Veress needle (or a 16–18 G intravenous cannula) is inserted through the abdominal wall paraumbilically respecting sterile conditions [15]. A 10–20 ml syringe is filled with saline and connected with the canula, and the plunger is removed. The appearance of bubbles shows a successful drainage of the capnoperitoneum. CO_2 is absorbed about 300 times faster than room air. Only gas-related events requiring an intervention should therefore be categorized as adverse events [15].

The endoscopist should try to reduce the CO_2 gas flow to the necessary minimum. The use of a low-flow CO_2 gas tube has been described helpful in this regard. In case of a pneumothorax with a volume of more than 30%, a thoracic drainage should be introduced for 2 or 3 days. In the rare case of capno-pericardium, a cardiac arrest may occur the way that anesthetists and endoscopists should be aware of this rare but possible complication [49].

Close anesthesiologic supervision of changes in airway pressures and hemodynamics are recommended, and an arterial line for monitoring of arterial blood gases can be considered [15, 50]. Important guiding parameters indicating the need for an intervention include significant abdominal distension, increased end-tidal CO_2, and peak airway pressure. Increasing minute ventilation is usually enough to manage an increase in end-tidal CO_2 levels associated with CO_2 insufflation [40]. Loeser et al. analyzed 173 consecutive POEM patients of a tertiary care single center in Germany over a 4-year period from an anesthesiologic standpoint [50]. During POEM, cardiorespiratory parameters increased from baseline: pmax 15.1 vs 19.8 cm H_2O,

etCO$_2$ 4.5 vs 5.5 kPa [34.0 vs 41.6 mmHg], MAP 73.9 vs 99.3 mmHg, and HR 67.6 vs 85.3 min(−1) ($p < 0.001$ for each). Hyperventilation [MV 5.9 vs 9.0 L.min(−1), $p < 0.001$] was applied to counteract iatrogenic hypercapnia. Individuals with tension capnoperitoneum are treated with percutaneous needle decompression (PND; $n = 55$). They had higher peak pmax values [22.8 vs 18.4 cm H_2O, $p < 0.001$] than patients who did not require PND. After PND, pmax [22.8 vs 19.9 cm H_2O, $p = 0.045$] and MAP [98.2 vs 88.6 mmHg, $p = 0.013$] decreased. Adverse events included pneumothorax ($n = 1$), transient myocardial ischemia ($n = 1$), and subcutaneous emphysema ($n = 49$). The latter precluded immediate extubation in eight cases. Postanesthesia care unit (PACU) stay was significantly longer in individuals with subcutaneous emphysema than in those without ($p < 0.001$). The authors concluded that carbon dioxide insufflation during POEM produced systemic CO_2 uptake and increased intra-abdominal pressure. Changes in cardiorespiratory parameters included increased pmax, etCO$_2$, MAP, and HR. Hyperventilation and percutaneous abdominal needle decompression helped to mitigate some of these changes. Subcutaneous emphysema was common in 28.3% of cases and did delay extubation and prolong PACU stay.

Bleeding

Bleeding is a common side effect during any of the different steps of POEM, especially during submucosal tunneling (Figs. 19.1, 19.2, 19.3, and 19.4). Careful stepwise dissection will allow vessels to be visualized and to be prophylactically treated using cautious coagulation with the electrocautery knife itself or by means of a "Coag Grasper" (Olympus, Center Valley, PA, USA) using "Soft Coag" or low wattage "Forced Coag" current. Caution should be applied in case bleeding originates from a vessel running along the mucosal surface side of the tunnel in order to

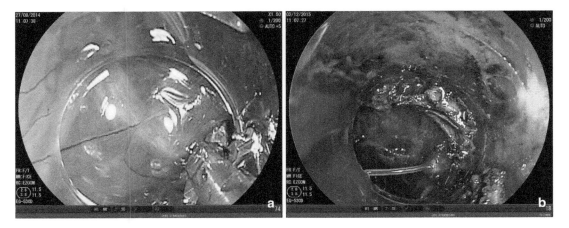

Fig. 19.3 2.5 mm arterial vessel crossing the submucosal tunnel (**a**). Secondary severe bleeding after to short sealing of the vessel ends by means of the coag-grasper (**b**)

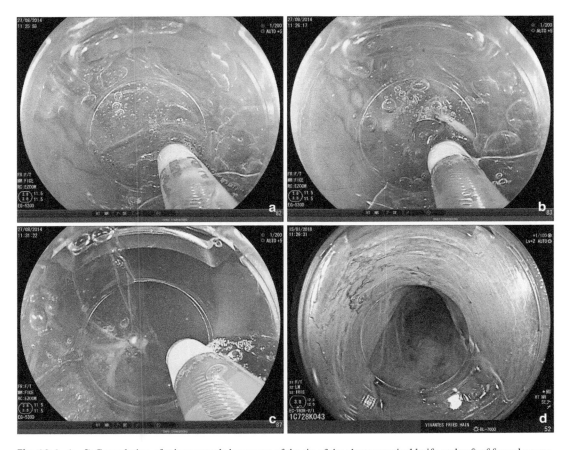

Fig. 19.4 (**a–d**) Coagulation of minor vessels by means of the tip of the electrosurgical knife and soft of forced coagulation current following the vessel course before transsection (**a–c**). Completed tunnel after dissection (**d**)

prevent secondary mucosal defects and perforation after coagulation. A gentle compression with the tip of the endoscope +/− cautious secondary coagulation is carried out in these cases. The placement of clips in the tunnel is usually avoided as secondary perforation of the covering mucosa should be feared.

Guidelines recommend to perform POEM without anticoagulant or antiplatelet therapy except for acetylsalicylic acid. It is recommended that all patients should have a blood type and antibody screening before starting the procedure [51, 52]. Postoperative bleeding apparently is infrequent. In a large series of Li et al. with 428 patients, delayed bleeding has been reported in 0.7% [53].

Secondary bleeding into the tunnel is infrequent (Fig. 19.5a, b). However, a massive hematoma in the tunnel can result in pressure necrosis of the mucosal flap with potentially disastrous consequences in case of wide perforation. A CT scan should be performed to discriminate a mere bleeding into the tunnel from additional mediastinal effusion. Li et al. reported on three patients (0.7%, 3/428) who experienced delayed bleeding in the submucosal tunnel after POEM. None of these patients had any predisposing factor to bleeding, such as hypertension, coagulation disorders, and antiplatelet/anticoagulant therapy before undergoing POEM. There were no special difficulties related to tunnel creation or myotomy performance

in these cases. In one patient, a small hematoma was observed by CT before any clinical manifestation occurred; this patient then reported progressive serious retrosternal pain from the first day after surgery and vomited fresh blood on the third day. Two other patients suddenly vomited large amounts of fresh blood on the first and third days after the intervention, respectively; no submucosal hematoma was observed on CT scans before hematemesis occurred in these two patients. Emergency esophago-gastroscopy was performed immediately on all three patients, revealing a hematoma in the submucosal tunnel. After removing the metal clips from the mucosal entry, a large quantity of blood clots were discovered inside the submucosal tunnel and were removed. In the first patient, the bleeding source could not be identified, and a Sengstaken–Blakemore tube was directly placed into the stomach and lower esophagus to compress the bleeding sites. In the other two patients, active bleeding points were identified and coagulated with a hemostatic forceps in the forced coagulation mode. Almost all of the bleeding spots were from the cut muscular edges. A PPI, antibiotics, and hemocoagulase were administered to all three patients. Intermittent balloon deflation was performed every 24 h. The Sengstaken–Blakemore tube gastric balloon was permanently deflated on the first day after placement, and the esophageal balloon was deflated on the second day after insertion.

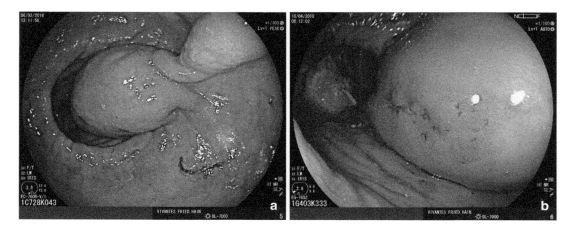

Fig. 19.5 (**a, b**) Enormous secondary hematoma at the level of the submucosal tunnel developing within the first 48 h post procedure possibly after repeat coughing

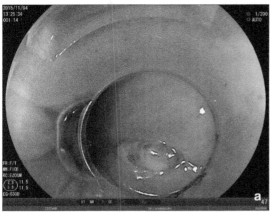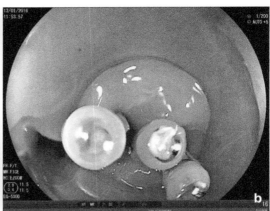

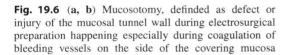

Fig. 19.6 (**a, b**) Mucosotomy, definded as defect or injury of the mucosal tunnel wall during electrosurgical preparation happening especially during coagulation of bleeding vessels on the side of the covering mucosa

(**a**) Adaptation of the mucosa left and right of the coagulation defect by means of three short arm clips (Hemoclip green; Olympus Tokyo, Japan)

Benech et al. from Lyon, France, reported on successful conservative management [54]. The patient had experienced massive epigastric pain shortly after the procedure and showed a drop in hemoglobin from 14.2 to 11.2 g/dl. We had a similar case, managed conservatively (Fig. 19.5a, b).

Perforation

After dissection of the muscular layer, even a small mucosal defect can become potentially dangerous. In case such a mucosotomy is detected during submucosal tunneling, closure should be performed immediately as otherwise a significant increase of the defect may occur (Fig. 19.6a, b) [38]. Preoperative edema of the mucosa is suggested a risk factor for mucosal injury during intervention. Mucosal edema makes closure difficult and promotes perforation. Edema has been seen in 8% of patients in a retrospective study of over 1600 patients [38]. The endoscopic tunnel should be created very close to the muscular layers to avoid injury to the mucosal flap and because of a lower vascularity adjacent to the muscle [55]. Most perforations happen at the level of the lower esophageal sphincter due to a narrowing at the cardia. If a mucosotomy is identified, it should be closed immediately with endoscopic clips. Larger mucosotomies have been closed

using a flexible endoscopic suturing device (OverStitch; Apollo Endosurgery, Austin, TX, United States) [56, 57]. Other salvage techniques used included fibrin glue and over-the-scope clips (OTSCs; Ovesco, Tuebingen, Germany) [58, 59]. In case of multiple ruptures which cannot be clipped, a covered retrievable stent may be used as rescue technique [60, 61].

Postprocedural Chest Pain

The most common periprocedural side effect is substernal chest pain. Data suggest an average mild to moderate chest pain after the procedure and during the following 3 days (4.6/10 immediately after POEM, 3.2–3.3/10 the following 2 days) [40]. As in tubular esophageal ESD, the application of a fentanyl patch, adapted to patients weight, age, and general condition, e.g., 25 mcg/g (12.5–50 mcg/h), applied at the beginning of the procedure, has been very valuable in our own experience over the last 5 years.

Infections and Pneumonia

In general index gastroscopy should be performed one to several days before the POEM procedure. In case signs of *Candida* esophagitis, a systemic antifungal treatment should be initiated immediately. Remaining material in the lower esophagus should be removed, and the patient is set on a strictly liquid diet 24–48 h before treatment. Single-shot antibiosis of, e.g., ceftriaxone plus metronidazole, is usually sufficient in a non-immunocompromised patient.

Sterility is still under debate as the endoscope is penetrating into a space in direct contact with the mediastinum and abdominal cavity. On the other hand, infectious complications have been reported less frequent as feared in the initial era of procedure [46, 47]. As a routine, we remove the endoscope with sterile gloves from the washing machine after reprocessing it shortly before the procedure. The same is done if a drying cabinet is used for storage. It is then placed into a tray with a sterile cloth inside and covered which a second sterile cloth until its use for the procedure. The use of a sterile coat and sterile gloves is recommended for the procedure [46, 47]. However, this practice varies from center to center and many units perform POEM with the endoscope processed and handled as for any other upper endoscopy. Single centers ask the patients to flush the mouth with chlorhexidine solution before the intervention [62].

Pleural Effusion

Pleural effusion is noticed in 5–40% of POEM patients. Depending on the size of effusion, laboratory findings plus clinical signs of infection (fever, etc.), antibiotics and early pleural drainage or just waiting for spontaneous absorption is indicated [42].

Reflux After POEM and LHM

The most common long-term adverse event with POEM seems to be gastroesophageal reflux (GER). As the premise behind the POEM procedure, similar to Heller myotomy, is to decrease lower esophageal sphincter pressure, it is not surprising that post-POEM GER is encountered [63]. Early studies were focused on technical fea-

sibility and safety, with a short duration of follow-up. Furthermore, a large proportion of the early literature came from Asia, where GER is less prevalent. Finally, the consequences of asymptomatic or proton pump inhibitor (PPI)-responsive GER after POEM had not been clear at the time.

When objective data are reviewed, such as erosive esophagitis in EGD and/or an abnormal acid exposure on a pH study, the prevalence of GER after POEM appears to be in recent studies high and varies between 20% and 46% after POEM [51, 63–65]. Barrett's metaplasia has been reported in first few cases as found earlier after Heller myotomy [66, 67].

In patients with a hiatal hernia, the risk for erosive esophagitis and GERD post-POEM seems increased [68]. If the rates can be compared to those seen with Heller myotomy plus partial fundoplication had been long time contradictory [69–71]. Kumbhari et al. note that when Heller myotomy was first introduced, it was not combined with an anti-reflux procedure and initially not deemed necessary [72]. Subsequently a high rate of GERD became evident, and a partial fundoplication became standard practice [70, 73, 74].

Kumbhari et al. analyzed results from seven tertiary academic centers (one Asian, two US, four European). POEM had been carried out in 467 patients during the 5-year study period. A total of 282 patients were included in the analysis. One hundred eighty-five patients were excluded because no pH study was performed at ≥3 months after POEM. A post-procedure DeMeester score of ≥14.72 was seen in 57.8% of patients. Multivariable analysis revealed female sex to be the only independent association (odds ratio 1.69, 95% confidence interval 1.04–2.74) with post-POEM GER. No intraprocedural variables were associated with GER. Upper GI endoscopy was available in 233 patients, 54 (23.2%) of whom were noted to have reflux esophagitis (majority Los Angeles grade A or B). GER was asymptomatic in 60.1%. The authors concluded that post-POEM GER was seen in the majority of patients. No intraprocedural variables could be identified to allow for potential alteration in procedural technique.

Repici et al. published a meta-analysis on gastroesophageal reflux disease after POEM as compared with laparoscopic Heller's myotomy plus fundoplication published until February 2017 [65]. They identified 17 and 28 prospective studies, including 1542 and 2581 subjects who underwent POEM and LHM, respectively. Pooled rate of post-procedure reflux symptoms was 19.0% (95% CI, 15.7–22.8%) after POEM and 8.8% (95% CI, 5.3–14.1%) after LHM, respectively. Pooled rate estimate of abnormal acid exposure at pH monitoring was 39.0% (95% CI, 24.5–55.8%) after POEM and 16.8% (95% CI, 10.2–26.4%) after LHM, respectively. Rate of post-POEM esophagitis was 29.4% (95% CI, 18.5–43.3%) after POEM and 7.6% (95% CI, 4.1–13.7%) after LHM. At meta-regression, heterogeneity was partly explained by POEM approach and study population. They concluded that the incidence of reflux-disease appears to be significantly more frequent after POEM than after LHM with fundoplication. pH monitoring and appropriate treatment after POEM should be considered in order to prevent long-term reflux-related adverse events [65].

However, long-term results after LHM indicate that the antireflux effect of the fundoplication might only be of temporary nature. In their editorial, Rosch et al. asked the question "Will Reflux Kill POEM?" [66]. Rosch discusses that only one small randomized controlled trial ($n = 43$) has been published showing reflux rates of 9.1% versus 47.6% in the groups of Heller myotomy with and without Dor fundoplication, respectively [73]. Kummerow Broman et al. published the long-term symptomatic follow-up results on part of this group in 2018 [75]. They collected patient-reported measures of dysphagia and gastroesophageal reflux using the Dysphagia Score and the Gastroesophageal Reflux Disease-Health-Related Quality of Life (GERD-HRQL) instrument. Patient-reported re-interventions for dysphagia were verified by obtaining longitudinal medical records. Among living participants, 27/41 (66%) all completed the follow-up study at a mean of 11.8 years postoperatively. Median Dysphagia Scores and GERD-HRQL scores were slightly worse for Heller than Heller plus Dor but were not statistically different (6 vs 3,

$p = 0.08$ for dysphagia; 15 vs 13, $p = 0.25$ for reflux). Five patients in the Heller group and six in Heller plus Dor underwent re-intervention for dysphagia with most occurring more than 5 years postoperatively. One patient in each group underwent redo Heller myotomy and subsequent esophagectomy. Nearly all patients (96%) stated that they would undergo operation again. The authors concluded that long-term patient-reported outcomes after Heller alone and Heller plus Dor for achalasia were comparable, providing support for either procedure [75].

There is no consensus on how to manage patients with symptomatic gastroesophageal reflux disease, but a primary attempt with low-dose PPIs seems to work well for most patients [8, 10, 32, 38–45]. In case of the necessity of a secondary fundoplication only a partial or "floppy" fundoplication is recommended in order to not impair esophageal emptying with secondary dysphagia again [8, 10, 32, 38–45]. Kumta et al. even reported one case of endoscopic fundoplication in an patient with gastroesophageal reflux symptoms refractory to proton pump inhibitors [76].

Training in POEM

Requirements to Perform POEM

The first step for a "POEM learner" is an excellent knowledge of the specific thoracic and abdominal anatomy and the different steps of the procedure [77]. The second step is usually an "ex vivo" and "in vivo" training in the porcine model similar to ESD training [78]. The first clinical POEM cases in patients should be accompanied by an expert endoscopist from an external POEM referral center [79].

The NOSCAR (Natural Orifice Surgery Consortium for Assessment and Research) has proposed the following prerequisites for an endoscopic team planning to perform POEM in the future [46]:

1. A multidisciplinary team encompassing endoscopists and surgeons.
2. "Ex vivo" experience with animal or cadaver models before planning to perform first POEMs in humans.

3. A local institutional review board approval.
4. All cases should be registered in an outcome registry maintained by the concerned scientific societies.

Clinical Training in POEM

In general, it is recommended to start with POEM after reaching the top level of the endoscopic learning pyramid [80]. However, until today there are no valid data if an endoscopist experienced, e.g., in endoscopic submucosal dissection (ESD) acquires competence in POEM faster than an endoscopist without this qualification. Mittal et al. state that most advanced endoscopy training programs in the United States do not provide formal training in submucosal endoscopy or POEM [7]. In Europe, POEM procedures have been limited to a few centers so far and have been performed by experienced endoscopists only. As the procedure is carried out in the thoracic cavity close to the mediastinum in case of complications such as infection, bleeding or perforation consequences may be severe. It seemed logic that an extensive experience in interventional endoscopy, especially in hemostasis and perforation closure, seems necessary as well as the need for a specialized surgical team in case of severe complications. Furthermore the number of patients concerned is limited.

The ASGE recommends that competence acquisition in a "major skill" like POEM should be performed at teaching institutions with appropriate numbers using a preceptorship model. A quorum of procedures required to assess POEM has not been defined so far. In centers familiar with POEM, clinical training is mostly started by an advanced fellow or experienced consultant [7].

Before starting POEM, an intensive study of the literature, watching videos, attending live demonstrations, and a hands-on training course are usually recommended. Early training steps of POEM include a progressive approach to the technique in "ex vivo" pig esophagi. Training in live pigs is a common next step to train the technique in an environment with natural GI motility and vascularization. However, the discrepancy of the tender muscle layer in pigs and the potentially hypertrophic muscle layer in humans has to be noted as significant difference and limitation (Fig. 19.7a, b). After having attended a systematic course with practical exposure to the technique, a visit to an expert center is recommended to observe and assist the performance of several procedures. A close student–teacher relationship and sufficient phases of watching the procedure seem important

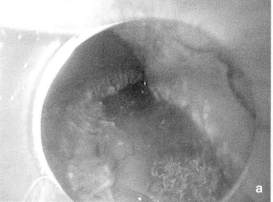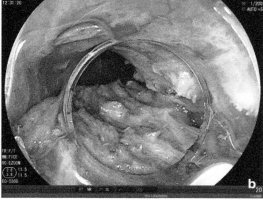

Fig. 19.7 Training for POEM in the animal model and situation in 'the real world': discrepancy in thickness of the tender muscular layer in the pig (**a**) and in a patient with achalasia Type III and enormous hypertrophy of the muscular layer (**b**)

Table 19.2 POEM training steps and protocol according to Dacha et al. [35]

Steps	Assessment parameters
Step 1: Dissection, establishing a submucosal tunnel	1. Able to identify the orientation of the submucosal tunnel, including the location of the mucosal layer and the location of the muscular layer 2. Able to judge need for more submucosal injection while performing submucosal dissection to prevent inadvertent complications 3. Able to secure hemostasis with a knife or a coagulation forceps 4. Able to perform all of the above without instructions and assistance from the mentor
Step 2: Myotomy inside the submucosal tunnel	1. Continue all above listed in step 1 2. Able to identify gastroesophageal junction 3. Able to identify circular muscular layer 4. Able to identify longitudinal muscular layer 5. Able to perform myotomy either on circular muscular layer or full-thickness myotomy 6. Able to perform all above without instructions or assistance from the mentor
Step 3: Creating a submucosal tunnel orifice	1. Continue all above listed in step 1 and step 2 2. Ability to raise a mucosal bleb with submucosal injection prior to performing mucosotomy incision 3. Able to enter submucosal tunnel efficiently after performing mucosotomy incision (2 and 3 should take no longer than 15 min) 4. Able to perform all of the above without instruction and assistance from the mentor
Other trainings	1. Ability to safely close mucosotomy incision with endoclips 2. Able to safely use a Veress needle to decompress symptomatic capnoperitoneum (even if it is not encountered) 3. Able to perform all the above without instruction and assistance from the mentor

before a student goes to unsupervised clinical procedure. A short course or workshop seems not to be a good platform to gather sufficient knowledge (see also below) [81]. Didactic training and hands-on fundamentals seminars are available, e.g., from the American Society for Gastrointestinal Endoscopy (ASGE) [82].

Mittal et al. suggest the following areas to be covered during training for POEM [7]:

1. Interpretation of high-resolution manometry and barium esophagram
2. Diagnostic endoscopic evaluation of the esophagus, gastroesophageal junction, and stomach
3. Appropriate site selection for mucosal entry
4. Identification of esophageal wall layers during submucosal dissection
5. Identification of dissection planes and orientation of mucosa and muscle layer during submucosal tunneling
6. Identification of the anatomical changes and structures at the gastroesophageal junction and cardia
7. Identification of circular and longitudinal muscle planes

8. Performance of selective circular vs full-thickness myotomy
9. Management of bleeding
10. Management of mucosal injury or perforation
11. Mucosotomy closure

A similar "checklist" for the single clinical training steps in POEM has been described by Dacha et al. [35] (Table 19.2).

Training in Porcine Models

For training purposes, first steps are usually performed in the pig model even though the pig is not optimal due to its thin muscular layer compared to a patient with spastic esophageal motor disorder (Fig. 19.7a, b). Training may include "ex vivo" porcine specimens with an esophagus left in its total length as well as training on live pigs under general anesthesia in the acute animal experiment. Table 19.3 shows advantages and disadvantages of both models.

Ren et al. as well as Chiu et al. described the learning curve for POEM in the early days of POEM including "ex vivo" and live porcine

Table 19.3 Advantages (+ to +++) and disadvantages (− to −−−) of the "ex vivo" and "in vivo" porcine model for the training of the POEM procedure

Model	Costs	Ethical concerns	Assessment of trainee performance	Reality of environment Training of complication management (bleeding/perforation, etc.)
Ex vivo porcine model	++	++	++	−−
Live pig model	−−	−−	++	++

models. Ren et al. trained the procedure in a total of five ex vivo porcine specimen before starting with the first patient (see below). Chiu et al. trained in two acute and seven survival pig models. Perforations occurred in 3/5 "ex vivo" specimen and in 1/7 survival animal models with acute fatal pneumomediastinum in one animal. The latter was attributed to the use of room air instead of CO_2 during the experiments. Both groups rated a training in "ex vivo" specimen and live pigs as very valuable [83, 84]. With the clinical experience in POEM of today, tutored experimental experience and clinical proctoring would have been strongly recommended.

Hernandez Mondragon described his personal preclinical learning curve for POEM in 50 procedures performed in the animal lab [85]. He started with 30 procedures using a mannequin containing an "en bloc" organ package of the esophagus, stomach, and duodenum from the pig cleaned, prepared, frozen, and then thawed 1 h before the procedure in 25 °C warm saline. In a second learning section, POEM was carried out in 20 pigs with a weight of 40–50 kg which were followed for 30 days. The learning process was defined as ability to perform the five steps of POEM, while mastery of the technique was considered a complication-free procedure. Mucosotomies (mucosal injuries with communication between the submucosal space and esophageal or gastric lumen) or free perforation by the endoscope were documented endoscopically and on the specimen. Additionally, the animal group included the incidence of hemorrhage or procedure-related death. Subcutaneous emphysema, pneumomediastinum, pneumoperitoneum, or bleeding during the procedure were considered as Adverse Event only if they could not be controlled by endoscopic measures or

medical maneuvers. The study seems to have been carried out meticulously but is hampered by its design with the same endoscopist performing procedures first "in vitro" and then "in vivo" with comparison of two sequential learning curves. The authors concluded that 16 "ex vivo" procedures and 10 in live pigs were necessary to perform the procedure without complications. After those numbers, the trainee gradually improved speed without scarifying safety [85]. The numbers given seem comparable to those recommended for the training in endoscopic submucosal dissection (ESD) where at least 25 preclinical resections "ex vivo" and "in vivo" are recommended [78, 86] (Fig. 19.3).

Clinical Learning Curve After Training

The role of prior experience of the trainee in tunneling techniques (ESD, etc.) and in the management of complications such as perforation and severe bleeding seems not completely clear so far. Werner et al. reported 24-month follow-up data of 80 patients who underwent POEM in a MC trial. More than half of the failures were reported during the first 10 procedures [39]. The authors concluded that there was a significant learning curve for POEM even for experienced interventional endoscopists. Kurian et al. analyzed their first 40 consecutive patients undergoing POEM. The learning curve plateau was at about 20 cases for an experienced endoscopist with no significant further increase in myotomy speed and length of procedure (LOP) thereafter. Patel et al. presented a paper about the personal learning curve of one of the first endoscopists performing POEM in the western world,

Stavros N. Stavropoulos from Mineola NY, USA. He described the grade of efficiency and mastery of POEM for 93 sequential procedures. The "efficiency" was reached when the procedure time started decreasing, and "mastery" was defined as plateau in procedure time (Fig. 19.8) [87]. In this analysis using penalized basis spline regression and CUSUM analysis, 40 procedures were required to gain "efficiency" and 60 procedures for "mastery" (Fig. 19.9). When the authors used adjusted regression analysis, only case number (operator experience) significantly affected procedure time (p <0.0001). The "trainee" had had prior experience in more than 60 upper and lower GI ESDs and a long experience in the management of complications such as severe bleeding or perforation [87].

Currently the optimal curriculum for POEM training is not clear. In every case, clinical proctoring at a high-volume institution seems an important step for successful clinical implementation of this technique [47]. Dacha et al.

recently reported on the successful clinical integration of advanced fellows after their third year fellowship and experience in hundreds of gastroscopies and colonoscopies and at least 100 ERCPs and 100 EUS procedures. All of them had participated actively in at least five upper or lower ESD cases. The authors did split the procedure in different training steps the trainees had to successfully complete (Table 19.3). All four trainees successfully completed step 1 after an average of 4.25 patients (range 3–6), step 2 with an average of 4.0 patients (range 3–5), and step 3 with an average of 5.0 patients (range 3–6). Three of the four trainees did in the following start performing POEM independently. For each step in POEM, such as dissection, hemostasis, and myotomy, trainees needed 3–6 patients to acquire the adequate skill and to complete the step without instructions from the mentor. Finally, each of the "learners" performed two cases of an entire POEM with the mentor but without instructions from the mentor. The authors therefore considered the total

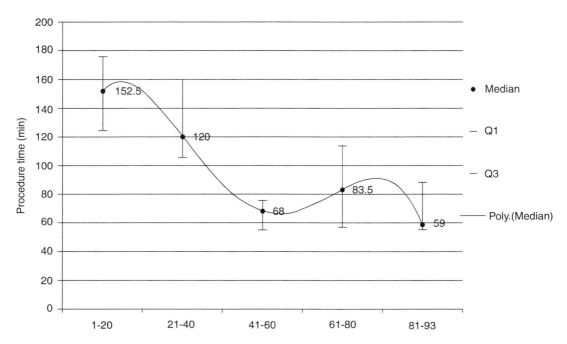

Fig. 19.8 Decrease of procedure time for POEM with increasing experience of a single endoscopist during his first 93 procedures. Sequential grouping of procedure time with median procedure time (interquartile range) in minutes. Adapted from Patel KS, Stavropoulos S. et al. [87]

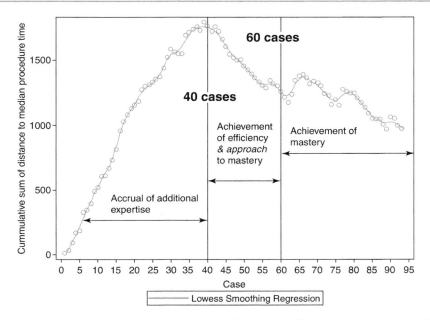

Fig. 19.9 Cumulative sum of distance to median procedure time presented as CUSUM plot for a single operator during his first 93 POEM procedures. The graph shows efficiency after 40 procedures and mastery after 60 procedures. From Patel KS, Stavros S et al. [87]

threshold number to be able to perform POEM independently about 20 cases per trainee [35].

POEM Training for All?

A study by Kishiki et al., published recently, reported on the learning progress of 65 participants in dedicated 1-day POEM training workshops at two US institutions [88]. Participants were mainly visceral surgeons in practice. Participants with more than 100 upper GI endoscopies were considered "experts," with less than 100 gastroscopies "novices." The authors called their project "into the fire." The 1-day training course included a hands-on pre−/posttest and a short quiz designed to assess participants' comprehension at the beginning and at the end of the course. Participants took part in lectures on patient selection, technique, troubleshooting, and discussion. Hands-on POEM training and competence assessment were evaluated on both "ex vivo" and "in vivo" porcine models using a new

metrics for POEM performance. The participants were stimulated to start thereafter the procedure at their home institution.

This approach seems risky in case the procedure is carried out without adequate proctoring and sufficient competence in the endoscopic management of complications [47]. Unfortunately, an additional qualification of the participants has not been reported but would be desirable. One hundred diagnostic gastroscopies correspond to the level of a first- to second-year GI-fellow who would by far not qualify for the procedure. A surgical resolution of endoscopically manageable problems cannot be considered adequate for an endoscopic procedure. Clinical education and proctorship in interventional endoscopy including the early recognition and management of complications, such as severe bleedings or perforations and the handling of patients under critical clinical situations, take a long learning curve and are impossible to be replaced by pure training on pig models and lectures [89].

References

1. Committee ASoP, Pasha SF, Acosta RD, Chandrasekhara V, Chathadi KV, Decker GA, et al. The role of endoscopy in the evaluation and management of dysphagia. Gastrointest Endosc. 2014;79(2):191–201.

2. Kantsevoy SV, Jagannath SB, Niiyama H, Chung SS, Cotton PB, Gostout CJ, et al. Endoscopic gastrojejunostomy with survival in a porcine model. Gastrointest Endosc. 2005;62(2):287–92.

3. Kalloo AN, Singh VK, Jagannath SB, Niiyama H, Hill SL, Vaughn CA, et al. Flexible transgastric peritoneoscopy: a novel approach to diagnostic and therapeutic interventions in the peritoneal cavity. Gastrointest Endosc. 2004;60(1):114–7.

4. Hochberger J, Lamade W. Transgastric surgery in the abdomen: the dawn of a new era? Gastrointest Endosc. 2005;62(2):293–6.

5. Inoue H, Minami H, Kobayashi Y, Sato Y, Kaga M, Suzuki M, et al. Peroral endoscopic myotomy (POEM) for esophageal achalasia. Endoscopy. 2010;42(4):265–71.

6. Pasricha PJ, Hawari R, Ahmed I, Chen J, Cotton PB, Hawes RH, et al. Submucosal endoscopic esophageal myotomy: a novel experimental approach for the treatment of achalasia. Endoscopy. 2007;39(9):761–4.

7. Mittal C, Wagh MS. Technical advances in Per-Oral Endoscopic Myotomy (POEM). Am J Gastroenterol. 2017;112(11):1627–31.

8. Haito-Chavez Y, Inoue H, Beard KW, Draganov PV, Ujiki M, Rahden BHA, et al. Comprehensive analysis of adverse events associated with per Oral endoscopic Myotomy in 1826 patients: an International Multicenter study. Am J Gastroenterol. 2017;112(8):1267–76.

9. Zhang X, Modayil RJ, Friedel D, Gurram KC, Brathwaite CE, Taylor SI, et al. Per-oral endoscopic myotomy in patients with or without prior Heller's myotomy: comparing long-term outcomes in a large U.S. single-center cohort (with videos). Gastrointest Endosc. 2018;87(4):972–85.

10. Teitelbaum EN, Dunst CM, Reavis KM, Sharata AM, Ward MA, DeMeester SR, et al. Clinical outcomes five years after POEM for treatment of primary esophageal motility disorders. Surg Endosc. 2018;32(1):421–7.

11. Muehldorfer SM, Schneider TH, Hochberger J, Martus P, Hahn EG, Ell C. Esophageal achalasia: intrasphincteric injection of botulinum toxin a versus balloon dilation. Endoscopy. 1999;31(7):517–21.

12. Wong I, Law S. Peroral endoscopic myotomy (POEM) for treating esophageal motility disorders. Ann Transl Med. 2017;5(8):192.

13. Crespin OM, Liu LWC, Parmar A, Jackson TD, Hamid J, Shlomovitz E, et al. Safety and efficacy of POEM for treatment of achalasia: a systematic review of the literature. Surg Endosc. 2017;31(5):2187–201.

14. Bechara R, Onimaru M, Ikeda H, Inoue H. Peroral endoscopic myotomy, 1000 cases later: pearls, pitfalls, and practical considerations. Gastrointest Endosc. 2016;84(2):330–8.

15. Nabi Z, Reddy DN, Ramchandani M. Adverse events during and after per-oral endoscopic myotomy: prevention, diagnosis, and management. Gastrointest Endosc. 2018;87(1):4–17.

16. Sanaka MR, Hayat U, Thota PN, Jegadeesan R, Ray M, Gabbard SL, et al. Efficacy of peroral endoscopic myotomy vs other achalasia treatments in improving esophageal function. World J Gastroenterol: WJG. 2016;22(20):4918–25.

17. Kahrilas PJ, Katzka D, Richter JE. Clinical practice update: the use of Per-Oral Endoscopic Myotomy in achalasia: expert review and best practice advice from the AGA Institute. Gastroenterology. 2017;153(5):1205–11.

18. Schlottmann F, Shaheen NJ, Madanick RD, Patti MG. The role of Heller myotomy and POEM for nonachalasia motility disorders. Dis Esophagus. 2017;30(4):1–5.

19. Khashab MA, Messallam AA, Onimaru M, Teitelbaum EN, Ujiki MB, Gitelis ME, et al. International multicenter experience with peroral endoscopic myotomy for the treatment of spastic esophageal disorders refractory to medical therapy (with video). Gastrointest Endosc. 2015;81(5):1170–7.

20. Khan MA, Kumbhari V, Ngamruengphong S, Ismail A, Chen YI, Chavez YH, et al. Is POEM the answer for management of spastic esophageal disorders? A systematic review and meta-analysis. Dig Dis Sci. 2017;62(1):35–44.

21. Parsa N, Khashab MA. POEM in the treatment of esophageal disorders. Curr Treat Options Gastroenterol. 2018;16:27.

22. Sharata AM, Dunst CM, Pescarus R, Shlomovitz E, Wille AJ, Reavis KM, et al. Peroral endoscopic myotomy (POEM) for esophageal primary motility disorders: analysis of 100 consecutive patients. J Gastrointest Surg. 2015;19(1):161–70; discussion 70

23. Teitelbaum EN, Rajeswaran S, Zhang R, Sieberg RT, Miller FH, Soper NJ, et al. Peroral esophageal myotomy (POEM) and laparoscopic Heller myotomy produce a similar short-term anatomic and functional effect. Surgery. 2013;154(4):885–91; discussion 91–2

24. Verlaan T, Rohof WO, Bredenoord AJ, Eberl S, Rosch T, Fockens P. Effect of peroral endoscopic myotomy on esophagogastric junction physiology in patients with achalasia. Gastrointest Endosc. 2013;78(1):39–44.

25. Peng L, Tian S, Du C, Yuan Z, Guo M, Lu L. Outcome of Peroral Endoscopic Myotomy (POEM) for treating achalasia compared with Laparoscopic Heller Myotomy (LHM). Surg Laparosc Endosc Percutan Tech. 2017;27(1):60–4.

26. Leeds SG, Burdick JS, Ogola GO, Ontiveros E. Comparison of outcomes of laparoscopic Heller myotomy versus per-oral endoscopic myotomy for

management of achalasia. Proc (Bayl Univ Med Cent). 2017;30(4):419–23.

27. Chan SM, Wu JC, Teoh AY, Yip HC, Ng EK, Lau JY, et al. Comparison of early outcomes and quality of life after laparoscopic Heller's cardiomyotomy to peroral endoscopic myotomy for treatment of achalasia. Dig Endosc. 2016;28(1):27–32.

28. Schneider AM, Louie BE, Warren HF, Farivar AS, Schembre DB, Aye RW. A matched comparison of Per Oral Endoscopic Myotomy to Laparoscopic Heller Myotomy in the treatment of achalasia. J Gastrointest Surg. 2016;20(11):1789–96.

29. Kumbhari V, Tieu AH, Onimaru M, El Zein MH, Teitelbaum EN, Ujiki MB, et al. Peroral endoscopic myotomy (POEM) vs laparoscopic Heller myotomy (LHM) for the treatment of type III achalasia in 75 patients: a multicenter comparative study. Endosc Int Open. 2015;3(3):E195–201.

30. Bhayani NH, Kurian AA, Dunst CM, Sharata AM, Rieder E, Swanstrom LL. A comparative study on comprehensive, objective outcomes of laparoscopic Heller myotomy with per-oral endoscopic myotomy (POEM) for achalasia. Ann Surg. 2014;259(6):1098–103.

31. Kahrilas PJ, Pandolfino JE. Treatments for achalasia in 2017: how to choose among them. Curr Opin Gastroenterol. 2017;33(4):270–6.

32. Inoue H, Sato H, Ikeda H, Onimaru M, Sato C, Minami H, et al. Per-Oral Endoscopic Myotomy: a series of 500 patients. J Am Coll Surg. 2015;221(2):256–64.

33. Perbtani YB, Mramba LK, Yang D, Suarez J, Draganov PV. Life after per-oral endoscopic Myotomy (POEM): long-term outcomes of quality of life and their association with Eckardt score. Gastrointest Endosc. 2018;87:1415.

34. Martinek J, Svecova H, Vackova Z, Dolezel R, Ngo O, Krajciova J, et al. Per-oral endoscopic myotomy (POEM): mid-term efficacy and safety. Surg Endosc. 2018;32(3):1293–302.

35. Dacha S, Wang L, Li X, Jiang Y, Philips G, Keilin SA, et al. Outcomes and quality of life assessment after per oral endoscopic myotomy (POEM) performed in the endoscopy unit with trainees. Surg Endosc. 2018;32:3046.

36. Li QL, Wu QN, Zhang XC, Xu MD, Zhang W, Chen SY, et al. Outcomes of per-oral endoscopic myotomy for treatment of esophageal achalasia with a median follow-up of 49 months. Gastrointest Endosc. 2018;87(6):1405–1412.e3.

37. Cotton PB, Eisen GM, Aabakken L, Baron TH, Hutter MM, Jacobson BC, et al. A lexicon for endoscopic adverse events: report of an ASGE workshop. Gastrointest Endosc. 2010;71(3):446–54.

38. Zhang XC, Li QL, Xu MD, Chen SY, Zhong YS, Zhang YQ, et al. Major perioperative adverse events of peroral endoscopic myotomy: a systematic 5-year analysis. Endoscopy. 2016;48(11):967–78.

39. Werner YB, Costamagna G, Swanstrom LL, von Renteln D, Familiari P, Sharata AM, et al. Clinical response to peroral endoscopic myotomy in patients with idiopathic achalasia at a minimum follow-up of 2 years. Gut. 2016;65(6):899–906.

40. Misra L, Fukami N, Nikolic K, Trentman TL. Peroral endoscopic myotomy: procedural complications and pain management for the perioperative clinician. Med Devices (Auckl). 2017;10:53–9.

41. Wang X, Tan Y, Zhang J, Liu D. Risk factors for gas-related complications of peroral endoscopic myotomy in achalasia. Neth J Med. 2015;73(2):76–81.

42. Ren Z, Zhong Y, Zhou P, Xu M, Cai M, Li L, et al. Perioperative management and treatment for complications during and after peroral endoscopic myotomy (POEM) for esophageal achalasia (EA) (data from 119 cases). Surg Endosc. 2012;26(11):3267–72.

43. Chung CS, Lin CK, Hsu WF, Lee TH, Wang HP, Liang CC. Education and imaging. Gastroenterology: pneumomediastinum and pneumoperitoneum after peroral endoscopic myotomy: complications or normal post-operative changes? J Gastroenterol Hepatol. 2015;30(10):1447.

44. Yang S, Zeng MS, Zhang ZY, Zhang HL, Liang L, Zhang XW. Pneumomediastinum and pneumoperitoneum on computed tomography after peroral endoscopic myotomy (POEM): postoperative changes or complications? Acta Radiol. 2015;56(10):1216–21.

45. Eleftheriadis N, Inoue H, Ikeda H, Onimaru M, Maselli R, Santi G. Submucosal tunnel endoscopy: Peroral endoscopic myotomy and peroral endoscopic tumor resection. World J Gastrointest Endosc. 2016;8(2):86–103.

46. Committee NPWP, Stavropoulos SN, Desilets DJ, Fuchs KH, Gostout CJ, Haber G, et al. Per-oral endoscopic myotomy white paper summary. Gastrointest Endosc. 2014;80(1):1–15.

47. American Society for Gastrointestinal Endoscopy PC, Chandrasekhara V, Desilets D, Falk GW, Inoue H, Romanelli JR, et al. The American Society for Gastrointestinal Endoscopy PIVI (Preservation and Incorporation of Valuable Endoscopic Innovations) on peroral endoscopic myotomy. Gastrointest Endosc. 2015;81(5):1087–100. e1

48. Akintoye E, Kumar N, Obaitan I, Alayo QA, Thompson CC. Peroral endoscopic myotomy: a meta-analysis. Endoscopy. 2016;48(12):1059–68.

49. Banks-Venegoni AL, Desilets DJ, Romanelli JR, Earle DB. Tension capnopericardium and cardiac arrest as an unexpected adverse event of peroral endoscopic myotomy (with video). Gastrointest Endosc. 2015;82(6):1137–9.

50. Loser B, Werner YB, Punke MA, Saugel B, Haas S, Reuter DA, et al. Anesthetic considerations for patients with esophageal achalasia undergoing peroral endoscopic myotomy: a retrospective case series review. Can J Anaesth. 2017;64(5):480–8.

51. Stavropoulos SN, Desilets DJ, Fuchs KH, Gostout CJ, Haber G, Inoue H, et al. Per-oral endoscopic myotomy white paper summary. Surg Endosc. 2014;28(7):2005–19.

52. Kumbhari V, Khashab MA. Peroral endoscopic myotomy. World J Gastrointest Endosc. 2015;7(5):496–509.

53. Li QL, Zhou PH, Yao LQ, Xu MD, Chen WF, Hu JW, et al. Early diagnosis and management of delayed bleeding in the submucosal tunnel after peroral endoscopic myotomy for achalasia (with video). Gastrointest Endosc. 2013;78(2):370–4.

54. Benech N, Pioche M, O'Brien M, Rivory J, Roman S, Mion F, et al. Esophageal hematoma after peroral endoscopic myotomy for achalasia in a patient on antiplatelet therapy. Endoscopy. 2015;47 Suppl 1 UCTN:E363–4.

55. Li QL, Zhou PH. Perspective on peroral endoscopic myotomy for achalasia: Zhongshan experience. Gut Liver. 2015;9(2):152–8.

56. Kurian AA, Bhayani NH, Reavis K, Dunst C, Swanstrom L. Endoscopic suture repair of full-thickness esophagotomy during per-oral esophageal myotomy for achalasia. Surg Endosc. 2013;27(10):3910.

57. Modayil R, Friedel D, Stavropoulos SN. Endoscopic suture repair of a large mucosal perforation during peroral endoscopic myotomy for treatment of achalasia. Gastrointest Endosc. 2014;80(6):1169–70.

58. Li H, Linghu E, Wang X. Fibrin sealant for closure of mucosal penetration at the cardia during peroral endoscopic myotomy (POEM). Endoscopy. 2012;44 Suppl 2 UCTN:E215–6.

59. Kumbhari V, Azola A, Saxena P, Modayil R, Kalloo AN, Stavropoulos SN, et al. Closure methods in submucosal endoscopy. Gastrointest Endosc. 2014;80(5):894–5.

60. Yang D, Zhang Q, Draganov PV. Successful placement of a fully covered esophageal stent to bridge a difficult-to-close mucosal incision during peroral endoscopic myotomy. Endoscopy. 2014;46 Suppl 1 UCTN:E467–8.

61. Ling T, Pei Q, Pan J, Zhang X, Lv Y, Li W, et al. Successful use of a covered, retrievable stent to seal a ruptured mucosal flap safety valve during per-oral endoscopic myotomy in a child with achalasia. Endoscopy. 2013;45 Suppl 2 UCTN:E63–4.

62. Khashab MA, Messallam AA, Saxena P, Kumbhari V, Ricourt E, Aguila G, et al. Jet injection of dyed saline facilitates efficient peroral endoscopic myotomy. Endoscopy. 2014;46(4):298–301.

63. Kumbhari V, Familiari P, Bjerregaard NC, Pioche M, Jones E, Ko WJ, et al. Gastroesophageal reflux after peroral endoscopic myotomy: a multicenter case-control study. Endoscopy. 2017;49(7):634–42.

64. Shiwaku H, Inoue H, Sasaki T, Yamashita K, Ohmiya T, Takeno S, et al. A prospective analysis of GERD after POEM on anterior myotomy. Surg Endosc. 2016;30(6):2496–504.

65. Repici A, Fuccio L, Maselli R, Mazza F, Correale L, Mandolesi D, et al. Gastroesophageal reflux disease after per-oral endoscopic myotomy as compared with Heller's myotomy with fundoplication: a systematic review with meta-analysis. Gastrointest Endosc. 2017;

66. Rosch T, Repici A, Boeckxstaens G. Will reflux kill POEM? Endoscopy. 2017;49(7):625–8.

67. Csendes A, Braghetto I, Burdiles P, Korn O, Csendes P, Henriquez A. Very late results of esophagomyotomy for patients with achalasia: clinical, endoscopic, histologic, manometric, and acid reflux studies in 67 patients for a mean follow-up of 190 months. Ann Surg. 2006;243(2):196–203.

68. Worrell SG, Alicuben ET, Boys J, DeMeester SR. Peroral Endoscopic Myotomy for achalasia in a thoracic surgical practice. Ann Thorac Surg. 2016;101(1):218–24. discussion 24-5

69. Rawlings A, Soper NJ, Oelschlager B, Swanstrom L, Matthews BD, Pellegrini C, et al. Laparoscopic Dor versus Toupet fundoplication following Heller myotomy for achalasia: results of a multicenter, prospective, randomized-controlled trial. Surg Endosc. 2012;26(1):18–26.

70. Khajanchee YS, Kanneganti S, Leatherwood AE, Hansen PD, Swanstrom LL. Laparoscopic Heller myotomy with Toupet fundoplication: outcomes predictors in 121 consecutive patients. Arch Surg. 2005;140(9):827–33; discussion 33–4

71. Schlottmann F, Luckett DJ, Fine J, Shaheen NJ, Patti MG. Laparoscopic Heller Myotomy versus Peroral Endoscopic Myotomy (POEM) for achalasia: a systematic review and meta-analysis. Ann Surg. 2018;267(3):451–60.

72. Richards WO, Sharp KW, Holzman MD. An antireflux procedure should not routinely be added to a Heller myotomy. J Gastrointest Surg. 2001;5(1):13–6.

73. Richards WO, Torquati A, Holzman MD, Khaitan L, Byrne D, Lutfi R, et al. Heller myotomy versus Heller myotomy with Dor fundoplication for achalasia: a prospective randomized double-blind clinical trial. Ann Surg. 2004;240(3):405–12; discussion 12–5

74. Torquati A, Lutfi R, Khaitan L, Sharp KW, Richards WO. Heller myotomy vs Heller myotomy plus Dor fundoplication: cost-utility analysis of a randomized trial. Surg Endosc. 2006;20(3):389–93.

75. Kummerow Broman K, Phillips SE, Faqih A, Kaiser J, Pierce RA, Poulose BK, et al. Heller myotomy versus Heller myotomy with Dor fundoplication for achalasia: long-term symptomatic follow-up of a prospective randomized controlled trial. Surg Endosc. 2018;32(4):1668–74.

76. Kumta NA, Kedia P, Sethi A, Kahaleh M. Transoral incisionless fundoplication for treatment of refractory GERD after peroral endoscopic myotomy. Gastrointest Endosc. 2015;81(1):224–5.

77. Onimaru M, Inoue H, Ikeda H, Sato C, Sato H, Phalanusitthepha C, et al. Greater curvature myotomy is a safe and effective modified technique in per-oral endoscopic myotomy (with videos). Gastrointest Endosc. 2015;81(6):1370–7.

78. Hochberger J, Kruse E, Wedi E, Buerrig KF, Dammer S, Koehler P, et al. Training in endoscopic mucosal resection and endoscopic submucosal dissection. In:

Cohen J, editor. Successful gastrointestinal endoscopy. Oxford, UK: Wiley-Blackwell; 2011. p. 204–37.

79. Stavropoulos SN, Modayil RJ, Friedel D, Savides T. The International Per Oral Endoscopic Myotomy Survey (IPOEMS): a snapshot of the global POEM experience. Surg Endosc. 2013;27(9):3322–38.

80. Hochberger J, Maiss J, Cohen J. Education and training in endoscopy. In: Wallace MB, Fockens P, Sung JJ, editors. Gastroenterological endoscopy. Stuttgart-New York: Thieme; 2018.

81. Committee ASoP, Faulx AL, Lightdale JR, Acosta RD, Agrawal D, Bruining DH, et al. Guidelines for privileging, credentialing, and proctoring to perform GI endoscopy. Gastrointest Endosc. 2017;85(2):273–81.

82. ASGE. ESD and POEM Course 2018. 2018. Available from: https://www.asge.org/home/education-meetings/advanced-education-training/clinical-courses/jges-masters-course-in-esd-with-optional-poem-add-on.

83. Ren Y, Tang X, Zhi F, Liu S, Wu J, Peng Y, et al. A stepwise approach for peroral endoscopic myotomy for treating achalasia: from animal models to patients. Scand J Gastroenterol. 2015;50(8):952–8.

84. Chiu PW, Wu JC, Teoh AY, Chan Y, Wong SK, Liu SY, et al. Peroral endoscopic myotomy for treatment of achalasia: from bench to bedside (with video). Gastrointest Endosc. 2013;77(1):29–38.

85. Hernandez Mondragon OV, Rascon Martinez DM, Munoz Bautista A, Altamirano Castaneda ML, Blanco-Velasco G, Blancas Valencia JM. The Per Oral Endoscopic Myotomy (POEM) technique: how many preclinical procedures are needed to master it? Endosc Int Open. 2015;3(6):E559–65.

86. Oyama T, Yahagi N, Ponchon T, Kiesslich T, Berr F. How to establish endoscopic submucosal dissection in Western countries. World J Gastroenterol: WJG. 2015;21(40):11209–20.

87. Patel KS, Calixte R, Modayil RJ, Friedel D, Brathwaite CE, Stavropoulos SN. The light at the end of the tunnel: a single-operator learning curve analysis for per oral endoscopic myotomy. Gastrointest Endosc. 2015;81(5):1181–7.

88. Kishiki T, Lapin B, Wang C, Jonson B, Patel L, Zapf M, et al. Teaching peroral endoscopic myotomy (POEM) to surgeons in practice: an "into the fire" pre/post-test curriculum. Surg Endosc. 2018;32(3):1414–21.

89. Committee AT, Adler DG, Bakis G, Coyle WJ, DeGregorio B, Dua KS, et al. Principles of training in GI endoscopy. Gastrointest Endosc. 2012;75(2):231–5.

Endoscopic Myotomy for Zenker's Diverticulum (Z-POEM)

20

Alessandro Fugazza, Roberta Maselli,
and Alessandro Repici

Introduction

Zenker's diverticulum (ZD) is a pulsion diverticulum that develops in an area of weakness of the posterior hypopharynx known as the Killian triangle. It is a relatively uncommon condition, with an overall prevalence estimated to be between 0.01% and 0.11% in the Western population, and occurs mainly in older patients (between the seventh and eighth decades) with a male predominance [1, 2].

The pathophysiology of ZD is not completely understood. The most widely accepted hypothesis is that an impaired relaxation of the cricopharyngeal muscle leads to chronically increased hypopharyngeal pressure facilitating the hernia-tion of the esophageal mucosa through the Killian triangle, thus resulting in a pulsion diverticulum [3–5].

ZD can be asymptomatic or can cause typical symptoms such as dysphagia, regurgitation, halitosis, chronic cough, foreign body sensation, aspiration pneumonia, and weight loss [6–8].

Symptoms are related to the accumulation of ingested material in the diverticular pouch and motor dysfunction with incomplete opening of the upper esophageal sphincter (UES) and are dependent on the size of the diverticulum. More rarely symptoms may be caused by extrinsic compression of the cervical esophagus by the diverticulum itself. As the diverticular sac enlarges, dysphagia may progressively increase leading to weight loss and malnutrition. Also aspiration pneumonia has been described as late-stage symptom in patients with severe impairment of swallowing capability and large diverticular pouch.

The diagnosis of ZD is based on clinical and radiographic findings, with barium esophagram being the confirmatory study [9] (Fig. 20.1). Even though barium study is important, dynamic continuous fluoroscopy at various stages of deglutition is also suggested as additional diagnostic procedure since static images may be insufficient in patients with small diverticulum. Moreover, evidence of overflow and aspiration can be clearly diagnosed with dynamic fluoroscopy.

Electronic Supplementary Material The online version of this chapter (https://doi.org/10.1007/978-3-030-21695-5_20) contains supplementary material, which is available to authorized users.

A. Fugazza (✉) · R. Maselli
Digestive Endoscopy Unit, Division of Gastroenterology, Humanitas Research Hospital, Rozzano, MI, Italy
e-mail: alessandro.fugazza@humanitas.it; roberta.maselli@humanitas.it

A. Repici
Digestive Endoscopy Unit, Division of Gastroenterology, Humanitas Research Hospital, Rozzano, MI, Italy

Humanitas University, Rozzano, MI, Italy
e-mail: alessandro.repici@hunimed.eu

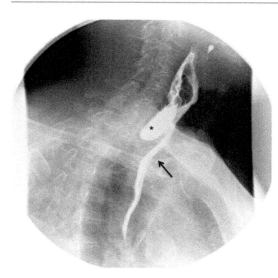

Fig. 20.1 Fluoroscopic image of a Zenker's diverticulum; asterisk, diverticular pouch; arrow, esophageal lumen

Treatment

The goal of the treatment of ZD is a cricopharyngeus muscle myotomy that may be realized surgically from the longitudinal layer of the muscle up to the submucosal plane or through the cutting of the septum between the diverticulum and the esophagus (septotomy) in case of transoral techniques [10, 11].

The decision on whether to use an open or transoral approach is related to several factors including anatomy and size of the diverticulum, patient's status and comorbidities, patient willingness, and finally local expertise.

In case of open surgery, the incision is usually performed along the anterior border of the sternocleidomastoid muscle, on the left of the neck, because the pouch expands preferentially in this location. Through this incision, the diverticulum is first exposed and then a contiguous tissue dissection is required to achieve adequate visualization of the neck of the diverticulum. At this point full-thickness careful myotomy is performed approximately 2 cm proximally into the constrictor to 5 cm distally into the proximal esophagus. The pouch is usually treated according to its size with either inversion or pexy. Only in case of

large pouch (>5 cm) the diverticulum is typically resected with closure of the opening by a linear stapling device. However, open surgery may be complicated by significant rates of morbidity and mortality, particularly because most patients with the disease are elderly and already have several comorbidities [12].

Transoral approach, which entails transoral division of the septum through rigid endoscope, or flexible endoscopy, has gained increased popularity in the last 20 years.

The rationale is that a septum containing the cricopharyngeal muscle divides the diverticulum sac from the esophagus. By dividing this wall, the cricopharyngeal muscle is incised and released from its high pressure, and the diverticulum is marsupialized thus becoming a unique cavity with the esophagus and eliminating food entrapment and relieving the outflow obstruction.

Septotomy performed by a rigid endoscope, first reported simultaneously in 1993 by Collard in Belgium [13] and Martin Hirsch in England [14], is based on a transoral single-stage cut and suture technique using a laparoscopic stapler introduced through a rigid endoscope. It is considered more suitable and preferable when compared with open surgery due to quicker diet resumption, lower adverse events rates, and shorter inpatient stay [15, 16].

However, approaches using rigid endoscopy have several limitations, including the need for general anesthesia and significant rates of intraoperative failure (5–10%), mainly in cases of small diverticular size (<3 cm) or because of restricted neck mobility or inadequate jaw opening preventing the advancement of the rigid diverticuloscope into the pharynx [15].

Flexible Endoscopic Myotomy

Flexible endoscopic (FE) myotomy, published for the first time in 1995 [17, 18], is less invasive than the two former techniques, can be performed without general anesthesia (necessary in the surgical approach), and does not require neck hyperextension (necessary for the rigid endoscopic procedure) [18–20]. The procedure can

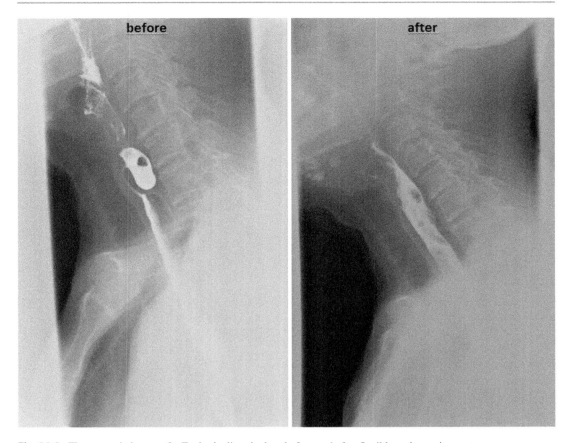

Fig. 20.2 Fluoroscopic image of a Zenker's diverticulum before and after flexible endoscopic myotomy

be safely performed in the endoscopy suite, in the inpatient or outpatient setting. Some centers offer the FE option to all ZD symptomatic patients, although most authors recommend reserving it for selected patients, especially high-risk elderly patients, poor surgical candidates who are expected to benefit the most from this technique [21].

The obvious advantages of FE over the conventional open surgical approach are the absence of cutaneous incision, shorter operative time, reduced postoperative discomfort, faster return to oral feeding, and shorter length of hospital stay [22].

FE septotomy involves an incision of the mucosa and the muscular fibers that form the diverticular septum. Flexible endoscopy shares the same principles and rationale as rigid endoscopy: the septum between the diverticulum and the esophagus contains the cricopharyngeal muscle, and by cutting the septum and creating a common cavity, a myotomy is automatically performed (Fig. 20.2).

Unfortunately, there is a lack of agreement on who are the best candidates for flexible endoscopic treatment. As a general principle, small–medium-sized (up to 5 cm) diverticula are best approached endoscopically either with rigid or flexible technique, while small-sized ZD (up to 3 cm) may be best amenable by flexible endoscopy because of the impossibility to properly accommodate the stapler which is currently longer than 3 cm. For large diverticula there may still be space for open surgical excision, especially in younger, good surgical candidates, even though long septum typically allows for long complete flexible myotomy with excellent resolution of symptoms (personal experience, no published data).

Since its introduction, many variations of the technique have been reported and a wide array of cutting devices have been used.

Technique

Patients are placed in a left lateral decubitus position under conscious or deep sedation. Differences in the sedation approach for these patients have been recorded in the published papers with several authors still preferring to perform this technique under general anesthesia [22] and some others being more keen to use propofol-based deep sedation in the majority of patients.

Antibiotic prophylaxis is not routinely administered.

The procedure is usually done with a standard flexible scope and begins with initial endoscopic examination of the pouch, estimation of the pouch and septum, and finally suctioning of possible retained material from the diverticulum. Prior to performing the procedure, it is a common practice to introduce a nasogastric or orogastric tube via a guidewire previously endoscopically advanced in the stomach. It serves to constantly recognize the esophageal lumen during myotomy. It allows enhanced visualization of the esophageal lumen and diverticulum, and it protects the anterior esophageal wall from injury from instruments used during myotomy [23].

Most frequently, a standard transparent cap or a dedicated hood with oblique design placed on the tip of the endoscope has been used with similar intentions [24] of enhancing visualization, improving scope stability, and stretching the septum at the time of its incision.

More rarely, instead of the orogastric tube, some experts use a soft diverticuloscope (Zenker's diverticulum overtube, ZDO-22-30; Cook Medical, Winston-Salem, North Carolina) to stabilize and visualize the septum (Fig. 20.3). The diverticuloscope is placed as an overtube on the endoscope and contains two distal flaps that serve to straddle the septum and safeguard the anterior esophageal wall and posterior diverticular wall.

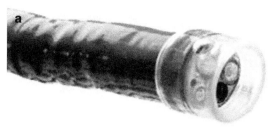
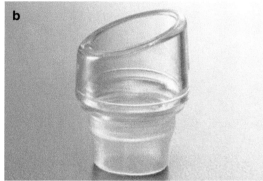
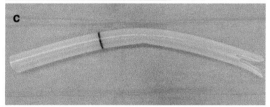

Fig. 20.3 (**a**) Standard transparent cap placed on the tip of the endoscope. (**b**) Dedicated hood with oblique design placed. (**c**) Soft diverticuloscope

Even though diverticuloscope may potentially improve the maneuverability with lower complication rates compared with the use of a transparent cap or no device, there are no significant differences in clinical outcomes with the use of one or other accessories [24–27].

However, it is worth noting that the diverticuloscope is only commercially available in Canada and Europe.

Regardless of different accessories that can be selected to improve septum exposure, different cutting techniques and devices can be used (needle knife, hook knife, monopolar forceps, argon plasma coagulation) depending on physicians' personal experience and preferences. The most commonly used devices are hook knife and the needle knife (Olympus Medical, Tokyo, Japan) [11, 17, 20, 25, 27, 28]. The technique with the needle knife of a single incision alongside the midline of the diverticular septum, through blended current coagulation, is shown in Video 20.1. The incision is distally directed toward the bottom of the pouch, by moving the tip of the endoscope, hence the tip of the needle.

Nevertheless using the hook knife (Olympus Medical, Tokyo, Japan), a potentially more complete myotomy can be achieved since the muscular fibers at the bottom of the septum may be gently pulled upward using the hook part of the knife before cutting, allowing very precise dissection [11, 29] (Fig. 20.4).

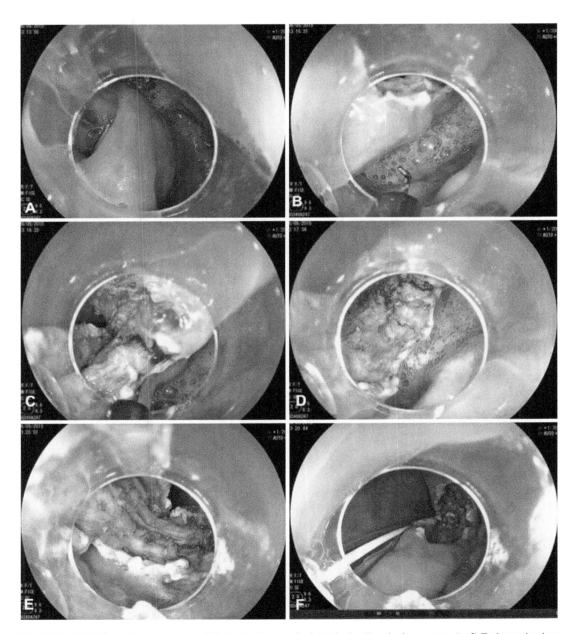

Fig. 20.4 (a) Endoscopic appearance of Zenker's diverticulum with orogastric tube in the lumen of the esophagus. (b) The hook knife used to perform the endoscopic incision in the diverticular septum. (c, d) Endoscopic view of the exposed muscular fibers of the cricopharyngeal muscle. (e, f) Septum completely divided

At the end of the cut, one or more endoclips are placed to prevent delayed perforation or bleeding.

Additional approaches used to divide the septum include monopolar and bipolar forceps, argon plasma coagulation, harmonic scalpels, and stapling devices, the latter two of which are advanced alongside the scope and not through the working channel of the scope. The optimal cutting technique remains quite elusive because of the lack of comparative trials among different endoscopic techniques.

More recently, some researchers reported a number of technique modifications such as the use of a stag beetle knife (SB Knife, Sumitomo Bakelite, Tokyo, Japan) with two insulated monopolar blades, which facilitates the procedure of "grasp and cut" [30], or using a stag beetle knife where two parallel incisions on the septum are performed to dissect the mucosa and the horizontal fibers of the cricopharyngeal muscle and the septum in between is removed with the aid of a polypectomy snare [31, 32].

Outcome

Available data from previous series suggest that adequate treatment can be provided in one to two treatment sessions with a quite high rate of clinical resolution of symptoms and a low rate of diverticular recurrence. Most of the studies report a clinical resolution rate of about 90%. However most of these studies are retrospective and comparison among different studies is biased by the lack of universally agreed formal definitions of clinical success.

Improvement in symptoms can be evaluated through different scores which try to include the different symptoms related to the diverticulum and make more reliable and standardized the evaluation of clinical outcome especially in the long term [33–35].

A recent meta-analysis showed that FE myotomy for ZD is effective and safe. The overall initial treatment success rate ranged from 56.4% to 100%, whereas the success rate of studies where a comprehensive evaluation of ZD symptoms

was carried out ranged from 56.4% to 96.6% [36].

In particular the meta-regression analyses for overall safety show that the cutting device, diverticulum size, or sedation was not associated with the outcomes of the procedure.

Adverse event rates ranged from 0% to 36.4%, with a median of 14.1%. The most frequently reported adverse event was perforation which occurred in 41 patients overall (6.5%).

Other common adverse events include hemorrhage, pneumonia, fever, emphysema, bleeding, and neck abscess.

Flexible endoscopy is associated with a clinical recurrence rate ranging from 0% to 32%, with a random effects pooled rate estimate of 11% [36]. The risk of recurrence of the symptoms is mainly related to the lack of the completeness of the incision which leaves a substantial amount of muscle active and responsible of recurrent symptoms. Changes in the motor activity of the esophagus (hypertonus), individual anatomical features of the diverticulum (such as a wide and deep diverticulum), and the diverticulum's relationship to the esophageal wall (a semi-lateral or lateral location) may also contribute to the likelihood of the disease recurrence.

Repeat endoscopic treatment, in case of treatment failure or symptoms recurrence, can easily and successfully be achieved with significant improvement in the majority of treated patients.

However, with the available literature, it is challenging to analyze the real recurrence rate since there exists a high heterogeneity across studies, with a mean follow-up duration which ranges from 7 months to 43 months [36].

Z-POEM

Recent advances in natural orifice transluminal endoscopic surgery (NOTES) have given rise to novel myotomy techniques including peroral endoscopic myotomy (POEM) [37].

Recently, some authors have reported a novel technique called the submucosal tunneling endoscopic septum division (STESD) [38–40] or so-called Z-POEM, inspired by the POEM technique.

The theoretical advantage is to completely dissect the muscular septum through a submucosal tunnel while maintaining the mucosal integrity. This procedure has the potential to reduce the risk of perforation and mediastinitis and the rate of recurrence [38].

The Z-POEM procedure includes four steps [38, 39]:

1. *Mucosal Incision*:
   Submucosal injection is performed 3 cm proximal to the diverticular septum, and a 1.5–2.0-cm longitudinal mucosal incision is performed for the tunnel entry.
2. *Submucosal Tunneling*:
   A submucosal longitudinal tunnel is created by using a technique similar to endoscopic submucosal dissection between the mucosal and muscular layers. Tunneling is performed at both sides of the septum and ends 1–2 cm distal to the bottom of the diverticulum, in the esophageal side, to ensure a satisfactory endoscopic view and enough working space for the myotomy.
3. *Septum Division*:
   Cricopharyngeal muscle fibers of the septum are dissected down to the bottom of the diverticulum and further into the normal esophageal muscle.
4. *Mucosal Closure*:
   The mucosal incision site is closed with several hemostatic clips.

However in the available literature, only case reports [38, 39] and case series [40] are available showing a potential promising approach in the treatment of a subgroup of patients with ZD.

Therefore further studies are required to validate this technique in terms of outcome and safety comparing it with classic FE myotomy.

Conclusion

Due to heterogeneity of data and lack of standardized protocols, a direct comparison of the various techniques is difficult. The literature is mainly based on retrospective case series or com-parative case series, and the optimal treatment modality has not yet been established. The choice between the different approaches depends on local expertise and preferences. However, based on retrospective literature results, appropriate technique selection dictated by the size of the diverticulum and the patient's conditions is necessary.

Prospective clinical studies are required to establish the best treatment for Zenker's diverticulum.

References

1. Wheeler D. Diverticula of the foregut. Radiology. 1947;49(4):476–82.
2. Maran AG, Wilson JA, Al Muhanna AH. Pharyngeal diverticula. Clin Otolaryngol Allied Sci. 1986;11(4):219–25.
3. Cook IJ, Gabb M, Panagopoulos V, Jamieson GG, Dodds WJ, Dent J, et al. Pharyngeal (Zenker's) diverticulum is a disorder of upper esophageal sphincter opening. Gastroenterology. 1992;103(4):1229–35.
4. Fulp SR, Castell DO. Manometric aspects of Zenker's diverticulum. Hepato-Gastroenterology. 1992;39(2):123–6.
5. Brueckner J, Schneider A, Messmann H, Golder SK. Long-term symptomatic control of Zenker diverticulum by flexible endoscopic mucomy-otomy with the hook knife and predisposing factors for clinical recurrence. Scand J Gastroenterol. 2016;51(6):666–71.
6. Bizzotto A, Iacopini F, Landi R, Costamagna G. Zenker's diverticulum: exploring treatment options. Acta Otorhinolaryngol Ital. 2013;33(4):219–29.
7. Dzeletovic I, Ekbom DC, Baron TH. Flexible endoscopic and surgical management of Zenker's diverticulum. Expert Rev Gastroenterol Hepatol. 2012;6(4):449–65; quiz 66
8. Negus VE. Pharyngeal diverticula; observations on their evolution and treatment. Br J Surg. 1950;38(150):129–46.
9. Mantsopoulos K, Psychogios G, Karatzanis A, Kunzel J, Lell M, Zenk J, et al. Clinical relevance and prognostic value of radiographic findings in Zenker's diverticulum. Eur Arch Otorhinolaryngol. 2014;271(3):583–8.
10. van Overbeek JJ. Pathogenesis and methods of treatment of Zenker's diverticulum. Ann Otol Rhinol Laryngol. 2003;112(7):583–93.
11. Repici A, Pagano N, Romeo F, Danese S, Arosio M, Rando G, et al. Endoscopic flexible treatment of Zenker's diverticulum: a modification of the needle-knife technique. Endoscopy. 2010;42(7):532–5.

12. Repici A. Endoscopic treatment of zenker diverticulum. Gastroenterol Hepatol. 2010;6(10):628–30.

13. Collard JM, Otte JB, Kestens PJ. Endoscopic stapling technique of esophagodiverticulostomy for Zenker's diverticulum. Ann Thorac Surg. 1993;56(3):573–6.

14. Martin-Hirsch DP, Newbegin CJ. Autosuture GIA gun: a new application in the treatment of hypopharyngeal diverticula. J Laryngol Otol. 1993;107(8):723–5.

15. Keck T, Rozsasi A, Grun PM. Surgical treatment of hypopharyngeal diverticulum (Zenker's diverticulum). Eur Arch Otorhinolaryngol. 2010;267(4):587–92.

16. Chang CY, Payyapilli RJ, Scher RL. Endoscopic staple diverticulostomy for Zenker's diverticulum: review of literature and experience in 159 consecutive cases. Laryngoscope. 2003;113(6):957–65.

17. Ishioka S, Sakai P, Maluf Filho F, Melo JM. Endoscopic incision of Zenker's diverticula. Endoscopy. 1995;27(6):433–7.

18. Mulder CJ, den Hartog G, Robijn RJ, Thies JE. Flexible endoscopic treatment of Zenker's diverticulum: a new approach. Endoscopy. 1995;27(6):438–42.

19. Mulder CJ, Costamagna G, Sakai P. Zenker's diverticulum: treatment using a flexible endoscope. Endoscopy. 2001;33(11):991–7.

20. Case DJ, Baron TH. Flexible endoscopic management of Zenker diverticulum: the Mayo Clinic experience. Mayo Clin Proc. 2010;85(8):719–22.

21. Ferreira LE, Simmons DT, Baron TH. Zenker's diverticula: pathophysiology, clinical presentation, and flexible endoscopic management. Dis Esophagus. 2008;21(1):1–8.

22. Aiolfi A, Scolari F, Saino G, Bonavina L. Current status of minimally invasive endoscopic management for Zenker diverticulum. World J Gastrointest Endos. 2015;7(2):87–93.

23. Perbtani Y, Suarez A, Wagh MS. Techniques and efficacy of flexible endoscopic therapy of Zenker's diverticulum. World J Gastrointest Endosc. 2015;7(3):206–12.

24. Rabenstein T, May A, Michel J, Manner H, Pech O, Gossner L, et al. Argon plasma coagulation for flexible endoscopic Zenker's diverticulotomy. Endoscopy. 2007;39(2):141–5.

25. Costamagna G, Iacopini F, Tringali A, Marchese M, Spada C, Familiari P, et al. Flexible endoscopic Zenker's diverticulotomy: cap-assisted technique vs. diverticuloscope-assisted technique. Endoscopy. 2007;39(2):146–52.

26. Mulder CJ. Zapping Zenker's diverticulum: gastroscopic treatment. Can J Gastroenterol. 1999;13(5):405–7.

27. Sakai P, Ishioka S, Maluf-Filho F, Chaves D, Moura EG. Endoscopic treatment of Zenker's diverticulum with an oblique-end hood attached to the endoscope. Gastrointest Endosc. 2001;54(6):760–3.

28. Vogelsang A, Preiss C, Neuhaus H, Schumacher B. Endotherapy of Zenker's diverticulum using the needle-knife technique: long-term follow-up. Endoscopy. 2007;39(2):131–6.

29. Rouquette O, Abergel A, Mulliez A, Poincloux L. Usefulness of the hook knife in flexible endoscopic myotomy for Zenker's diverticulum. World JGastrointest Endosc. 2017;9(8):411–6.

30. Ramchandani M, Nageshwar Reddy D. New endoscopic "scissors" to treat Zenker's diverticulum (with video). Gastrointest Endosc. 2013;78(4):645–8.

31. Battaglia G, Antonello A, Realdon S, Cesarotto M, Zanatta L, Ishaq S. Flexible endoscopic treatment for Zenker's diverticulum with the SB knife. Preliminary results from a single-center experience. Digestive endoscopy. 2015;27(7):728–33.

32. Goelder SK, Brueckner J, Messmann H. Endoscopic treatment of Zenker's diverticulum with the stag beetle knife (sb knife) – feasibility and follow-up. Scand J Gastroenterol. 2016;51(10):1155–8.

33. Dakkak M, Bennett JR. A new dysphagia score with objective validation. J Clin Gastroenterol. 1992;14(2):99–100.

34. McHorney CA, Robbins J, Lomax K, Rosenbek JC, Chignell K, Kramer AE, et al. The SWAL-QOL and SWAL-CARE outcomes tool for oropharyngeal dysphagia in adults: III. Documentation of reliability and validity. Dysphagia. 2002;17(2):97–114.

35. Costamagna G, Iacopini F, Bizzotto A, Familiari P, Tringali A, Perri V, et al. Prognostic variables for the clinical success of flexible endoscopic septotomy of Zenker's diverticulum. Gastrointest Endosc. 2016;83(4):765–73.

36. Ishaq S, Hassan C, Antonello A, Tanner K, Bellisario C, Battaglia G, et al. Flexible endoscopic treatment for Zenker's diverticulum: a systematic review and meta-analysis. Gastrointest Endosc. 2016;83(6):1076–89 e5.

37. Inoue H, Minami H, Kobayashi Y, Sato Y, Kaga M, Suzuki M, et al. Peroral endoscopic myotomy (POEM) for esophageal achalasia. Endoscopy. 2010;42(4):265–71.

38. Li QL, Chen WF, Zhang XC, Cai MY, Zhang YQ, Hu JW, et al. Submucosal tunneling endoscopic septum division: a novel technique for treating Zenker's diverticulum. Gastroenterology. 2016;151(6):1071–4.

39. Brieau B, Leblanc S, Bordacahar B, Barret M, Coriat R, Prat F, et al. Submucosal tunneling endoscopic septum division for Zenker's diverticulum: a reproducible procedure for endoscopists who perform peroral endoscopic myotomy. Endoscopy. 2017;49(6):613–4.

40. Cai M, Xu M, Li Q, Chen W, Zhu Y, Zhang D, et al. Preliminary results of submucosal tunneling endoscopic septum division in the treatment of esophageal diverticulum. Zhonghua Wei Chang Wai Ke Za Zhi. 2017;20(5):530–4.

Per-Oral Endoscopic Pyloromyotomy (G-POEM) and Per-Rectal Endoscopic Myotomy (PREM)

21

Amol Bapaye and Amit Maydeo

Per-oral Endoscopic Pyloromyotomy (G-POEM, POEP, POP)

Introduction

Gastroparesis is defined as a clinical syndrome of objectively delayed gastric emptying in the absence of mechanical obstruction and cardinal symptoms including early satiety, post-prandial fullness, nausea, vomiting, bloating, and abdominal pain [1, 2]. Prevalence in the general population varies from 0.2% to 5% [1]. Gastroparesis significantly affects quality of life (QOL) [3]. Hospitalizations, emergency room visits, and doctor consultations for gastroparesis have shown a significant rise; and it has also been shown to be associated with increased morbidity and mortality [4, 5].

The common etiological factors for gastroparesis include diabetes (types I and II), post-viral

infections, and post-operative or idiopathic causes. Gastroparesis has also been reported in patients with thyroid disorders, Parkinson's disease, paraneoplastic syndromes, and early scleroderma [1, 6].

Pharmacological therapy for gastroparesis is limited. Metoclopramide is the only drug that is USFDA-approved; and it has a black box warning due to the risk of tardive dyskinesia and a recommendation that it should not be used continuously for more than 3 months [7].

Endoscopic and surgical interventions for gastroparesis have revolved around relaxation, distension, or destruction of the pyloric sphincter. Intra-pyloric injection of botulinum toxin, though initially thought effective, was later proved to have results similar to placebo in two controlled trials [8, 9]. Surgical pyloroplasty was shown to be effective to alleviate symptoms in patients with refractory gastroparesis [10]. Similarly, trans-pyloric stent placement has shown good short-term clinical benefit, although stent migration is frequently noted and may necessitate re-interventions [11, 12].

Gastric electrical stimulation is a promising alternative; however, data is still evolving and the device is FDA-approved for only humanitarian use under research protocol settings [13]. Also, the procedure is invasive, requiring surgical implantation of the device and necessitating hospitalization.

Electronic Supplementary Material The online version of this chapter (https://doi.org/10.1007/978-3-030-21695-5_21) contains supplementary material, which is available to authorized users.

A. Bapaye (✉)
Shivanand Desai Center for Digestive Disorders, Deenanath Mangeshkar Hospital and Research Center, Pune, India

A. Maydeo
Baldota Institute of Digestive Sciences, Global Hospital, Mumbai, India

© Springer Nature Switzerland AG 2020
M. S. Wagh, S. B. Wani (eds.), *Gastrointestinal Interventional Endoscopy*,
https://doi.org/10.1007/978-3-030-21695-5_21

All the above mentioned interventions for gastroparesis have either shown limited success or have limited applicability. Based on the success of surgical pyloroplasty (invasive) and transpyloric stenting (migration risk), gastric per-oral endoscopic pyloromyotomy (G-POEM) was described since it provides a minimally invasive and yet effective dehiscence of the pyloric sphincter.

Principle of G-POEM

G-POEM is based on principles of submucosal tunneling endoscopy. After Inoue et al. described the first human series of per-oral endoscopic myotomy (POEM) for achalasia cardia in 2010 [14], Khashab et al. conceptualized and performed pyloromyotomy through a submucosal gastric tunnel in 2013 using the same principle of the submucosal tunneling approach [12]. One year earlier, Kawai et al. had hypothesized and described this technique in porcine models [15]. The submucosal tunnel with the mucosal flap valve permits access to the submucosal and deeper muscle layers of the stomach and pylorus, at the same time protecting against a full-thickness perforation. An endoscopic submucosal pyloromyotomy can thus be achieved safely without the risk of a full-thickness perforation.

Patient Selection and Pre-procedure Workup

Symptomatology of Gastroparesis

Diagnosis of gastroparesis is mainly clinical and based on symptoms. The common symptoms reported include nausea, vomiting, and post-prandial bloating. Pain is less frequent although it has been reported. Severe cases may present with malnutrition, weight loss, and/or dehydration.

Gastroparesis Cardinal Symptom Index (GCSI)

The Gastroparesis Cardinal Symptom Index (GCSI) is a clinical score that is calculated to assess the severity of symptoms. GCSI is based on three sub-scales – post-prandial fullness/early satiety (four items), nausea/vomiting (three items), and bloating (two items); each item is being scored from 0 to 5. The total score is calculated and correlates with symptom severity (Table 21.1) [16].

EGD and Imaging

Although most patients would have undergone an EGD earlier during the evaluation, EGD is important to rule out mechanical factors contributing to the gastric outlet obstruction, e.g., duodenal or pyloric ulcers, infiltrating malignancy, or extrinsic compression from surrounding structures.

Table 21.1 Gastric Cardinal Symptom Index[a]

	Symptom	None	Very mild	Mild	Moderate	Severe	Very severe
1	Nausea (feeling sick to your stomach as if you were going vomit or throw up)	0	1	2	3	4	5
2	Retching (heaving as if to vomit, but nothing comes up)	0	1	2	3	4	5
3	Vomiting	0	1	2	3	4	5
4	Stomach fullness	0	1	2	3	4	5
5	Not able to finish a normal-sized meal	0	1	2	3	4	5
6	Feeling excessively full after meals	0	1	2	3	4	5
7	Loss of appetite	0	1	2	3	4	5
8	Bloating (feeling like you need to loosen your clothes)	0	1	2	3	4	5
9	Stomach or belly visibly larger	0	1	2	3	4	5

For each symptom, please circle the number that best describes how severe the symptom has been during the past 2 weeks. If you have not experienced this symptom, circle 0. If the symptom has been very mild, circle 1. If the symptom has been mild, circle 2. If it has been moderate, circle 3. If it has been severe, circle 4. If it has been very severe, circle 5. Please be sure to answer every question
Please rate the severity of the following symptoms during the past 2 weeks
[a]This questionnaire asks you about the severity of symptoms you may have related to your gastrointestinal problem. There are no right or wrong answers. Please answer each question as accurately as possible

EGD can also assess the amount of gastric food stasis, which must be cleared before performing G-POEM.

CECT of the abdomen is often performed to rule out compression by extrinsic mass lesions and/or to also rule out proximal bowel obstruction which may sometimes mimic the symptoms of gastroparesis.

Gastric Emptying Scintigraphy (GES)
The conventional test for assessment of gastroparesis is gastric emptying scintigraphy (GES). GES is performed using a ^{99m}Tc-sulfur colloid-labeled solid meal and is reported as the percent gastric retention at 1, 2, and 4 h [1]. More than 30% gastric retention is considered clinically significant. Patients must stop prokinetics or other medications that can interfere with gastric motility before they are subjected to GES.

EndoFlip and Pyloric Manometry
EndoFlip estimates the distensibility of the pylorus, whereas pyloric manometry can estimate the extent of pylorospasm. These tests, although described, are not routinely available, and their role in clinical management is unclear and uncommon.

Other less frequently performed tests include wireless motility capsule (WMC) (that measures pH, pressure, and temperature and assesses gastric emptying by the acidic gastric residence time) and breath testing (using 13C-octanoate or spirulina) [1].

Other Biochemical and Metabolic Workups
Patients must be evaluated for their diabetic status, presence of possible hypothyroidism, and other metabolic workups to identify the potential etiology of gastroparesis. Investigations to assess for fitness for general anesthesia are required; and metabolic abnormalities, especially electrolyte nutritional imbalance, must be optimally corrected before the patient can be scheduled for G-POEM.

Although not mandatory, most centers may offer a therapeutic trial of diet modulation, prokinetics, or even a trans-pyloric stent placement to assess symptom relief before scheduling G-POEM.

Technique and Variations of G-POEM

G-POEM is a relatively new and evolving procedure. The technique is therefore also evolving, and many operators are likely to have their own preferences when performing this procedure. The description that follows is one that the authors perform on a regular basis. Suitable variations based on individual anatomy and circumstances may be implemented depending on the operator's understanding and training of the subject.

It is also important to note that G-POEM is a complex flexible endoscopic surgical procedure using the principles of third space endoscopy with inherent risks; and written, pictorial, and video descriptions cannot be a substitute for appropriate supervised training and credentialing for performance of third space endoscopy techniques.

Prerequisites and Preliminary Considerations
1. G-POEM is performed under general anesthesia.
2. Patients must be fasting overnight at least for 12 h; those with significant gastric stasis may require longer periods of fasting. A screening EGD is performed to confirm that the stomach is empty of all food and fluid residue.
3. In patients with significant gastric solid food residue, it may be necessary to clean the stomach by nasogastric or endoscopic lavage 1 or 2 days prior to G-POEM.
4. Unlike POEM, G-POEM may be performed in either the supine or the left lateral position. We prefer the supine position in most situations except when the stomach is grossly dilated, wherein the position of the antrum and pylorus is more accessible in the left lateral position.

Instrumentation
1. High-definition gastroscope (GIF-HQ190, Olympus Corp., Tokyo, Japan).
2. Transparent distal attachment (Olympus) – various shapes are available; our preference is the straight cap.
3. Carbon dioxide insufflator.

4. Endoscope flushing pump.
5. Injector needle 25G with short bevel.
6. Injectate – normal saline stained with indigo carmine or methylene blue solution. Do ensure that the solution is light sky blue in color and is not very dark, as a dark solution hampers dissection and hemostasis within the tunnel.
7. Diathermy settings – ERBE Vio II™ (200D or 300D) or Vio III™ workstation (ERBE GmBH, Tubingen, Germany):
   (a) Incision – EndoCut™ effect, 2; cut duration, 3; cut interval, 3
   (b) Submucosal dissection – spray coagulation, 50W; effect, 2. Or forced coagulation, 60W; effect, 2
   (c) Coagulation – soft coagulation, 80W; effect, 4
   (d) Myotomy – spray coagulation, 50W; effect, 2. Or forced coagulation, 60W; effect, 2
8. Alternatively, ESG 400™ (Olympus) diathermy can also be used.
9. Knife – a choice of knives is available. The most commonly used knives are the HybridKnife™ (ERBE GmBH) or the triangular tip (TT) Knife™ (Olympus). The HybridKnife™ has to be used in conjunction with the ERBEJet™ injector workstation that has the ability for high-pressure injection resulting in rapid mucosal elevation, and the knife can inject and cut using the same instrument. An injector version of the TT Knife™ is also available in some countries – TT-J Knife™ (Olympus). The TT-J Knife™ permits injection and cutting using the same instrument similar to the HybridKnife.
10. Insulated tip (IT)-2™ Knife (Olympus) – for dissection at the pylorus and myotomy.
11. Hemostatic forceps – Coagrasper™ (Olympus).
12. Closure devices:
   (a) Mucosal clips (Olympus, Boston Scientific Corporation, Cook, or similar).
   (b) Over-the-scope clips (OTSC™ clip, Ovesco, Germany) or Padlock™ (US Endoscopy, USA) are preferred by some operators.
   (c) Endoscopic suturing (OverStitch™, Apollo Endosurgery Inc., USA) is also an alternative if closure is difficult using clips.

The G-POEM Procedure (Video 21.1)

1. The air pump on the endoscope processor is turned off and carbon dioxide is used for insufflation.
2. After a screening EGD, the endoscope is withdrawn into the gastric antrum.
3. A mucosal incision site is selected approximately 3–5 cm proximal to the pylorus.
4. Submucosal injection is performed using a 23 or 25G injector needle to raise a sizeable submucosal cushion (Fig. 21.1). It is recommended to inject approximately 20–25 ml of injectate to raise this cushion. Smaller volumes may also be used but the elevation can disappear rapidly and make entry into the submucosal tunnel difficult.
5. A longitudinal mucosal incision approximately 15–20 mm in length is made using either the HybridKnife™ or TT Knife™ and the diathermy settings are done as described above. Gastric mucosa is thicker than esophageal mucosa and therefore the cut should be deep enough for the blue-stained submucosa to be visible (Fig. 21.2). A good mucosal

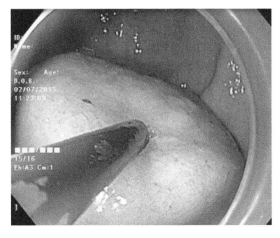

Fig. 21.1 Submucosal cushion created in the distal antrum approximately 6 cm proximal to the pylorus

incision is one that cuts the mucosa and muscularis mucosae so that the mucosal edges separate and the stained submucosa is visible.

6. Some workers prefer a transverse incision to a longitudinal one because it is easier to close the incision using the OverStitch™ device (Apollo Endosurgery Inc., USA).

7. Using the principle of POEM, the mucosal edges are undermined to create space in the submucosa, especially toward the apex of the incision. Care must be taken to ensure that the muscle layer is not damaged during this step; otherwise there is a risk of full-thickness perforation (Fig. 21.3).

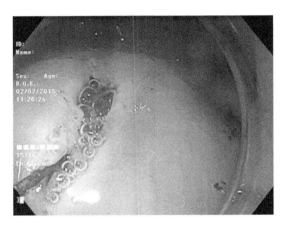

Fig. 21.2 A triangular tip knife is used to make a longitudinal incision on the elevated mucosa

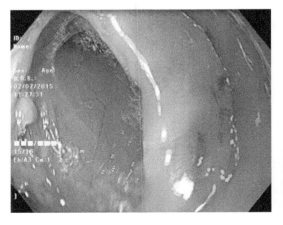

Fig. 21.3 The mucosal edges are undermined by dissecting the submucosa, thereby creating space to introduce the endoscope into the tunnel

8. Once adequate space has been created, the gastroscope is gently maneuvered using rotatory and pushing movement using the big wheel and shaft so that the scope enters the submucosal space. The stomach is a much roomier organ than the esophagus, and therefore the scope may require some maneuvering before one can enter the tunnel. A simple trick is to tip the scope down in such a manner that the mucosal flap disappears from the screen and then the scope is pushed further. This prevents the scope from slipping out into the gastric cavity.

9. Once inside the tunnel, dissection is continued in a plane close to the muscle layer so that the circular muscle fibers are clearly visible. Gastric submucosa is much thicker and fibrotic as compared to esophageal submucosa which is supple. Point to note is that if the circular muscle fibers are not seen, it is likely that the plane of dissection is superficial and needs correction (Fig. 21.4).

10. Gastric submucosa is also quite vascular. Submucosal vessels in the stomach often require formal coagulation using Coagrasper™ rather than contact coagulation by the knife.

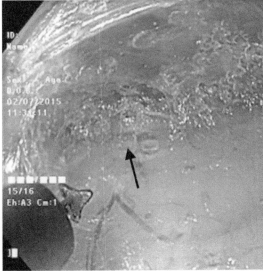

Fig. 21.4 Submucosal dissection is performed in a direction perpendicular to the circular muscle fibers (arrow)

11. Dissection is performed in a direction perpendicular to the circular muscle fibers. Stomach is a roomy organ and your tunnel needs to narrow down and point toward the pylorus. Unless the direction of dissection is carefully monitored, it is easy to lose direction. Frequently withdrawing the endoscope from the tunnel into the gastric lumen to check the direction of dissection is helpful.

12. Tunnel length for G-POEM is much shorter as compared to esophageal POEM; and unless the direction is wayward, one should reach the pylorus quite quickly.

13. Identification of the pylorus/pyloric ring – this is the most crucial step of the procedure (Fig. 21.5). As dissection progresses toward the pylorus, the circular muscle fibers start narrowing down to form a tight ring at the pylorus. A change in the mucosa is also seen, which becomes initially more adherent and then suddenly thins out beyond the ring. This is the undersurface of the duodenal mucosa as seen from the tunnel. Dissection at the level of the pyloric ring can be difficult as the duodenal mucosa is firmly adherent to the circular muscle; repeated injections and patient dissection are the key to circumvent this problem.

14. The duodenal mucosa is seen almost vertical in relation to the pyloric ring (Fig. 21.5). Care should be taken at this point to prevent injury to the duodenal mucosa. It is recommended to change to an IT-2 Knife™ at this point to minimize this risk. The dissection is continued for another 5 mm (it is not necessary and not recommended to continue tunneling beyond the pyloric ring as in esophageal POEM wherein the tunnel is continued for 2–3 cm beyond the gastroesophageal junction).

15. The endoscope is withdrawn and is passed across the pylorus into the duodenal bulb to confirm mucosal staining at the pylorus and just beyond it (Fig. 21.6).

16. Once adequacy of the tunnel has been confirmed, the endoscope is reintroduced into the tunnel. A full-thickness pyloromyotomy is performed using the IT-2 Knife™ by hooking the instrument onto the pyloric muscular ring and pulling it from distal to proximal (Fig. 21.7). This direction of myotomy is important to prevent inadvertent duodenal mucosal injury. The pyloric ring can be quite thick; full-thickness myotomy must be ensured to achieve the desired result.

17. Pyloromyotomy should be approximately 2–3 cm in length; it is not recommended to perform a longer myotomy due to the risk of

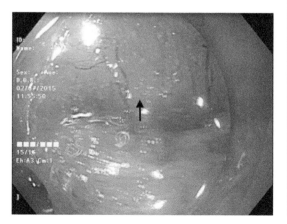

Fig. 21.5 Pyloric ring seen through the submucosal tunnel. The duodenal mucosa is seen stretched vertically beyond the ring (arrow)

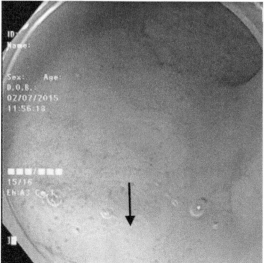

Fig. 21.6 Confirm adequacy of the submucosal tunnel by inspecting the blue staining of the duodenal mucosa beyond the pylorus (arrow)

damage to the gastric pacemaker situated in the antrum. On completion of the pyloromyotomy, the duodenal mucosa can be seen prolapsing into the tunnel (Fig. 21.8).

18. Care should be taken to avoid damage to the branches of the gastro-epiploic vessels which are in close relation to the pylorus at this location. Bleeding from these vessels can be brisk and severe, and the vessels can continue to bleed into the peritoneal cavity if left unattended.

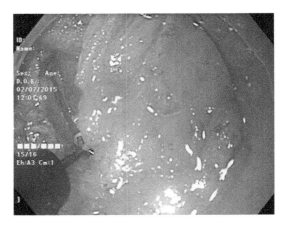

Fig. 21.7 Full-thickness myotomy is performed using the IT-2 Knife™. The insulated ceramic tip of the instrument protects against inadvertent duodenal mucosal injury

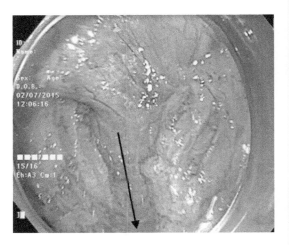

Fig. 21.8 Completed pyloromyotomy as seen from the submucosal tunnel. Note the prolapsing duodenal mucosa after myotomy (arrow). A short myotomy approximately 2 cm in length is recommended (thick arrow)

19. Once myotomy is completed and hemostasis has been confirmed, the endoscope is again withdrawn and passed into the duodenal bulb to rule out mucosal injury. While passing across the pylorus, one may feel reduction in the resistance to the scope, in spite of the distal cap attached to it, though this is less clearly appreciable as compared to esophageal POEM wherein the gastro-esophageal junction is wide open after the myotomy.

20. Closure of the mucosal incision is the final step of G-POEM. As in esophageal POEM, this can be achieved by applying serial mucosal clips, the first clip being applied beyond the distal incision angle and then progressing proximally to approximate the mucosal edges (Figs. 21.9, and 21.10). As compared to esophageal POEM, the mucosal edges in G-POEM tend to separate laterally and are difficult to approximate. The incision also frequently elongates to some extent, possibly because the gastric mucosa has folds and is loosely attached to the submucosa. To prevent clips from slipping, care must be taken to ensure an adequate bite of

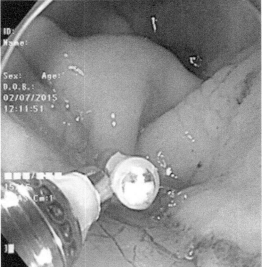

Fig. 21.9 The first clip is applied just beyond the distal angle of the incision. This lifts the mucosal edges and facilitates subsequent clip placement

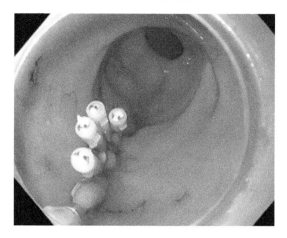

Fig. 21.10 Completed closure of mucosal incision by serial clips

the mucosa and to apply the clips close to one another so that the tension is distributed evenly. Several clips may be necessary to achieve an optimum closure.

21. In case of severe tension on the mucosal edges, alternative techniques like OTSC clips or OverStitch™ closure may be considered. It is imperative that the mucosal closure is secure, failing which, there may be a risk of leakage of gastric contents and peritoneal contamination.

22. In very severe cases when the operator is unsure about the secureness of the mucosal closure, a nasogastric tube may be inserted to decompress the stomach post-procedure. Alternatively, a triple lumen nasojejunal tube is placed temporarily to aspirate the stomach as well as achieve feeding into the intestine.

Post-procedure Care and Instructions

1. Patients are maintained nil orally for at least 24 h post-procedure, longer in cases when security of mucosal closure is suspect.

2. Intravenous broad-spectrum antibiotics are administered for 48 h post-procedure.

3. Some workers prescribe proton pump inhibitors in the post-operative period; however there is no clear justification for their routine use. Although their use may reduce risk of post-operative hemorrhage, acid secretion is suppressed and thus may increase the risk of post-operative infection.

4. Patients are monitored for hemodynamic and respiratory instability, which may indicate ongoing hemorrhage, infection, or peritonitis. It is important to note that hemorrhage after G-POEM may not always occur inside the gastric lumen and therefore may not present as hematemesis, but may present as progressive abdominal distension, pain, and hemodynamic instability indicating an ongoing intraperitoneal bleeding.

5. Most patients do not complain of significant post-procedure pain. Analgesic requirements are minimal and often on demand. Most post-operative pain is due to gaseous distension that disappears within a few hours. Care must be taken while administering narcotic analgesics to patients with diabetic gastroparesis since this may further affect their gastric dysmotility.

6. It is our policy to get a hematocrit estimation 12 h post-procedure. A dropping hematocrit indicates ongoing blood loss and needs prompt evaluation.

7. An upper GI series using either barium or water-soluble contrast medium is performed after 24 h to rule out a leak.

8. After confirming absence of a leak, patients are instructed to start liquids and soft low-residue diet is gradually initiated within 48 h.

9. Patients are usually discharged on the second post-operative day with instructions to contact the unit in case of emergency.

10. Patients are advised to continue soft diet for 8–10 days, after which they can resume normal diet.

11. The first follow-up visit is usually scheduled between 4 and 6 weeks. In addition to GCSI estimation, an EGD and a GES are repeated at follow-up to assess the response to G-POEM.

Adverse Events and Technical Challenges

G-POEM is an endoscopic surgical procedure and carries potential risk of adverse events. If performed following the instructions detailed above and adhering to surgical principles, it is a remarkably safe procedure with minimal adverse events and quick recovery. However, the following potential adverse events have been reported and are possible:

1. Capnoperitoneum – Mild capnoperitoneum is common and almost invariable during G-POEM due to the insufflated CO2 gas that escapes through the tunnel into the peritoneal cavity. Most often it is insignificant and asymptomatic.

2. Tension capnoperitoneum with resultant respiratory compromise and rising end-tidal CO2 (*Et-CO2*) – This can occur due to over-insufflation during tunneling or myotomy. If the respiratory compromise is mild, the procedure can be halted for some time, the endoscope is withdrawn, and the anesthetist hyperventilates the patient so that the carbon dioxide is washed out. In case of severe respiratory distress, abdominal paracentesis can be performed using a wide-bore needle (16G) to decompress the abdomen and improve ventilation. In most situations, ventilation will improve using these measures. In the rare event that the patient continues to remain unstable, the procedure may have to be aborted. Significant capnoperitoneum reported as adverse event was reported on one occasion by Khashab et al. and on two occasions by Gonzalez et al. in their series [17, 18].

3. Hemorrhage – Gastric submucosa is vascular and bleeding can occur during the procedure and must be suitably arrested. Significant post-procedure hemorrhage is uncommon if optimum measures for hemostasis have been undertaken during the procedure. It can occur due to rebleeding from one of the submucosal vessels, or from subserosal vessels during myotomy. It is important to note that post-procedure bleeding may not always become clinically evident by presenting with hematemesis but may rarely continue within the peritoneal cavity and present as hemorrhagic shock. Appropriate resuscitation measures including transfusion of blood products may be required. Repeat EGD with reentry into the tunnel after removal of the clips, evacuation of blood clots, and arrest of bleeding source may be required if ongoing bleeding is suspected. Surgical exploration or interventional radiology support may also be required if endoscopic measures fail to stop the bleeding. Schlomovitz et al. reported bleeding in one patient that was treated by hemoclips; and Kahaleh et al. reported bleeding inside the tunnel that required coagulation using Coagrasper™ forceps [19, 20].

4. Infection and peritonitis – G-POEM breaches the integrity of the gastrointestinal tract. Although the submucosal flap valve technique has been shown to be exceedingly safe against leakage of bowel contents, peritoneal contamination or infection can occur. The integrity of the mucosal closure is paramount. Broad-spectrum antibiotics may usually be adequate for mild infections; however surgical exploration and peritoneal drainage may be required for severe cases. The risk of infection appears to be infrequent however, with no study to date reporting significant infection or peritonitis.

5. Gastric ulcer – Pre-pyloric ulcer has been occasionally reported as an adverse event after G-POEM [17, 20]. The mechanism is poorly understood but may be related to devascularization of the mucosal flap during tunneling. Khashab et al. reported severe atrophic gastritis as a possible contributory factor, whereas Kahaleh et al. reported that the ulcer was possibly a residual mucosal defect. Therapy using proton pump inhibitors and sucralfate was adequate.

Apart from these specific issues, adverse events related to anesthesia, intubation, and the endoscopic procedure are potentially possible. G-POEM however appears to be a safe procedure with a low overall incidence of adverse events of 6–7% in most series.

Status of G-POEM

G-POEM was conceptualized and reported by Kawai et al. in a porcine model in 2012 [15]. Subsequently, Khashab et al. reported the first successful human G-POEM in 2013 in a patient with refractory diabetic gastroparesis [12]. The initial 2 years saw several case reports and short case series being published endorsing the safety and feasibility of this procedure. G-POEM was reported for various indications – Chaves et al. and Chung et al. reported it for early post-operative gastroparesis, whereas we reported it for delayed post-operative gastroparesis [21–23]. Mekaroonkamol et al. reported a successful series of three patients of varying etiologies – idiopathic, post-infectious, and post-operative gastroparesis [24]. There was also a case report of combined POEM and G-POEM for recurrent

achalasia and refractory gastroparesis wherein POEM was preceded by the G-POEM so as to mitigate the risk of severe reflux because of gastroparesis [25]. Pham et al. have reported this procedure in a patient with primary pyloric stenosis [26]. Shlomovitz et al. demonstrated successful G-POEM in six out of seven patients and also documented normalization of gastric emptying in five patients [19].

In the last 2 years, larger patient series have been reported in the form of single- or multi-center studies. Current literature on G-POEM is summarized in Table 21.2. The first multicenter study by Khashab et al. demonstrated success of G-POEM in a retrospective cohort of 30 patients [17]. Adverse events were few (6.7%) and length of hospital stay was short (mean 3.3 days). Symptom improvement was seen in 26/30 (86%) patients during a median follow-up of 5.5 months, and patients with symptoms of nausea and vomiting responded the most. The study concluded that G-POEM was safe and effective in the treatment of refractory gastroparesis.

Another recently published multicenter study of 33 patients by Kahaleh et al. has seconded these observations [20]. They reported 85% clinical success at the end of a median of 11.5 months.

Table 21.2 Summary of current G-POEM literature

	N	Technical success (%)	Procedure time (min)	Clinical success (%)	GES improved	Adverse events	Follow-up (months)
Shlomovitz (2015) [19]	7	100	90–120	86 (6/7)	80 (4/5)	1 – bleeding (clips)	6.5 ± 2.1
Khashab (2016)	30	100	72 (35–223)	86 (26/30)	47 (14/30)	1 capnoperitoneum, 1 ulcer	5.5
Gonzalez (2016)	12	100	51 (32–105)	85 (10/12)	75 (9/12)	2 capnoperitoneum	5
Mekaroonkamol (2016) [24]	3	100	74 (55–93)	100 (3/3)	100 (3/3)	Nil	3
Gonzalez (2017) [18]	29	100	47 (32–118)	79 (3 months) 69 (6 months)	55 (16/29)	1 bleeding (clips), 1 abscess (conservative)	10 ± 6.4
Dacha (2017) [27]	16	100	49.7 ± 22.1	81 (13/16)	75 (12/16)	Nil	6
Rodriguez (2017)	47	100	41.2 ± 28.5	66 (31/47)	34 (16/47)	1 death (cardiac disease, unrelated to procedure)	3
Kahaleh (2018) [20]	33	100	77.6 (37–255)	85 (28/33)	100	1 bleeding (clips), 1 ulcer	11.5

Mean GCSI scores and gastric emptying times on GES improved significantly from 33 and 222.4 min before G-POEM to 0.8 and 143.6 min post-procedure, respectively ($p < 0.00001$ and $p \leq 0.05$). Mean length of hospital stay in these studies was 3.3 (range 1–12) and 5.4 (range 1–14) days, respectively. Both studies concluded that G-POEM was safe and effective for the treatment of refractory gastroparesis.

A single-center study by Dacha et al. evaluated outcomes at 1, 6, and 12 months post-G-POEM. GCSI scores improved from an average of 3.40 ± 0.50 pre-procedure (16 patients) to 1.48 ± 0.95 (P Z .0001) at 1-month (16 patients), 1.36 ± 0.9 ($P < .01$) at 6-month (13 patients), and 1.46 ± 1.4 ($P < .01$) at 12-month (6 patients) follow-up; and SF36 questionnaire demonstrated a significant improvement in quality of life in several domains that was sustained through 6-month follow-up. Mean 4-h gastric retention on GES decreased from $62.9\% \pm 24.3\%$ to $17.6\% \pm 16.7\%$ ($P = .007$) after G-POEM [27].

A prospective multicenter study by the Johns Hopkins group is currently underway, and interim results recently presented in abstract form reported 73% clinical success rates at 1- to 3-month follow-up [28]. It would be interesting to evaluate the final outcomes of this study, particularly as, in addition to GCSI, the study also includes several additional symptom scores for a more comprehensive assessment of symptom relief.

G-POEM technique has also evolved over time. In contrast to the triangular tip or hook knife to perform pyloromyotomy, most workers now prefer an insulated tip (IT)-2 Knife™ for performing the myotomy to protect the duodenal mucosa from inadvertent injury. Identification of the pylorus can sometimes be challenging. Xue et al. in a non-randomized study of 14 patients demonstrated significant reduction in procedure times (36 min $\pm$ 13 vs. 56 min $\pm$ 13, $p = 0.01$) by performing a fluoroscopy-guided G-POEM, wherein a clip at the pyloric ring was used as a landmark to create an adequate submucosal tunnel [29].

G-POEM has been described for refractory gastroparesis. However, gastroparesis is a complex disorder wherein impaired gastric dysmotility and pylorospasm both play a variable role in its pathophysiology. Impaired gastric body motility is likely the primary cause for diabetic gastroparesis (autonomic neuropathy), whereas pylorospasm may be an important factor in postoperative gastroparesis (after vagal injury or vagotomy). It is therefore essential to identify which patients are most likely to benefit by G-POEM [30].

Gonzalez et al. in a single-center study of 29 patients have attempted to answer this question [18]. They reported inferior results of G-POEM for diabetic gastroparesis as compared with either post-surgical or idiopathic gastroparesis (57% vs. 80% and 93% at 3 months; 43% vs. 50% and 92% at 6 months). Diabetes and female sex were found to be predictors of failure in univariate analysis. Although this was not subsequently confirmed in multivariate analysis (possibly owing to small sample size), the study raised concerns about efficacy of G-POEM in patients with diabetes [18]. The study by Dacha et al. reported all three failures in their series occurring in diabetic patients [27]. This has raised significant concern about the efficacy of G-POEM in diabetics, with even a suggestion that other modalities like gastric electrical stimulation may be more suitable in diabetics [18]. However, a recent study published in abstract form reported no significant difference in outcomes of G-POEM for diabetic versus non-diabetic gastroparesis; and duration of illness was the only factor showing significant correlation with outcomes, with patients with long-standing symptoms reporting inferior results [31].

An important issue that requires consideration in long-term follow-up is the incidence of duodenogastric biliary reflux that can occur after G-POEM. Based on the POEM experience, where reflux was initially under-reported but has later emerged as a significant post-POEM concern, reflux after G-POEM could face a similar fate. The long-term consequences of this reflux are currently unknown but can be somewhat ascertained from that of patients undergoing pyloroplasty or gastro-jejunostomy. One must remember that reflux after POEM is treatable, whereas that after G-POEM is currently impossible to treat. It is possible that the symptom benefit provided by G-POEM may outweigh the negative consequences of reflux in these difficult-to-treat patients.

To conclude, data on G-POEM is still evolving. Current data suggests that it is a safe and effective procedure and demonstrates sustained efficacy at 1 year. Future studies are needed to further establish the role of G-POEM in clinical practice and particularly to identify patients who are most likely to benefit by this procedure.

Per-rectal Endoscopic Myotomy (PREM)

Introduction

Hirschsprung's disease (HD) is a congenital disorder characterized by the absence of intrinsic ganglion cells in submucosal and myenteric plexuses of the hindgut and presents with constipation, intestinal obstruction, and/or megacolon. The incidence is 1 in 2000 to 5000 live births; and it is often associated with trisomy 21. The disease commonly affects the recto-sigmoid region (short-segment HD), although ultrashort- (rectal involvement) and long-segment (proximal to sigmoid) variants have also been described less frequently [32, 33]. The disease is commonly diagnosed in infancy, although few skip detection till adulthood. The pathophysiology of HD is explained by failure of relaxation of the aganglionic distal bowel segment leading to a functional bowel obstruction. Longer the aganglionic segment, more severe is the obstruction.

The standard treatment of HD consists of a single- or multi-stage surgical or laparoscopic pull-through procedure with or without diverting colostomy. Several variants of the pull-through operation have been described – Swenson's, Duhamel's and modified Duhamel's, and Soave's or the Boley Scot or modified Soave's procedures [32–34]. During the last two decades, laparoscopic pull-through approaches have been described, often as single-stage procedures, thereby eliminating the need for a diverting colostomy [35–37]. Although it is the gold standard for over six decades, the pull-through operation has several drawbacks. They are multi-stage surgical procedures performed in neonates and infants and carry a high morbidity. Anal incontinence is reported in up to 55.7% patients and fecal soiling in 37.8%. Significantly inferior functional bowel scores and quality-of-life (QOL) scores have regularly been reported following these surgical procedures. Understandably, psycho-social problems are often reported in these children [33, 38–40]. Residual aganglionosis is frequent and requires repeat interventions [33, 40, 41]. HD in patients more than 1 year presents a further surgical challenge due to significant proximal bowel dilatation, resulting in difficulty in performing the pull-through surgery resulting in post-operative morbidity [40, 41].

Transanal posterior anorectal myectomy (PARM) was described nearly four decades ago by Hamdy and Scobie as a lesser invasive procedure for short-segment adult HD and to treat residual aganglionosis following pull-through surgery [42–46]. The procedure had limited applicability because of the limited extent of myectomy possible via the transanal approach. To improve results, low anterior resection and PARM were reported by Lernau et al., again with limited results [47].

Evolution, Philosophy, and Development of PREM

PREM is based on submucosal tunneling endoscopy and the mucosal flap valve as described for POEM and G-POEM [12, 14]. As described earlier, the aganglionic segment in HD is spastic and fails to relax in response to peristalsis. If this segment can be opened by performing a myotomy, the spasticity can disappear and therefore the functional obstruction can be alleviated. PARM was described using this same hypothesis; however, the extent of myotomy or myectomy through the transanal approach was limited. Using the principles of third space endoscopy and submucosal tunneling, a longer myotomy of a desired predetermined length can be achieved.

Wang et al. in an abstract form reported successful transanal endoscopic myotomy (PAEM) for internal anal sphincter achalasia in an animal model [48]. Based on these results, per-rectal endoscopic myotomy (PREM) was conceptualized by one of the current authors (A.B.) [49]. The first human PREM was performed successfully for a 24-year-old adult HD patient wherein a 20-cm-long full-thickness myotomy was achieved [49]. Subsequently, we also reported the first successful pediatric PREM in an 8-year-old child [50].

Patient Selection and Pre-procedure Workup

Clinical Profile

Constipation in the post-natal or neonatal period or early infancy is the commonest presenting symptom. Older children may present with history of refractory constipation since birth, history of neonatal surgery or colostomy, abdominal distension, visible colonic or bowel loop, failure to thrive, and/or delayed milestones. Adult patients may be even more difficult to identify – often presenting as severe refractory constipation.

Diagnosis

1. Barium enema (BE) – This is the most commonly performed imaging procedure for diagnosis of HD. The characteristic appearance is that of a dilated proximal colon (usually sigmoid) tapering to a narrow, spastic rectum (Fig. 21.11a, b). The conical zone is almost invariably appreciated on BE and is pathognomonic of HD. It generally corresponds to the transition zone at the junction of ganglionic and aganglionic segments.

2. Anorectal high-resolution manometry (HRM) – HRM is often used to rule out other defecation disorders like obstructive defecation syndrome (ODS) or anal stricture. The characteristic feature is absence of a recto-anal inhibitory reflex (RAIR), which is seen in ODS but is absent in HD. Since HRM requires

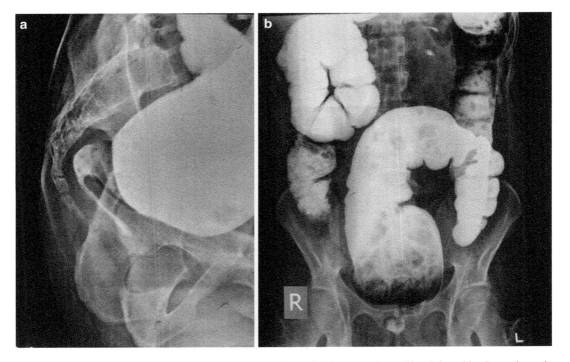

Fig. 21.11 Barium enema in HD – left lateral (**a**) and AP views (**b**) demonstrating a dilated sigmoid colon and spastic rectum. Note the conical transition zone between the dilated and spastic segment

a conscious and cooperative patient, it is often used in older children or adults but cannot be used in neonates. If the child is under anesthesia or sedation, high resting intra-rectal pressures can indirectly indicate a spastic rectal segment.

3. Colonoscopy or sigmoidoscopy – It is mandatory to rule out any obstructive lesion in the rectum or sigmoid colon. Colonoscopy also is required for mapping of the aganglionic segment.

Colonoscopy

Patients with HD are severely constipated and require a special regimen of bowel preparation before colonoscopy can be attempted. In adults, up to 10 l of polyethylene glycol (PEG) solution may be used over a 2- to 3-day period with the patient consuming only clear liquids during this time. Younger patients may require up to 50–75 ml/kg body weight of the solution administered through a nasogastric tube for effective cleansing. Despite such aggressive bowel preparation, patients may still harbor large stool masses that may require washing, breaking down, and evacuation at the time of the procedure. Care must be taken to prevent electrolyte imbalance and hypoglycemia during the bowel preparation, especially in smaller children.

During colonoscopy, the scope must be passed beyond the spastic segment into the dilated proximal segment. The mucosa is examined for stasis ulcers, frequently seen because of the large stool masses, which may require breaking down and evacuation. Any other pathology must also be looked for. Once the colon is reasonably clear of fecal contents, mapping is performed.

Colonoscopic Mapping of the Aganglionic Segment

Accurate mapping of the aganglionic segment is crucial to the success of PREM. Mapping is performed by taking serial deep submucosal biopsies starting in the dilated colon proximal to the conical zone and moving distally up to the lower rectum. Biopsies are generally recommended at approximately 3- to 5-cm intervals by endoscopic mucosal resection (EMR) technique [49]. We

generally recommend the biopsies to be taken on the anterior wall of the rectum and sigmoid so that the posterior wall remains clean for the subsequent PREM. A cap or band EMR technique has been described and is effective to achieve adequate samples [49–51].

Technique (Video 21.2) – After ensuring that the colon is clean of stool residue, a submucosal cushion is raised on the anterior colonic or rectal wall starting proximally in the dilated bowel segment using a normal saline solution stained with indigo carmine or methylene blue (Fig. 21.12a). Using either a cap or band EMR technique and a polypectomy snare, a mucosal disk along with submucosa is resected and retrieved (Fig. 21.12b, c). The procedure is repeated every 3–5 cm by gradually withdrawing the endoscope from proximal to distal. The last biopsy must be taken at least 3–4 cm inside the anorectal junction. This is because the distal 2–3 cm of the rectum demonstrates physiological aganglionosis [32] and may therefore lead to confusion during reporting.

The specimens are serially labeled according to their distance from the anal verge and subjected to histopathological examination. Immunohistochemistry (IHC) staining is performed on these samples to identify ganglion cells located in the deep submucosa (Fig. 21.13a–c). Starting from the most proximal sample, the pathologist must report the distalmost location where ganglia were identified and the first sample where they could not be demonstrated. The region between these two locations is the transition zone. For the myotomy to be effective, it must extend at least 2–3 cm proximal to this location.

The PREM Procedure

PREM is a new and evolving procedure. To date, the only reports of PREM are from the author's (A.B.) center. As is true for every procedure that is evolving, the technique often changes as experience grows. The description that follows represents our current understanding of this procedure and its technicalities. We present the basic steps

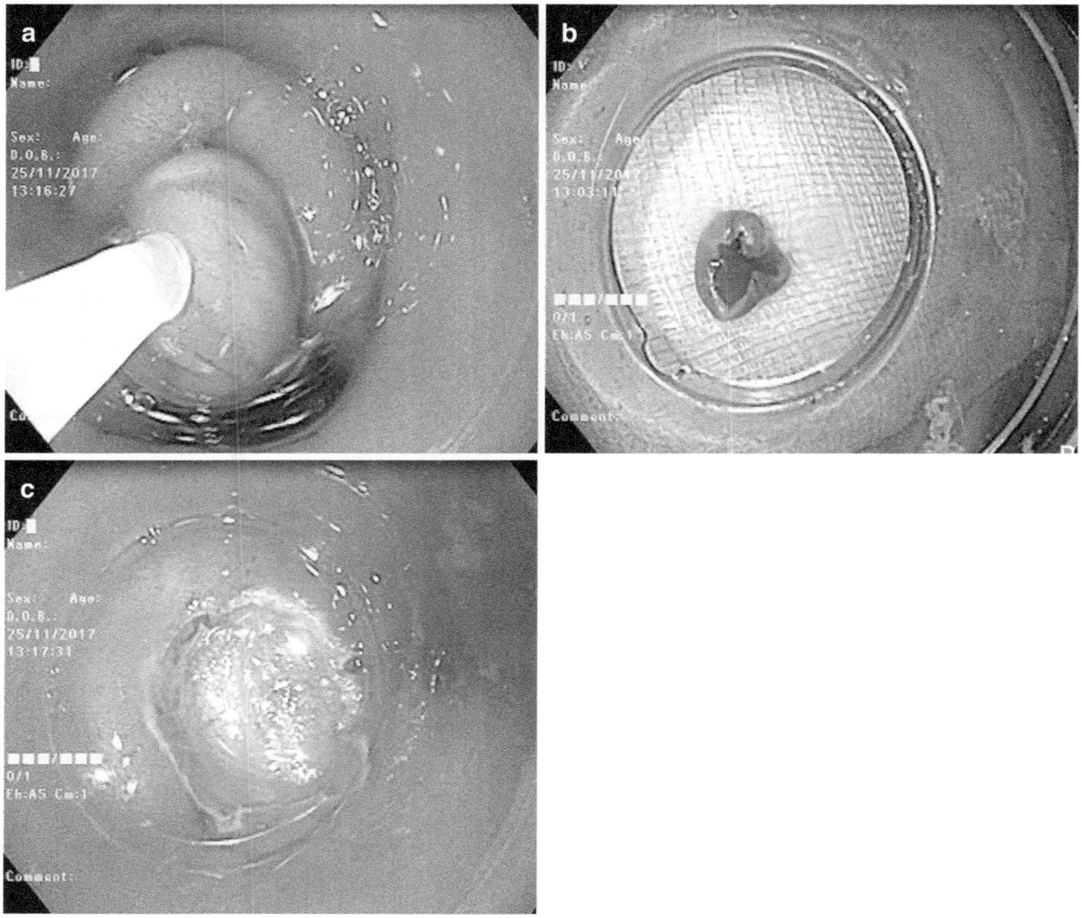

Fig. 21.12 (**a**) Submucosal cushion raised by injection of normal saline stained with methylene blue. (**b**) Retrieved EMR specimen. Note the large disk of mucosa with substantial submucosa in the biopsy specimen. (**c**) Inspection of ulcer base post-EMR shows blue-stained deep submucosa without muscle injury

and precautions that should be undertaken while performing this procedure. We believe that as more centers perform PREM, this technique will further evolve and is likely to change.

Pre-procedure Preparation

1. Optimum bowel preparation is crucial for the success of PREM. Preparation should be even more stringent as compared to the initial colonoscopy at the time of biopsy, because it would be disastrous if stool residue enters the tunnel.
2. Bowel disinfection is desirable. We recommend oral rifaximin in a dose of 20–25 mg/kg/day administered for 3 days pre-PREM.

3. PREM is performed under general anesthesia.
4. The patient is positioned in the prone position with slight elevation of the pelvic girdle and the buttocks strapped laterally (Fig. 21.14). This is because PREM is performed by the posterior approach by creating a tunnel along the sacral hollow. With the patient in supine position, it is often impossible or extremely difficult to angulate the endoscope adequately to enter the tunnel in such an angulated position. Also, the patients' legs interfere with the endoscope handling and assistance. The prone position is therefore more convenient; and the pelvic girdle elevation empties the

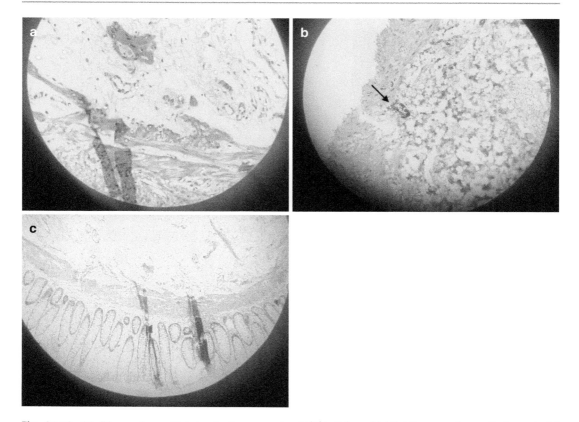

Fig. 21.13 (**a**) Biopsy from dilated colonic segment (10X), H&E stain – ganglion cells in submucosa. (**b**) Biopsy from dilated colonic segment (10X), IHC cal-retinin stain – highlighting ganglion cells (arrow). (**c**) Biopsy from spastic segment (10X), H&E stain – absent ganglion cells in submucosa

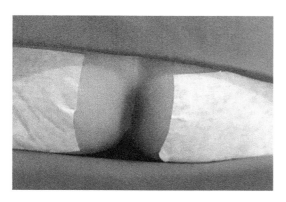

Fig. 21.14 Patient position for PREM. Note the elevated pelvis and the buttocks strapped laterally

rectum of stool and fluid and maintains a reasonably clean field of dissection.
5. Intravenous broad-spectrum antibiotics (e.g., third-generation cephalosporin and metronidazole) are administered at the time of induc-tion of anesthesia and continued for 72 h post-PREM.
6. Ensure and ascertain the exact length of myotomy to be performed based on the report of the serial biopsies taken earlier.

Instrumentation

Instrumentation for PREM is same as G-POEM. Few differences exist as follows:

1. We prefer a standard high-definition gastroscope to colonoscope due to superior and easier handling of the equipment and instruments.
2. Clip-and-line technique is often required to gain entry into the submucosal tunnel (Video 21.3).
3. Diathermy settings must be lower as compared to G-POEM to prevent inadvertent

injury as rectal and colonic submucosa is thin and rectal mucosa is delicate.

4. A Dual Knife™ may be preferred over TT Knife™ in infants due to the thin submucosal layer and risk of mucosal injury.

The PREM Procedure (Video 21.4)

1. Ensure that the air on the endoscope processor is turned off and that only carbon dioxide insufflation is used.

2. PREM is performed by the posterior approach by creating a tunnel along the sacral hollow following the curve.

3. Using an injector needle (25G), submucosal elevation is achieved within a centimeter of the anorectal junction (Fig. 21.15). The rectal mucosa and wall are thin; care must be taken to avoid deep injection.

4. Using a triangular tip knife (TT Knife-J™, Olympus), a 10- to 15-mm mucosal incision is performed on the elevated area (Fig. 21.16). The incision may be longitudinal or horizontal; we prefer longitudinal since it is easier to close using clips.

5. A hemoclip with a string attached is applied to the apex of the incision and the string is pulled to achieve retraction of the mucosal flap (Video 21.3). This enables submucosal dissection and entry into the submucosal tunnel. Once the endoscope is stabilized within the tunnel, the clip may be removed.

6. Submucosal dissection is continued like that described for POEM or G-POEM, maintaining a direction perpendicular to the circular muscle fibers (Fig. 21.17). In infants and small children, the submucosa can be thin. A Dual Knife™ with a shorter knife tip may be used instead of a triangular tip knife that has a longer cutting tip.

7. As dissection proceeds cranially, the circular muscle layer veers off to the left as

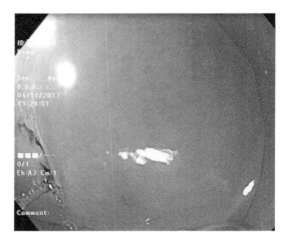

Fig. 21.16 Longitudinal incision inside the anorectal junction using a TT-J Knife™

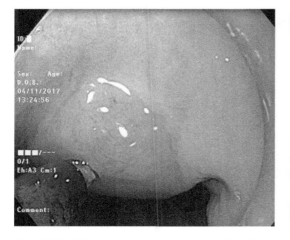

Fig. 21.15 Submucosal elevation by methylene blue-stained normal saline just inside anorectal junction

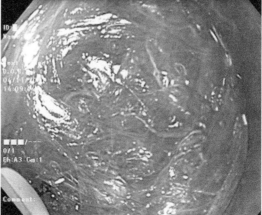

Fig. 21.17 Submucosal tunnel for PREM. Note the thin submucosa and direction of dissection perpendicular to the circular muscle fibers

the recto-sigmoid junction is reached. The tunnel must therefore also be directed to follow this direction (Fig. 21.18a). Care must be taken to avoid injury to the mucosa or to the muscle layers at this point. Frequent withdrawal into the lumen to inspect the mucosa and the direction and extent of the tunnel is mandatory (Fig. 21.18b).

8. The tunnel is completed using the above steps. Tunnel must extend well into the dilated proximal segment for adequacy of myotomy.

9. Once the desired length of tunnel has been achieved, full-thickness myotomy is commenced. Myotomy is performed using an insulated tip (IT) Knife™ or TT Knife™ (Olympus) and is performed in a cranial to caudal direction (Fig. 21.19). Myotomy must be commenced at the proximal end of the submucosal tunnel. Distally, the myotomy is extended within 1 cm of the mucosal incision as compared to other tunneling techniques wherein a 2- to 3-cm distance between mucosal entry and myotomy is maintained (Fig. 21.20). This is because of two factors – it

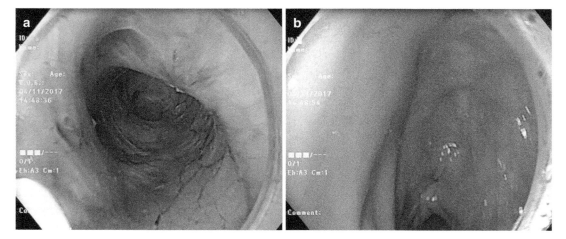

Fig. 21.18 (**a**) Rectal lumen curves to the left and the tunnel creation must follow this direction. (**b**) Luminal view of completed submucosal tunnel in the rectum

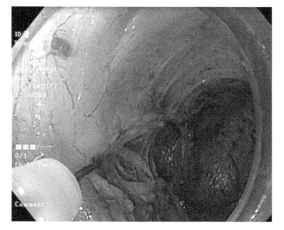

Fig. 21.19 Full-thickness myotomy in cranial to caudal direction starting at the apex of the submucosal tunnel

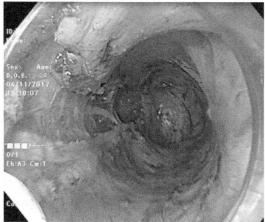

Fig. 21.20 Completed full-thickness myotomy

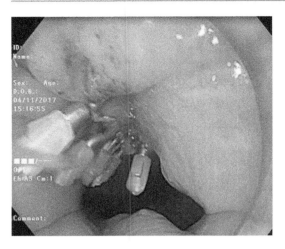

Fig. 21.21 Mucosal incision closure achieved by serial hemoclips

is imperative to divide the circular muscle fibers of the rectum in their entire length up to the internal anal sphincter to ensure release of the spasticity. Also, because the tunnel in PREM is from distal to proximal, chances of contamination due to rectal contents entering the tunnel are unlikely.

10. Care must be taken during myotomy to avoid injury and bleeding from peri-rectal vessels and within the tunnel; and optimum hemostasis must be achieved.

11. The mucosal incision is closed using multiple hemoclips (Fig. 21.21).

Post-Procedure Care and Instructions

1. Patients are maintained fasting until presence of peristalsis is confirmed, after which clear liquids can be slowly commenced and stepped up to standard diet.

2. Intravenous antibiotics are continued for 72 h.

3. Analgesics are rarely, if ever, required.

4. Stool softener/mild laxative like lactulose is prescribed to maintain a soft stool consistency.

5. Patients are discharged once they tolerate oral diet.

6. First follow-up visit is usually scheduled at 2 weeks. Laxatives are continued till the first follow-up and may then be discontinued or tapered depending on stool frequency and

consistency. It must be remembered that the proximal dilated colon is quite flaccid and may require up to 3–6 months to regain its tone and function, and small doses of laxatives may be required till then.

7. At follow-up, patients are asked about their stool frequency, stool consistency, need for straining, incontinence or urgency if any, and QOL scores.

8. Barium or water-soluble contrast enema and/or anorectal HRM may be repeated at around 12 weeks to objectively assess reduction in proximal colonic dilatation and intra-rectal pressures. The RAIR is unlikely to recover as the rectum remains aganglionic; however the rectal capacity improves thereby improving defecation.

Status of PREM

PREM is a very recent addition to the basket of third space endoscopy procedures, having been described only about 1 year ago. To date, only two case reports of PREM have been published, both from our center (A.B.) – one for an adult and another for a pediatric patient [49, 50]. A further case report of a 2-year-old infant undergoing PREM was presented as part of conference proceedings [52]. The current follow-up on these three patients is 30 months, 18 months, and 8 months, respectively. All three patients report regular (daily) bowel movement with minimal occasional laxative use; and there are no reported episodes of incontinence, diarrhea, or enterocolitis.

At the time of writing this manuscript, we have information on two more PREM procedures – on patients aged 18 months and 4 years. Both patients underwent full-thickness myotomy 17 and 14 cm in length, respectively. At follow-up periods of 7 and 3 months, both patients remain well and report daily stool passage with minimal laxative use and no incontinence.

Although these are very early times for PREM, the initial results reported in these above case reports are encouraging. The procedure is safe and has been shown to be effective in a small cohort of patients. This is important especially because PREM offers a minimally invasive endoscopic treatment option for an otherwise significantly morbid surgical procedure with long-term sequelae and sub-optimal outcomes.

However, PREM faces several challenges before it could be considered as a mainstream accepted procedure for treatment of HD. The prevalence of HD is low – approximately one in every 2000–5000 live births [32]. Also, prevalence of HD is very low in Western countries like Europe and North America; and most recent studies have been reported from Asian or African countries [32, 33]. HD patients are primarily treated by pediatric surgeons, pediatricians, or neonatologists, specialties that have limited exposure to endoscopic techniques and technological advances. Interdisciplinary interaction can help to improve this situation.

For PREM to progress to a clinically acceptable procedure like POEM, it needs to be accepted and performed by interventional endoscopists across the globe. Endoscopists are encouraged to evaluate the efficacy and applicability of PREM in multicenter prospective trials, followed by possibly a randomized trial that compares PREM to surgical (laparoscopic) pull-through procedure. Until such a time, however, PREM may remain a promising although under-evaluated and underutilized treatment option for HD.

References

1. Camilleri M, Parkman HP, Shafi MA, Abell TL, Gerson L, American College of G. Clinical guideline: management of gastroparesis. Am J Gastroenterol. 2013;108(1):18–37; quiz 8. https://doi.org/10.1038/ajg.2012.373.
2. Camilleri M, Bharucha AE, Farrugia G. Epidemiology, mechanisms, and management of diabetic gastroparesis. Clin Gastroenterol Hepatol. 2011;9(1):5–12; quiz e7. https://doi.org/10.1016/j.cgh.2010.09.022.
3. Parkman HP, Hasler WL, Fisher RS, American GA. American Gastroenterological Association technical review on the diagnosis and treatment of gastroparesis. Gastroenterology. 2004;127(5):1592–622.
4. Wang YR, Fisher RS, Parkman HP. Gastroparesis-related hospitalizations in the United States: trends, characteristics, and outcomes, 1995–2004. Am J Gastroenterol. 2008;103(2):313–22. https://doi.org/10.1111/j.1572-0241.2007.01658.x.
5. Talley NJ, Young L, Bytzer P, Hammer J, Leemon M, Jones M, et al. Impact of chronic gastrointestinal symptoms in diabetes mellitus on health-related quality of life. Am J Gastroenterol. 2001;96(1):71–6. https://doi.org/10.1111/j.1572-0241.2001.03350.x.
6. Goldblatt F, Gordon TP, Waterman SA. Antibody-mediated gastrointestinal dysmotility in scleroderma. Gastroenterology. 2002;123(4):1144–50.
7. Rao AS, Camilleri M. Review article: metoclopramide and tardive dyskinesia. Aliment Pharmacol Ther. 2010;31(1):11–9. https://doi.org/10.1111/j.1365-2036.2009.04189.x.
8. Arts J, Holvoet L, Caenepeel P, Bisschops R, Sifrim D, Verbeke K, et al. Clinical trial: a randomized-controlled crossover study of intrapyloric injection of botulinum toxin in gastroparesis. Aliment Pharmacol Ther. 2007;26(9):1251–8. https://doi.org/10.1111/j.1365-2036.2007.03467.x.
9. Friedenberg FK, Palit A, Parkman HP, Hanlon A, Nelson DB. Botulinum toxin A for the treatment of delayed gastric emptying. Am J Gastroenterol. 2008;103(2):416–23. https://doi.org/10.1111/j.1572-0241.2007.01676.x.
10. Hibbard ML, Dunst CM, Swanstrom LL. Laparoscopic and endoscopic pyloroplasty for gastroparesis results in sustained symptom improvement. J Gastrointest Surg. 2011;15(9):1513–9. https://doi.org/10.1007/s11605-011-1607-6.
11. Clarke JO, Sharaiha RZ, Kord Valeshabad A, Lee LA, Kalloo AN, Khashab MA. Through-the-scope transpyloric stent placement improves symptoms and gastric emptying in patients with gastroparesis. Endoscopy. 2013;45(Suppl 2 UCTN):E189–90. https://doi.org/10.1055/s-0032-1326400.
12. Khashab MA, Stein E, Clarke JO, Saxena P, Kumbhari V, Chander Roland B, et al. Gastric peroral endoscopic myotomy for refractory gastroparesis: first human endoscopic pyloromyotomy (with video). Gastrointest Endosc. 2013;78(5):764–8. https://doi.org/10.1016/j.gie.2013.07.019.
13. O'Grady G, Egbuji JU, Du P, Cheng LK, Pullan AJ, Windsor JA. High-frequency gastric electrical stimulation for the treatment of gastroparesis: a meta-analysis. World J Surg. 2009;33(8):1693–701. https://doi.org/10.1007/s00268-009-0096-1.
14. Inoue H, Minami H, Kobayashi Y, Sato Y, Kaga M, Suzuki M, et al. Peroral endoscopic myotomy (POEM) for esophageal achalasia. Endoscopy. 2010;42(4):265–71. https://doi.org/10.1055/s-0029-1244080.
15. Kawai M, Peretta S, Burckhardt O, Dallemagne B, Marescaux J, Tanigawa N. Endoscopic pyloromyotomy: a new concept of minimally invasive surgery for pyloric stenosis. Endoscopy. 2012;44(2):169–73. https://doi.org/10.1055/s-0031-1291475.
16. Revicki DA, Rentz AM, Dubois D, Kahrilas P, Stanghellini V, Talley NJ, et al. Gastroparesis cardinal symptom index (GCSI): development and

validation of a patient reported assessment of severity of gastroparesis symptoms. Qual Life Res. 2004;13(4):833–44. https://doi.org/10.1023/B:QURE.0000021689.86296.e4.

17. Khashab MA, Ngamruengphong S, Carr-Locke D, Bapaye A, Benias PC, Serouya S, et al. Gastric per-oral endoscopic myotomy for refractory gastroparesis: results from the first multicenter study on endoscopic pyloromyotomy (with video). Gastrointest Endosc. 2017;85(1):123–8. https://doi.org/10.1016/j.gie.2016.06.048.

18. Gonzalez JM, Benezech A, Vitton V, Barthet M. G-POEM with antro-pyloromyotomy for the treatment of refractory gastroparesis: mid-term follow-up and factors predicting outcome. Aliment Pharmacol Ther. 2017;46(3):364–70. https://doi.org/10.1111/apt.14132.

19. Shlomovitz E, Pescarus R, Cassera MA, Sharata AM, Reavis KM, Dunst CM, et al. Early human experience with per-oral endoscopic pyloromyotomy (POP). Surg Endosc. 2015;29(3):543–51. https://doi.org/10.1007/s00464-014-3720-6.

20. Kahaleh M, Gonzalez JM, Xu MM, Andalib I, Gaidhane M, Tyberg A, et al. Gastric per-oral endoscopic myotomy for the treatment of refractory gastroparesis: a multicenter international experience. Endoscopy. 2018; https://doi.org/10.1055/a-0596-7199.

21. Bapaye A, Dubale N, Pujari R, Kulkarni A, Jajoo Naval R, Vyas V, et al. Peroral endoscopic pyloromyotomy for delayed postoperative gastroparesis. Endoscopy. 2015;47(S 01):E581–E2. https://doi.org/10.1055/s-0034-1393368.

22. Chung H, Dallemagne B, Perretta S, Lee SK, Shin SK, Park JC, et al. Endoscopic pyloromyotomy for post-esophagectomy gastric outlet obstruction. Endoscopy. 2014;46(Suppl 1 UCTN):E345–6. https://doi.org/10.1055/s-0034-1377599.

23. Chaves DM, de Moura EG, Mestieri LH, Artifon EL, Sakai P. Endoscopic pyloromyotomy via a gastric submucosal tunnel dissection for the treatment of gastroparesis after surgical vagal lesion. Gastrointest Endosc. 2014;80(1):164. https://doi.org/10.1016/j.gie.2014.03.045.

24. Mekaroonkamol P, Li LY, Dacha S, Xu Y, Keilin SD, Willingham FF, et al. Gastric peroral endoscopic pyloromyotomy (G-POEM) as a salvage therapy for refractory gastroparesis: a case series of different subtypes. Neurogastroenterol Motil. 2016;28(8):1272–7. https://doi.org/10.1111/nmo.12854.

25. Bapaye A, Mahadik M, Pujari R, Vyas V, Dubale N. Per-oral endoscopic pyloromyotomy and per-oral endoscopic myotomy for coexisting refractory gastroparesis and recurrent achalasia cardia in a single patient. Gastrointest Endosc. 2016;84(4):734–5. https://doi.org/10.1016/j.gie.2016.04.001.

26. Pham KD, Viste A, Dicko A, Hausken T, Hatlebakk JG. Peroral endoscopic pyloromyotomy for primary pyloric stenosis. Endoscopy. 2015;47(Suppl 1):E637–8. https://doi.org/10.1055/s-0034-1393675.

27. Dacha S, Mekaroonkamol P, Li L, Shahnavaz N, Sakaria S, Keilin S, et al. Outcomes and quality-of-life assessment after gastric per-oral endoscopic pyloromyotomy (with video). Gastrointest Endosc. 2017;86(2):282–9. https://doi.org/10.1016/j.gie.2017.01.031.

28. Sanaei O, Chaves D, Aadam AA, de Moura EG, Baptista A, El Zein MH, et al. Sa1948 gastric peroral endoscopic myotomy (G-POEM) for the treatment of refractory gastroparesis: interim results from the first international prospective trial. Gastrointest Endosc. 2018;87(6):AB261–AB2. https://doi.org/10.1016/j.gie.2018.04.1562.

29. Xue HB, Fan HZ, Meng XM, Cristofaro S, Mekaroonkamol P, Dacha S, et al. Fluoroscopy-guided gastric peroral endoscopic pyloromyotomy (G-POEM): a more reliable and efficient method for treatment of refractory gastroparesis. Surg Endosc. 2017;31(11):4617–24. https://doi.org/10.1007/s00464-017-5524-y.

30. Bapaye A. Third-space endoscopy – can we see light at the end of the tunnel? (Editorial). Endoscopy. 2018;50:1047–8. https://doi.org/10.1055/a-0637-9050.

31. Mekaroonkamol P, Patel V, Shah R, Li T, Li B, Tao J, et al. 838 Duration of the disease, rather than the etiology of gastroparesis, is the key predictive factor for clinical response after gastric per oral endoscopic pyloromyotomy (GPOEM). Gastrointest Endosc. 2018;87(6):AB119–AB20. https://doi.org/10.1016/j.gie.2018.04.1311.

32. Wyllie R. Motility disorders and Hirschsprung disease. In: Kliegman R, Behrman R, Jenson H, Stanton B, editors. Nelson textbook of pediatrics. 18th ed. Philadelphia, PA: Saunders Elsevier; 2008. p. 1565–7.

33. Sharma S, Gupta DK. Hirschsprung's disease presenting beyond infancy: surgical options and postoperative outcome. Pediatr Surg Int. 2012;28(1):5–8. https://doi.org/10.1007/s00383-011-3002-5.

34. Pini Prato A, Gentilino V, Giunta C, Avanzini S, Parodi S, Mattioli G, et al. Hirschsprung's disease: 13 years' experience in 112 patients from a single institution. Pediatr Surg Int. 2008;24(2):175–82. https://doi.org/10.1007/s00383-007-2089-1.

35. Georgeson KE, Fuenfer MM, Hardin WD. Primary laparoscopic pull-through for Hirschsprung's disease in infants and children. J Pediatr Surg. 1995;30(7):1017–21; discussion 21-2

36. Langer JC. Laparoscopic and transanal pull-through for Hirschsprung disease. Semin Pediatr Surg. 2012;21(4):283–90. https://doi.org/10.1053/j.sempedsurg.2012.07.002.

37. Thomson D, Allin B, Long AM, Bradnock T, Walker G, Knight M. Laparoscopic assistance for primary transanal pull-through in Hirschsprung's disease: a systematic review and meta-analysis. BMJ Open. 2015;5(3):e006063. https://doi.org/10.1136/bmjopen-2014-006063.

38. Bai Y, Chen H, Hao J, Huang Y, Wang W. Long term outcome and quality of life after Swenson

procedure for Hirschsprung's disease. J Pediatr Surg. 2002;37:639–42.

39. Nurko S. Complications after gastrointestinal surgery: a medical perspective. In: Walker W, Durie P, Hamilton J, Walker-Smith J, Watkins J, editors. Pediatric gastrointestinal disease. Patholhysiology, diagnosis, management. 4th ed. St. Louis: Mosby; 2004. p. 2111–38.

40. Ekenze SO, Ngaikedi C, Obasi AA. Problems and outcome of Hirschsprung's disease presenting after 1 year of age in a developing country. World J Surg. 2011;35(1):22–6. https://doi.org/10.1007/s00268-010-0828-2.

41. Friedmacher F, Puri P. Residual aganglionosis after pull-through operation for Hirschsprung's disease: a systematic review and meta-analysis. Pediatr Surg Int. 2011;27(10):1053–7. https://doi.org/10.1007/s00383-011-2958-5.

42. Hamdy MH, Scobie WG. Anorectal myectomy in adult Hirschsprung's disease: a report of six cases. Br J Surg. 1984;71(8):611–3.

43. Kaymakcioglu N, Yagci G, Can MF, Demiriz M, Peker Y, Akdeniz A. Role of anorectal myectomy in the treatment of short segment Hirschsprung's disease in young adults. Int Surg. 2005;90(2):109–12.

44. Pattana-arun J, Ruanroadroun T, Tantiphalachiva K, Sahakitrungruang C, Attithansakul P, Rojanasakul A. Internal sphincter myectomy for adult Hirschsprung's disease: a single institute experience. J Med Assoc Thail. 2010;93(8):911–5.

45. Abbas Banani S, Forootan H. Role of anorectal myectomy after failed endorectal pull-through in Hirschsprung's disease. J Pediatr Surg. 1994;29(10):1307–9.

46. Kimura K, Inomata Y, Soper RT. Posterior sagittal rectal myectomy for persistent rectal achalasia after the Soave procedure for Hirschsprung's disease. J Pediatr Surg. 1993;28(9):1200–1.

47. Lernau OZ, Nissan S. Low anterior resection with a long posterior anorectal myectomy and sphincterectomy for Hirschsprung's disease. J Pediatr Surg. 1980;15(5):613–4.

48. Wang L, Cai Q, Fan C, Ren W, Yu J. Mo1628 a new potential method per anus endoscopic myotomy for treatment of internal anal sphincter achalasia. Gastrointest Endosc. 2013;77(5):AB451. https://doi.org/10.1016/j.gie.2013.03.376.

49. Bapaye A, Wagholikar G, Jog S, Kothurkar A, Purandare S, Dubale N, et al. Per rectal endoscopic myotomy for the treatment of adult Hirschsprung's disease: first human case (with video). Dig Endosc. 2016;28(6):680–4. https://doi.org/10.1111/den.12689.

50. Bapaye A, Bharadwaj T, Mahadik M, Ware S, Nemade P, Pujari R, et al. Per-rectal endoscopic myotomy (PREM) for pediatric Hirschsprung's disease. Endoscopy. 2018;50(6):E644–E5. https://doi.org/10.1055/a-0583-7570.

51. Nabi Z, Chavan R, Shava U, Sekharan A, Reddy DN. A novel endoscopic technique to obtain rectal biopsy specimens in children with suspected Hirschsprung's disease. VideoGIE. 2018;3(5):157–8. https://doi.org/10.1016/j.vgie.2018.02.008.

52. Bapaye A, Mahadik M, Kumar Korrapati S, Nemade P, Pujari R, Date S, et al. Per rectal endoscopic myotomy (PREM) for infantile Hirschsprung's disease. Endoscopy. 2018;50(04):OP209V. https://doi.org/10.1055/s-0038-1637246.

Part IV

Endoscopic Anti-reflux Therapies

Zaheer Nabi and D. Nageshwar Reddy

Introduction

Gastroesophageal reflux disease (GERD) is defined as troublesome symptoms and/or complications due to reflux of stomach contents [47]. GERD is a chronic condition which not only impairs the quality of life (QOL) but also predisposes to Barrett's esophagus and esophageal adenocarcinoma [41].

The prevalence of GERD is rising mainly due to a global upsurge in obesity [38]. The pooled prevalence of GERD from population-based studies is 13.3% (95% CI 12.0–14.6%) [8].

Proton pump inhibitors (PPIs) and lifestyle modifications have been the cornerstone of medical management of GERD. Unfortunately, about 30–40% of these patients especially those with regurgitation do not respond well to PPIs. Refractory GERD has been defined as symptoms caused by the reflux of gastric contents that do not respond to a stable double dose of a PPI over a 12-week treatment period [45]. The response to heartburn in patients with erosive and non-erosive GERD is 56–77% and 37–61%, respectively. In contrast, regurgitation responds in only 26–44% patients [17]. Reflux symptoms in non-responders are associated with psychological distress and reduced QOL [53]. The standard of care in these patients has been laparoscopic fundoplication (partial or total). However, adverse events like dysphagia and gas bloat are potential concerns. Moreover, surgery is not preferred by all, and therefore, minimally invasive therapeutic modalities are required to bridge the gap between PPIs and surgery.

Endoscopic Anti-Reflux Therapies (EARTs)

A plethora of endoscopic anti-reflux therapies (EARTs) has been evaluated for the management of GERD. These include injection implants, application of radiofrequency energy, endoscopic suturing, and endoscopic fundoplication (Table 22.1). The rise and fall of EARTs has been well appreciated over the last few decades. Some of these EARTs could not withstand the test of time and were withdrawn either due to lack of efficacy or serious adverse events (AEs).

Z. Nabi (✉)
Department of Gastroenterology, Asian Institute of Gastroenterology, Hyderabad, India

D. N. Reddy
Asian Institute of Gastroenterology, Hyderabad, India

© Springer Nature Switzerland AG 2020
M. S. Wagh, S. B. Wani (eds.), *Gastrointestinal Interventional Endoscopy*,
https://doi.org/10.1007/978-3-030-21695-5_22

Table 22.1 Endoscopic anti-reflux modalities

	Equipment/ device	Pros	Cons	Adverse events	Current status
Injectable implants	Enteryx Gatekeeper Plexiglas	Short-term efficacy +	Serious adverse events (including death)	Dysphagia, chest pain, pneumothorax, pneumomediastinum, perforation, severe bleeding leading to death	Withdrawn
Radiofrequency application	Stretta	Safe Large experience Office procedure Randomized trials+	Mixed results Less impressive objective improvement	0.93% Mucosal erosions/lacerations, gastroparesis	SAGES (moderate evidence, strong recommendation) ASGE (low evidence)
Endoscopic suturing, plication and mucosal resection					
Endoscopic suturing	EndoCinch	Good short-term results, no serious AEs	Lack of reduction in esophageal acid exposure Loss of efficacy in long term	Mild adverse events (pain, nausea)	Withdrawn
Transoral fundoplication	EsophyX™	Long-term data available Randomized Trials+	Loss of efficacy in long term pH normalization less impressive (30–40%)	2.4% Perforation, bleeding Pneumothorax Epigastric pain	SAGES (moderate evidence, strong recommendation) ASGE (low evidence)
Endoscopic stapling	MUSE™	Effective in short term (up to 4 years)	Limited long-term data No Randomized trial	Serious adverse events in initial cases Pneumothorax, pneumoperitoneum, esophageal leaks, perforation, bleeding,	Preliminary data Long-term studies and Randomized trials required
Endoscopic full thickness plication	GERDx	Effective in short term (3 months)	Only one study with new device No long-term data	Pneumonia, empyema, severe pain, hematoma	Preliminary data Further evaluation required
Endoscopic mucosal resection	ARMS (anti-reflux mucosectomy)	Safe and easy No special equipment	Technique not standardized Long-term data not available	Bleeding Dysphagia	Preliminary data Further evaluation required

Endoscopic Anti-Reflux Therapies: Modalities of the Past

Endoscopic Injection of Bulking Agents

EARTs of yesteryears include injection of bulking agents (Enteryx, Gatekeeper Reflux Repair System, Plexiglas, Durasphere) and endoscopic suturing (EndoCinch and NDO plicator) to boost the anti-reflux barrier.

The injectable bulking agents which have been used for sphincter augmentation are made of biocompatible non-resorbable co-polymers. These include ethylene-vinyl-alcohol copolymer (Enteryx), hydrogel cylinder-shaped prostheses (Gatekeeper System), and polymethyl methacrylate (Plexiglas). Initial studies evaluating sphincter augmentation with injectable bulking agents showed encouraging results [6, 10, 11, 14, 25, 44]. In a randomized sham controlled trial, implantation of Enteryx was more effective in reducing PPI dependency and symptoms of GERD [6]. In contrast, another multicenter randomized trial concluded that injectable prosthesis (Gatekeeper System) was no better than control group with respect to improvement in symptoms or objective parameters like esophageal acid exposure [12]. However, most of the other studies were non-randomized with small patient population and short follow-up periods. Besides, there was no significant improvement in objective parameters like esophageal acid exposure [20]. Nevertheless, the predominant reason for discontinuation of these agents was occurrence of serious AEs including several deaths. Serious AEs reported with the use of injectable implants include pneumothorax, pneumomediastinum, free perforation, esophageal abscess, atelectasis, pleural effusion, pericardial effusion requiring surgery, para-esophageal collection, visceral artery embolization, fatal haemorrhage, and sepsis [6, 12, 13, 19]. These AEs were attributed to uncontrolled depth of injection and migration of injected particles (embolization). Subsequently, some modifications were introduced like increasing the size of particles (40–125 microns) and modification of injection catheter [16, 27] to reduce embolization and accurately localize the depth of injection, respectively. However, despite these proposed improvisations, injectable techniques did not pick up again.

Endoscopic Suturing and Plication

Unwillingness for an invasive procedure and accompanying AEs associated with laparoscopic fundoplication have propelled the development of minimally invasive endoscopic options which mimic surgical fundoplication.

Various plication and suturing devices that have been evaluated for GERD include endoscopic suturing device (EndoCinch, Ethicon Endo-Surgery, Cincinnati, OH), endoscopic full thickness plication device (the Plicator, *NDO* Surgical, Inc., Mansfield, MA), transoral incisionless fundoplication device (EsophyX, EndoGastric Solutions, Redmond, WA), and ultrasonic surgical endostapler (MUSE, Medigus, Omer, Israel). All of these work on the same principle, i.e., enforcing the GEJ with sutures or plicators to reduce reflux events.

EndoCinch was the earliest of these devices to be evaluated (FDA approval in year 2000) with reasonable outcomes in short term. However, long-term results were disappointing and primarily attributable to suture loss. In addition, lack of significant improvement in objective parameters suggested that the device requires modifications for subsequent clinical use [33, 42, 43]. In a well-conducted prospective trial, more than 80% of patients had lost at least one suture at 18-month follow-up. Corresponding to the same, a short-term efficacy of 71% at 3 months could not be maintained at 18 months when efficacy was only 20% [43]. As of now EndoCinch device has been discontinued by the manufacturer and is no longer available for commercial use.

The Plicator device was next to be approved in 2003. The device soon underwent revision a few years later (2007) due to serious technical failure requiring surgical removal. Several studies confirmed the efficacy of the Plicator device in improving symptoms, esophageal acid exposure, and PPI dependence [36, 37,

40]. In the subsequent years, a key modification in the technique where multiple plicator implants were used instead of one was shown to improve the results with this device [28, 48, 49]. For unclear reasons, the manufacturers withdrew the device from market. More recently, the Plicator technology has been taken over by another manufacturer (GERDX, G-SURG, GmbH, Seeon-Seebruck, Germany) and is being further evaluated in clinical trials (NCT03322553).

Endoscopic Anti-Reflux Therapies: The Present

The currently available EARTs include transoral incisionless fundoplication (TIF) device (EsophyX, EndoGastric Solutions, Redmond, WA), ultrasonic surgical endostapler (MUSE, Medigus, Omer, Israel), endoscopic full thickness plication device (GERDX, G-SURG, GmbH, Seeon-Seebruck, Germany), and radiofrequency energy (Stretta).

Endoscopic Fundoplication

Transoral fundoplication using EsophyX device is among the well-studied anti-reflux devices. In randomized studies, improvement in GERD-HRQL and discontinuation of PPIs have been more or less uniform with this device [22]. However, improvement in objective pH parameters like normalization of esophageal acid exposure time and DeMeester score is less impressive. Like EndoCinch, the loss of sutures and deterioration of GEJ flap valve were found in one study and may be partly responsible for loss of response with this device as well [51].

The other endoscopic fundoplication devices including GERDx and MUSE are more recent and long-term results are awaited [18, 50].

Radiofrequency Energy Application (Stretta)

Application of RFA to GEJ or Stretta (Mederi Therapeutics, Greenwich, Connecticut) is the old-est (FDA approval in year 2000) of currently available EARTs. Over 15,000 patients have been treated with this device. Ease of application, no requirement of general anesthesia, minimal impact on future anti-reflux therapies, and excellent safety profile (<1% AE) have enabled it to sustain among the various disappearing endoscopic therapies for GERD. Multiple studies have revealed the safety and efficacy of RFA for the management of GERD [7, 29, 35, 46, 52]. In addition, several non-randomized studies have reported reasonable (although inferior) outcomes of RFA when compared to surgical fundoplication for the management of typical and atypical symptoms of GERD [5, 21, 30, 31, 54, 55]. Despite excellent outcomes in multiple short- and long-term studies, RFA has not gained a worldwide acceptance as expected. The skepticism regarding the efficacy of Stretta is not absolutely unreasonable. Among the vast number of studies published on Stretta, there are only five randomized trials with maximum follow-up duration of 12 months [1–4, 26]. Moreover, important outcome parameters like HRQL, PPI use, and heartburn were not measured in all of them. Consequently, a meta-analysis comprising of these four RCTs ($n = 92$) concluded that RFA is no better than placebo or sham therapy [32]. This is in contrast with the results from another recent systematic review and meta-analysis which encompassed 23 cohort studies in addition to the four RCTs ($n = 2468$) included in the previous meta-analysis. This review concluded the efficacy of RFA with significant reduction in the use of PPIs and improvement in esophageal acid exposure time, heartburn symptoms, and HRQL [9]. The long-term maintenance of efficacy with Stretta was confirmed in two single-arm studies with follow-up duration of 8 and 10 years, respectively [7, 35]. In the prospective study by Noar and colleagues, GERD-HRQL was normalized in 72% at 10-years follow-up [35]. PPI discontinuation was achieved in 41% at 10 years and 79% at 8 years in these studies [7, 35].

In conclusion, RFA treatment leads to improvement in symptoms and HRQL and allows elimination or reduction in doses of PPIs. However, the improvement in objective parameters like esophageal acid exposure, basal lower esophageal sphincter pressure, and erosive esophagitis is not impressive. Large, randomized, and sham controlled studies with long-term follow-up are required to establish the role of RFA in the management algorithm of GERD. Also, the impact of second session of RFA on treatment outcomes needs to be studied. One study did report improved results with a second session of RFA in initial non-responders [2].

Endoscopic Anti-reflux mucosectomy (ARMS)

ARMS is an endoscopic technique in which mucosal resection is performed along the lesser curvature side of gastric cardia to reshape the mucosal flap valve. Initial results published by Inoue and colleagues demonstrated the feasibility and safety of ARMS [23]. More recently, the same group has demonstrated reasonable outcomes in a relatively large cohort of patients with refractory GERD (DDW 2017). There was significant improvement in QOL, esophageal acid exposure time, and endoscopic appearance of gastric flap valve, and PPIs could be discontinued in 61% of patients at one-year follow-up. Certain important questions need to be addressed before wider clinical adoption of ARMS. The technique is not standardized and the extent of mucosectomy is mainly based on the subjective judgment of the operator. Too much resection may lead to stricture, whereas too less will be unrewarding. Second, the impact of mucosectomy on the feasibility of subsequent EARTs is not known. As of now, the available data is limited and ongoing randomized trials (NCT03259191) may clarify the role of ARMS in the management of GERD.

Endoscopic Anti-Reflux Therapies: Lessons Learned

Goals and Patient Selection

The objective benefit from EARTs is not unequivocal. The results are not absolutely concordant between randomized trials and cohort studies as discussed above. Moreover, there is discrepancy in the response rates between symptoms and 24-hour pH metrics. Improved patient outcomes

(GERD-HRQL) have been reported despite a lack of improvement in esophageal acid exposure times in many of the studies. This discrepancy can be attributed to either high placebo or sham response rates or poor correlation between symptom response and esophageal acid exposure in these patients. This brings us back to the argument – what should be the goal of anti-reflux therapies: normalization of esophageal acid exposure or symptom relief? The proponents of EART would argue that normalization of esophageal acid exposure may not be required to relieve troublesome symptoms of GERD or healing of esophagitis. Moreover, the improvement in GERD-HRQL and reduction in use of PPI are more relevant goals from a patient's perspective. On the other hand, normalization of esophageal acid exposure is an important objective parameter and cannot be ignored altogether. Lack of normalization in the majority would raise concerns regarding the mode of action as well as long-term durability of these procedures. This in turn implies that further modifications in technique or anti-reflux devices or both may be required. In conclusion, a reasonable goal would be improvement in quality of life with elimination of troublesome regurgitation and heartburn, abolition or reduction in requirement of PPI, and a reasonable improvement in esophageal acid exposure.

Appropriate patient selection is paramount for achieving optimal outcomes with EARTs in patients with GERD. An important question is that which patients qualify for EARTs. Broadly speaking two categories of patients appear to be appropriate candidates for EARTs. These include patients in whom symptoms of GERD are adequately controlled on PPIs but unwilling to continue them for long term. The second group is patients in whom symptoms are inadequately controlled on PPIs, i.e., refractory GERD, but are reluctant to undergo a surgical procedure. These patients should be subsequently investigated so that they can gain optimum benefits from EARTs. In addition, the cause of refractoriness to PPIs should be actively sought. A proportion of these patients are non-compliant to lifestyle modifications and adequate PPI dosage and, therefore, are not refractory in true sense.

The currently available EARTs are better avoided in those with large hiatal hernia (>2 cm),

Hill's grade III/IV flap valve, severe esophagitis (Los Angeles grade C and D), poor symptom correlation on pH-impedance, psychological comorbidity, functional heartburn, ineffective esophageal peristalsis analysis, and high BMI [34].

Endoscopic Anti-Reflux Therapies – Wait or Ready for Prime Time

The emergence and persistence of some of the EARTs is partly due to unwillingness of the patients to undergo surgery and adverse events related to total fundoplication procedure. However, this argument may not hold absolutely if emerging surgical options like magnetic sphincter augmentation and electrical stimulation therapy are considered [15, 39]. These procedures, though invasive, have been shown to be associated with reduced rate of typical AEs associated with total fundoplication procedure like dysphagia and gas bloat. Therefore, EARTs are likely to face wider range of competitors in the near future (Fig. 22.1).

EARTs have the potential to control the troublesome symptoms of GERD, which are adequately or inadequately controlled by PPIs. The presently available EARTs are at different phases of development. While some of these have been extensively evaluated, the evidence is more limited for others. For some endoscopic therapies like ARMS, the technique is yet to be standardized. For others like MUSE and GERDx, long-term data and randomized trials are required. Among the currently available EARTs, transoral fundoplication (EsophyX) and application of radiofrequency energy (Stretta) procedure have been available for more than a decade now. Based on the available evidence, these EARTs have found a recommendation from three societal guidelines. The updated guidelines by the Society of American Gastrointestinal and Endoscopic Surgeons (SAGES) and American Society of Gastrointestinal Endoscopy (ASGE) recommend TIF and Stretta in appropriately selected patients with GERD (SAGES, strong recommendation, moderate quality of evidence; ASGE, low quality of evidence). Recent evidence-based guidelines by the Japanese Society of Gastroenterology mention that EARTs are safe and effective in short term (recommendation NA, evidence level B) [24].

Summary

The management of GERD in PPI non-responders remains a challenge. EARTs have the potential to bridge the gap between medical and surgical treatment of GERD. But skepticism regarding safety, long-term efficacy, and improvement in objective parameters remains. Some of the EARTs have sustained their existence due to decent safety and short-term efficacy. An ideal EART should be safe and durable and withstand the test of time. Improvement in devices and techniques, appropriate patient selection, and setting of realistic targets should improve the outcomes in patients with GERD.

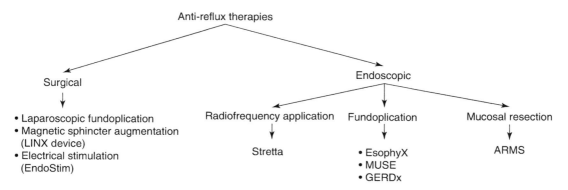

Fig. 22.1 Endoluminal and surgical treatment options for gastroesophageal reflux disease

References

1. Arts J, Bisschops R, Blondeau K, Farre R, Vos R, Holvoet L, Caenepeel P, Lerut A, Tack J. A double-blind sham-controlled study of the effect of radio-frequency energy on symptoms and distensibility of the gastro-esophageal junction in GERD. Am J Gastroenterol. 2012;107(2):222–30. https://doi.org/10.1038/ajg.2011.395.

2. Aziz AM, El-Khayat HR, Sadek A, Mattar SG, McNulty G, Kongkam P, Guda MF, Lehman GA. A prospective randomized trial of sham, single-dose Stretta, and double-dose Stretta for the treatment of gastroesophageal reflux disease. Surg Endosc. 2010;24(4):818–25. https://doi.org/10.1007/s00464-009-0671-4.

3. Corley DA, Katz P, Wo JM, Stefan A, Patti M, Rothstein R, Edmundowicz S, Kline M, Mason R, Wolfe MM. Improvement of gastroesophageal reflux symptoms after radiofrequency energy: a randomized, sham-controlled trial. Gastroenterology. 2003;125(3):668–76.

4. Coron E, Sebille V, Cadiot G, Zerbib F, Ducrotte P, Ducrot F, Pouderoux P, Arts J, Le Rhun M, Piche T, Bruley des Varannes S, Galmiche JP, Consortium de Recherche Independant sur le Traitement et L'exploration du Reflux Gastro-oesophagien et de Le. Clinical trial: radiofrequency energy delivery in proton pump inhibitor-dependent gastro-oesophageal reflux disease patients. Aliment Pharmacol Ther. 2008;28(9):1147–58. https://doi.org/10.1111/j.1365-2036.2008.03790.x.

5. Das B, Reddy M, Khan OA. Is the Stretta procedure as effective as the best medical and surgical treatments for gastro-oesophageal reflux disease? A best evidence topic. Int J Surg. 2016;30:19–24. https://doi.org/10.1016/j.ijsu.2016.03.062.

6. Deviere J, Costamagna G, Neuhaus H, Voderholzer W, Louis H, Tringali A, Marchese M, Fiedler T, Darb-Esfahani P, Schumacher B. Nonresorbable copolymer implantation for gastroesophageal reflux disease: a randomized sham-controlled multicenter trial. Gastroenterology. 2005;128(3):532–40.

7. Dughera L, Navino M, Cassolino P, De Cento M, Cacciotella L, Cisaro F, Chiaverina M. Long-term results of radiofrequency energy delivery for the treatment of GERD: results of a prospective 48-month study. Diagn Ther Endosc. 2011;2011:507157. https://doi.org/10.1155/2011/507157.

8. Eusebi LH, Ratnakumaran R, Yuan Y, Solaymani-Dodaran M, Bazzoli F, Ford AC. Global prevalence of, and risk factors for, gastro-oesophageal reflux symptoms: a meta-analysis. Gut. 2017; https://doi.org/10.1136/gutjnl-2016-313589.

9. Fass R, Cahn F, Scotti DJ, Gregory DA. Systematic review and meta-analysis of controlled and prospective cohort efficacy studies of endoscopic radiofrequency for treatment of gastroesophageal reflux disease. Surg Endosc. 2017; https://doi.org/10.1007/s00464-017-5431-2.

10. Feretis C, Benakis P, Dimopoulos C, Dailianas A, Filalithis P, Stamou KM, Manouras A, Apostolidis N. Endoscopic implantation of Plexiglas (PMMA) microspheres for the treatment of GERD. Gastrointest Endosc. 2001;53(4):423–6. https://doi.org/10.1067/mge.2001.113912.

11. Fockens P, Bruno MJ, Gabbrielli A, Odegaard S, Hatlebakk J, Allescher HD, Rosch T, Rhodes M, Bastid C, Rey J, Boyer J, Muehldorffer S, van den Hombergh U, Costamagna G. Endoscopic augmentation of the lower esophageal sphincter for the treatment of gastroesophageal reflux disease: multicenter study of the Gatekeeper reflux repair system. Endoscopy. 2004;36(8):682–9. https://doi.org/10.1055/s-2004-825665.

12. Fockens P, Cohen L, Edmundowicz SA, Binmoeller K, Rothstein RI, Smith D, Lin E, Nickl N, Overholt B, Kahrilas PJ, Vakil N, Abdel Aziz Hassan AM, Lehman GA. Prospective randomized controlled trial of an injectable esophageal prosthesis versus a sham procedure for endoscopic treatment of gastroesophageal reflux disease. Surg Endosc. 2010;24(6):1387–97. https://doi.org/10.1007/s00464-009-0784-9.

13. Fry LC, Monkemuller K, Malfertheiner P. Systematic review: endoluminal therapy for gastro-oesophageal reflux disease: evidence from clinical trials. Eur J Gastroenterol Hepatol. 2007;19(12):1125–39. https://doi.org/10.1097/MEG.0b013e3282f16a21.

14. Ganz RA, Fallon E, Wittchow T, Klein D. A new injectable agent for the treatment of GERD: results of the Durasphere pilot trial. Gastrointest Endosc. 2009;69(2):318–23. https://doi.org/10.1016/j.gie.2008.07.034.

15. Ganz RA, Peters JH, Horgan S, Bemelman WA, Dunst CM, Edmundowicz SA, Lipham JC, Luketich JD, Melvin WS, Oelschlager BK, Schlack-Haerer SC, Smith CD, Smith CC, Dunn D, Taiganides PA. Esophageal sphincter device for gastroesophageal reflux disease. N Engl J Med. 2013;368(8):719–27. https://doi.org/10.1056/NEJMoa1205544.

16. Ganz RA, Rydell M, Termin P. Accurate localization of tissue layers in the esophagus by using a double-lumen injection catheter: implications for the Enteryx procedure. Gastrointest Endosc. 2006;63(3):468–72. https://doi.org/10.1016/j.gie.2005.11.044.

17. Gyawali CP, Fass R. Management of gastroesophageal reflux disease. Gastroenterology. 2017; https://doi.org/10.1053/j.gastro.2017.07.049.

18. He S, Feussner H, Nennstiel S, Bajbouj M, Huser N, Wilhelm D. Endoluminal sphincter augmentation with the MUSE system and GERDX system in the treatment of gastroesophageal reflux disease: a new impact? Surg Technol Int. 2017;30:131–40.

19. Helo N, Wu A, Moon E, Wang W. Visceral artery embolization after endoscopic injection of Enteryx for gastroesophageal reflux disease. J Radiol Case Rep. 2014;8(9):21–4. https://doi.org/10.3941/jrcr.v8i9.1861.

20. Hogan WJ. Clinical trials evaluating endoscopic GERD treatments: is it time for a moratorium

on the clinical use of these procedures? Am J Gastroenterol. 2006;101(3):437–9. https://doi.org/10.1111/j.1572-0241.2006.00523.x.

21. Hu Z, Wu J, Wang Z, Zhang Y, Liang W, Yan C. Outcome of Stretta radiofrequency and fundoplication for GERD-related severe asthmatic symptoms. Front Med. 2015;9(4):437–43. https://doi.org/10.1007/s11684-015-0422-y.

22. Huang X, Chen S, Zhao H, Zeng X, Lian J, Tseng Y, Chen J. Efficacy of transoral incisionless fundoplication (TIF) for the treatment of GERD: a systematic review with meta-analysis. Surg Endosc. 2017;31(3):1032–44. https://doi.org/10.1007/s00464-016-5111-7.

23. Inoue H, Ito H, Ikeda H, Sato C, Sato H, Phalanusitthepha C, Hayee B, Eleftheriadis N, Kudo SE. Anti-reflux mucosectomy for gastroesophageal reflux disease in the absence of hiatus hernia: a pilot study. Ann Gastroenterol. 2014;27(4):346–51.

24. Iwakiri K, Kinoshita Y, Habu Y, Oshima T, Manabe N, Fujiwara Y, Nagahara A, Kawamura O, Iwakiri R, Ozawa S, Ashida K, Ohara S, Kashiwagi H, Adachi K, Higuchi K, Miwa H, Fujimoto K, Kusano M, Hoshihara Y, Kawano T, Haruma K, Hongo M, Sugano K, Watanabe M, Shimosegawa T. Evidence-based clinical practice guidelines for gastroesophageal reflux disease 2015. J Gastroenterol. 2016;51(8):751–67. https://doi.org/10.1007/s00535-016-1227-8.

25. Johnson DA, Ganz R, Aisenberg J, Cohen LB, Deviere J, Foley TR, Haber GB, Peters JH, Lehman GA. Endoscopic implantation of enteryx for treatment of GERD: 12-month results of a prospective, multicenter trial. Am J Gastroenterol. 2003;98(9):1921–30. https://doi.org/10.1111/j.1572-0241.2003.08109.x.

26. Kalapala R, Shah H, Nabi Z, Darisetty S, Talukdar R, Nageshwar Reddy D. Treatment of gastroesophageal reflux disease using radiofrequency ablation (Stretta procedure): an interim analysis of a randomized trial. Indian J Gastroenterol. 2017; https://doi.org/10.1007/s12664-017-0796-7.

27. Kamler JP, Lemperle G, Lemperle S, Lehman GA. Endoscopic lower esophageal sphincter bulking for the treatment of GERD: safety evaluation of injectable polymethylmethacrylate microspheres in miniature swine. Gastrointest Endosc. 2010;72(2):337–42. https://doi.org/10.1016/j.gie.2010.02.035.

28. Koch OO, Kaindlstorfer A, Antoniou SA, Spaun G, Pointner R, Swanstrom LL. Subjective and objective data on esophageal manometry and impedance pH monitoring 1 year after endoscopic full-thickness plication for the treatment of GERD by using multiple plication implants. Gastrointest Endosc. 2013;77(1):7–14. https://doi.org/10.1016/j.gie.2012.07.033.

29. Liang WT, Wang ZG, Wang F, Yang Y, Hu ZW, Liu JJ, Zhu GC, Zhang C, Wu JM. Long-term outcomes of patients with refractory gastroesophageal reflux disease following a minimally invasive endoscopic procedure: a prospective observational study. BMC Gastroenterol. 2014a;14:178. https://doi.org/10.1186/1471-230X-14-178.

30. Liang WT, Wu JN, Wang F, Hu ZW, Wang ZG, Ji T, Zhan XL, Zhang C. Five-year follow-up of a prospective study comparing laparoscopic Nissen fundoplication with Stretta radiofrequency for gastroesophageal reflux disease. Minerva Chir. 2014b;69(4):217–23.

31. Liang WT, Yan C, Wang ZG, Wu JM, Hu ZW, Zhan XL, Wang F, Ma SS, Chen MP. Early and midterm outcome after laparoscopic fundoplication and a minimally invasive endoscopic procedure in patients with gastroesophageal reflux disease: a prospective observational study. J Laparoendosc Adv Surg Tech A. 2015;25(8):657–61. https://doi.org/10.1089/lap.2015.0188.

32. Lipka S, Kumar A, Richter JE. No evidence for efficacy of radiofrequency ablation for treatment of gastroesophageal reflux disease: a systematic review and meta-analysis. Clin Gastroenterol Hepatol. 2015;13(6):1058–67. e1051. https://doi.org/10.1016/j.cgh.2014.10.013.

33. Montgomery M, Hakanson B, Ljungqvist O, Ahlman B, Thorell A. Twelve months' follow-up after treatment with the EndoCinch endoscopic technique for gastro-oesophageal reflux disease: a randomized, placebo-controlled study. Scand J Gastroenterol. 2006;41(12):1382–9. https://doi.org/10.1080/00365520600735738.

34. Nabi Z, Reddy DN. Endoscopic management of gastroesophageal reflux disease: revisited. Clin Endosc. 2016;49(5):408–16. https://doi.org/10.5946/ce.2016.133.

35. Noar M, Squires P, Noar E, Lee M. Long-term maintenance effect of radiofrequency energy delivery for refractory GERD: a decade later. Surg Endosc. 2014;28(8):2323–33. https://doi.org/10.1007/s00464-014-3461-6.

36. Pleskow D, Rothstein R, Kozarek R, Haber G, Gostout C, Lo S, Hawes R, Lembo A. Endoscopic full-thickness plication for the treatment of GERD: five-year long-term multicenter results. Surg Endosc. 2008;22(2):326–32. https://doi.org/10.1007/s00464-007-9667-0.

37. Pleskow D, Rothstein R, Lo S, Hawes R, Kozarek R, Haber G, Gostout C, Lembo A. Endoscopic full-thickness plication for the treatment of GERD: a multicenter trial. Gastrointest Endosc. 2004;59(2):163–71.

38. Richter JE, Rubenstein JH. Presentation and epidemiology of gastroesophageal reflux disease. Gastroenterology. 2017; https://doi.org/10.1053/j.gastro.2017.07.045.

39. Rodriguez L, Rodriguez PA, Gomez B, Netto MG, Crowell MD, Soffer E. Electrical stimulation therapy of the lower esophageal sphincter is successful in treating GERD: long-term 3-year results. Surg Endosc. 2016;30(7):2666–72. https://doi.org/10.1007/s00464-015-4539-5.

40. Rothstein R, Filipi C, Caca K, Pruitt R, Mergener K, Torquati A, Haber G, Chen Y, Chang K, Wong D, Deviere J, Pleskow D, Lightdale C, Ades A, Kozarek R, Richards W, Lembo A. Endoscopic full-thickness plication for the treatment of gastroesophageal reflux disease: a randomized, sham-controlled trial.

Gastroenterology. 2006;131(3):704–12. https://doi.org/10.1053/j.gastro.2006.07.004.

41. Savarino E, Marabotto E, Bodini G, Pellegatta G, Coppo C, Giambruno E, Brunacci M, Zentilin P, Savarino V. Epidemiology and natural history of gastroesophageal reflux disease. Minerva Gastroenterol Dietol. 2017;63(3):175–83. https://doi.org/10.23736/S1121-421X.17.02383-2.

42. Schiefke I, Neumann S, Zabel-Langhennig A, Moessner J, Caca K. Use of an endoscopic suturing device (the "ESD") to treat patients with gastroesophageal reflux disease, after unsuccessful EndoCinch endoluminal gastroplication: another failure. Endoscopy. 2005a;37(8):700–5. https://doi.org/10.1055/s-2005-870128.

43. Schiefke I, Zabel-Langhennig A, Neumann S, Feisthammel J, Moessner J, Caca K. Long term failure of endoscopic gastroplication (EndoCinch). Gut. 2005b;54(6):752–8. https://doi.org/10.1136/gut.2004.058354.

44. Schumacher B, Neuhaus H, Ortner M, Laugier R, Benson M, Boyer J, Ponchon T, Hagenmuller F, Grimaud JC, Rampal P, Rey JF, Fuchs KH, Allgaier HP, Hochberger J, Stein HJ, Armengol JA, Siersema PD, Deviere J. Reduced medication dependency and improved symptoms and quality of life 12 months after enteryx implantation for gastroesophageal reflux. J Clin Gastroenterol. 2005;39(3):212–9.

45. Sifrim D, Zerbib F. Diagnosis and management of patients with reflux symptoms refractory to proton pump inhibitors. Gut. 2012;61(9):1340–54. https://doi.org/10.1136/gutjnl-2011-301897.

46. Torquati A, Houston HL, Kaiser J, Holzman MD, Richards WO. Long-term follow-up study of the Stretta procedure for the treatment of gastroesophageal reflux disease. Surg Endosc. 2004;18(10):1475–9. https://doi.org/10.1007/s00464-003-9181-y.

47. Vakil N, van Zanten SV, Kahrilas P, Dent J, Jones R, Global Consensus G. The Montreal definition and classification of gastroesophageal reflux disease: a global evidence-based consensus. Am J Gastroenterol. 2006;101(8):1900–20.; quiz 1943. https://doi.org/10.1111/j.1572-0241.2006.00630.x.

48. von Renteln D, Brey U, Riecken B, Caca K. Endoscopic full-thickness plication (Plicator) with two serially placed implants improves esophagitis

and reduces PPI use and esophageal acid exposure. Endoscopy. 2008;40(3):173–8. https://doi.org/10.1055/s-2007-995515.

49. von Renteln D, Schiefke I, Fuchs KH, Raczynski S, Philipper M, Breithaupt W, Caca K, Neuhaus H. Endoscopic full-thickness plication for the treatment of gastroesophageal reflux disease using multiple Plicator implants: 12-month multicenter study results. Surg Endosc. 2009;23(8):1866–75. https://doi.org/10.1007/s00464-009-0490-7.

50. Weitzendorfer M, Spaun GO, Antoniou SA, Tschoner A, Schredl P, Emmanuel K, Koch OO. Interim report of a prospective trial on the clinical efficiency of a new full-thickness endoscopic plication device for patients with GERD: impact of changed suture material. Surg Laparosc Endosc Percutan Tech. 2017;27(3):163–9. https://doi.org/10.1097/SLE.0000000000000396.

51. Witteman BP, Conchillo JM, Rinsma NF, Betzel B, Peeters A, Koek GH, Stassen LP, Bouvy ND. Randomized controlled trial of transoral incisionless fundoplication vs. proton pump inhibitors for treatment of gastroesophageal reflux disease. Am J Gastroenterol. 2015;110(4):531–42. https://doi.org/10.1038/ajg.2015.28.

52. Wolfsen HC, Richards WO. The Stretta procedure for the treatment of GERD: a registry of 558 patients. J Laparoendosc Adv Surg Tech A. 2002;12(6):395–402. https://doi.org/10.1089/109264202762252640.

53. Yadlapati R, Tye M, Keefer L, Kahrilas PJ, Pandolfino JE. Psychosocial distress and quality of life impairment are associated with symptom severity in PPI non-responders with normal impedance-pH profiles. Am J Gastroenterol. 2017; https://doi.org/10.1038/ajg.2017.263.

54. Yan C, Liang WT, Wang ZG, Hu ZW, Wu JM, Zhang C, Chen MP. Comparison of Stretta procedure and toupet fundoplication for gastroesophageal reflux disease-related extra-esophageal symptoms. World J Gastroenterol. 2015;21(45):12882–7. https://doi.org/10.3748/wjg.v21.i45.12882.

55. Zhang C, Wu J, Hu Z, Yan C, Gao X, Liang W, Liu D, Li F, Wang Z. Diagnosis and anti-reflux therapy for GERD with respiratory symptoms: a study using multichannel intraluminal impedance-pH monitoring. PLoS One. 2016;11(8):e0160139. https://doi.org/10.1371/journal.pone.0160139.

Transoral Incisionless Fundoplication (TIF) for Treatment of Gastroesophageal Reflux Disease

Pier Alberto Testoni, Sabrina Gloria Giulia Testoni, Giorgia Mazzoleni, and Lorella Fanti

Introduction

Gastroesophageal reflux disease (GERD) is a very common disorder that can be currently treated by medical therapy and surgical or endoscopic transoral fundoplication. Medical therapy represents the most common approach: proton pump inhibitors relieve symptoms and improve the patient's quality of life in the majority of cases. However, concerns related to potential side effects of continuous long-term medication, drug intolerance or unresponsiveness, and the need of high dosages for long periods to treat symptoms or prevent recurrences have increased in the recent years. Moreover, medical therapy may be inadequate to treat symptoms occurring in presence of weakly acidic reflux and has high cost in the long term for either patients or health-care system, if started at the young age and maintained for many years.

Electronic Supplementary Material The online version of this chapter (https://doi.org/10.1007/978-3-030-21695-5_23) contains supplementary material, which is available to authorized users.

P. A. Testoni (✉) · S. G. G. Testoni · G. Mazzoleni · L. Fanti
IRCCS San Raffaele Scientific Institute, Vita-Salute San Raffaele University, Division of Gastroenterology and Gastrointestinal Endoscopy, Milano (MI), Italy
e-mail: testoni.pieralberto@hsr.it;
testoni.sabrinagloriagiulia@hsr.it;
mazzoleni.giorgia@hsr.it; fanti.lorella@hsr.it

On the other hand, laparoscopic fundoplication, although still considered the gold-standard approach for GERD refractory to medical treatment, is associated with the risk of long-term adverse events such as long-lasting dysphagia (5–12%), inability to vomit or belch, gas/bloat syndrome (19%), excessive flatulence, diarrhea, or functional dyspepsia related to delayed gastric emptying [1–5]. In fact, patients suffering from mild GERD are in general reluctant to undergo surgical repair of the valve, considering the risk of persistent side effects and its invasiveness.

In the last 10 years, transoral incisionless fundoplication (TIF) has been shown to be an effective and promising therapeutic option as alternative to medical and surgical therapy. TIF reconfigures the tissue to obtain a full-thickness gastroesophageal valve from inside the stomach, by serosa-to-serosa plications which include the muscle layers: the new valve is capable to boost the barrier function of the LES with less patient discomfort and possibly fewer technique-related complications and side effects, compared to surgery.

TIF has been shown to achieve long-lasting improvement of esophageal and extra-esophageal GERD-related symptoms (up to 10 years), cessation or marked reduction of proton pump inhibitor (PPI) medication in 75–90% of patients, and improvement of functional findings, measured by either pH or impedance monitoring. TIF may be performed by using the EsophyX® device

(EndoGastric Solutions, Redmond, WA, USA) or the Medigus ultrasonic surgical endostapler (MUSE™, Medigus, Omer, Israel).

The endoluminal platform with the greatest global experience thus far is the TIF performed by using the EsophyX® device (EndoGastric Solutions, Redmond, WA, USA), with over 17,000 procedures performed to date. EsophyX® constructs an omega-shaped valve 3–5 cm long, in a 250°–300° circumferential pattern around the gastroesophageal junction, by deploying multiple non-absorbable polypropylene fasteners through the two layers (esophagus and stomach) under endoscopic vision of the operator. TIF with this device has proved good, durable, long-term follow-up data from multiple investigators that have used the TIF-2 methodology. The device has been recently updated and improved in a new-generation instrument: the EsophyX Z®.

The newest endoluminal fundoplication device to gain FDA approval was the Medigus endoscopic stapling system (Medigus, Omer, Israel). Medigus ultrasonic surgical endostapler (MUSE™) staples the fundus of the stomach to the esophagus below the diaphragm using multiple sets of metal stitches placed under an ultrasound-guided technique and creates an anterior fundoplication functionally similar to standard surgical Dor-Thal operation. Differently from EsophyX®, the new valve is constructed under ultrasonic control. In the case of sliding hiatal hernia, the procedure can be performed only if the hernia can be reduced below the diaphragm.

Techniques for TIF

Pre-procedure Evaluation

Pre-operative upper GI endoscopy is mandatory to determine the distance between the incisor teeth and both the esophago-gastric junction (EGJ) and the diaphragmatic hiatus and the greatest transverse dimension of the hiatus under full gastric distension. In fact, with the current TIF technique, only a hiatal hernia not exceeding 3.0 cm in length can be fully reduced below the diaphragm, while a plication performed in a hiatus with a transverse dimension >3.0 cm can end up in the thorax, a situation that reduces the efficacy of the newly created valve. Prior to the procedure, all patients should undergo esophageal manometry to exclude primary motility disorders and 24-h pH-impedance monitoring to avoid the inclusion of patients with functional heartburn. High-resolution manometry should be preferred for a more accurate recognition of esophageal motor disorders. If the MUSE™ device is used, barium swallow should be performed in cases of hiatal hernia to assess the reducibility of the hernia, since irreducibility is a contraindication to the procedure.

Transoral Fundoplication by EsophyX® Device

The EsophyX® device is composed of (a) a handle, wherein controls are located; (b) an 18-mm-diameter chassis through which control channels run and a standard front-view 9-mm-diameter endoscope can be inserted; (c) the tissue invaginator, constituted of side holes located on the distal part of the chassis, to which external suction can be applied; (d) the tissue mold, which can be brought into retroflection and pushes tissue against the shaft of the device; (e) a helical screw, which is advanced into the tissue and permits retraction of the tissue between the tissue mold and the shaft; (f) two stylets, which penetrate through the plicated tissue and the tissue mold, over which polypropylene H-shaped fasteners can be deployed; and (g) a cartridge containing 20 fasteners. The updated device, EsophyX Z®, is characterized by a fastener deployment similar to a surgical stapler firing mechanism with a reduction of control complexity and dual fastener deployment and is improved by managing trailing leg. The crossing profile has been reduced with elimination of tissue mold elbow and increase of tissue mold lateral stiffness; and the tissue mold tip covers stylets during deployment.

Details of the first- and second-generation EsophyX® devices are illustrated in the Fig. 23.1.

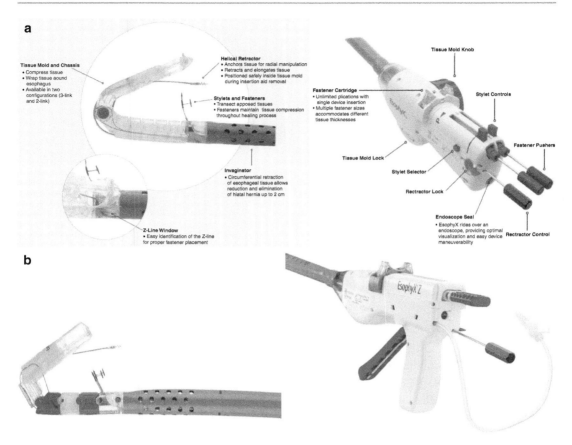

Fig. 23.1 The EsophyX® device. (**a**) The first-generation device; (**b**) the second-generation device. (Courtesy of EndoGastric Solutions, Inc., Redmond, WA, USA) (**a**) ©2015 EndoGastric Solutions, Inc. (**b**) ©2015 EndoGastric Solutions, Inc

The procedure is performed by two operators: one controls the device and the other one operates the endoscope. The device is inserted transorally with the patient in the left lateral or supine position, under general anesthesia. Hypopharyngeal perforation has been reported in this phase of the procedure if the device is introduced without an adequate caution; in difficult cases, the device can be gently rotated to pass the upper esophageal sphincter. The risk of this complication is reduced with the second-generation device, because of its smaller diameter.

Once into the stomach, air or CO2 is insufflated to distend the gastric cavity and permits an adequate vision of the gastric fundus and EGJ; CO2 is preferable, because it leads to a faster and more sustained gastric insufflation and induces less discomfort to patients. With the endoscope placed in retroflexion position, the lesser curve is located at the 12 o' clock position and the greater curve at the 6 o' clock in the patient placed in left decubitus. Once the tissue mold is retroflexed, it is closed against the EsophyX® device, rotated to 11 or 1 o' clock position (lesser curve), and pulled back to place its tip just inside the esophageal lumen. At this point, the helical screw is advanced to engage tissue under direct vision just below the Z-line, the shaft of the device is advanced caudally, the tissue mold is opened, and the helical screw cable is freed from the tissue mold. Then, a tension is applied to helical retractor while a slight opening and closing of the tissue mold allows the fundus to slide through the tissue mold; in this phase the stomach is being

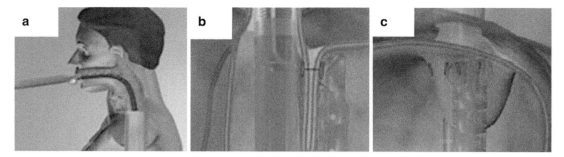

Fig. 23.2 Schematic representation of the EsophyX® procedure (**a**) The EsophyX® device enters the esophagus through the mouth and is positioned at the gastroesophageal junction. (**b**) The device wraps the fundus around the distal esophagus and fastens a tissue fold; this step is then repeated multiple times to reconstruct a robust tight valve (**c**). (Courtesy of EndoGastric Solutions, Inc., Redmond, WA, USA)

desufflated. Failure to desufflate the stomach during this phase of the procedure limits the size of the fundoplication.

After completing this maneuver, both helical retractor and tissue mold are locked in place, suction is applied to the tissue invaginator for approximately half a minute, and the device is then advanced caudally into the stomach, which has been re-insufflated. The latter maneuver ensures that esophago-gastric plication is performed in an intra-abdominal position and reduces hiatal hernia, when present.

Plication is carried out by deploying multiple polypropylene, H-shaped fasteners advanced over two stylets, one anterior and the other posterior. The fastener deployment process initiates on the far posterior and anterior sides of the esophago-gastric valve adjacent to the lesser curvature and then is extended to the greater curvature by rotating the tissue mold axially to slide the stomach over the esophagus, resulting in circumferential tightening and a new valve circumference of >240°. The stylet is advanced under direct endoscopical vision through the tissue mold until its tip is seen by the operator. The fastener is then advanced over the stylet and deployed to create a serosa-to-serosa plication. Once the tip of the fastener becomes visible at the tissue mold, the stylet is pulled back while the fastener is maintained in place; by this way, the leading leg of the fastener is derailed and the fastener is deployed. Fourteen fasteners allowing 7 plications are needed to construct a satisfactory circumferential gastroesophageal valve; however, the higher the number of fasteners deployed, the more continent the newly created valve is [6].

Details of the EsophyX® technique are shown in the Fig. 23.2. Please include a step-by-step video showing each step of the EsophyX technique.

Endoscopic pre- and post-procedural findings are reported in Fig. 23.3.

Besides the standard procedure, two modified techniques have been reported over time to create the fundoplication. The technique we used in the last years engages tissue by advancing the helical screw just below the Z-line on the far posterior and anterior sides of the esophago-gastric valve adjacent to the lesser curvature (11 and 1 o' clock position). Before inserting the stylet, a torque is applied by rotation (clockwise and counter-clockwise at 11 and 1 o' clock, respectively) of the tissue mold locked; such a maneuver allows part of the fundus to rotate around the esophageal wall and more tissue to be engaged by the stylet. Four fasteners for each site are deployed, at 1 and 11 o' clock position, and two fasteners for each site in the middle part of the valve, at 4, 6, and 8 o' clock position, to reinforce and prolong caudally the plication. This technique increased by 30% the success rate of the procedure. With the standard TIF technique, 11/27 patients (40.7%) did not take PPI therapy at 12 months; with the application of the rotational TIF technique, 14/22 patients (63.6%) were full responders [7].

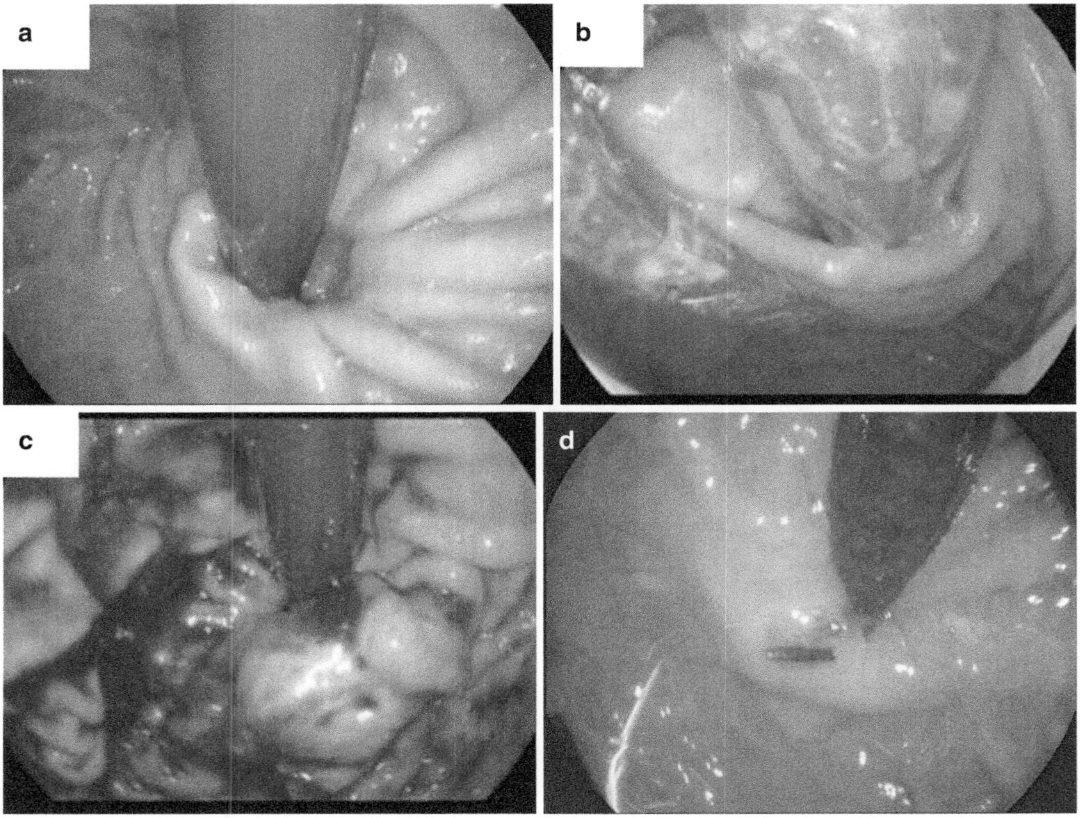

Fig. 23.3 Endoscopic findings of the gastroesophageal valve before and after the TIF procedure by EsophyX® device (**a**) The gastroesophageal valve before the procedure by EsophyX® device. (**b**) The "Bell Roll" maneuver to create the new gastroesophageal valve. (**c**) The gastroesophageal valve immediately after the EsophyX® procedure. (**d**) The gastroesophageal valve 6 months after the EsophyX® procedure. (Authors' cases)

Bell R et al. have developed a rotational fundoplication, the so-called "Bell Roll" maneuver [8]. The helical retractor is engaged at 12 o' clock and the tissue mold is placed at 6 o' clock. The device, with the tissue mold partially closed against the fundus of the stomach, is pulled cranially by 1–3 cm into the esophagus, depending on the depth of the plication intended; tension is then applied to the helical retractor to advance caudally the EGJ while the stomach is desufflated; at this time, the tissue mold locked is rotated toward the lesser curve by a radial motion of the handle of the device to the 12 o' clock position. This maneuver rolls the fundus over and around the distal esophagus to the 1 o' clock position.

At the end of the plication, an immediate endoscopy is performed to evaluate the pharynx, the esophageal lumen, and the gastric fundus and the fundoplication.

Transoral Fundoplication by MUSE™

The MUSE™ device includes the endostapler and a console connected with the endostapler, containing a controller for the camera, ultrasonic range finder and various sensors, a pump for insufflation and irrigation, a suction system, power, and controls for the LED.

The endostapler has (a) a handle, wherein controls are located; (b) an insertion tube

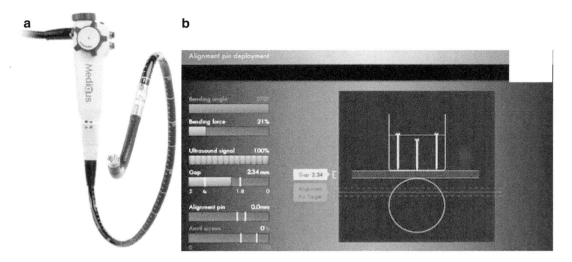

Fig. 23.4 The Medigus surgical ultrasonic endostapler device (MUSE™). (Courtesy of Medigus, Omer, Israel) (**a**) The MUSE™ device. (**b**) The console connected with the endostapler, containing a controller for the camera, ultrasonic range finder, and various sensors (banding angle, banding force, alignment pin, anvil screws, gap)

15.5 mm in diameter, 66 cm long, containing the suction, insufflation/irrigation channels, and electrical and mechanical cables which operate the device; (c) a rigid section 66 mm in length that contains the cartridge (each cartridge contains five standard 4.8-mm titanium staples, the ultrasound mirror, one alignment pin funnel, and two anvil screw funnels); and (d) the distal tip, similar to that of an endoscope, with suction, irrigation, illumination (via LED), and visualization (via miniature camera) capabilities. The anvil, alignment pin, anvil screw, and ultrasound are all designed to ensure proper alignment and positioning of the device during stapling. The distal tip may be articulated in one direction to align with the rigid section and cartridge, with a bending radius of 26 and 40 mm.

Details of the device are illustrated in Fig. 23.4.

The procedure can be performed by one operator in experienced hands. The patient is placed in the supine position, under general anesthesia with endotracheal intubation. Positive end expiratory pressure (PEEP) of at least 5 mm Hg (7.5 cm H2O) is administered. After a preliminary endoscopic assessment of the esophagus and stomach and once no contraindications are found, an overtube is placed. Then, the endostapler is inserted transorally through the overtube and gently advanced into the stomach under direct vision; passing the rigid section across the pharyngo-esophageal junction may encounter some resistance. To avoid applying excessive force and risk of injury to the esophagus, the overtube may be withdrawn approximately 5 cm and then advanced with the endostapler as a unit. This maneuver can be repeated until the system reaches the esophageal midbody. Flexing the neck may make passage easier.

Once into the stomach, distended by insufflation of air or CO2, the stapler is advanced until the tip is approximately 5 cm past the EGJ and then retroflexed by 180° to obtain an adequate vision of the gastric fundus and EGJ to select stapling location.

The most important stapling location is the leftmost location, which is typically performed first. This is the anchoring point for the fundus and should be placed as far to the left of the esophagus as possible. At times, depending on anatomy, it may be easier to perform the first stapling in a more central location. The additional stapling locations should be within 60°–180° as long as the rightmost stapling should not be done

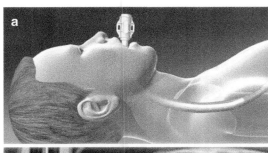

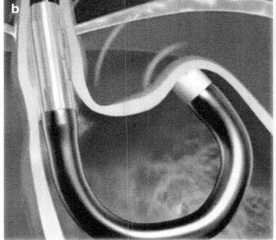

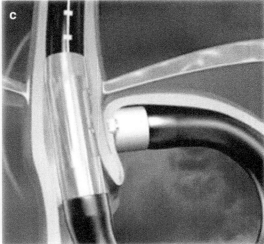

Fig. 23.5 Schematic representation of the Medigus ultrasonic surgical endostapler (MUSE™) procedure (**a**) The endostapler is inserted transorally through the overtube and gently advanced into the stomach under direct vision. (**b**) Once into the stomach, distended by insufflation of air or CO_2, the stapler is advanced until the tip is approximately 5 cm past the EGJ and then retroflexed by 180° to obtain an adequate vision of the gastric fundus and EGJ to select stapling location. Tissue clamping and stapling are performed under ultrasonic guidance. (**c**) This step is then repeated at least twice to reconstruct a robust tight valve. The additional stapling locations should be within 60°–180° of the valve circumference. (Courtesy of Medigus, Omer, Israel)

on the lesser curve, because stapling in the lesser curve may attach the antrum to the esophagus and open the esophago-gastric junction rather than close it. Additional staplings may be placed between the leftmost and rightmost. Once the correct location for stapling has been identified, all the procedures are performed under ultrasound guidance. Subsequent phases of the procedure include clamping tissue, deploying alignment pin, advancing anvil screw, stapling, and retrieving anvil screws [9].

Details of the MUSE™ technique are shown in Fig. 23.5.

Endoscopic pre- and post-procedural findings after TIF with MUSE™ are reported in Fig. 23.6.

Post-operative Care

Antiemetic prophylaxis with at least two drugs (according to the ASA recommendations for interventions with high risk of post-procedure nausea and vomiting) and full muscle relaxation throughout the procedure are mandatory for TIF. Antiemetic prophylaxis is maintained i.v. for 24 h, while broad-spectrum antibiotic therapy is maintained i.v. for 48 h and then by oral route over a 5-day period.

Almost all patients complain of transient pharyngeal irritation, as a result of insertion and manipulation of the device, and some have mild to moderate epigastric pain in the 6 h after

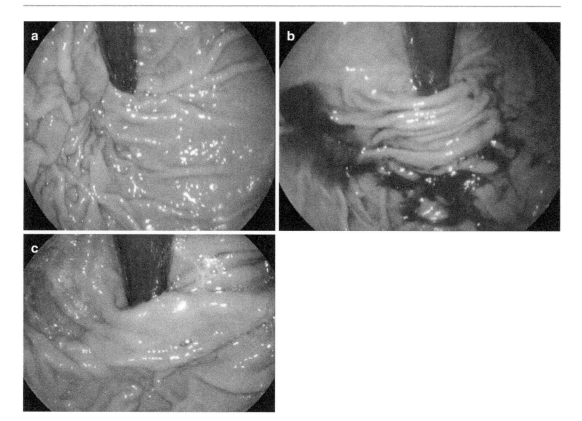

Fig. 23.6 Endoscopic findings of gastroesophageal valve before and after the TIF procedure by Medigus ultrasonic surgical endostapler (MUSE™) (**a**) The gastroesophageal valve before the TIF procedure by Medigus ultrasonic surgical endostapler (MUSE™). (**b**) The gastroesophageal valve immediately after the TIF procedure by Medigus ultrasonic surgical endostapler (MUSE™).(**c**) The gastroesophageal valve 6 months after the TIF procedure by Medigus ultrasonic surgical endostapler (MUSE™). (Authors' cases)

the procedure. Pain persisting for 2–4 days may require analgesics and should be considered for esophageal or gastric leak; CT scan and hydrosoluble contrast x-ray investigation should be carried out in these cases. Dysphagia or gas bloating is generally not reported by patients. White blood cell count may be slightly increased after the procedure. At discharge, patients were instructed to follow a liquid diet for the first 2 weeks and a soft diet for the next 4 weeks. PPI were discontinued 7 days after the procedure.

Patients were also asked to refrain from vigorous exercise for 4 weeks.

Complications

The overall complication rate reported in studies so far available for TIF by EsophyX® ranges from 3% to 10%. Sixteen studies (4 RCTs and 12 prospective observational trials) reported the occurrence of severe adverse events [10]. As a whole, 19 severe adverse events occurred in a total of 781 patients who underwent TIF, with a mean incidence rate of 2.4%. Severe adverse events included seven cases of perforation, five cases of bleeding requiring blood transfusions, four cases of pneumothorax, and one involving severe epigastric pain. Mediastinal abscess as a consequence of esophageal perforation has been reported in less than 2% of cases. Bleeding occurred at the site of the helical retractor insertion. No procedure-related deaths occurred.

The finding of free air in the abdomen immediately after the procedure is not always a sign of clinically relevant complications.

In the three studies so far published on TIF by MUSE™ device, minor side effects such as chest pain, sore throat, transient atelectasis, shoulder pain, and belching were reported in 5.5–22% of patients. Major complications were reported in 6.2% of cases (4 out of 64 patients) and were pneumothorax (one case), pneumothorax and esophageal leak (one case), and bleeding (one case). Patients with pneumothorax and esophageal leak and with bleeding required intervention [11–14].

No late complications or long-lasting side effects were reported for both TIF techniques.

Outcomes

To date, 14 observational non-randomized prospective studies and 5 randomized controlled trials have been published on TIF performed by EsophyX® [10]. Three observational prospective studies and two abstracts have been published on TIF performed by MUSE™.

Among the observational studies on EsophyX® procedure, two provided results in 3 months (32 pts) [4, 15], nine in 6 months (439 pts) [7, 16–23], seven in 12 months (329 pts) [6, 7, 14, 16, 17, 22–24], and three in 24 months (81 pts) [7, 23–25] and 36 months (105 pts) [20, 23, 24], and only one showed results after 4, 5, and 6 years of follow-up [23]. In all studies but three, TIF was proven to discontinue anti-reflux medications or markedly decrease their dose; three studies raised concerns about the effectiveness of the procedure [15, 17, 26]. Results at 3 years have been published recently in the TEMPO randomized trial with a crossover arm: regurgitation and atypical GERD symptoms were eliminated in 90% and 88% of patients, respectively [27].

Sixteen studies assessed symptoms by means of the GERD health-related quality of life (HRQL); 11 evaluated pre- and post-procedure pH +/− impedance recordings.

Six- and 12-month outcomes after TIF showed that 75% to 84% and 53% to 85% of patients had either discontinued PPI use or halved the dose of PPI therapy, respectively. Normalization of esophageal acid exposure, in terms of total acidic refluxes, number of refluxates, and DeMeester score, was reported in 37–89% of patients.

Two years after TIF, daily high-dosage PPI dependence was eliminated in 75–93% of patients.

In the three observational series reporting 3-year outcomes, discontinuation of daily PPI ranged from 74% to 84% of cases.

Only one study assessed outcomes 6 years after TIF in 14/50 patients who undergone the procedure. High-dosage PPI dependence was eliminated in 86% of patients, and approximately half of them completely stopped PPI use [23], providing evidence of the lasting effect of TIF on symptoms and PPI usage. The long-term efficacy of TIF was maintained in the 12 patients of the same prospective series followed up to 10 years: 91.7% patients had either stopped or halved their PPI therapy. Intention-to-treat analysis of the effect of TIF on PPI use at 10 years showed that 78.6% of patients had stopped or halved PPI therapy, while 35.7% had completely discontinued it.

The mean GERD-HRQL scores off PPI therapy and mean heartburn and regurgitation scores still remained significantly lower than before treatment and did not differ compared to the 3, 5-, 7.5-, and 10-year scores. Results are summarized in Fig. 23.7 and Table 23.1.

Unsuccessful outcomes of TIF occurred mainly between 6 and 12 months after the procedure, while between 12 and 36 months, the results did not substantially differ. Six- to ten-year results were substantially similar to those reported at 36 months.

These findings show that an appropriate patient selection plays a pivotal role in achiev-

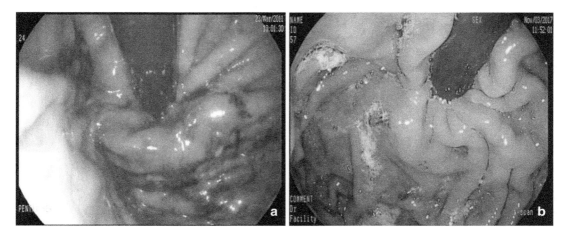

Fig. 23.7 Endoscopic findings of gastroesophageal valve before, immediately after, and 24 months after the TIF procedure by EsophyX® (**a**) The gastroesophageal valve immediately after the TIF procedure by EsophyX®. (**b**) The gastroesophageal valve 6 years after TIF by EsophyX®. (Authors' cases)

Table 23.1 PPI consumption and outcomes up to 10 years after TIF by EsophyX®

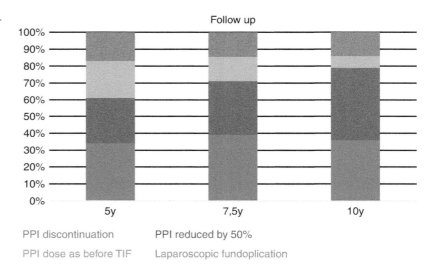

Follow up

PPI discontinuation   PPI reduced by 50%

PPI dose as before TIF   Laparoscopic fundoplication

ing clinical success after TIF and confirm that factors negatively affecting post-operative outcomes play a role early in the post-operative period in most patients. Operator's experience plays an important role in TIF outcomes, too. All TIF failures observed in our series occurred in patients who underwent the procedure early in the operator's learning curve. A retrospective study in 124 unselected patients carried out in two community hospitals and reporting, respectively, 75% and 80% of patients free of typical and atypical GERD symptoms over a mean follow-up of 7 months confirmed that the opera-

tor's experience plays a major role in successful outcomes [28].

In the six RCTs comparing the esophageal acid exposure time with the control, TIF significantly reduced intra-esophageal acid exposure time in GERD patients without PPI therapy [27, 29–33]. TIF showed similar efficacy with respect to esophageal acid exposure time, compared with PPIs, and significantly improved patients' acid exposure time compared with sham groups.

Three RCTs evaluated the total reflux episodes before and after TIF procedure [20, 29, 31].

Patients undergoing endoscopic fundoplication yielded significant reduction in reflux episodes compared with those who did not.

Three RCTs [27, 31, 32] reported the incidence of acid reflux episodes before and after TIF therapy. Patients undergoing endoscopic fundoplication showed no significant differences from those who received PPI therapy.

Unsuccessful outcomes after TIF were reported in three studies. Two series found worsening of distal esophageal acid exposure in 66.7% of cases and persisting of GERD symptoms in 68% of cases, respectively, in small series with a short follow-up (12 months) [17, 26]. An open-label study comparing TIF with robot-assisted Nissen fundoplication in PPI-refractory GERD patients reported complete symptom remission and normalization of esophageal acid exposure time in 30% and 100% of patients after TIF and 50% and 100% after Nissen fundoplication [15]. These data suggest that, in a challenging clinical setting such as PPI refractoriness, Nissen fundoplication seems more effective than TIF by EsophyX®.

In case of failure of TIF, surgical fundoplication has been shown to be feasible, without technical difficulties or increased morbidity. Surgical revision after TIF failure was reported in 8.1–18.0% of cases [7, 24, 34, 35]. In two studies Nissen fundoplication induced complete disappearance of symptoms in all cases of TIF failure (respectively, 9 and 11 patients) [35, 36]. In our series, however, only one out of the four patients who undergone Nissen fundoplication for persisting GERD symptoms after TIF stopped acid-suppressive therapy [7]: this finding may depend upon the particular subset of patients who underwent TIF in our series, those who had only a mild impairment of the gastroesophageal junction and suffered from GERD-related symptoms that could have been generated by a number of complex mechanisms, including increased esophageal sensitivity to refluxate.

On the other hand, re-intervention after laparoscopic fundoplication has been reported in up to 14% of cases [1] and TIF has been found effective after failed surgery [37].

Only five studies so far assessed outcomes after TIF performed by MUSE™ technique (anterior fundoplication). A pilot study assessed GERD-related symptoms and PPI use up to 5 years after the procedure in 13 subjects: GERD-related symptom score at 6 months was normalized in 92% of cases, and PPI use was completely stopped or reduced by half in 77% of cases (54% off PPI completely). PPI therapy was abolished or reduced by half in 82% of patients at 12 months and in 73% at 36 months; this rate persisted and was unchanged for up to 5 years [11].

In a multicenter, prospective international study enrolling 66 patients with a 6-month follow-up, GERD-related symptom scores improved by more than 50% in 73% of patients, and 85% were no longer using PPI or had their daily dose markedly reduced by more than 50%; 64.6% of patients discontinued PPI medication. At 24-h pH recording, the total time with esophageal pH < 4.0 decreased significantly from baseline [12].

Another study assessed efficacy and safety of TIF performed by MUSE™ in 37 patients at baseline, 6 months, and up to 4 years post-procedure in a single center [13]. The proportions of patients who remained off daily PPI were 83.8% (31/37) at 6 months and 69.4% (25/36) at 4 years post-procedure. GERD health-related quality of life (HRQL) scores (off PPI) were significantly decreased from baseline to 6 months and 4 years post-procedure. The daily dosage of GERD medications, measured as omeprazole equivalents (mean ± SD, mg), decreased from 66.1 ± 33.2 at baseline to 10.8 ± 15.9 at 6 months and 12.8 ± 19.4 at 4 years post-procedure ($P < 0.01$). Two abstracts presented at DDW in 2017 reported the discontinuation of PPI therapy in 76% of patients at 6 months in a multicenter study and in 74% and 79% of patients at 6 and 12 months in a single-center study.

There were no post-procedure side effects commonly seen after laparoscopic fundoplication such as gas bloating, inability to belch or vomit, dysphagia, or diarrhea.

Factors Affecting Outcomes After TIF

Analysis of factors that could influence the results of endoluminal transoral fundoplication has been so far assessed only for the EsophyX® technique.

In our series, from the technical point of view, the number of fasteners deployed and the rotational technique applied were associated with a good outcome; a larger number of fasteners raised the probability of being a responder by about fourfold [7]. Another study reported the number of satisfactory fasteners as critical point for the success of the procedure, too [8].The rotational technique raised the probability of being a responder by one half, confirming other recent reports [8, 21]. Among patient-related factors affecting post-operative outcomes in our series, pre-operative Hill grades III and IV, hiatal hernia larger than 2 cm, and ineffective esophageal motility were associated with a higher rate of unsuccessful results. The defective clearance of refluxate could induce an epithelial sensitization that might produce symptoms, even in presence of low-volume gastroesophageal reflux [38]. A univariate and multivariate analysis of pre-operative factors influencing symptomatic outcomes of TIF by EsophyX® was performed on data from 158 consecutive patients [39]. Predictors of successful outcomes for patients with typical symptoms have been found such as age ≥ 50 years, a GERD health-related quality of life score (GERD-HRQL) on PPIs ≥15, a reflux symptom index >13 on PPIs, and a gastroesophageal reflux symptom score ≥ 18 on PPIs. Age and GERD-HRLQ remained significant predictors also at the multivariate analysis. For patients with atypical GERD symptoms, only a GERD-HRQL score ≥ 15 on PPIs was associated with successful outcomes.

Conclusions

In the last years TIF has become a relatively common procedure for treating pathological gastroesophageal reflux. Most of the interventions have been performed in clinical trials including patients with typical gastroesophageal reflux symptoms responsive or partially responsive to PPI therapy, without hiatal hernia or with small hiatal hernia (<3 cm), who refused life-long medical therapy, or were intolerant to PPIs, or required high dosage of antisecretory maintenance therapy. Patients with grade C and D esophagitis, according to Los Angeles classification, and Barrett's esophagus were excluded from these studies.

In the majority of studies, TIF was done by EsophyX® device and was proven effective in the short term, eliminating the daily dependence from PPIs in 75–85% of patients. Similar results were obtained for TIF done with Medigus endostapler, but in few studies so far.

In the three series reporting 3-year outcomes, results did not differ from those at 1 and 2 years and persisted up to 6 years; results at 6 years have been maintained up to 10 years, in the few cases in whom such a long clinical follow-up has been obtained.

Troublesome procedure-related persisting side effects were not reported in all the published studies, with both techniques.

Overall outcomes showed that transoral fundoplication can be an effective and safe alternative therapeutic option to surgery in a selected subset of patients, as those recruited in the published studies. In available series with 3-year follow-up, post-TIF results were slightly inferior to those reported in patients operated by Nissen fundoplication, but similar to those with surgical posterior partial (Toupet) or anterior partial (Dor-Thal) fundoplication, without any of the surgery-related side effects such as dysphagia and gas bloat. In a longer follow-up (6–10 years), TIF outcomes are substantially comparable with those of Nissen fundoplication, although reported only in few cases.

Currently, based on clinical results, TIF may be offered as a routine alternative to surgery in patients suffering from gastroesophageal reflux disease and grade A–B esophagitis, if present, with the sole limitation of the length and reducibility of hiatal hernia, which is at present the only limiting factor affecting the choice of the intervention. TIF may also be offered to patients who have some risk of developing persistent post-surgical side effects. To date, data supporting the efficacy of TIF in the treatment of severe grades of esophagitis or symptoms associated with oropharyngeal reflux are lacking.

However, as for all new procedures introduced in clinical practice, despite favorable short-/medium-term outcomes, questions still arise about the long-term efficacy of the techniques, mainly for the MUSE™ one, in controlling symptoms and persistence over time of the newly created valve. Therefore, randomized controlled trials are warranted in order to establish the role of TIF in the management of GERD patients and which, among the two techniques, could be more effective and safe.

References

1. Lundell L, Miettinen P. Continued (5 years) follow up of a randomized clinical study comparing antireflux surgery and omeprazole in GERD. J Am Coll Surg. 2001;192:171–82.
2. Draaisma WE, Rijnhart-de Jong HG, Broeders IAMJ, Smout AJ, Furnee EJ, Gooszen HG. Five-year subjective and objective results of laparoscopic and conventional Nissen fundoplication. Ann Surg. 2006;244:34–41.
3. Smith CD. Surgical therapy for gastroesophageal reflux disease: indications, evaluation and procedures. Gastrointest Endosc Clin N Am. 2009;19:35–48.
4. Broeders JA, Draaisma WA, Bredenoord AJ, Smout AJ, Broeders IA, Gooszen HG. Long-term outcome of Nissen fundoplication in non-erosive and erosive gastro-esophageal reflux disease. Br J Surg. 2010;97:845–52.
5. Alemanno G, Bergamini C, Prosperi P, Bruscino A, Leahu A, Somigli R, Martellucci J, Valeri A. A long-term evaluation of the quality of life after laparoscopic Nissen-Rossetti anti-reflux surgery. J Minim Access Surg. 2017;13:208–14.
6. Cadiere GB, Rajan A, Germay O, Himpens J. Endoluminal fundoplication by a transoral device for the treatment of GERD: a feasibility study. Surg Endosc. 2008;22:333–42.
7. Testoni PA, Vailati C, Testoni S, Corsetti M. Transoral incisionless fundoplication (TIF 2.0) with Esophyx for gastroesophageal reflux disease: long-term results and findings affecting outcome. Surg Endosc. 2012;26:1425–35.
8. Bell RC, Cadière GB. Transoral rotational esophagogastric fundoplication: technical, anatomical, and safety considerations. Surg Endosc. 2011;25:2387–99.
9. Kauer WK, Roy-Shapira A, Watson D, Sonnenschein M, Sonnenschein E, Unger J, Voget M, Stein HJ. Preclinical trial of a modified gastroscope that performs a true anterior fundoplication for the endoluminal treatment of gastroesophageal reflux disease. Surg Endosc. 2009;23:2728–31.
10. Huang X, Chen S, Zhao H, Zeng X, Lin J, Tseng Y, Chen J. Efficacy of transoral incisionless fundoplication (TIF) for the treatment of GERD: a systematic review with meta-analysis. Surg Endosc. 2017;31:1032–44.
11. Roy-Shapira A, Bapaye A, Date S, Pujari R, Dorwat S. Trans-oral anterior fundoplication: 5-year follow-up of pilot study. Surg Endosc. 2015;29(12):3717–21.
12. Zacheri J, Roy-Shapira A, Bonavina L, Bapaye A, Kiesslich R, Schoppmann SF, Kessler WR, Selzer DJ, Broderick RC, Lehman GA, Horgan S. Endoscopic anterior fundoplication with the Medigus ultrasonic surgical endostapler (MUSE) for gastroesophageal reflux: 6-month results from a multi-center prospective trial. Surg Endosc. 2015;29:220–9.
13. Kim HJ, Kwon CI, Kessler WR, Selzer DJ, McNulty G, Bapaye A, Bonavina L, Lehman GA. Long-term follow-up results of endoscopic treatment of gastroesophageal reflux disease with the MUSE™ endoscopic stapling device. Surg Endosc. 2016;30:3402–8.
14. Demyttenaere SV, Bergman S, Pham T, Anderson J, Dettorre R, Melvin WS, Mikami DJ. Transoral incisionless fundoplication for gastro-esophageal reflux disease in an unselected patient population. Surg Endosc. 2010;24:854–8.
15. Frazzoni M, Conigliaro R, Manta R, Melotti G. Reflux parameters as modified by EsophyX or laparoscopic fundoplication in refractory GERD. Aliment Pharmacol Ther. 2011;34:67–75.
16. Cadière GB, Buset M, Muls V, Rajan A, Rösch T, Eckardt AJ, Weerts J, Bastens B, Costamagna G, Marchese M, Louis H, Mana F, Sermon F, Gawlicka AK, Daniel MA, Devière J. Antireflux transoral incisionless fundoplication using EsophyX: 12-month results of a prospective multicenter study. World J Surg. 2008;32:1676–88.
17. Repici A, Fumagalli U, Malesci A, Barbera R, Gambaro C, Rosati R. Endoluminal fundoplication (ELF) for GERD using Esophyx: a 12-month follow-up in a single-center experience. J Gastrointest Surg. 2010;14:1–6.
18. Testoni PA, Corsetti M, Di Pietro S, Castellaneta AG, Vailati C, Masci E, Passaretti S. Effect of transoral incisionless fundoplication on symptoms, PPI use, and pH-impedance refluxes of GERD patients. World J Surg. 2010;34:750–7.
19. Petersen R, Filippa L, Wassenaar EB, Martin AV, Tatum R, Oelschlager BK. Comprehensive evaluation of endoscopic fundoplication using the Esophyx device. Surg Endosc. 2012;26:1021–7.
20. Witteman PBL, Strijkers R, de Vries E, Toemen L, Conchillo JM, Hameeteman W, Dagnelie PC, Koek GH, Bouvy ND. Transoral incisionless fundoplication

for treatment of gastroesophageal reflux diseases in clinical practice. Surg Endosc. 2012;26:3307–15.

21. Bell RC, Mavrelis PG, Barnes WE, Dargis D, Carter BJ, Hoddinott KM, Sewell RW, Trad KS, DaCosta Gill B, Ihde GM. A prospective multicenter registry of patients with chronic gastro-esophageal reflux disease receiving transoral incisionless fundoplication. J Am Coll Surg. 2012;215:794–809.

22. Wilson EB, Barnes WE, Mavrelis PG, Carter BJ, Bell RCW, Sewell RW, Ihde GM, Dargis D, Hoddinott KM, Shughoury AB, Gill BD, Fox MA, Turgeon DG, Freeman KD, Gunsberger T, Hausmann MG, Leblanc KA, Deljkich E, Trad KS. The effects of transoral incisionless fundoplication on chronic GERD patients: 12-month prospective multicenter experience. Surg Laparosc Endosc Percutan Tech. 2014;24:36–46.

23. Testoni PA, Testoni S, Mazzoleni G, Vailati C, Passaretti S. Long-term efficacy of transoral incisionless fundoplication with Esophyx (TIF 2.0) and factors affecting outcomesin GERD patients followed for up to 6 years: a prospective single-center study. Surg Endosc. 2015;29:2770–80.

24. Muls V, Eckardt AJ, Marchese M, Bastens B, Buset M, Devière J, Louis H, Rajan A, Daniel MA, Costamagna G. Three-year results of a multicenter prospective study of transoral incisionless fundoplication. Surg Innov. 2013;20(4):321–30.

25. Cadière GB, Van Sante N, Graves JE, Gawlicka AK, Rajan A. Two-year results of a feasibility study on antireflux transoral incisionless fundoplication using Esophyx. Surg Endosc. 2009;23:957–64.

26. Hoppo T, Immanuel A, Schuchert M, Dubrava Z, Smith A, Nottle P, Watson DI, Jobe BA. Transoral incisionless fundoplication 2.0 procedure using EsophyX™ for gastroesophageal reflux disease. J Gastrointest Surg. 2010;14:1895–901.

27. Trad K, Fox MA, Simoni G, Shughoury AB, Mavrelis PG, Raza M, Helse JA, Barnes WE. Transoralfundopliication offers durable symptom control for chronic GERD: 3-year report from the TEMPIO randomized trail with a crossover arm. Surg Endosc. 2017;31:2498–508.

28. Barnes WE, Hoddinott KM, Mundy S, et al. Transoral incisionless fundoplication offers high patient satisfaction and relief of therapy-resistant typical and atypical symptoms of GERD in community practice. Surg Innov. 2011;18:119–29.

29. Hunter GJ, Kahrilas PJ, Bell RC, Wilson EB, Trad KS, Dolan JP, Perry KA, Oelschlager BK, Soper NJ, Snyder BE, Burch MA, Melvin WS, Reavis KM, Turgeon DG, Hungness ES, Diggs BS. Efficacy of transoral fundoplication vs omeprazole for treatment of regurgitation in a randomized controlled trial. Gastroenterology. 2015;148:324–33.

30. Hakansson B, Montgomery M, Cadiere GB, Rajan A, Bruley des Varannes S, Lerhun M, Coron E, Tack J, Bischops R, Thorell A, Arnelo U, Lundell L. Randomised clinical trial: transoral incisionless fundoplication vs. sham intervention to control chronic GERD. Aliment Pharmacol Ther. 2015;42:1261–70.

31. Rinsma NF, Farre´ R, Bouvy ND, Masclee AM, Conchillo JM. The effect of endoscopic fundoplication and proton pump inhibitors on baseline impedance and heartburn severity in GERD patients. Neurogastroenterol Motil. 2015;27:220–8.

32. Trad KS, Barnes WE, Simoni G, Shughoury AB, Mavrelis PG, Raza M, Heise JA, Turgeon DG. Fox MA (2015) Transoral incisionless fundoplication effective in eliminating GERD symptoms in partial responders to proton pump inhibitor therapy at 6 months: the TEMPO randomized clinical trial. Surg Innov. 2015;22:26–40.

33. Trad KS, Simoni G, Barnes WE, Shughoury AB, Raza M, Heise JA, Turgeon DG, Fox MA, Mavrelis PG. Efficacy of transoral fundoplication for treatment of chronic gastroesophageal reflux disease incompletely controlled with high-dose proton-pump inhibitors therapy: a randomized, multicenter, open label, crossover study. BMC Gastroenterol. 2014;14:174.

34. Svoboda P, Kantorová I, Kozumplík L, Scheer P, Radvan M, Radvanová J, Krass V, Horálek F. Our experience with transoral incisionless plication of gastroesophageal reflux disease: NOTES procedure. Hepatogastroenterology. 2011;109:1208–13.

35. Fumagalli Romario U, Barbera R, Repici A, Porta M, Malesci A, Rosati R. Nissen fundoplication after failure of endoluminal fundoplication: short-term results. J Gastrointest Surg. 2011;15:439–43.

36. Furnée EJ, Broeders JA, Draaisma WA, Schwartz MP, Hazebroek EJ, Smout AJ, van Rijn PJ, Broeders IA. Laparoscopic Nissen fundoplication after failed Esophyx fundoplication. Br J Surg. 2010;97:1051–5.

37. Bell RCW, Hufford RJ, Fearon J, Freeman KD. Revision of failed traditional fundoplication using Esophyxtransoral fundoplication. Surg Endosc. 2013;27:761–7.

38. Kim KY, Kim GH, Kim DU, Wang SG, Lee BJ, Lee JC, Park DY, Song GA. Is ineffective esophageal motility associated with gastropharyngeal reflux disease? World J Gastroenterol. 2008;14:6030–5.

39. Bell RC, Fox MA, Barnes WE, Mavrelis PG, Sewell RW, Carter BJ, Ihde GM, Trad KS, Dargis D, Hoddinott KM, Freeman KD, Gunsberger T, Hausmann MG, Gill BD, Wilson E. Univariate and multivariate analysis of preoperative factors influencing symptomatic outcomes of transoral fundoplication. Surg Endosc. 2014;28:2949–58.

Radiofrequency Ablation (RFA) and Anti-Reflux MucoSectomy (ARMS) for Gastroesophageal Reflux Disease

Bryan Brimhall, Amit Maydeo, Mihir S. Wagh, and Hazem Hammad

Gastroesophageal reflux disease (GERD) has been treated traditionally by lifestyle modifications, medications, and at times surgical interventions. The incidence of GERD has been increasing overall, particularly in North America and East Asia [1]. Up to 20–30% of patients with erosive reflux and 40% of patients with non-erosive reflux do not respond to the mainstay of therapy, proton pump inhibitors (PPI) [2]. Other options such as anti-reflux surgery (open or laparoscopic fundoplica-tion) have been utilized if PPI therapy is not effective, but surgical fundoplication patients restart PPI therapy approximately a quarter of the time in long-term follow-up. After surgery, 15% and 30% of patients have re-intervention following laparoscopic or conventional fundoplication, respectively [3, 4]. In the recent past, multiple other endoscopic options for therapy have been introduced including: magnetic sphincter augmentation (MSA) otherwise known as the LINX system (Torax Medical Inc., Shoreview, MN, USA); radiofrequency ablation, also known as the Stretta system (Mederi Therapeutics, Norwalk, CT, USA); transoral incisionless fundoplication (TIF) (EsophyX; EndoGastric Solutions, Redmond, WA, USA); Medigus Ultrasonic Surgical Endostapler (Medigus, Omer, Israel); and endoscopic full-thickness plication (GERDx System; G-SURG GmbH, Seeon-Seebruck, Germany) [4–6]. Many of these previously mentioned interventions have been discussed in other chapters of this textbook. Herein, we will focus on radiofrequency ablation and anti-reflux mucosectomy (ARMS).

Electronic Supplementary Material The online version of this chapter (https://doi.org/10.1007/978-3-030-21695-5_24) contains supplementary material, which is available to authorized users.

B. Brimhall
Division of Gastroenterology, University of Colorado, Boulder, CO, USA

A. Maydeo
Baldota Institute of Digestive Sciences, Global Hospital, Mumbai, India

M. S. Wagh
Interventional Endoscopy, Division of Gastroenterology, University of Colorado-Denver, Aurora, CO, USA
e-mail: mihir.wagh@cuanschutz.edu

H. Hammad (✉)
Division of Gastroenterology and Hepatology, Section of Therapeutic Endoscopy, University of Colorado Anschutz Medical Center and Veterans Affairs Eastern Colorado Health Care System, Aurora, CO, USA
e-mail: Hazem.Hammad@ucdenver.edu

Radiofrequency Ablation (Stretta)

Radiofrequency ablation for treatment of GERD, also known as the Stretta system (Mederi Therapeutics, Norwalk, CT, USA), was approved by the FDA in 2000. It uses application of radiofrequency energy via a 20 French soft tip balloon

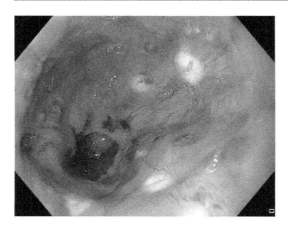

Fig. 24.1 Endoscopy after Stretta procedure showing the thermal effect on the lower esophageal tissue. (Images courtesy of Steven Edmundowicz, MD)

catheter system to the lower esophageal sphincter muscle and gastric cardia [7]. Multiple doses of energy are applied (through four built-in needles) by changing the position of the balloon catheter system in relation to the Z line and rotating the balloon catheter (Fig. 24.1). Radiofrequency energy is usually delivered with low power (5 watts) with a thermocouple system that avoids high temperatures at both the muscularis (>85 °C) and mucosal levels (>50 °C). Water irrigation is also used to avoid overheating that could result in mucosal injury [4]. Previously proposed mechanisms of action have included fibrosis of the submucosa and muscularis at the gastroesophageal junction, but more recent data argues against the fibrosis theory and propose that the low energy delivered induces muscle fiber proliferation and muscle fiber volume increase with subsequent physiological barrier creation [7–11].

Corley et al. evaluated patients with both symptoms of GERD and pathologic esophageal acid exposure randomized to either RFA ($n = 35$) or sham therapy ($n = 29$). They showed improvement in daily heartburn symptoms between RFA and sham (61% v 33%, $p = 0.005$), and $a > 50\%$ improvement in GERD quality of life score (61% v 30%, $p = 0.03$). However, at 6 months there was no difference seen in daily medication use after a medication withdrawal protocol (55% v 61%, $p = 0.67$) and no difference in esophageal acid exposure [12].

The second randomized trial performed by Aziz et al. included patients that had 6 months of

heartburn and a GERD health-related quality of life (GERD-HRQL) score of >18 when all medications (excluding antacids) were stopped for 10 days. The first arm was a single Stretta procedure, the 2nd arm was a "sham" procedure where patients underwent sedated endoscopy and the Stretta catheter was placed but no energy was delivered, and the third arm received the Stretta procedure, but in those who did not have a 75% improvement in GERD-HRQL scoring, then a repeat Stretta procedure was performed. The primary endpoint was improvement in GERD-HRQL from baseline. The study revealed that GERD-HRQL improved in the sham and treatment arm comparing pre- and post endoscopy scores. The degree of GERD-HRQL improvement was greater in the treatment group compared to the sham group, but this finding was not significant. Acid exposure time for the sham procedure group was not significant pre and post (9.9 min +/− 2.6 to 8.2 ± 3.1, $p > 0.05$) although it was reduced for both the single Stretta (9.4 min +/− 3.4 to 6.7 ± 2.8, $p < 0.01$) and double Stretta procedure groups (8.8 min +/− 2.8 to 5.2 ± 2.4, $p < 0.01$). Mean lower esophageal sphincter pressure at 12 months was also significantly increased in both single (11.6 ± 3.2 to 16.2 ± 4.5 mmHg, $p < 0.01$) and double treatment (12.2 ± 3.7 to 19.6 ± 2.9 mmHg, $p < 0.01$) arms compared to sham (14.1 ± 2.6 to 15.9 ± 3.2 mmHg, $p > 0.05$) [13].

Arts et al. looked at 22 GERD patients with a complete or partial response to high dose PPI therapy with long-standing history of established GERD with typical symptoms and pathological esophageal pH monitoring (>4% of time pH < 4) in a double-blind, sham-controlled, crossover radiofrequency trial [11]. These patients all had symptom assessment, endoscopy, manometry, 24-h esophageal pH monitoring, and a distensibility test of the GEJ completed prior to the study and after 3 months. In the first group of 11 patients that underwent Stretta therapy first followed by sham, they had a significant decrease in symptom scores (14.7 ± 1.5 v 8.3 ± 1.9, $p < 0.005$), but at 3 months when they underwent the sham procedure as part of the crossover, there was no additional significant difference observed (7.8 ± 2.1). In the second group who underwent sham therapy first, their symptoms did not improve significantly (16.1 ± 2.5 v 15.6 ± 2.2), but at 3 months when they underwent the Stretta procedure, there was a significant difference seen (7.2 ± 1.6, $p < 0.05$). At follow-up endoscopy at 3 and 6 months post Stretta procedure, there was no difference seen in number of patients with erosive esophagitis or the grade of esophagitis in comparison to pre-Stretta therapy. At 3 and 6 months, there was no difference observed in pathologic esophageal acid exposure or proton pump inhibitor used pre- and post Stretta procedure in either group. There was no significant difference seen in lower esophageal pressure, esophageal distensibility, or esophageal motility in the two groups prior to Stretta and at 3 and 6 months post procedure. This study did show a decrease in compliance at the gastroesophageal junction after the Stretta procedure (17.8 ± 3.6 v 7.4 ± 3.4 ml/mm Hg, $p < 0.05$) which reversed to pre-Stretta levels with administration of Sildenafil 50 mg, a smooth muscle relaxant which argues against fibrosis as the etiology of improvement of symptom scores as discussed earlier [11].

Coron et al. describe their experience in 43 patients in a randomized controlled trial comparing Stretta and proton pump inhibitor therapy [14]. All patients were using PPI therapy prior to the study. Primary endpoint evaluated at 6 months was the ability to stop or decrease PPI therapy to <50% of the effective dose required at baseline. At 6 months there was a significant improvement in patients that could either stop PPI therapy or reduce dose to <50% in favor of Stretta therapy (78% v 40%, $p = 0.01$), but this did not hold true at 12 months (56% v 35%, $p = 0.16$). HRQL scores were not different between groups, and there was no significant change in regard to esophageal acid exposure between baseline and 6 months after Stretta therapy [14].

Randomized controlled trials showing efficacy of the Stretta procedure are limited. There have been systemic reviews that have shown improvement in heartburn and GERD-HRQL scores. In one systematic review that included 20 articles (2 randomized controlled trial, 18 cohort studies) and 1441 patients in total, GERD symptoms and patient satisfaction based on mean Likert scores improved significantly (1.43 ± 4.1 to 4.07 ± 3.1, $p = 0.0006$) as well as GERD-HRQL scores (26.11 ± 27.2 to 9.25 ± 23.7, $p = 0.0001$). In this same analysis, DeMeester scores improved significantly (44.37 ± 93 to 28.53 ± 33.4, $p = 0.0074$) as well as esophageal acid exposure time (10.29% ± 17.8% to 6.51% ± 12.5%, $p = 0.0003$) [15].

A more recent meta-analysis performed by Lipka et al. with 165 patients, which only included randomized controlled trials of Stretta in comparison with either sham procedure [3] or PPI therapy [1], showed no difference between Stretta and sham therapies in regard to esophageal pH values (mean difference 1.56; 95% CI, −2.56 to 5.69; $p = 0.46$), augmentation of lower esophageal sphincter pressure (−0.3; 95% CI, −2.66 to 2.02; $P = 0.79$), HRQL score (−5.24; 95% CI, −12.95 to 2.46; $P = 0.18$), or the ability to stop the use of proton pump inhibitors (relative risk 0.87; 95% CI, 0.75–1.00; $P = 0.06$) [16].

Adverse events encountered with Stretta are usually mild and can include chest pain (50%), transient fever, and esophageal ulcers. Gastroparesis has been reported which has been thought to be due to inadvertent vagal nerve injury [4, 7]. Radiofrequency ablation therapy (Stretta) is currently lacking stringent long-term objective data, and it is difficult to recommend at this time based on this available data.

Anti-reflux Mucosectomy (ARMS)

In 2003, Satodate et al. reported a case of circumferential mucosal resection of the distal esophagus and gastric cardia for treatment of high-grade dysplasia in a patient with Barrett's esophagus [17]. The patient prior to resection had a DeMeester score of 5 with a significant hiatal hernia (flap valve grade 3). Resection included 2 cm of the gastric cardia to ensure adequate margins. On follow-up, the patient was noted to form a scar at the level of the gastric cardia and had subsequent normalization of acid exposure on 24-h pH monitoring [18]. The patient did require multiple balloon dilations for initial stricture formation, but he remained asymptomatic from a GERD standpoint. This patient prompted Professor Inoue and the Tokyo

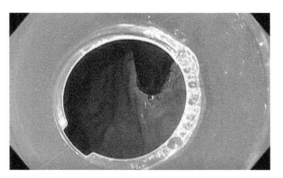

Fig. 24.2 Gastroesophageal junction/cardia prior to ARMS being performed

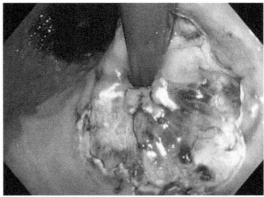

Fig. 24.3 Resection area after ARMS

group to investigate whether mucosectomy for GERD in the absence of a hiatus hernia was feasible for treatment of refractory GERD.

Inoue et al. selected PPI refractory GERD patients without a sliding hiatal hernia in the presence or absence of Barrett's esophagus at their institution in Japan for study inclusion [19]. To evaluate the severity of GERD symptoms, the DeMeester score was applied [20]. Upper endoscopy was performed to evaluate the size and grade of any hiatal hernia and presence of esophagitis and/or Barrett's (Fig. 24.2). All patients also underwent esophageal testing with manometry, 24-h pH monitoring and Bilitec. Gastroesophageal flap valve grading (grade 1–4) was used to describe the size and grade of any hiatal hernia [21].

In the first 2 ARMS patients, circumferential resection was performed to resect Barrett's with high-grade dysplasia. The subsequent eight patients had crescentic ARMS performed with either piecemeal endoscopic mucosal resection (EMR) (two patients) or endoscopic submucosal dissection (ESD) (six patients) which included 1 cm of the esophagus and 2 cm of the gastric cardia along the lesser curvature as measured from the gastric side. The procedure was conducted by first marking the mucosal resection site with an electrocautery knife followed by injection of saline and indigo carmine dye into the submucosa for lifting prior to 270-degree resection completed with either EMR or ESD (Figs. 24.2, 24.3, and 24.4 and Video 24.1). Patients were allowed water the day after the

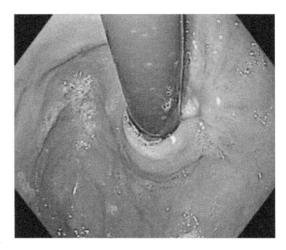

Fig. 24.4 Follow-up endoscopy 1 month after ARMS showing scar in the lesser curvature with improved flap valve

procedure, followed by a soft diet on the second day and a normal diet thereafter starting on the third day. PPI therapy was continued in all patients for 40 days after ARMS was completed and then stopped. Esophageal testing was then completed 2 months after the initial procedure for comparison.

The group reported no complications in any of the ten patients. DeMeester scores improved significantly for heartburn (2.7–0.3, $p = 0.0022$), regurgitation (2.5–0.3, $p = 0.0022$), and overall total score (5.1–0.8, $p = 0.0022$). Flap valve score was also significantly improved after intervention (3.2–1.2, $p = 0.0152$) [19]. In the first two patients with 10 and 3 years of follow-up, respectively, they reported no recurrence of symptoms, esophagitis, or Barrett's esophagus. In the subsequent eight patients that had ARMS completed without evidence of Barrett's, the pH <4 improved significantly from 29.1% of the time to 3.1% of the time ($p = 0.01$) although they reported that half of the patients refused pH evaluation after the ARMS which limits this data. Procedure time on average was 76 min (42–124, $N = 3$) in piecemeal EMR patients and 127 min (98–176, $N = 7$) for ESD. In all ten patients, PPI therapy was discontinued at 40 days successfully. Inoue et al. suggest that scar formation following mucosal defect as the underlying mechanism for preventing gastroesophageal reflux in addition to a possible remodeling of the mucosal flap valve well (Fig. 24.4).

Inoue et al. have also published an abstract with 67 consecutive patients who have undergone ARMS therapy [22]. Similar to previous, semi-circumferential mucosectomy in the gastric cardia was completed centered at the lesser curve. F scale improved from 26.8 to 8.3 ($p < 0.01$), and the GERD Q score was reduced from 9.9 to 5.7 ($p < 0.01$) at 2 months post therapy. In 24-h pH impedance monitoring percent time, clearance of pH (total) was improved from 22.8% to 7.0% ($p < 0.05$). PPI therapy was discontinued in 55% of patients and reduced in 23% of patients at two-month follow-up. At 1 year following ARMS intervention, PPI non-use was 61%.

In addition to Inoue et al., other groups have reported their findings. Bapaye et al. reported on 12 patients with refractory GERD, defined as symptoms greater than 1 year, and daily PPI usage for >6 months with absence of hiatal hernia >3 cm who underwent ARMS with a cap EMR technique [23]. They followed patients for 4–6 weeks post ARMS. Mean GERD-HRQL improved from 40 to 12 which they reported as significant as well as mean DeMeester score improvement from 28 to 9. They did report two adverse events which were both muscle injuries treated with endoclip placement. At 4 weeks follow-up, 9/12 (75%) patients had discontinued PPI use and 2/12 (16.7%) had a 50% reduction in PPI usage.

Chuttani and colleagues have reported on a novel variation of ARMS which they term the Cardia Ligation Endoscopic Anti-Reflux (CLEAR) procedure [24]. This variation of the ARMS procedure involved band ligation of the gastric cardia in lieu of mucosal resection in an attempt to decrease procedure-related adverse events. The initial results in two patients appear promising.

ARMS is a novel endoscopic therapy that holds promise for severe GERD without hiatal hernia in patients failing lifestyle modifications and medical therapy. Short-term data shows excellent results but long-term data is still lacking. There is one current trial (Clinicaltrials.gov identifier NCT03259191) that is enrolling at the time of this publication with the goal of obtaining long-term follow-up. Benefits of ARMS include the fact that no proprietary equipment is needed and that no artificial prosthesis is left in place like some other endoscopic GERD interventions. The techniques of EMR/ESD are practiced more widely and the hope that these techniques will be easily transferable to ARMS therapy. Questions that need to be addressed in long-term trials for ARMS include what is the ideal amount and location of tissue to be resected for the procedure to be efficacious but not cause adverse events such as dysphagia. There also needs to be a comparison of lesser and greater curvature resection. Lesser curvature has been proposed as being better in the idea that a more acute angle is formed by scarring, but this has not been tested to date. Even with these questions, endoscopic therapy for refractory GERD is promising, and the ARMS technique holds great promise.

References

1. El-Serag HB, Sweet S, Winchester CC, et al. Update on the epidemiology of gastro-oesophageal reflux disease: a systematic review. Gut. 2014;63:871–80.
2. Katz PO, Gerson LB, Vela MF. Guidelines for the diagnosis and management of gastroesophageal reflux disease. Am J Gastroenterol. 2013;108:308–28; quiz 329
3. Broeders JA, Rijnhart-de Jong HG, Draaisma WA, et al. Ten-year outcome of laparoscopic and

conventional nissen fundoplication: randomized clinical trial. Ann Surg. 2009;250:698–706.

4. Nabi Z, Reddy DN. Endoscopic management of gastroesophageal reflux disease: revisited. Clin Endosc. 2016;49:408–16.

5. Triadafilopoulos G. Endoscopic options for gastroesophageal reflux: where are we now and what does the future hold? Curr Gastroenterol Rep. 2016;18:47.

6. Triadafilopoulos G, Clarke JO, Hawn M. Precision GERD management for the 21st century. Dis Esophagus. 2017;30:1–6.

7. Pandolfino JE, Krishnan K. Do endoscopic antireflux procedures fit in the current treatment paradigm of gastroesophageal reflux disease? Clin Gastroenterol Hepatol. 2014;12:544–54.

8. Noar M, Squires P. Radiofrequency energy delivery to the lower esophageal sphincter: toward a precise understanding of Stretta technology. Clin Gastroenterol Hepatol. 2015;13:406–7.

9. Kim MS, Holloway RH, Dent J, et al. Radiofrequency energy delivery to the gastric cardia inhibits triggering of transient lower esophageal sphincter relaxation and gastroesophageal reflux in dogs. Gastrointest Endosc. 2003;57:17–22.

10. Tam WC, Schoeman MN, Zhang Q, et al. Delivery of radiofrequency energy to the lower oesophageal sphincter and gastric cardia inhibits transient lower oesophageal sphincter relaxations and gastro-oesophageal reflux in patients with reflux disease. Gut. 2003;52:479–85.

11. Arts J, Bisschops R, Blondeau K, et al. A double-blind sham-controlled study of the effect of radiofrequency energy on symptoms and distensibility of the gastroesophageal junction in GERD. Am J Gastroenterol. 2012;107:222–30.

12. Corley DA, Katz P, Wo JM, et al. Improvement of gastroesophageal reflux symptoms after radiofrequency energy: a randomized, sham-controlled trial. Gastroenterology. 2003;125:668–76.

13. Aziz AM, El-Khayat HR, Sadek A, et al. A prospective randomized trial of sham, single-dose Stretta, and double-dose Stretta for the treatment of gastroesophageal reflux disease. Surg Endosc. 2010;24:818–25.

14. Coron E, Sebille V, Cadiot G, et al. Clinical trial: radiofrequency energy delivery in proton pump inhibitor-dependent gastro-oesophageal reflux disease patients. Aliment Pharmacol Ther. 2008;28:1147–58.

15. Perry KA, Banerjee A, Melvin WS. Radiofrequency energy delivery to the lower esophageal sphincter reduces esophageal acid exposure and improves GERD symptoms: a systematic review and meta-analysis. Surg Laparosc Endosc Percutan Tech. 2012;22:283–8.

16. Lipka S, Kumar A, Richter JE. No evidence for efficacy of radiofrequency ablation for treatment of gastroesophageal reflux disease: a systematic review and meta-analysis. Clin Gastroenterol Hepatol. 2015;13:1058–67.e1.

17. Satodate H, Inoue H, Yoshida T, et al. Circumferential EMR of carcinoma arising in Barrett's esophagus: case report. Gastrointest Endosc. 2003;58:288–92.

18. Satodate H, Inoue H, Fukami N, et al. Squamous reepithelialization after circumferential endoscopic mucosal resection of superficial carcinoma arising in Barrett's esophagus. Endoscopy. 2004;36:909–12.

19. Inoue H, Ito H, Ikeda H, et al. Anti-reflux mucosectomy for gastroesophageal reflux disease in the absence of hiatus hernia: a pilot study. Ann Gastroenterol. 2014;27:346–51.

20. DeMeester TR, Johnson LF. The evaluation of objective measurements of gastroesophageal reflux and their contribution to patient management. Surg Clin North Am. 1976;56:39–53.

21. Hill LD, Kozarek RA, Kraemer SJ, et al. The gastroesophageal flap valve: in vitro and in vivo observations. Gastrointest Endosc. 1996;44:541–7.

22. Inoue H, Sumi K, Tatsuta T, et al. 998 Clinical results of antireflux mucosectomy (ARMS) for refractory gerd. Gastrointest Endosc;85:AB120.

23. Bapaye A, Reddy Gangireddy SS, Mahadik M, et al. 999 Anti-reflux mucosectomy (ARMS) for refractory gerd and initial clinical experience. Gastrointest Endosc;85:AB120.

24. Chuttani R, de Moura DT, Cohen J. 852 Clear: cardia ligation anti-reflux procedure for gerd. Gastrointest Endosc;85:AB110.

Part V

Endoscopic Tissue Apposition

Olaya I. Brewer Gutierrez and Stuart K. Amateau

Introduction

For decades surgeons and gastroenterologists have desired a set of tools to perform minimally invasive extraluminal endoscopic interventions, a so-called tool box of instruments to push the boundaries of conventional endoscopy. A critical instrument for such procedures would be a closure device to manage the iatrogenic defects, prompting the development of an endoscopic suturing "machine" in the mid-1980s [1, 2]. Animal and cadaveric studies soon followed with early iterations of endoscopic suturing devices including the EndoCinch (Bard, Inc., Billerica, Mass) and the Sew-Right Device (Wilson-Cook Medical, Inc., Winston Salem, N.C.). Subsequently, these devices were utilized to tighten the lower esophageal sphincter in patients with reflux; however, results were variable and demonstrated poor durability [3]. Moreover, the systems were far from facile and device development continued. The invention of the Eagle Claw II system through a collaborative effort of the Apollo Group and Olympus Medical (Tokyo Japan) provided the basic design subsequently optimized by Apollo Endosurgery (San Diego, CA) and incorporated into the OverStitch [4].

The Overstitch endoscopic suturing system (Apollo Endosurgery, Austin, Texas) provided several critical technological leaps forward, including full thickness bites, the flexibility to deploy running or interrupted sutures, and the capability of reloading sutures without the removal of the device from the patient. The OverStitch is the only current Federal Food and Drug Administration (FDA) device approved for endoscopic suturing in the United States and produced in its current form since 2011. The device is a purpose-built single-use design which is traditionally mounted onto a double channel therapeutic Olympus gastroscope (GIF 2TH180/160). Recognized applications of endoscopic suturing within the foregut and hindgut include tissue apposition to manage perforation, defect closure, fistula, anastomotic leaks, and bleeding as well as stent fixation, as well as bariatric interventions such as post Roux-en-Y gastric bypass outlet reduction (transoral outlet reduction, TORe) and endoscopic sleeve gastroplasty (ESG) [5]. While these topics are discussed in detail elsewhere, the present chapter is intended to discuss proper, optimized basic endoscopic suturing technique, suture patterns, as well as the necessary equipment and assembly.

O. I. Brewer Gutierrez
Johns Hopkins Medical Institution, Department of Medicine, Division of Gasroenerology and Hepatology, Baltimore, MD, USA
e-mail: obrewer1@jhmi.edu

S. K. Amateau (✉)
University of Minnesota Medical Center, Department of Medicine, Division of Gastroenterology and Hepatology, Minneapolis, MN, USA
e-mail: amateau@umn.edu

© Springer Nature Switzerland AG 2020
M. S. Wagh, S. B. Wani (eds.), *Gastrointestinal Interventional Endoscopy*,
https://doi.org/10.1007/978-3-030-21695-5_25

Preprocedure Planning

Most endoscopists consider endoscopic suturing an advanced technique and therefore should be performed by individuals capable of complex luminal endoscopy with an understanding of basic suturing techniques. Moreover, there should be a basic appreciation of the inherent risks of iatrogenic complication when passing a metal device seated at the tip of an endoscope that has the potential for deep to full thickness bites of tissue, including perforation and hemorrhage, respectively. Frequently, endoscopists who utilize the device first observe colleagues or mentors in vivo and practice ex vivo prior to their first in human experience.

To simplify the procedure, an understanding of the particular task at hand is critical. This may involve diagnostic imaging and or multidisciplinary discussion. For instance, management of a suspect sleeve gastrectomy leak should first involve knowledge that these typically occur at the apex of the suture line and are frequently associated to downstream stenosis. This will prompt the endoscopist to first obtain an oral contrasted radiologic study which should then be reviewed with a minimally invasive surgeon to allow consideration of various management decisions ranging from continued observation, placement of percutaneous drains, endoscopic management, or re-do surgical intervention. Clearly, given the broad application of endoscopic suturing, each clinical scenario requires similar thought and assessment to achieve successful outcomes.

Available Equipment

Beyond endoscopic skill and pre-procedure planning, knowledge of the primary device and associated equipment is essential (Fig. 25.1). The current iteration of the OverStitch endoscopic suturing system is designed specifically for the Olympus double channel therapeutic gastroscope, both the most modern 2 T 180 as well as its predecessor the 2 T 160 (Fig. 25.1a). The system itself comprises an apparatus that mounts to the front of the two working channels with a lever facing rightward that controls the position, be it open or closed, of the needle body and anchor by

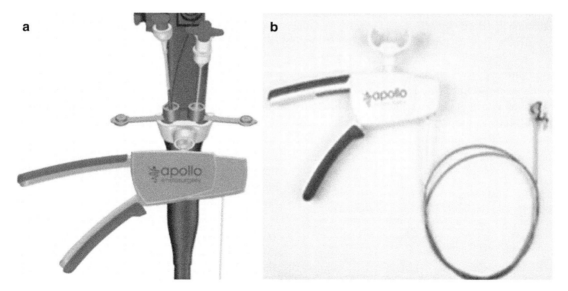

Fig. 25.1 Demonstrations of the Overstitch endoscopic suturing device including (**a**) the Olympus double channel therapeutic gastroscope with needle driver attached, (**b**) OverStitch system with handle and needle driver (needle anchor not shown), (**c**) working ends of the device with components labeled, (**d**) polypropylene and polydioxanone suture, (**e**) suture cinch device, (**f**) distal end of tissue helix device, and (**g**) overtube demonstrating specialized end inflation catheter both designed to retain gas insufflation. (Used with permission from Apollo Endosurgery)

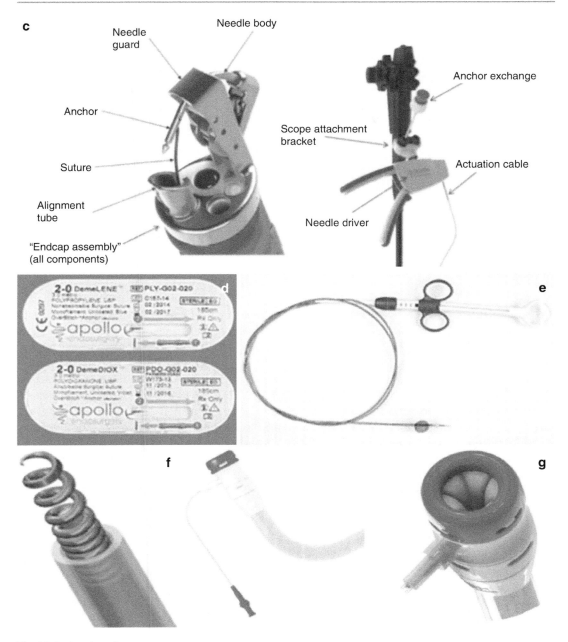

Fig. 25.1 (continued)

transducing tension across a metal articulation cable which runs along the flexible insertion tube (Fig. 25.1b). The needle body itself sits on a metal endcap assembly designed to seat snugly with the distal tip and allow passage of devices through both working channels while not obscuring the light guides, objective lens, or nozzles (Fig. 25.1c). Two purpose built 2-0 sutures are available, one being non-absorbable polypropylene and the other absorbable polydioxanone, and depending on the application sufficient quantities should be ensured (Fig. 25.1d). An anchor exchange apparatus is used to position these sutures across the larger 3.7 (rightward) working channel in range of needle driver. While the distal biting end of each suture becomes one of the tags allowing durable tightening, a unique device called the suture cinch is required to both cut the suture and provide the opposing tag for durable deployment (Fig. 25.1e). Two noncritical accessory devices have also been developed. To assist in positioning tissues within the path of the needle driver, a tissue helix may be utilized through the smaller 2.8 mm (leftward) working channel (Fig. 25.1f). As the device is relatively blunt and rigid, and affixed to the distal end of the endoscope, a specialized overtube is available and designed to allow safe passage across the hypopharynx and proximal esophagus while maintaining gas insufflation (Fig. 25.1g).

Patient and Procedure Preparation

Frequently, endoscopic suturing procedures are performed under general anesthesia given the complexity of the related procedures, and the large caliber of devices passed per os along the esophagus. Beyond improving patient tolerance, endotracheal intubation secures the airway and allows for supine positioning with fear of pulmonary aspiration if desired for adjunct fluoroscopy. If supine position is utilized, the endoscopist will need to appreciate the possibility of decreased device response due to angulation and restriction of the tension cable. It is recommended to perform a diagnostic endoscopy to assess the area of interest and ensure the pre-procedure plan of action remains appropriate and feasible. If a foregut procedure is being performed, during this assessment, the overtube may be positioned by loading the device over the proximal end of the insertion tube, passage of the distal end into the stomach, and then careful advancement of the overtube along the insertion tube until such point as the bulbous proximal end abuts the bite block. Care should be taken to cease passage if resistance is experienced as this rarely may indicate invagination of the esophageal wall between the overtube and insertion

tube, which may then result in esophageal perforation. This device also incorporates a catheter through which air may be inserted to inflate a proximal circumferential balloon designed to assist in maintaining insufflation. Moreover, the catheter may be affixed to the bite block with a hemostat or similar device to prevent outward migration with movement of the endoscope.

Suture Device Equipment Set-Up

While initially preparing and passing the system within the patient, the handle of the needle driver should be in the closed position to keep the sharp needle end of the suturing arm housed within the alignment tube and to minimize the profile of the device. The primary OverStitch system is first mounted on the Olympus dual channel therapeutic gastroscope using the scope attachment bracket at the level of the biopsy channels with a 90° angle and rocked firmly to lock the needle driver handle in rightward position onto the scope (Fig. 25.2a). With the needle driver in the closed position, the actuation cable is guided alongside the flexible insertion tube and the endcap assembly seated onto the distal end of the gastroscope, ensuring optimal alignment so as to avoid obscuring the endoscopic component (Fig. 25.2b). Next, with the suture arm now open, choose the desired suture and load its blunt end within the anchor exchange device provided with the system. The operator or assistant should press these devices together firmly until a "click" is perceived, be it audible and or tactile (Fig. 25.2c). The suture should then be run loosely along the anchor exchange, and the distal end of the anchor passed through the larger 3.7 mm rightward working channel until the distal end is several centimeters beyond the alignment tube so as to provide necessary slack, or play, allowing critical mobility while manipulating the device and suturing. The anchor and suture are then withdrawn so as to have the metal end of the suture just within the alignment tube. The needle driver handle should then be closed to move the suture arm just above

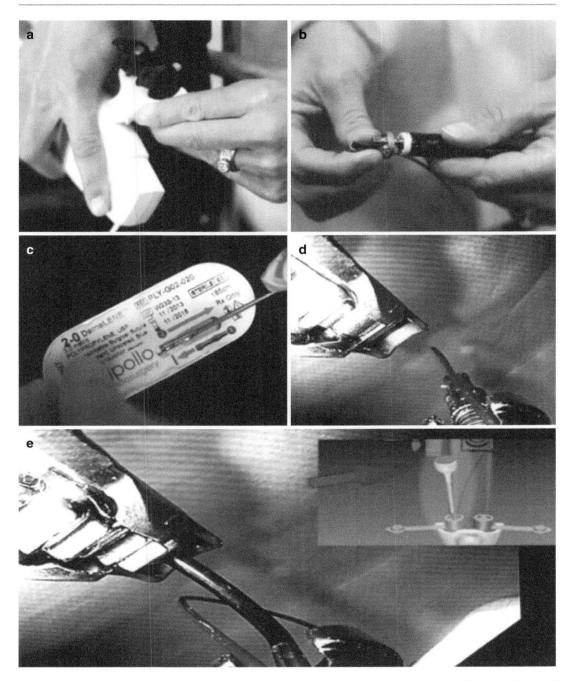

Fig. 25.2 (**a**) Attachment of the system handle to the endoscope. (**b**) The handle of the needle driver is placed on a 90° angle at the level of the biopsy channels of the scope. (**c**) The suture is loaded into the anchor exchange catheter. (**d**) The suture is threaded into the 3.7 mm gastroscope channel and once advanced beyond the needle tower is then pulled back to create a suture loop or "slack". (**e**) The needle driver handle is closed so the curved body of the needle is facing the endoscopic channel and the anchor exchange catheter is pushed aligned to the curved body of the needle until resistance or a "click" is heard. Then the blue button of the anchor exchange (inset with arrow) catheter is pushed down and slightly pulled back about 1 cm simultaneously so the suture is transferred from the anchor exchange catheter to the curved body of the needle; the exchange catheter is released and the suture handle opened. (Used with permission from Apollo Endosurgery)

the alignment tube (Fig. 25.2d). Next, the suture is loaded onto the curved needle body by again pushing the anchor exchange firmly toward the needle until resistance is met again, or a tactile click is appreciated. This represents proper insertion of the suture with the arm, though at this stage the suture also remains attached to the exchange anchor. Therefore, to release the suture from the exchange, the operator now presses the blue button at the proximal end of the exchange device and in tandem pulls gently on the exchange. Care should always be taken when pressing the release button of the exchange, as this will either release the suture to the needle or "fire" the distal end of the suture from the system to allow cinching. With the suture on the needle body, the first tissue bite may follow (Fig. 25.2e). This first suture may be loaded to the suture arm either ex vivo or in vivo; however, the former is preferred to ensure appropriate functionality of the overall system. Of course, a major advantage of this iteration of the suturing device is its ability to reload sutures without removal of the device and therefore allowing the operator to maintain constant visualization of the target.

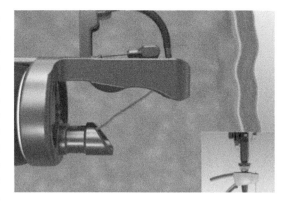

Fig. 25.3 Suture loaded on the needle body which is in open position prior to initial tissue bite. (Used with permission from Apollo Endosurgery)

General Endoscopic Suturing Technique

The following steps depict the general endoscopic suturing technique. These steps are the same with minimal variations depending on the type of procedure to be performed.

- *Step 1:* Carefully advance the dual channel therapeutic gastroscope with attached OverStitch device with the arm in closed position per os, with or without overtube, or per rectum into range of the targeted tissues of the foregut, midgut, or hindgut. With the endoscope in range, begin to plan the methods needed to achieve the desired outcome. This includes identifying what is to be apposed, the type of stitch pattern, and the sequence of sutures. For instance, the location of the first

bite may in large part be determined by the decision of suture pattern and particulars of positioning. Importantly, given the nuance of over-under-under-over suture technique found with most patterns, the first bite usually involves the distal edge to be approximated, while the second is the proximal, as this will naturally allow this sequence. As the suture is loaded on the needle arm, the driver handle may then be opened to ready for the first bite. Meanwhile, the exchange catheter remains within the 3.7 mm working channel ready to recapture the suture as below (Fig. 25.3).

- *Step 2:* While it is possible to position the needle guard and body appropriately to obtain a full thickness bite, it is recommended to utilize the tissue helix assist device to allow full control of the manipulated tissue. To do so, the device is passed through the secondary 2.8 mm leftward working channel of the therapeutic gastroscope with the distal metal spiral contained within the catheter; this may involve pulling back the blue cross on the proximal end of the device. With the helix catheter visualized endoscopically, the assistant exposes the metal spiral by pushing on the blue cross (Fig. 25.4).
- *Step 3:* The helix is then advanced onto the tissue target, and the assistant begins to turn the blue cross clockwise 3–4 times, while the

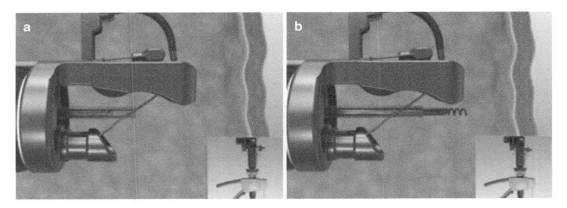

Fig. 25.4 The helix is passed through the endoscope (**a**) with the spiral contained within the catheter and (**b**) then is exposed in proximity of tissue target. (Used with permission from Apollo Endosurgery)

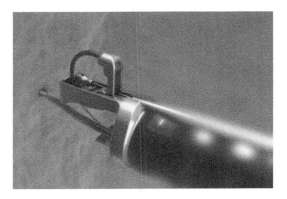

Fig. 25.5 Helix engaged and within targeted tissue. (Used with permission from Apollo Endosurgery)

endoscopist pushes the catheter toward the tissue (Fig. 25.5). Frequently, though not always, the endoscopist will appreciate a subtle tissue bounce, and this will help ensure full thickness suturing.

- *Step 4:* The helix catheter is then slightly withdrawn pulling the grasped tissue toward the tip of the endoscope into path of the loaded needle arum. The endoscopist may or may not slightly push forward the insertion tube or even use suction to improve alignment of the target (Fig. 25.6).
- *Steps 5 and 6:* Next, with the tissue well within the alignment with the arm, the operator closes the needle driver handle to advance the anchor and suture though the tissues held

by the helix. Without delay the anchor exchange is advanced forward to come in contact with the suture on the needle arm. As previous, a tactile click will usually, though not always, be appreciated suggesting appropriate engagement of the anchor exchanger with the suture on the needle arm (Fig. 25.7). Of importance, the suture has not yet been exchanged, and the helix remains connected with the tissue.

- *Step 7:* Without pressing the blue button of the exchanger, gently pull the anchor exchange back to disengage the suture from the needle arm (Fig. 25.8). Again the helix remains engaged with tissues until the next step.
- *Step 8:* The assistant next turns the helix counter clockwise a minimum of 4 rotations to release the tissue, again frequently associated with a subtle tissue bounce. The entire helix spiral should be visualized endoscopically and the catheter withdrawn slightly toward the endoscope. The assistant should then pull back on the blue cross to retract the helix, and the catheter may then be withdrawn entirely into the working channel.
- *Step 9:* While both the sharp end of the suture is detached from the needle body and the helix from the tissue, the tissue remains engaged with the needle body until it is placed into the open position using the handle. However, in

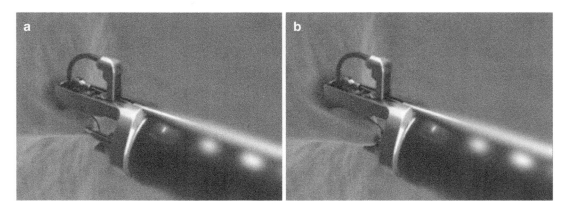

Fig. 25.6 Sequences (**a**, **b**) demonstrating use of the helix to pull tissues into the path of the needle arm. (Used with permission from Apollo Endosurgery)

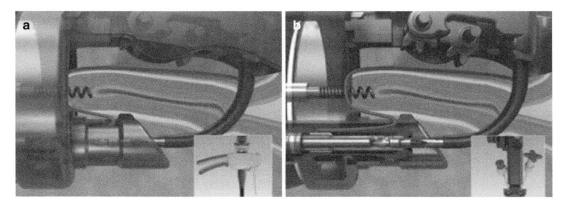

Figs. 25.7 (**a**) The needle arm bites the tissue held by the helix and (**b**) the exchange is engaged with the needle arm and suture. (Used with permission from Apollo Endosurgery)

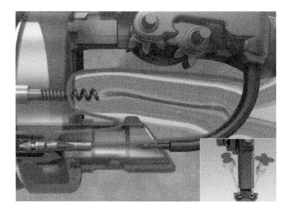

Fig. 25.8 Demonstration of the anchor exchanger recapturing the suture from the needle arm. (Used with permission from Apollo Endosurgery)

the open position, the endoscopist attempts to create some distance from the target area using the slack created while initially loading the suture with the exchanger (Fig. 25.9).

- *Step 10:* With the first full thickness bite completed, the endoscopist next passes the suture back to the needle body to allow the process to continue. Each step above is repeated to achieve the desired suture throw.

- *Steps 1b–10b:* The above steps are then repeated taking various bites of tissue appropriate for the chosen suture technique, be it interrupted, running, purse-string, or horizontal mattress (as described below), and the desired outcome achieved (Fig. 25.10).

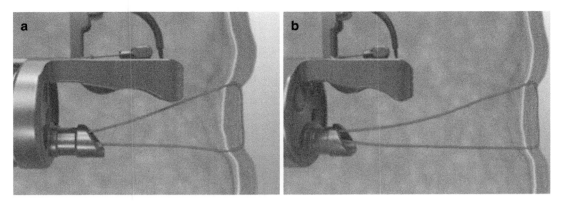

Fig. 25.9 Progressive distancing (**a, b**) from the target area in preparation to reload the suture. (Used with permission from Apollo Endosurgery)

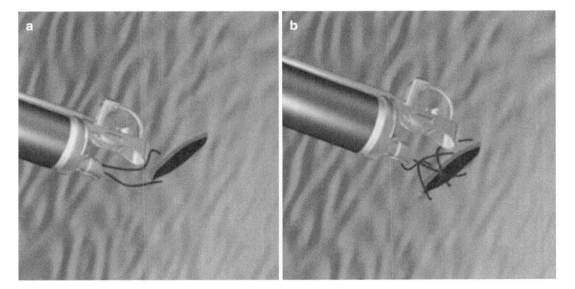

Fig. 25.10 Schematic of (**a**) a simple running suture to (**b**) close a small defect. (Used with permission from Apollo Endosurgery)

Cinching and Cutting

After completing the desired suture throw, which will have various nuances for each of the different techniques, the suture has to be cinched tight to achieve apposition and then cut to allow removal of excess suture material.

- *Step 1:* The sharp biting end of the suture needs to be thrown or released from the device com-

pletely. This follows the last bite of tissue and another exchange of the suture back to the anchor exchange device. The needle driver then needs to be opened to clear the alignment tube, the anchor exchange passed fully out of the tube, and the blue button now depressed, again not while engaged with the needle arm, thereby releasing the sharp end away from the device. This sharp end serves as one of the two "T-tags" and allows knotless suture tightening (Fig. 25.11).

- *Step 2:* The operator may now remove the anchor exchange leaving the single "loose" end of the suture across the alignment tube and through the working channel. A suture cinch is then loaded by passing a small length of the free end suture through the golden loop. The tab is then carefully removed, thereby pulling the suture through a small pinhole at the apex of the distal end of the cinch. These steps may be performed by either the operator or the assistant, depending on the team's particular dynamics. With the device essentially loaded as a short exchange, the endoscopist

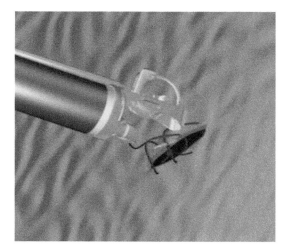

Fig. 25.11 Schematic of a running suture with biting end released and now functioning as a tag for knotless tightening. (Used with permission from Apollo Endosurgery)

passes the cinch along the suture as one would any other short exchange device (Fig. 25.12).

- *Step 3:* The endoscopist then passes the loaded cinch device over the suture as they would a short exchange device, holding slight back tension to avoid bunching the suture within the 3.7 mm working channel (Fig. 25.13).
- *Step 4.* The cinch is passed over the suture, out the channel, and across the alignment tube into a position appropriate for the suture technique employed as the distal most end is the second proximal tag allowing for knotless tightening. This may involve placement of the distal end across the defect or toward the pole opposite of the sharp initial tag.
- *Step 5.* With the distal end of the cinch in position, the operator continues to apply counter tension to the free end of the suture. It should be appreciated that recognizing the appropriate level of tightness for each suture technique takes experience, as malfunction such as premature break may occur if too tight, and laxity may occur if too loose. Many operators choose to vary tension by consecutive wraps of the suture around their right pointer finger. Regardless, with the suture appropriately tight, the assistant releases the safety spacer by opening their hand and then cuts the suture to release the second tension tag by closing their hand, bringing their thumb and 2nd/3rd fingers together (Fig. 25.14). The cinch catheter and excess suture, now released, are removed in tandem.

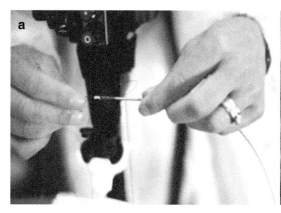
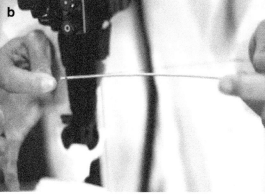

Fig. 25.12 (**a**) Passage of the loose end of the suture through the loop tag of the cinch followed by (**b**) removal of the gold pull tab allowing loading of the suture through the distal end of the cinch device. (Used with permission from Apollo Endosurgery)

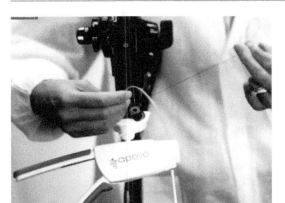

Fig. 25.13 Image showing passage of the cinch over the suture with the offhand applying back tension. (Used with permission from Apollo Endosurgery)

Suture Patterns and Techniques

The current iteration of the endoscopic suturing device allows the endoscopist to replicate suture techniques that traditionally require open or laparoscopic surgery without the need to remove the endoscope to reload fresh suture material. Moreover, the utilization of bipolar tags overcomes the hurdle of securing the suture by traditional knot technique which would require multiple articulating devices. This allows the endoscopist to secure devices as well as close partial or full thickness defects, both of which are beyond the reliable capability of hemostatic or over the scope clips [6]. While there are tens of modified variations of basic suture techniques,

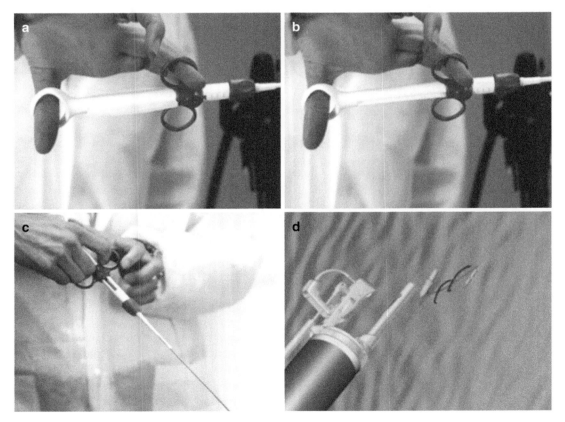

Fig. 25.14 Images demonstrating the cinch and cut maneuver, including (**a**) starting hand position, (**b**) removal of the safety tab by extending the thumb away from the other digits, (**c**) combined cinch and cut by closing the fingers toward one another, and (**d**) schematic demonstrating a simple running suture with both tags found within the lumen. (Used with permission from Apollo Endosurgery)

three common strategies are utilized endoscopically including simple interrupted stitching, simple running, and figure-of-8 technique. Ex vivo evaluation of the performance of these three techniques demonstrated significantly improved water tightness with the figure-of-8 technique, while the there was no significant difference in burst pressure or procedure time required [7]. These core strategies will be reviewed in more detail below; however, it should be noted that modified versions of the horizontal mattress and purse string suture have also been described in the endoscopic setting.

Interrupted suture Interrupted sutures represents the first suture typically mastered by the operator as it is the simplest and usually applicable, though not always ideal, in most clinical scenarios. The technique involves a full thickness bite on one side of the defect followed by another at the opposite approximated side and a third bite near the first bite (Fig. 25.15). This third bite differs from the two typically required for wound closure as tags are used rather than a traditional knot. The suture is then released from the device completely, cinched, and cut under moderate tension. As noted above, given the desired sequence of over-under-under-over

technique, the first bite usually involves the distal edge to be approximated, while the second is the proximal, as this will naturally allow this order. This process is repeated using sutures approximating each side as close to the suture proceeding as feasible until the defect is closed. This allows decreased tissue drag during tightening of the suture compared to other techniques such as the running suture. Moreover, there is little risk of suture crossing and entanglement, and any suture failure would result in limited dehiscence of the approximation rather than complete separation of tissues. Therefore, this technique is ideal of stent fixation and endoscopic bariatric procedures such as sleeve creation and gastrojejunal anastomotic modification. However, as approximation of the defect edges occurs immediately with the tightening of the first suture, complete closure of defects may be limited at the edges or between larger gaps between suture as visualization and positioning becomes increasingly difficult and inaccurate. Moreover, there is an appreciable increase in cost proportionate to the number of sutures.

Running suture A continuous pattern of suture, or running suture, involves closure of a defect with a single suture and single cinch. The technique is initiated with an interrupted suture pattern as described above; rather than cinch after the third bite, the fourth bite of tissue occurs a short distance from the second and the fifth across the defect from the fourth to approximate the edges (Fig. 25.16). This continues along the length of the defect through the last region of approximation where the suture may be thrown, cinched, and cut with or without another pattern of interrupted suture. This technique typically improves endoscopic visualization and requires less suture and cinch material. Suture drag, however, increases due to increased resistance with multiple bites; however, this may be in part addressed by careful slow tightening throughout the process. The technique is overall more complex than interrupted sutures and therefore more prone to user error such as with entanglement of the thread with the needle body or inability to

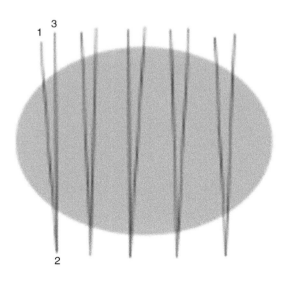

Fig. 25.15 Schematic demonstrating interrupted suture pattern with the first and third bites at the more distal edge, biting over to under, and the second, under to over

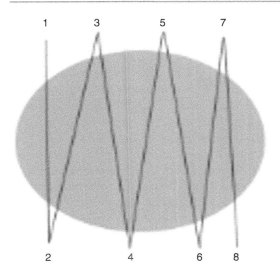

Fig. 25.16 Schematic demonstrating running suture pattern with odd bites on the more distal edge, biting over to under, and even bites on the more proximal, biting under to over

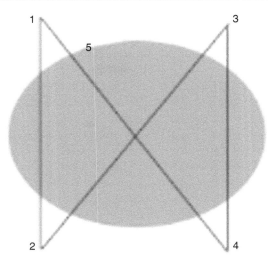

Fig. 25.17 Schematic demonstrating figure-8 pattern with odd bites on the distal edge and even on proximal edge, with the last (5th) bite at the site of the first

create sufficient slack to continue the stitch. Moreover, any error or malfunction such as premature throw, suture breakage, or malalignment of the needle body will result in complete loss of apposition and require restarting the approximation, perhaps now with increased blood in the field. Similarly, with delayed suture failure, the entire approximation will release as opposed to techniques where multiple sutures are utilized for closure. To address this scenario, one may consider a running suture with subsequent interrupted sutures serving as so-called retention threads.

Figure-of-8 A technique utilizing the advantages, while avoiding many of the disadvantages, of both the interrupted suture and the running stitch is the figure-of-8. As its name implies, the endoscopist creates a pattern which schematically appears as the number 8 to approximate the edges of tissues (Fig. 25.17). To do so, the first bite of tissue is taken near the edge of the defect and the second on the opposite side of the defect in near approximation. The third is on the same side as the first though slightly along the axis of the defect and the fourth directly across from the third to achieve

approximation. A fifth bite is then taken in the same location as the first, completing the "8" and the suture thrown. Tension is applied and the suture cinched and cut with the second tag desired on the other side (within) the defect. This may be applied with an individual suture to close smaller defects, or subsequent figure-of-8 sutures may be utilized in side by side fashion to close larger defects. As noted above, ex vivo data suggest improved water tightness without sacrificing burst pressure characteristics or increasing procedure length. The technique is frequently preferred for oversewing fistulae and for approximating ulcerations with visible vessels. However, the technique is certainly more technically challenging than interrupted sutures and increases the risk of entanglement with the needle body. Also, as with running sutures, if only one suture is utilized, there is a greater likelihood of clinical failure with any slack or suture break or erosion.

Other Suture Techniques

Endoscopists have also utilized baseball, horizontal mattress, and purse string patterns. While little data exists regarding these techniques for endoscopic management of disease, understanding these patterns may prove useful to the operator in various clinic situations. Briefly, the horizontal mattress is a complex modification of the running suture. Here, the first and second bites are on opposite sides of the defect; however, the next bite is on the same edge as the second slightly along the axis of the defect. The fourth bite is on the opposite edge of and across from the third. The fifth bite is then on the opposite edges of the fourth just downstream from the third; however, BEFORE the tissue is bit, the thread between the first and third is purposefully intertwined. And the technique continues down the axis of the defect until approximation is achieved. While this stitch may improve water tightness and increase burst pressure, these theoretical advantages need to be weighed against the increased risk of entanglement and continued disadvantage of clinical failure with malfunction of the suture. A purse string has also been described for closure of defects. Here consecutive full thickness bites are taken around the circumference of the defect until the last stitch meets the first. Tension would tighten the defect like the string of an ancient purse of gold and subsequently be held in position by the tags. However, this technique has the same disadvantages of running suture and perhaps has less performance on burst and water tightness.

Technical Complications and Troubleshooting

While the current iteration of endoscopic suturing device has addressed a number of obstacles found in previous designs, the procedure continues to present challenges to even the most experienced of operators. As with any endoscopic procedure, visualization of the target may be challenging, and therefore it is highly recommended that a diagnostic evaluation precedes loading the device. This will allow for an understanding of endoscopic position and anatomic location as well as the opportunity to optimize the field, such as with clearing remnant food or blood. Furthermore, in terms of bleeding, it is quite likely that a full thickness bite results in acute bleeding which further obscures the view. Therefore, conceptualizing the pattern and placement of bites is recommended before the first pass of the needle.

Subtle changes to scope position and rotation may either ease or complicate the procedure. This may lead to entrapment (or release) of the suture from the arm or malposition of the anchor exchange (Fig. 25.18). To undo over-rotation and align the device toward the appropriate position of the bite, deflect the tip downward (big wheel away) with subtle deflection either left or right (small wheel). Frequently, release from needle body entrapment also requires creation or reduction of slack on the thread, and at times even incomplete closure of the needle driver so as to not lead to another bite or misalignment, but allowing for a decreased profile. The thread may also entangle around the alignment tube. To resolve this scenario, one may carefully push out the anchor with slight counter tension on the endoscope insertion tube to loosen the suture and undo the loop. Similar techniques may be used to reverse crisscrossed suture.

The quality of tissue in the region of defect also plays a major role in the technical success of the procedure. Situations where healthy tissue exists, such as with creation of an endoscopic sleeve, allows the operator to create greater tension with each suture throw without increased risk of suture tearing through the bites of tissue. Moreover, the same is typical for fresh iatrogenic defects. However, with long-standing fistulae or leaks or regions involved with ischemia, such as with ulceration and anastomoses, involved tissues tend to be friable and sutures fail with only minimal tension. In these clinical situations, the region to be approximated should be expanded to include healthier tissues. This may involve increased suture and procedure time; however, overall outcomes would be expected to improve.

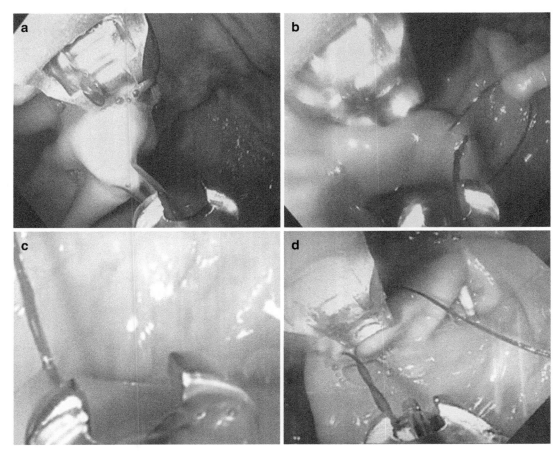

Fig. 25.18 In vivo endoscopic images of hurdles experienced with endoscopic suture including (**a**) entrapment of the needle body, (**b**) malpositioning of the anchor exchange, (**c**) entrapment of the alignment tube, and (**d**) crisscross suture. (Used with permission from Apollo Endosurgery)

Conclusions

Endoscopic suturing represents a critical pathway toward the continued evolution of the endoscopist from a diagnostician to an interventionist. As found in associated chapters, the documented applications of this technique continue to expand, from simple adjunct fixation techniques to critical defect closures minimizing clinical morbidity, to rounding out the toolbox of pioneering natural orifice transluminal endoscopic surgery (NOTES) procedures. While the current iteration of the commercially available endoscopic suturing device allows a range of suture patterns with reasonable burst pressures and water tightness, limitations still exist, including the need for a highly skilled endoscopist, risks of iatrogenic complications, and requirement for a dual channel gastroscope. Next generation devices already in the pipeline address these shortcomings, with the ultimate goal of developing safer, simpler, more widely applicable endoscopic suturing devices.

Acknowledgments Figures 25.1, 25.2, 25.3, 25.4, 25.5, 25.6, 25.7, 25.8, 25.9, 25.10, 25.11, 25.12, 25.13, 25.14 and 25.18 were used with permission of Apollo Endosurgery.

References

1. Swain CP, Mills TN. An endoscopic sewing machine. Gastrointest Endosc. 1986;32:36–8.
2. Melzer A, Schurr MO, Lirici MM, et al. Future trends in endoscopic suturing. Endosc Surg Allied Technol. 1994;2(1):78–82.
3. Fennerty MB. Endoscopic suturing for treatment of GERD. Gastrointest Endosc. 2003;57:390–5.
4. Hu B, Chung SC, Sun LC, Kawashima K, et al. Eagle Claw II: a novel endosuture device that uses a curved needle for major arterial bleeding: a bench study. Gastrointest Endosc. 2005;62:266–70.
5. Stavropoulos SN, Modayil R, Friedel D. Current applications of endoscopic suturing. World J Gastrointest Endosc. 2015;7(8):777–89.
6. Lee WC, Ko WJ, Cho JH, et al. Endoscopic treatment of various gastrointestinal tract defects with an over-the-scope clip: case series from a tertiary referral hospital. Clin Endosc. 2014;47:178–82.
7. Halvax P, Diana M, Nagao Y, et al. Experimental evaluation of the optimal suture pattern with a flexible endoscopic suturing system. Surg Innov. 2017;24(3):201–4.

Roupen Djinbachian and Daniel von Renteln

Endoscopic Clips

History of Endoscopic Clips

Endoscopic clips were first introduced in Japan in 1975 by Hayashi et al. and Kumarata et al. as a means of treating gastrointestinal hemorrhage and marking intestinal lesions for subsequent surgery [1, 2]. Originally, two clips were developed: a light "type A" clip for bleeding peptic ulcer treatment and a larger "type B" clip for post-polypectomy hemostasis [1]. Through this collaboration, Olympus Optical Co., Ltd. filed the first endoscopic clip patent, paving the way for a new era of interventional endoscopy [3]. Endoscopic clips initially had poor adherence to the target site (falling after 72 hours) and required a complicated multistep procedure to be deployed [1], hampering their widespread adoption. This led Lehman et al. to describe

them as "cumbersome and probably not practical for routine use" in a 1985 paper published in *Gastrointestinal Endoscopy* [4]. However, these clips saw subsequent incremental improvements over the following years that simplified their deployment procedure and expanded their capabilities to the point where they are now standard endoscopic tools for treating GI bleeding, GI perforations, and many other emerging indications.

In 1985 Hachisu et al. described what was referred as a "J-clip" (Olympus Co., Tokyo, Japan), a reloadable clip that can be loaded on the tip of the clipping apparatus and manipulated through moving two sliders on the handle of the device. This greatly simplified the opening, closing, and release of the clip into a two-step process, to the point where an endoscopist could conceivably perform the procedure without any assistance [5]. The authors followed up by describing the closing of Mallory-Weiss tears, peptic ulcers, and Dieulafoy's lesions among others. In 1993 the first instance of endoscopic closure of a perforation using a clip was described by Binmoeller et al. [6]. Endoscopic clips were further improved by Hachisu et al. in 1996 by imparting onto them the capacity to rotate during the procedure. This allowed hemostasis to be performed more easily and reliably [7]. Two years later in 1998, Rodella et al. described the first clipping of anastomotic leakages occurring post-gastric surgery [8].

R. Djinbachian
Division of Internal Medicine, Montreal University Hospital Center (CHUM), Montreal, Canada

Montreal University Research Center (CRCHUM), Montreal, Canada

D. von Renteln (✉)
Division of Internal Medicine, Montreal University Research Center (CRCHUM), Montreal, Canada

Division of Gastroenterology, Montreal University Hospital Center (CHUM), Montreal, Canada

© Springer Nature Switzerland AG 2020
M. S. Wagh, S. B. Wani (eds.), *Gastrointestinal Interventional Endoscopy*,
https://doi.org/10.1007/978-3-030-21695-5_26

In subsequent years, numerous new clip types by different companies were introduced. While the first endoscopic clip devices were reusable and needed to be manually reloaded with disposable clips for every use, the first preloaded single-use disposable clips only appeared in 2002 with the introduction of QuickClip from Olympus Corporation [9]. This greatly improved the convenience of using endoscopic clips. The following year, the TriClip (Cook Medical Inc., Bloomington, Indiana, USA) and the Resolution clip (Boston Scientific Corporation, Marlborough, Massachusetts, USA) were introduced [9]. The TriClip's primary feature was the inclusion of three prongs meant to facilitate grasping, while the Resolution clip could be opened and closed five times as long as the clip was not released—a feature missing from the QuickClip and the TriClip at the time. In 2005 the Olympus Corporation followed up with the QuickClip2, a rotatable version of the original QuickClip. In 2016 Boston Scientific launched the Resolution 360, a clip with one-to-one rotation capabilities. The devices were all considered safe and effective and provided endoscopists with new tools for a wide range of applications such as GI perforation, diverticular bleeding, and peptic ulcer bleeding.

Endoscopic Clips Currently Available

The indications for current available clips described here are based on the United States Food and Drug Administration's online medical device database [10]. Details are summarized in Table 26.1.

Boston Scientific

Resolution Clip

Indications for the clip include: bleeding ulcers, hemostasis of upper GI mucosal/submucosal lesions less than 3 cm, arteries less than 2 mm, polyps less than 1.5 cm in diameter, diverticula, closure of GI perforations less than 2 cm that can be treated conservatively, endoscopic marking, anchoring jejunal feeding tubes, and prophylaxis for delayed bleeding.

The clip has a span of 11 mm and can be opened and closed up to five times. It can be rotated, but the response is not one-to-one, and the clip is rated as magnetic resonance imaging (MRI) conditional.

Resolution 360

Indications for the clip include: bleeding ulcers, hemostasis of upper GI mucosal/submucosal lesions less than 3 cm, arteries less than 2 mm, polyps less than 1.5 cm in diameter, diverticula, closure of GI perforations less than 2 cm that can be treated conservatively, endoscopic marking, anchoring jejunal feeding tubes, and prophylaxis for delayed bleeding.

The clip has a span of 11 mm and can be opened and closed up to five times. It can be rotated with a one-to-one response and is rated as MRI conditional (Fig. 26.1).

ConMed

DuraClip

Indications for the clip include: bleeding ulcers, hemostasis of upper GI mucosal/submucosal lesions less than 3 cm, polyps less than 1.5 cm in

Table 26.1 Comparison of current clips

	Span (mm)	MRI compatible	Rotatable	Can be reopened
Resolution Clip[1]	11	Up to 3 Tesla, 2500 Gauss/cm	Yes	Up to 5 times
Resolution 360[1]	11	Up to 3 Tesla, 2500 Gauss/cm	1–1	Up to 5 times
DuraClip[2]	11	MR safe	1–1	Unlimited
Instinct[3]	16	Up to 3 Tesla, 1600 Gauss/cm	1–1	Up to 5 times
QuickClip2[4]	7.5, 11	No	1–1	No
QuickClip Pro[4]	11	Up to 3 Tesla, 1800 Gauss/cm	Yes	Unlimited
OTSC[5]	11, 12, 14	Up to 3 Tesla, 720 Gauss/cm	No	No
Padlock Clip[6]	9.5–14	Up to 3 Tesla[7]	No	No

1 Boston Scientific, *2* ConMed, *3* cook medical, *4* Olympus, *5* Ovesco, *6* US endoscopy, *7* Gauss/cm not available

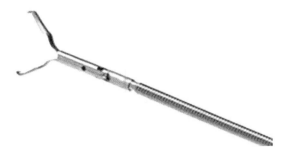

Fig. 26.1 Resolution 360. (Image courtesy of Boston Scientific. Reprint with kind permission. Unauthorised use not permitted)

diameter, diverticula, and closure of GI perforations less than 2 cm that can be treated conservatively.

The clip has a span of 11 mm and can be opened and closed in an unlimited amount of times. It can be rotated with a one-to-one response and is rated as MRI safe.

Cook Medical

Instinct Clip

Indications for the clip include: bleeding ulcers, hemostasis of upper GI mucosal/submucosal lesions less than 3 cm, arteries less than 2 mm, polyps less than 1.5 cm in diameter, and endoscopic marking.

The clip has a span of 16 mm and can be opened and closed up to five times. It can be rotated with a one-to-one response and is rated as MRI conditional.

Olympus

QuickClip2

Indications for the clip include: bleeding ulcers, hemostasis of upper GI mucosal/submucosal lesions less than 3 cm, arteries less than 2 mm, polyps less than 1.5 cm in diameter, diverticula, closure of GI perforations less than 2 cm that can be treated conservatively, and endoscopic marking.

The clip comes with either a span of 7.5 or 11 mm and cannot be reopened. It can be rotated with a one-to-one response but is not rated as safe for MRI use.

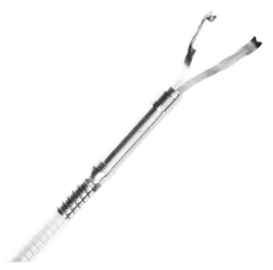

Fig. 26.2 QuickClip Pro. (Image courtesy of Olympus. Reprint with kind permission. Unauthorised use not permitted)

QuickClip Pro

Indications for the clip include: bleeding ulcers, hemostasis of upper GI mucosal/submucosal lesions less than 3 cm, arteries less than 2 mm, polyps less than 1.5 cm in diameter, diverticula, closure of GI perforations less than 2 cm that can be treated conservatively, and endoscopic marking.

The clip has a span of 11 mm and can be opened and closed in an unlimited amount of times. It can be rotated but the response is not one-to-one and the clip is rated as MRI conditional (Fig. 26.2).

Ovesco

Over-the-Scope Clip (OTSC)

Indications for the clip include: bleeding ulcers, hemostasis of upper GI mucosal/submucosal lesions less than 3 cm, arteries less than 2 mm, polyps less than 1.5 cm in diameter, diverticula, closure of GI perforations less than 2 cm that can be treated conservatively, and endoscopic marking.

The clip comes with either a span of 11, 12, or 14 mm and is mounted over the scope. It cannot be reopened and can be removed using a special tool provided by Ovesco Endoscopy (Tübingen,

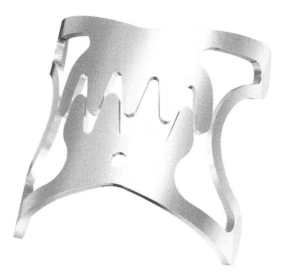

Fig. 26.3 Over-the-scope clip. (Image courtesy of Ovesco. Reprint with kind permission. Unauthorised use not permitted)

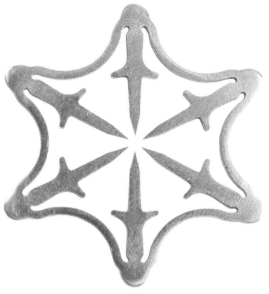

Fig. 26.4 Padlock Clip. (Image courtesy of US Endoscopy. Reprint with kind permission. Unauthorised use not permitted)

Germany) but cannot be reapplied after removal. The clip is rated MRI conditional (Fig. 26.3).

US Endoscopy

Padlock Clip

Indications for the clip include: bleeding ulcers, hemostasis of upper GI mucosal/submucosal lesions less than 3 cm, arteries less than 2 mm, polyps less than 1.5 cm in diameter, diverticula, closure of GI perforations less than 2 cm that can be treated conservatively, and endoscopic marking.

The clip comes with spans of 9.5 or 11 mm for the Padlock clip and spans of 11–14 mm for the Padlock Pro-Select clip. This clip is mounted over the scope. It cannot be reopened. It can be removed but cannot be reapplied after removal. The clip is rated MRI conditional (Fig. 26.4).

Indications for Clips

Indications for Bleeding

Acute Bleeding
Ulcer Bleeding

Peptic ulcers represent the most common cause of upper GI bleed (around 60%) [11], and they

require emergency endoscopic intervention to achieve prompt hemostasis. The mortality rate for patients hospitalized for upper GI bleed has been placed between 4.5% and 8.2% [12], making it a significant risk for patients. Endoscopic treatment is recommended for the treatment of ulcers with high-risk stigmata (Classed Forrest Ia and Ib) [13], whereas ulcers with an adherent clot should have the clot removed to evaluate the underlying lesion and treated accordingly [13, 14].

Endoscopic clip use for ulcer treatment has the added benefit of allowing the approximation of the ulcer margin [15]. Its effectiveness could be compromised by the presence of fibrosis at the base or around the ulcer, making it more rigid and more difficult to place the clips. Furthermore, ulcers located on the posterior wall of the duodenal bulb can make it harder to deploy clips effectively [16]. During the treatment of the ulcer, clots are usually removed prior to clipping to better visualize the target site of clip application. The clip is then opened and pointed at the base of a visible vessel, then pressed over it. Suction is then applied to capture more targets in before closing the clip. Finally, the clip is closed and deployed, bringing the tissues together and closing the lesion. More than one clip can be required to achieve proper hemostasis depending on the severity of the ulcer.

An over-the-scope clip could also be used for peptic ulcer hemostasis but requires an en-face approach, whereas through-the-scope clips could be used either en-face or tangentially with similar efficacy [17]. Applying an over-the-scope clip on an ulcer requires pressing the end of the endoscope over the lesion and turning the provided hand wheel clockwise. The open clip presently resting over the scope immediately releases and closes the tissue, aiming to achieve hemostasis.

Clips have been shown to be more effective than injection monotherapy for ulcer hemostasis, with a 78% reduction in bleeding recurrence and need for surgery [18], but are of comparable efficacy to thermo-coagulation [18, 19]. Clips do, however, have a lower risk of perforation when compared to thermo-coagulation, making them a very attractive alternative. Clips could also be used in combination with epinephrine injections to halt bleeding, although this did not show a statistically significant difference in preventing rebleeding compared to clipping monotherapy [18]. Epinephrine injections can be performed either before or after clip placement. Injections after clipping would however be preferable, since injecting prior to clipping would cause the target tissues to swell and may cause the clip to fall off prematurely as the swelling subsides.

Over-the-scope clips have also been shown to be effective in treating peptic ulcer bleeding [20]. A 2017 prospective randomized multicenter trial has shown in its preliminary results that the OTSC was superior than through-the-scope clip and epinephrine injection combination therapy [21]. Further studies still need to be performed, but the OTSC shows real promise in supplanting standard therapies for peptic ulcer bleeding.

Diverticular Bleeding

Diverticular hemorrhages are the most common cause of lower GI bleeds, constituting about 40% of total hospitalizations for LGIB [22, 23]. Although most bleeds resolve spontaneously, endoscopic intervention is sometimes required to stem the bleeding.

There are many options to endoscopically stop diverticular bleeds through clipping. Clips can be applied to close the diverticulum or directly on a bleeding vessel within it. Multiple clips could also be applied one next to each other to close a particularly large diverticulum. For bleeding occurring from a diverticular dome, a clip could be positioned so that one prong lay inside the diverticulum and the other on the outside. Closing the clip then cuts off supply from the vessel leading to the bleeding site [24]. The American College of Gastroenterology currently recommends clipping as the first-line hemostatic technique for diverticular bleeding [25].

Over-the-scope techniques have also been described for the closing of diverticular bleeding [26], where the clip is positioned center on the diverticulum with each prong resting on one edge of the diverticulum. Suction is performed to grab as much tissue as possible and the clip is released, clamping down behind the diverticulum bleeding area. This cuts off the blood supply to achieve hemostasis [27].

Clipping has been proven effective in managing acute diverticular bleeding [25]. It may be preferable to other hemostatic methods because of its lower risk for perforation and its ability to minimize tissue damage [25]. The rate of hemorrhage after clipping was shown to be about 17% [24, 28] with no early bleeding recurrence (defined as <30 days). Clips could be used in this case as markings to determine whether the hemorrhage was de novo or reoccurring. Current guidelines therefore suggest performing hemostasis (preferably clipping) if a non-bleeding visible vessel, a difficult-to-remove adherent clot, or active bleeding is found during colonoscopy [25].

Dieulafoy's Lesions

Dieulafoy's lesions account for less than 6% of non-variceal upper gastrointestinal bleeding [29, 30]. They are associated with a 5% mortality rate due to exsanguination [31], posing a real risk to patient safety, and therefore require prompt hemostasis to improve outcomes. Clipping is one such option to achieve hemostasis in these patients.

Hemoclipping was found to be more effective than epinephrine injection for Dieulafoy lesion hemostasis and significantly reduced the chance of bleeding recurrence following treatment [32]. The success rate of clips for treatment of these lesions is well above 90% with a very little risk of rebleeding [32–34]. Clipping is therefore very useful as a first-line treatment for Dieulafoy's lesions. One downside to this method is that some lesions are in hard-to-reach places, such as the lesser curvature of the stomach, the fundus or on the posterior bulb of the duodenal wall. A skilled endoscopist is therefore needed to deploy and successfully use the clip for these lesions. Finally, clips and endoscopic band ligation were similarly effective in treating Dieulafoy's lesions [30]. Both methods can be considered for such cases.

Successful over-the-scope clip treatment for Dieulafoy bleeding has been described [17, 35, 36]; however, more research needs to be done to compare its efficacy to existing through-the-scope clips and other hemostatic methods.

Mallory-Weiss Syndrome

Mallory-Weiss tears are an uncommon cause of upper GI hemorrhage. They constitute around 5% of all causes of upper GI bleeding [37, 38]. Mechanical hemostasis through clipping offers a practical solution for treating both these tears and the bleeding associated with them.

Endoscopic clipping has been found to be effective for the treatment of Mallory-Weiss tears [37–39], with an efficacy similar to endoscopic band ligation [40]. The advantages of using mechanical clipping for the treatment of Mallory-Weiss syndrome hemorrhage include the ability to stop the bleeding as well as closing the physical tear responsible for that bleeding [39]. It may also be a preferable technique to thermo-coagulation, as the esophageal wall is thin and more prone to full thickness perforation, especially if the mucosal wall is already torn.

Over-the-scope clips can also treat Mallory-Weiss tears, with multiple reports showing successful application of the devices to halt bleeding [17, 41]. It is slowly becoming another tool in the endoscopist's armamentarium to manage these types of lesions.

Prophylaxis

Post-Polypectomy

Post-polypectomy bleeding is an important complication after polyp removal, with an incidence rate between 3% and 8% [42, 43] and delayed bleeding usually occurring within 14 days after polypectomy [44]. Although immediate bleeding can be successfully treated using clipping, current practice can include prophylactic clipping of certain lesions to prevent future hemorrhage. For pedunculated polyp bleeding, the best way to achieve hemostasis is to deploy the clip across the stalk or to clip the base of the polyp. This effectively cuts off the blood supply from the feeding vessel. For sessile polyps, the bleeding region should be clipped first and the lesion on the mucosa entirely closed afterward. Multiple clips could be used for either of these procedures to achieve the desired effect [45].

Categories to stratify polyps for prophylactic clipping are dependent on polyp size (small/mid-sized polyps and large polyps) and polyp morphology (pedunculated/flat polyps).

Small and Mid-Sized Polyps Small polyps are defined as up to 1 cm in diameter, and mid-sized polyps can be defined as smaller than 2 cm in diameter. In patient populations presenting these types of polyps, prophylactic post-polypectomy clipping tends to be ineffective in decreasing subsequent bleeding episodes [46, 47].

There is still the possibility that prophylaxis could be useful for patients at high risk of GI bleeding. A meta-analysis showed that patients on uninterrupted Clopidogrel therapy had a higher risk of delayed bleeding post-polypectomy. However, the included studies had varying or unknown rates of concomitant Clopidogrel and Aspirin (ASA) use [48]. The effect of Clopidogrel alone on post-polypectomy bleeding is controversial [48–50], but a 2015 meta-analysis showed that Clopidogrel alone did increase the incidence of delayed post-polypectomy bleeding [51]. The literature also shows that dual antiplatelet therapy increases the chance of delayed post-polypectomy bleeding [50, 51].

Current guidelines recommend stopping Clopidogrel but not ASA therapy 5 days prior to the procedure or postponing procedures if Clopidogrel cannot be stopped [52, 53]. The effect of prophylactic clipping in these patients has not yet been studied extensively but could potentially eliminate the need to stop antiplatelet therapy prior to procedures. It could also potentially prevent the occurrence of delayed bleeding when antiplatelet or anticoagulation therapy is resumed after polypectomies. One study showed that prophylactic clipping in patients on antiplatelet or anticoagulation therapy was more cost-effective that prophylactic clipping on patients not taking these medications [54].

Large Polyps Large polyps are defined as 2 cm or larger in diameter. While post-polypectomy clipping has become a more common practice among endoscopists, the efficacy of the practice for prophylaxis in large polyps is subject to controversy. Multiple studies show no added benefit for prophylactic use of clipping in this scenario [47, 55], but these studies are limited by their retrospective nature and the inclusion of some small polyps in their analyses. Two randomized control studies on large polyps showed conflicting results when determining the effectiveness of prophylactic clipping in decreasing the incidence of delayed bleeding [56, 57]. Further studies on exclusively large polyps also show mixed results [58, 59].

It is nevertheless important to note that prophylactic clipping of large polyps could be of use in certain patient populations with high risk of bleeding post-polypectomy. In one study, patients with the following factors were determined to be at high risk of delayed bleeding post procedure: patients older than 75, ASA class of three or more, lesion size of 4 cm or more, Aspirin treatment, and right-sided lesions [60]. These patients might qualify for prophylactic clipping. Accumulating many of these factors raises risk of bleeding up to 40% for the high-risk group. Basing the decision to clip on a score calculated from these factors has been proposed to reduce post-polypectomy hemorrhagic complications [60].

There is as of yet insufficient evidence to recommend general prophylactic clipping of polyps, but prospective randomized control trials are underway to better understand the value of prophylactic clipping in high-risk patients and for large non-pedunculated polyps [61].

Flat and Pedunculated Polyps Polyp morphology can play a role in determining the probability of bleeding post procedure. Pedunculated polyps were found to be a risk factor for post-polypectomy hemorrhages [62, 63], particularly for pedunculated polyps with large stalks [62]. A larger polyp base was associated with a richer vascularization of the stalk; additionally, while small stalks have linear vessels running through them, larger stalks present with a more irregular pattern to the vessels [62]. This makes these polyps more likely to bleed post polypectomy.

A prospective randomized study has shown no benefit in prophylactic clipping of large pedunculated polyps [64]. A multicenter prospective randomized study also found that the efficacy of clipping was the same as that of endoloop for prophylaxis [65]. A 2016 meta-analysis by Park et al. showed that prophylactic clipping reduced the occurrence of early bleeding in pedunculated polyps [47]. Theoretically, clipping large pedunculated polyps might seem attractive due to the increased risk of bleeding associated with their removal; however, the data is insufficient to recommend this practice.

The efficacy of prophylactic clipping monotherapy on flat polyps is also indeterminate. However, one study showed that combined mechanical and injection therapy did not decrease the risk of early post-polypectomy bleeding in flat polyps [47]. Further research is underway to elucidate the benefits of post-prophylactic clipping on these large flat polyps [61].

Indications for Perforation

Perforations are a rare complication of endoscopic manipulation of the GI tract, with an incidence of 1 in 1000 for therapeutic colonoscopies and 1 in 1400 for nontherapeutic colonoscopies [66]. Although the proportion of

Table 26.2 Indications for perforation closure

Clips	Indicated for perforation
Resolution Clip[1]	Up to 2 cm
Resolution 360[1]	Up to 2 cm
DuraClip[2]	Up to 2 cm
Instinct[3]	No
QuickClip2[4]	Up to 2 cm
QuickClip Pro[4]	Up to 2 cm
OTSC[5]	Up to 2 cm
Padlock Clip[6]	Up to 2 cm

1 Boston Scientific, *2* ConMed, *3* Cook Medical, *4* Olympus, *5* Ovesco, *6* US Endoscopy

iatrogenic perforations is low, the large number of endoscopies performed throughout the world makes it a real risk in absolute terms. Historically, the treatment of choice for these perforations was surgical closure of the lesions, involving invasive procedures and long recovery times. However, endoscopic clips have become an efficient alternative treatment, removing the need for surgery (Table 26.2).

Surgical rescue of iatrogenic gastrointestinal perforations has a morbidity rate of 36% and mortality of 7% [67]. Clipping of perforations has a success rate of around 90% with through-the-scope clips and around 88% with over-the-scope clips [68]. Endoscopic clips are therefore an effective alternative to surgical repair for perforations depending on the size of the lesion, with large perforations (>1 cm) proving more difficult to close than smaller ones [68].

One study performed on a porcine model ($N = 8$) showed a 25% rate of leakage for endoluminal closure of large perforations [69], while a second study on a similar model indicated difficulty in closing widely spaced incision sites [70]. It is therefore unclear if perforations larger than 1 cm can be reliably closed with through-the-scope clips. In the case of larger gastric perforations, a second technique has proven successful, where either the greater or lesser omentum is suctioned and used as a patch in conjunction with clip application [71–73]. For large lesions, standard clips also have the shortcoming of poor bite depth for tissue acquisition; an over-the-scope clip could therefore be beneficial to grasp the muscularis layer more tightly and provide a solid

closure of the perforation. This technique has proven effective for perforations up to 3 cm in size and could be promising as a first-line approach for iatrogenic perforations followed by surgery if unsuccessful [74]. Since endoscopic clipping, if successful, does not carry the same risk of complications as surgery, it is recommended to favor this procedure whenever an endoscopist is comfortable enough and adequately trained to perform it.

Fistulae

Gastrointestinal fistulae present a unique challenge for endoscopists. The tissues forming these fistulae tend to be scarred, fibrotic, and less malleable than normal gastrointestinal tissue, requiring more force to approximate the lesion and form a proper closure. Through-the-scope clip monotherapy has been used to successfully close these fistulae [8, 75]. A clip and cautery combination has also been attempted with moderate success in three patients [76]. However, patients in these studies did not undergo long-term follow-ups to establish persisting closure of fistulae and therefore show no data on the reoccurrence of these lesions after treatment. One retrospective study suggests that less than 20% of patients experience lasting treatment success 2 years post-endoclip closure [76].

Studies involving through-the-scope treatment of fistulae have been limited to small patient sample sizes, with a lack of large studies or long follow-up periods. While treating fistulae with these methods seems to be successful in the short term, there is no guarantee that it will result in lasting definitive closure over a longer term. To date, no endoscopic clip has specifically been approved for the treatment of fistulae, although most are approved for the treatment of perforations up to 2 cm.

One method to prevent treatment failure post-clipping involves the use of over-the-scope clips. These clips provide a better approximation of tissues and closure strength which can be very useful when dealing with chronic fibrotic fistulae. So far, multiple case series have studied the performance of over-the-scope clips for this indication (Table 26.3), but reported sample sizes remain

Table 26.3 OTSC performance for fistulae

Study author and date	Type of study	Number of cases	Follow-up period	Initial success (%)	Recurrence rate after initial success (%)
Haito-Chavez et al. (2014) [77]	Retrospective	91	Median of 121 days	90.6	57.1
Mercky et al. (2014) [78]	Retrospective	30	Average of 10.4 months	100	47
Baron et al. (2012) [79]	Retrospective	28	1 month	96	32
Winder et al. (2016) [80]	Retrospective	22	Median of 4.7 months	n.s.[1]	22.7
Law et al. (2013) [81]	Retrospective	21	Median of 148 days	95	67
Surace et al. (2011) [82]	Prospective	19	8 months	n.s.[1]	58
Mennigen et al. (2013) [83]	Retrospective	14	Median of 5.5 months	100	21
Manta et al. (2011) [84]	Prospective	12	1–3 months	92	[a]
Von Renteln et al. (2010) [85]	Prospective	4	2 months	50	[a]
Parodi et al. (2010) [86]	Prospective	4	1–2 weeks	100	[a]
Goenka et al. (2017) [87]	Prospective	3	1–2 months	66	[a]
Dişibeyaz et al. (2012) [88]	Prospective	3	0–18 days	33	[a]

[1] not specified
[a]No long-term follow-up available

small. The OTSC proves to be very successful at initial fistulae closure but the recurrence rate is between 32 and 67% in the three largest reported studies [77–79]. The OTSC seems to be somewhat successful for treating fistulae (Table 26.3), but larger prospective studies with long-term follow-ups need to be performed to be able to better understand its efficacy.

Per Oral Endoscopic Myotomy

A further use for endoscopic clips is the closing of submucosal tunnel incision sites during POEM techniques. The opening is typically closed with multiple clips to prevent leakage of gastric content in the tunnel or mediastinum [89–91]. Clips are also used to close perforations that may occur during tunnel creation [89]. The use of over-the-scope clips has been described for the closure of initial orifice and may allow for better full thickness closure [92].

Securing Tubes and Stents

Feeding Tubes

Another use for endoclips is the securing of feeding tubes on the jejunal mucosa to prevent migration back into the stomach. This technique typically involves blindly inserting the feeding tube in the stomach and then grasping the suture loops with the clip. The clip is then pulled back in the endoscope, and the scope is advanced to the ligament of Treitz where the clip is opened again and secured on the intestinal wall [93, 94]. This technique can also be used to secure feeding tubes to the gastric or duodenal wall and is successful in preventing migration [94, 95].

Stents

A possible complication to the application of stents is their migration from their original location. The securing of stents with clips has previously been covered in literature for the esophagus [96, 97] and the small bowel [98] with little to no subsequent migration.

Miscellaneous Indications

PEG Tube Removal

The opening left behind after removal of percutaneous endoscopic gastrotomy (PEG) tubes is usually allowed to heal naturally. Refractory persistence of fistulae is a known complication of such procedures. These lesions can be successfully closed using standard clips [99, 100]. Over-the-scope closure has also been described in the literature with good results [101–103]. Clip retention is an important factor for the healing of these refractory lesions; therefore over-the-scope clips could provide an added benefit by adhering to the mucosa for a longer period of time when compared to standard clip therapy.

Endoscopic Marking of Lesions

Endoscopic clips can be used as markers for different indications. In one instance, a clip has been used to mark vascular malformation in the small intestine for subsequent angiography [104]. Clips have also been used as markers to assist surgeons in determining the extent of resection for lesions [1, 105], although this indication has largely been taken over by the use of tattoos, limiting the role of clips as tools for surgical marking.

General Safety

Endoscopic clips are safe with very few reported complications. As of yet, no studies have been undertaken to determine the rate of complication due to clips, most likely due to the feasibility problems of gathering a sample size large enough to accurately capture such a rare complication. Perforations are one of the risks of endoscopy, but these are not exclusive to clips and would be more applicable to traumatic techniques such as thermo-coagulation. The perforation rate for therapeutic colonoscopies is around 0.1% [106]; therefore we can project that the proportion caused by clips is much lower than that rate. One incidence of abdominal aortic aneurism rupture has been described in the literature, although the correlation between the clipping and the complication is unclear [107]. An incidence of small bowel occlusion has been reported after misapplication of an OTSC [79]. However, Ovesco clips can be removed after their application, so it is still possible to rescue the occlusion after such a misapplication.

Future Directions

The potential for new indications for endoscopic clip use is vast. Clips show promise for further expansion in the domain of perforation treatment. The OTSC has shown to be particularly effective in the closure of large perforations [74]. It is likely that this technique will become more common, reducing the need for surgical salvage repair of iatrogenic perforations.

Expanding the indication for the size of perforation closure is also an avenue that could be explored in the future. Currently, most clips are indicated for perforations up to 2 cm with the OTSC showing potential for larger perforation closure. Larger clip sizes could prove useful to address this gap in perforation closure indications.

Endoscopic full thickness resection using the OTSC is a newer technique that has been performed successfully on porcine models [108] and has started to be utilized on patient populations [109, 110]. The further development of this technique is expected, expanding endoscopic treatment for difficult to resect lesions (i.e., muscular biopsies, submucosal fibrosis, non-lifting sign, or superficial submucosal infiltration of gastrointestinal cancers).

Randomized control trials should be conducted to compare the OTSC to standard through-the-scope clips for different indications. A cost-benefit analysis for its application also needs to be performed since it is more expensive than through-the-scope clips but would potentially require fewer total clips to perform the same procedure.

Post-polypectomy prophylactic clipping is still controversial in its efficacy for preventing delayed bleeding post procedure. An international multicenter randomized trial called the Large Polyp Study (LPS) on polyps larger than 2 cm is currently in progress to try to answer the controversy around this practice [61].

Standard clips are evolving to become better tools for endoscopists to use. Expansion in MRI safety, better responses to rotation, and the ability to reapply clips after misapplication are among the things that will be improved in the coming years.

Combination therapies for gastrointestinal bleeding also need to be reassessed due to the changing landscape of available techniques. Through-the-scope clips have evolved through the years, over-the-scope clips are increasing in popularity, and HemoSpray could potentially be a good additive therapy alongside standard clips or over-the-scope clips for a multitude of hemostasis indications. It would therefore be beneficial to perform studies comparing standard clip monotherapy, over-the-scope clip monotherapy, and combination therapies with or without HemoSpray for all clipping indications to update our current first-line recommendations.

Endoscopic Glues

History of Endoscopic Glues

Tissue adhesive use for endoscopic therapy was described for the first time by Martin et al. in 1977 [111]. The adhesive in question was a tri-fluoroisopropyl cyanoacrylate polymer (Flucrylate) used to successfully stop upper GI bleeding in five out of six initial patients presenting with massive bleeding from upper GI ulcers, varices, and esophagitis. However, further experiments performed the following years in canine gastric ulcer models showed that the adhesive was ineffective in arresting bleeding [112, 113] and was even described as "unpredictable as an adjunctive treatment" [113]. In 1979 Fibrin glues made their first appearance in a paper by Linscheer et al. that described successfully spraying thrombin and fibrinogen solutions on a canine ulcer model to arrest bleeding [114]. Five years later, butyl-cyanoacrylate was used for the first time to obturate esophageal varices [115]. That same feat was performed in 1989 with a combination of fibrin glue and sclerotherapy [116] and in 1992 with fibrin glue monotherapy [117].

Endoscopic glues progressively saw more testing in the following years, with descriptions of application on Dieulafoy's lesions [118], bleeding tumors [119], post-polypectomy bleeding [120], and fistulae [121]. A collagen-fibrin sealant was developed in 2002 [122] but failed to find much traction as a general use glue for endoscopy. Through the years, endoscopic glues failed to find as much widespread use as hemostatic clips for the treatment of bleeding and perforations.

Types of Endoscopic Glues

Cyanoacrylates

Cyanoacrylates are a type of synthetic glue that solidify upon contact with water or blood [123]. They can be mixed with oils such as lipiodol to slow down the solidification rate, thus rendering the glue easier to apply through the endoscope channel [124]. Injecting the glue comes with the risk of embolization into vessels. Small amounts of glue (0.5–1 ml) must therefore be used per injection to mitigate that risk [123]. Cyanoacrylates can also block endoscopic channels when released inside the endoscope. It is therefore recommended to coat the working channel and the tip of the endoscope with oil before applying the glue, and to flush the endoscope with saline after glue application [124]. An added precaution could also involve removing the entire endoscope and cleaning the injection needle with alcohol before removing the needle through the endoscope [125].

Fibrin Glues

Fibrin glues are composed of a solution of fibrinogen and factor XIII alongside a second solution of thrombin. When these solutions are applied consecutively, a fibrin polymer clot is formed on a bleeding site that mimics physiological coagulation [124]. Fibrin glues can also cause clots inside channels if the two solutions are released in the endoscope, but the risks of blockage are lower than with cyanoacrylates [125]. Double-lumen catheters could be used to inject both solutions at the same time so that they only combine distally [125].

Indications for Endoscopic Glues

Varices

Variceal bleeding is a severe and deadly complication that occurs in patients with cirrhosis. Its inhospital mortality rate in the 1980s was around 40% [126] but decreased significantly over the decades with the appearance of new treatment modalities including endoscopic hemostasis. The inhospital mortality rate in the 2000s decreased to about 15% [126]. Urgent endoscopic intervention via methods such as band ligation and glue obliteration is paramount for treating these bleeding varices.

The treatment of varices with endoscopic glues involves injecting the glue into the varices to solidify and form a cast. The mucosa then sloughs off, and the cast slowly extrudes into the gastric lumen over the next 3 months [127].

Gastric Varices

Gastric varices are a main indication for treatment using endoscopic glue techniques. A randomized controlled trial ($N = 37$) showed that cyanoacrylate injection was of similar efficacy to alcohol sclerotherapy for treating acute bleeding from gastric varices [128]. It is, however, more effective in achieving gastric variceal eradication [128]. Two RCTs showed that cyanoacrylates were either more effective [129] or equal to [130] band ligation for achieving initial hemostasis. However, both studies show that acrylate glue therapy was more successful in preventing rebleeding rates [129, 130].

Fibrin glues were also shown to be successful in treating gastric varices in multiple studies [131–133]. However, no RCT have yet been performed to compare their efficacy to other hemostasis methods, and no studies have compared their performance with cyanoacrylate glues. Cyanoacrylates have so far been the most popular method of treating gastric varices with a proven track record and high-quality studies backing their use (128130). It is therefore recommended to favor this method when dealing with gastric varices.

Cyanoacrylates can also be used effectively to treat gastric varices to prevent first-time hemorrhages. They have proven more effective when compared to beta blockers for gastric variceal bleeding prophylaxis [134, 135].

Esophageal Varices

Cyanoacrylate glues have been used successfully for the treatment of esophageal varices [136, 137], but other methods such as band ligation have been subject to more research to establish their efficacy and safety for this indication. It is possible, however, to use glue injection as a rescue therapy when bleeding is refractory to band ligation treatment. No study has yet attempted to compare glue injection to band ligation for esophageal variceal hemorrhage.

Per Oral Endoscopic Myotomy

The closure of POEM openings can be accomplished by using cyanoacrylate glues [138] and is a cheap and effective way of doing so when compared to clips, which can become expensive if using OTSC. However, one downside of this method is the likely loss of strong mechanical closure forces compared to closure using clips. Mucosal perforations during POEM procedures have also been closed successfully using either cyanoacrylate monotherapy [139] or in combination with the OTSC [140]. The data so far is insufficient to recommend using glues over other techniques. Glues are a cheaper alternative but clips theoretically provide a stronger closure of lesions.

Fistulae

Endoscopic glues can also be effective for the treatment of gastrointestinal fistulae [121]. Fibrin glue has been shown to reduce the healing time of fistulae with a faster re-initiation of oral feeding [141]. It was found to be an effective second-line treatment for patients who are resistant to conservative management of their fistulae [142, 143]. Two studies did not make the distinction between fistulae and anastomotic leakages in their data but showed that fibrin glue is effective for both indications [144] and that a vicryl plug could be used effectively as a combination therapy alongside fibrin glues [145]. Cyanoacrylates can also be used for the treatment of fistulae [146], although the data has been limited to a few reported cases.

Fibrin glues show promise in the closing of fistulae as a first- or second-line treatment and are an inexpensive technique compared to clips. They do, however, require multiple sessions to achieve full healing of the fistula and would therefore be less convenient than a single clipping session. It is unclear whether fibrin glues would still be an effective treatment in high-output fistulae. Glues have also shown to be ineffective in chronically infected, neoplastic, or radiation-treated tissues [147]. Studies determining the efficacy of fibrin glues suffer from low sample sizes, so large multicenter prospective studies are needed to validate their indication for the treatment of fistulae.

Non-variceal Bleeding

Endoscopic treatment of non-variceal bleeding using glues has been tried for Dieulafoy's lesions [118], bleeding tumors [119], post-polypectomy bleeding [120], and peptic ulcers [111]. However, clipping is currently the standard therapy for these lesions and has proven to be successful without the risk of embolization into arteries. Glues have very limited use for non-variceal GI bleeding.

Safety of Endoscopic Glues

A potential complication of endoscopic glue therapy is the injection of products into veins or arteries causing thrombosis or embolization. A case of portal and splenic vein thrombosis after Histoacryl injection has been described in the literature [148]. Multiple cases of cerebrovascular complications [149] and pulmonary emboli [150] following cyanoacrylate injection have also been reported. In some cases, embolization of injected glues resulted in death [149, 151]. Given the potential severity of the complications associated with glue injection, it is recommended to proceed with caution when administering cyanoacrylates and to limit the amounts of glue to 0.5–1 ml per injection [123].

Inadvertent injection of glues in the working channel of endoscopes could result in a blockage, requiring often endoscope repair. It is possible to remove some obstructions from the endoscope by pushing instruments such as biopsy forceps through the channel [152], but not all blockages can be cleared this way. This can delay procedures and require the reapplication of endoscopes in the GI tract, increasing the chances of overall complications.

Future Directions

Endoscopic glues have been around in the endoscopist's armamentarium for a long time. Their indications have so far been limited to the treatment of gastric varices and fistulae. Endoscopic glue has recently been used for POEM procedures to close the mucosal incision site or seal mucosal perforations. Research in this area and future expansion of this technique will likely remain limited.

References

1. Hayashi T. The study on stanch clips for the treatment by endoscopy. Gastroenterol Endosc. 1975;17(1):92–101.
2. 処置用ファイバースコープ(Gastrofiberscope for Treatment: T. G. F. Olympus)の使用経験―特に粘膜下病変の診断を中心に. 胃と腸. 1974;9(3):355–64.
3. Komiya O. Surgical instrument for clipping any affected portion of a body cavity. Google Patents; 1976.
4. Lehman GA, Maveety PR, O'Connor KW. Mucosal clipping—utility and safety testing in the colon. Gastrointest Endosc. 1985;31(4):273–6.
5. Hachisu T, Nakao T, Suzuki N. The endoscopic clipping hemostasis against upper gastrointestinal bleeding (a device of the improved clip and its clinical study). Gastroenterol Endosc. 1985;27(2):276.
6. Binmoeller KF, Grimm H, Soehendra N. Endoscopic closure of a perforation using metallic clips after snare excision of a gastric leiomyoma. Gastrointest Endosc. 1993;39(2):172–4.
7. Katon RM. Experimental control of gastrointestinal hemorrhage via the endoscope: a new era dawns. Gastroenterology. 1996;70(2):272–7.
8. Rodella L, Laterza E, De Manzoni G, Kind R, Lombardo F, Catalano F, et al. Endoscopic clipping of anastomotic leakages in esophagogastric surgery. Endoscopy. 1998;30(05):453–6.
9. Chuttani R, Barkun A, Carpenter S, Chotiprasidhi P, Ginsberg GG, Hussain N, et al. Endoscopic clip application devices. Gastrointest Endosc. 2006;63(6):746–50.

10. Available from: https://www.accessdata.fda.gov/scripts/cdrh/cfdocs/cfPMN/pmn.cfm.

11. Longstreth GF. Epidemiology of hospitalization for acute upper gastrointestinal hemorrhage: a population-based study. Am J Gastroenterol. 1995;90(2):206–10.

12. Srygley FD, Gerardo CJ, Tran T, Fisher DA. Does this patient have a severe upper gastrointestinal bleed? JAMA. 2012;307(10):1072–9.

13. Hwang JH, Fisher DA, Ben-Menachem T, Chandrasekhara V, Chathadi K, Decker GA, et al. The role of endoscopy in the management of acute non-variceal upper GI bleeding. Gastrointest Endosc. 2012;75(6):1132–8.

14. Cipolletta L, Cipolletta F, Marmo C, Piscopo R, Rotondano G, Marmo R. Mechanical methods to endoscopically treat nonvariceal upper gastrointestinal bleeding. Tech Gastrointest Endosc. 2016;18(4):191–7.

15. Tang SJ. Endoscopic treatment of upper gastrointestinal ulcer bleeding. Video J EncyclGI Endoscop. 2013;1(1):143–7.

16. Jang JY. Recent developments in the endoscopic treatment of patients with peptic ulcer bleeding. Clin Endosc. 2016;49(5):417–20.

17. Mori H, Kobara H, Masaki T. Rapid over-the-scope-clip emergency hemostasis guidewire-assisted method for proximal colon Dieulafoy massive bleeding. Dig Endosc. 2017;29(1):127–8.

18. Laine L, McQuaid KR. Endoscopic therapy for bleeding ulcers: an evidence-based approach based on meta-analyses of randomized controlled trials. Clin Gastroenterol Hepatol. 2009;7(1):33–47.

19. Sung JJY, Tsoi KKF, Lai LH, Wu JCY, Lau JYW. Endoscopic clipping versus injection and thermo-coagulation in the treatment of non-variceal upper gastrointestinal bleeding: a meta-analysis. Gut. 2007;56(10):1364–73.

20. Manno M, Mangiafico S, Caruso A, Barbera C, Bertani H, Mirante VG, et al. First-line endoscopic treatment with OTSC in patients with high-risk non-variceal upper gastrointestinal bleeding: preliminary experience in 40 cases. Surg Endosc. 2016;30(5):2026–9.

21. Schmidt A, Goelder S, Messmann H, Goetz M, Kratt T, Meining A, et al. 62 over-the-scope-clips versus standard endoscopic therapy in patients with recurrent peptic ulcer bleeding and a prospective randomized, multicenter trial (sting). Gastrointest Endosc. 2017;85(5):AB50.

22. Schuetz A, Jauch K-W. Lower gastrointestinal bleeding: therapeutic strategies, surgical techniques and results. Langenbeck's Arch Surg. 2001;386(1):17–25.

23. Longstreth GF. Epidemiology and outcome of patients hospitalized with acute lower gastrointestinal hemorrhage: a population-based study. Am J Gastroenterol. 1997;92(3):419–24.

24. Yen EF, Ladabaum U, Muthusamy VR, Cello JP, McQuaid KR, Shah JN. Colonoscopic treatment of acute diverticular hemorrhage using endoclips. Dig Dis Sci. 2008;53(9):2480–5.

25. Strate LL, Gralnek IM. ACG clinical guideline: management of patients with acute lower gastrointestinal bleeding. Am J Gastroenterol. 2016;111(4):459–74.

26. Soriani P, Tontini GE, Vavassori S, Neumann H, Pastorelli L, Vecchi M, et al. Over-the-scope clipping in recurrent colonic diverticular bleeding. Endoscopy. 2016;48(S 01):E306–E7.

27. Probst A, Braun G, Goelder S, Messmann H. Endoscopic treatment of colonic diverticular bleeding using an over-the-scope clip. Endoscopy. 2016;48(S 01):E160–E.

28. Strate LL, Naumann CR. The role of colonoscopy and radiological procedures in the management of acute lower intestinal bleeding. Clin Gastroenterol Hepatol. 2010;8(4):333–43.

29. Lee YT, Walmsley RS, Leong RWL, Sung JJY. Dieulafoy's lesion. Gastrointest Endosc. 2003;58(2):236–43.

30. Ahn D-W, Lee SH, Park YS, Shin CM, Hwang J-H, Kim J-W, et al. Hemostatic efficacy and clinical outcome of endoscopic treatment of Dieulafoy's lesions: comparison of endoscopic hemoclip placement and endoscopic band ligation. Gastrointest Endosc. 2012;75(1):32–8.

31. Lara LF, Sreenarasimhaiah J, Tang SJ, Afonso BB, Rockey DC. Dieulafoy lesions of the GI tract: localization and therapeutic outcomes. Dig Dis Sci. 2010;55(12):3436–41.

32. Park CH, Sohn YH, Lee WS, Joo YE, Choi SK, Rew JS, et al. The usefulness of endoscopic hemoclipping for bleeding Dieulafoy lesions. Endoscopy. 2003;35(5):388–92.

33. Park CH, Joo YE, Kim HS, Choi SK, Rew JS, Kim SJ. A prospective, randomized trial of endoscopic band ligation versus endoscopic hemoclip placement for bleeding gastric Dieulafoy's lesions. Endoscopy. 2004;36(8):677–81.

34. Chung IK, Kim EJ, Lee MS, Kim HS, Park SH, Lee MH, et al. Bleeding Dieulafoy's lesions and the choice of endoscopic method: comparing the hemostatic efficacy of mechanical and injection methods. Gastrointest Endosc. 2000;52(6):721–4.

35. Gómez V, Kyanam Kabir Baig KR, Lukens FJ, Woodward T. Novel treatment of a gastric Dieulafoy lesion with an over-the-scope clip. Endoscopy. 2013;45(S 02):E71-E.

36. Chaer RA, Helton WS. Dieulafoy's disease. J Am Coll Surg. 2003;196(2):290–6.

37. Rockall TA, Logan RF, Devlin HB, Northfield TC. Incidence of and mortality from acute upper gastrointestinal haemorrhage in the United Kingdom. Steering committee and members of the national audit of acute upper gastrointestinal haemorrhage. BMJ. 1995;311(6999):222–6.

38. Yamaguchi Y, Yamato T, Katsumi N, Morozumi K, Abe T, Ishida H, et al. Endoscopic hemoclipping for upper GI bleeding due to Mallory-Weiss syndrome. Gastrointest Endosc. 2001;53(4):427–30.

39. Shimoda R, Iwakiri R, Sakata H, Ogata S, Ootani H, Sakata Y, et al. Endoscopic hemostasis with metallic hemoclips for iatrogenic Mallory-Weiss tear

caused by endoscopic examination. Dig Endosc. 2009;21(1):20–3.

40. Cho YS, Chae HS, Kim HK, Kim JS, Kim BW, Kim SS, et al. Endoscopic band ligation and endoscopic hemoclip placement for patients with Mallory-Weiss syndrome and active bleeding. World J Gastroenterol. 2008;14(13):2080–4.

41. Sharma M, Lingampalli R, Jindal S, Somani P. Management of a Dieulafoy ulcer bleed with an over-the-scope clip. VideoGIE. 2017;2(8):199–200.

42. Kim HS, Kim TI, Kim WH, Kim YH, Kim HJ, Yang SK, et al. Risk factors for immediate postpolypectomy bleeding of the colon: a multicenter study. Am J Gastroenterol. 2006;101(6):1333–41.

43. Qumseya BJ, Wolfsen C, Wang Y, Othman M, Raimondo M, Bouras E, et al. Factors associated with increased bleeding post-endoscopic mucosal resection. J Dig Dis. 2013;14(3):140–6.

44. Watabe H, Yamaji Y, Okamoto M, Kondo S, Ohta M, Ikenoue T, et al. Risk assessment for delayed hemorrhagic complication of colonic polypectomy: polyp-related factors and patient-related factors. Gastrointest Endosc. 2006;64(1):73–8.

45. Hokama A, Kishimoto K, Kinjo F, Fujita J. Endoscopic clipping in the lower gastrointestinal tract. World J Gastrointest Endosc. 2009;1(1):7–11.

46. Shioji K, Suzuki Y, Kobayashi M, Nakamura A, Azumaya M, Takeuchi M, et al. Prophylactic clip application does not decrease delayed bleeding after colonoscopic polypectomy. Gastrointest Endosc. 2003;57(6):691–4.

47. Park CH, Jung YS, Nam E, Eun CS, Park DI, Han DS. Comparison of efficacy of prophylactic endoscopic therapies for postpolypectomy bleeding in the colorectum: a systematic review and network meta-analysis. Am J Gastroenterol. 2016;111(9):1230–43.

48. Gandhi S, Narula N, Mosleh W, Marshall JK, Farkouh M. Meta-analysis: colonoscopic postpolypectomy bleeding in patients on continued clopidogrel therapy. Aliment Pharmacol Ther. 2013;37(10):947–52.

49. Hui AJ, Wong RMY, Ching JYL, Hung LCT, Sydney Chung SC, Sung JJY. Risk of colonoscopic polypectomy bleeding with anticoagulants and antiplatelet agents: analysis of 1657 cases. Gastrointest Endosc. 2004;59(1):44–8.

50. Singh M, Mehta N, Murthy UK, Kaul V, Arif A, Newman N. Postpolypectomy bleeding in patients undergoing colonoscopy on uninterrupted clopidogrel therapy. Gastrointest Endosc. 2010;71(6):998–1005.

51. Shalman D, Gerson LB. Systematic review with meta-analysis: the risk of gastrointestinal haemorrhage post-polypectomy in patients receiving anti-platelet, anti-coagulant and/or thienopyridine medications. Aliment Pharmacol Ther. 2015;42(8):949–56.

52. Veitch AM, Vanbiervliet G, Gershlick AH, Boustiere C, Baglin TP, Smith L-A, et al. Endoscopy in patients on antiplatelet or anticoagulant therapy, including direct oral anticoagulants: British Society of Gastroenterology (BSG) and European Society of Gastrointestinal Endoscopy (ESGE) guidelines. Endoscopy. 2016;48(04):385–402.

53. Acosta RD, Abraham NS, Chandrasekhara V, Chathadi KV, Early DS, Eloubeidi MA, et al. The management of antithrombotic agents for patients undergoing GI endoscopy. Gastrointest Endosc. 2016;83(1):3–16.

54. Parikh ND, Zanocco K, Keswani RN, Gawron AJ. A cost-efficacy decision analysis of prophylactic clip placement after endoscopic removal of large polyps. Clin Gastroenterol Hepatol. 2013;11(10):1319–24.

55. Quintanilla E, Castro JL, Rabago LR, Chico I, Olivares A, Ortega A, et al. Is the use of prophylactic hemoclips in the endoscopic resection of large pedunculated polyps useful? A prospective and randomized study. J Interv Gastroenterol. 2012;2(2):99–104.

56. Liaquat H, Rohn E, Rex DK. Prophylactic clip closure reduced the risk of delayed postpolypectomy hemorrhage: experience in 277 clipped large sessile or flat colorectal lesions and 247 control lesions. Gastrointest Endosc. 2013;77(3):401–7.

57. Dokoshi T, Fujiya M, Tanaka K, Sakatani A, Inaba Y, Ueno N, et al. A randomized study on the effectiveness of prophylactic clipping during endoscopic resection of colon polyps for the prevention of delayed bleeding. Biomed Res Int. 2015;2015:490272.

58. Lim SH, Levenick JM, Mathew A, Moyer MT, Dye CE, McGarrity TJ. Su1687 neither prophylactic clips nor ablation prevent post-polypectomy bleeding, results from 334 large (>2cm) polyp resections using endocut. Gastrointest Endosc. 2016;83(5):AB395.

59. Zhang Q-S, Han B, Xu J-H, Gao P, Shen Y-C. Clip closure of defect after endoscopic resection in patients with larger colorectal tumors decreased the adverse events. Gastrointest Endosc. 2015;82(5):904–9.

60. Albeniz E, Fraile M, Ibanez B, Alonso-Aguirre P, Martinez-Ares D, Soto S, et al. A scoring system to determine risk of delayed bleeding after endoscopic mucosal resection of large colorectal lesions. Clin Gastroenterol Hepatol. 2016;14(8):1140–7.

61. Pohl H. Clipping after polyp resection: uncertainties of a randomized trial. Gastrointest Endosc. 2015;82(5):910–1.

62. Dobrowolski S, Dobosz M, Babicki A, Głowacki J, Nałęcz A. Blood supply of colorectal polyps correlates with risk of bleeding after colonoscopic polypectomy. Gastrointest Endosc. 2006;63(7):1004–9.

63. Kim HS, Kim TI, Kim WH, Kim Y-H, Kim HJ, Yang S-K, et al. Risk factors for immediate postpolypectomy bleeding of the colon: a multicenter study. Am J Gastroenterol. 2006;101(6):1333–41.

64. Quintanilla E, Castro JL, Rábago LR, Chico I, Olivares A, Ortega A, et al. Is the use of prophylactic hemoclips in the endoscopic resection of large pedunculated polyps useful? A prospective and randomized study. J Intervent Gastroenterol. 2012;2(4):183–8.

65. Ji JS, Lee SW, Kim TH, Cho YS, Kim HK, Lee KM, et al. Comparison of prophylactic clip and endoloop application for the prevention of postpolypectomy

bleeding in pedunculated colonic polyps: a prospective, randomized, multicenter study. Endoscopy. 2014;46(7):598–604.

66. Panteris V, Haringsma J, Kuipers EJ. Colonoscopy perforation rate, mechanisms and outcome: from diagnostic to therapeutic colonoscopy. Endoscopy. 2009;41(11):941–51.

67. Iqbal CW, Cullinane DC, Schiller HJ, Sawyer MD, Zietlow SP, Farley DR. Surgical management and outcomes of 165 colonoscopic perforations from a single institution. Arch Surg. 2008;143(7):701–7.

68. Verlaan T, Voermans RP, van Berge Henegouwen MI, Bemelman WA, Fockens P. Endoscopic closure of acute perforations of the GI tract: a systematic review of the literature. Gastrointest Endosc. 2015;82(4):618–28.e5.

69. Raju GS, Ahmed I, Brining D, Xiao S-Y. Endoluminal closure of large perforations of colon with clips in a porcine model (with video). Gastrointest Endosc. 2006;64(4):640–6.

70. Merrifield BF, Wagh MS, Thompson CC. Peroral transgastric organ resection: a feasibility study in pigs. Gastrointest Endosc. 2006;63(4):693–7.

71. Tsunada S, Ogata S, Ohyama T, Ootani H, Oda K, Kikkawa A, et al. Endoscopic closure of perforations caused by EMR in the stomach by application of metallic clips. Gastrointest Endosc. 2003;57(7):948–51.

72. Minami S, Gotoda T, Ono H, Oda I, Hamanaka H. Complete endoscopic closure of gastric perforation induced by endoscopic resection of early gastric cancer using endoclips can prevent surgery (with video). Gastrointest Endosc. 2006;63(4):596–601.

73. Ikehara H, Gotoda T, Ono H, Oda I, Saito D. Gastric perforation during endoscopic resection for gastric carcinoma and the risk of peritoneal dissemination. Br J Surg. 2007;94(8):992–5.

74. Voermans RP, Le Moine O, von Renteln D, Ponchon T, Giovannini M, Bruno M, et al. Efficacy of endoscopic closure of acute perforations of the gastrointestinal tract. Clin Gastroenterol Hepatol. 2012;10(6):603–8.

75. Raymer GS, Sadana A, Campbell DB, Rowe WA. Endoscopic clip application as an adjunct to closure of mature esophageal perforation with fistulae. Clin Gastroenterol Hepatol. 2003;1(1):44–50.

76. Fernandez-Esparrach G, Lautz DB, Thompson CC. Endoscopic repair of gastrogastric fistula after Roux-en-Y gastric bypass: a less-invasive approach. Surg Obes Relat Dis. 2010;6(3):282–8.

77. Haito-Chavez Y, Law JK, Kratt T, Arezzo A, Verra M, Morino M, et al. International multicenter experience with an over-the-scope clipping device for endoscopic management of GI defects (with video). Gastrointest Endosc. 2014;80(4):610–22.

78. Mercky P, Gonzalez J-M, Aimore Bonin E, Emungania O, Brunet J, Grimaud J-C, et al. Usefulness of over-the-scope clipping system for closing digestive fistulas. Dig Endosc. 2015;27(1):18–24.

79. Baron TH, Wong Kee Song LM, Ross A, Tokar JL, Irani S, Kozarek RA. Use of an over-the-scope clipping device: multicenter retrospective results of the first U.S. experience (with videos). Gastrointest Endosc. 2012;76(1):202–8.

80. Winder JS, Kulaylat AN, Schubart JR, Hal HM, Pauli EM. Management of non-acute gastrointestinal defects using the over-the-scope clips (OTSCs): a retrospective single-institution experience. Surg Endosc. 2016;30(6):2251–8.

81. Law R, Irani S, Wong Kee Song LM, Baron TH. Sa1480 delayed outcomes following fistula closure using the over-the-scope clip (OTSC). Gastrointest Endosc. 2013;77(5):AB221.

82. Surace M, Mercky P, Demarquay J-F, Gonzalez J-M, Dumas R, Ah-Soune P, et al. Endoscopic management of GI fistulae with the over-the-scope clip system (with video). Gastrointest Endosc. 2011;74(6):1416–9.

83. Mennigen R, Colombo-Benkmann M, Senninger N, Laukoetter M. Endoscopic closure of postoperative gastrointestinal leakages and fistulas with the over-the-scope clip (OTSC). J Gastrointest Surg. 2013;17(6):1058–65.

84. Manta R, Manno M, Bertani H, Barbera C, Pigo F, Mirante V, et al. Endoscopic treatment of gastrointestinal fistulas using an over-the-scope clip (OTSC) device: case series from a tertiary referral center. Endoscopy. 2011;43(6):545–8.

85. von Renteln D, Denzer UW, Schachschal G, Anders M, Groth S, Rösch T. Endoscopic closure of GI fistulae by using an over-the-scope clip (with videos). Gastrointest Endosc. 2010;72(6):1289–96.

86. Parodi A, Repici A, Pedroni A, Blanchi S, Conio M. Endoscopic management of GI perforations with a new over-the-scope clip device (with videos). Gastrointest Endosc. 2010;72(4):881–6.

87. Goenka MK, Rai VK, Goenka U, Tiwary IK. Endoscopic management of gastrointestinal leaks and bleeding with the over-the-scope clip: a prospective study. Clin Endosc. 2017;50(1):58–63.

88. Dişibeyaz S, Köksal AŞ, Parlak E, Torun S, Şaşmaz N. Endoscopic closure of gastrointestinal defects with an over-the-scope clip device. A case series and review of the literature. Clin Res Hepatol Gastroenterol. 2012;36(6):614–21.

89. Stavropoulos SN, Desilets DJ, Fuchs K-H, Gostout CJ, Haber G, Inoue H, et al. Per-oral endoscopic myotomy white paper summary. Gastrointest Endosc. 2012;80(1):1–15.

90. Ponsky JL, Marks JM, Pauli EM. How I do it: Per-oral endoscopic myotomy (POEM). J Gastrointest Surg. 2012;16(6):1251–5.

91. von Renteln D, Inoue H, Minami H, Werner YB, Pace A, Kersten JF, et al. Peroral endoscopic myotomy for the treatment of achalasia: a prospective single center study. Am J Gastroenterol. 2012;107(3):411–7.

92. Saxena P, Chavez YH, Kord Valeshabad A, Kalloo AN, Khashab MA. An alternative method for mucosal flap closure during peroral endoscopic myotomy

using an over-the-scope clipping device. Endoscopy. 2013;45(07):579–81.

93. Faigel DO, Kadish SL, Ginsberg GG. The difficult-to-place feeding tube: successful endoscopic placement using a mucosal clip. J Parenter Enter Nutr. 1996;20(4):306–8.

94. Frizzell E, Darwin P. Endoscopic placement of jejunal feeding tubes by using the resolution clip: report of 2 cases. Gastrointest Endosc. 2006;64(3):454–6.

95. Schrijver AM, Siersema PD, Vleggaar FP, Hirdes MMC, Monkelbaan JF. Endoclips for fixation of nasoenteral feeding tubes: a review. Dig Liver Dis. 2011;43(10):757–61.

96. Vanbiervliet G, Filippi J, Karimdjee BS, Venissac N, Iannelli A, Rahili A, et al. The role of clips in preventing migration of fully covered metallic esophageal stents: a pilot comparative study. Surg Endosc. 2012;26(1):53–9.

97. Sriram PV, Das G, Rao GV, Reddy DN. Another novel use of endoscopic clipping: to anchor an esophageal endoprosthesis. Endoscopy. 2001;33(8):724–6.

98. Kim ID, Kang DH, Choi CW, Kim HW, Jung WJ, Lee DH, et al. Prevention of covered enteral stent migration in patients with malignant gastric outlet obstruction: a pilot study of anchoring with endoscopic clips. Scand J Gastroenterol. 2010;45(1):100–5.

99. Chryssostalis A, Rosa I, Pileire G, Ozenne V, Chousterman M, Hagège H. Closure of refractory gastrocutaneous fistula using endoclipping. Endoscopy. 2005;37(09):924.

100. Thurairajah P, Hawthorne AB. Endoscopic clipping of a nonhealing gastrocutaneous fistula following gastrostomy removal. Endoscopy. 2004;36(09):834.

101. Turner JK, Hurley JJ, Ketchell I, Dolwani S. Over-the-scope clip to close a fistula after removing a percutaneous endoscopic gastrostomy tube. Endoscopy. 2010;42(S 02):E197–E8.

102. Magalhães RK, Barrias S, Rolanda C, Salgado M, Magalhães MJ, Simões V, et al. Successful endoscopic closure of gastrocutaneous fistula using an over-the-scope clip. Can J Gastroenterol Hepatol. 2014;28(5):238.

103. Singhal S, Changela K, Culliford A, Duddempudi S, Krishnaiah M, Anand S. Endoscopic closure of persistent gastrocutaneous fistulae, after percutaneous endoscopic gastrostomy (PEG) tube placement, using the over-the-scope-clip system. Ther Adv Gastroenterol. 2015;8(4):182–8.

104. Gölder S, Strotzer M, Grüne S, Zülke C, Schölmerich J, Messmann H. Combination of colonoscopy and clip application with angiography to mark vascular malformation in the small intestine. Endoscopy. 2003;35(06):551.

105. Hachisu T, Miyazaki S-I, Hamaguchi K-I. Endoscopic clip-marking of lesions using the newly developed HX-3L clip. Surg Endosc. 1989;3(3):142–7.

106. Qadeer MA, Dumot JA, Vargo JJ, Lopez AR, Rice TW. Endoscopic clips for closing esophageal perforations: case report and pooled analysis. Gastrointest Endosc. 2007;66(3):605–11.

107. Shimoda R, Iwakiri R, Sakata H, Ogata S, Kikkawa A, Ootani H, et al. Evaluation of endoscopic hemostasis with metallic hemoclips for bleeding gastric ulcer: comparison with endoscopic injection of absolute ethanol in a prospective, randomized study. Am J Gastroenterol. 2003;98(10):2198–202.

108. von Renteln D, Schmidt A, Vassiliou MC, Rudolph H-U, Caca K. Endoscopic full-thickness resection and defect closure in the colon. Gastrointest Endosc. 2010;71(7):1267–73.

109. Fahndrich M, Sandmann M. Endoscopic full-thickness resection for gastrointestinal lesions using the over-the-scope clip system: a case series. Endoscopy. 2015;47(1):76–9.

110. Schmidt A, Bauerfeind P, Gubler C, Damm M, Bauder M, Caca K. Endoscopic full-thickness resection in the colorectum with a novel over-the-scope device: first experience. Endoscopy. 2015;47(8):719–25.

111. Martin TR, Onstad GR, Silvis SE. Endoscopic control of massive upper gastrointestinal bleeding with a tissue adhesive (MBR 4197). Gastrointest Endosc. 1977;24(2):74–6.

112. Gilbert DA, Protell RL, Silverstein FE, Auth DC. Endoscopic treatment of nonvariceal upper gastrointestinal bleeding. J Clin Gastroenterol. 1980;2(2):139–44.

113. Protell RL, Silverstein FE, Gulacsik C, Martin TR, Dennis MB, Auth DC, et al. Failure of cyanoacrylate tissue glue (Flucrylate, MBR4197) to stop bleeding from experimental canine gastric ulcers. Am J Dig Dis. 1978;23(10):903–8.

114. Linscheer WG, Fazio TL. Control of upper gastrointestinal hemorrhage by endoscopic spraying of clotting factors. Gastroenterology. 1979;77(4):642–6.

115. Gotlib J, Demma I, Fonsecca A, Habib N, Houssin D, Bismuth H. Resultats a 1 an du traitement endoscopique electif des hemorragies par rupture de varices oesophagiennes chez le cirrhotique. Gastroenterol Clin Biol. 1984;8:133.

116. Kitano S, Hashizume M, Yamaga H, Wada H, Iso Y, Iwanaga T, et al. Human thrombin plus 5 per cent ethanolamine oleate injected to sclerose oesophageal varices: a prospective randomized trial. Br J Surg. 1989;76(7):715–8.

117. Snobl J, Van Buuren H, Van Blankenstein M. Endoscopic injection using thrombin: an effective and safe method for controlling oesophagogastric variceal bleeding. Gastroenterology. 1992;102:A891.

118. Yoshida T, Adachi K, Tanioka Y, Sasaki T, Ono S, Hanada H, et al. Dieulafoy's lesion of the esophagus correctly diagnosed and successfully treated by the endoscopic injection of N-butyl-2-cyanoacrylate. Endoscopy. 2004;36(02):183–5.

119. Rosa A, Sequeira C, Nunes A, Gregório C, Leite J, Leitão M, et al. Histoacryl in the endoscopic

treatment of severe arterial tumor bleeding. Endoscopy. 2000;32(12):S69-S.

120. Venezia P. Drug targets in colonoscopic polypectomy: biological sealants with special reference to fibrin-glue (tissucol). Curr Drug Targets Immune Endocr Metabol Disord. 2005;5(3):339–45.

121. Hwang TL, Chen MF. Randomized trial of fibrin tissue glue for low output enterocutaneous fistula. Br J Surg. 1996;83(1):112.

122. Milkes DE, Friedland S, Lin OS, Reid TR, Soetikno RM. A novel method to control severe upper GI bleeding from metastatic cancer with a hemostatic sealant: the CoStasis surgical hemostat. Gastrointest Endosc. 2002;55(6):735–40.

123. Seewald S, Sriram PVJ, Naga M, Fennerty MB, Boyer J, Oberti F, et al. Cyanoacrylate glue in gastric variceal bleeding. Endoscopy. 2002;34(11):926–32.

124. Bhat YM, Banerjee S, Barth BA, Chauhan SS, Gottlieb KT, Konda V, et al. Tissue adhesives: cyanoacrylate glue and fibrin sealant. Gastrointest Endosc. 2013;78(2):209–15.

125. Bhat YM. Tissue adhesives for endoscopic use. Gastroenterol Hepatol. 2014;10(4):251–3.

126. Carbonell N, Pauwels A, Serfaty L, Fourdan O, Lévy VG, Poupon R. Improved survival after variceal bleeding in patients with cirrhosis over the past two decades. Hepatology. 2004;40(3):652–9.

127. Tan PC, Hou MC, Lin HC, Liu TT, Lee FY, Chang FY, et al. A randomized trial of endoscopic treatment of acute gastric variceal hemorrhage: N-butyl-2-cyanoacrylate injection versus band ligation. Hepatology. 2006;43(4):690–7.

128. Sarin SK, Jain AK, Jain M, Gupta R. A randomized controlled trial of cyanoacrylate versus alcohol injection in patients with isolated fundic varices. Am J Gastroenterol. 2002;97(4):1010–5.

129. Lo GH, Lai KH, Cheng JS, Chen MH, Chiang HT. A prospective, randomized trial of butyl cyanoacrylate injection versus band ligation in the management of bleeding gastric varices. Hepatology. 2001;33(5):1060–4.

130. Tan P-C, Hou M-C, Lin H-C, Liu T-T, Lee F-Y, Chang F-Y, et al. A randomized trial of endoscopic treatment of acute gastric variceal hemorrhage: N-Butyl-2-Cyanoacrylate injection versus band ligation. Hepatology. 2006;43(4):690–7.

131. Heneghan MA, Byrne A, Harrison PM. An open pilot study of the effects of a human fibrin glue for endoscopic treatment of patients with acute bleeding from gastric varices. Gastrointest Endosc. 2002;56(3):422–6.

132. Datta D, Vlavianos P, Alisa A, Westaby D. Use of fibrin glue (beriplast) in the management of bleeding gastric varices. Endoscopy. 2003;35(8):675–8.

133. Yang WL, Tripathi D, Therapondos G, Todd A, Hayes PC. Endoscopic use of human thrombin in bleeding gastric varices. Am J Gastroenterol. 2002;97(6):1381–5.

134. Mishra SR, Sharma BC, Kumar A, Sarin SK. Primary prophylaxis of gastric variceal bleeding comparing cyanoacrylate injection and beta-blockers: a randomized controlled trial. J Hepatol. 2011;54(6):1161–7.

135. Mishra SR, Chander Sharma B, Kumar A, Sarin SK. Endoscopic cyanoacrylate injection versus beta-blocker for secondary prophylaxis of gastric variceal bleed: a randomised controlled trial. Gut. 2010;59(6):729–35.

136. Gotlib J-P. Endoscopic obturation of esophageal and gastric varices with a cyanoacrylic tissue adhesive. Can J Gastroenterol. 1990;4(9):637–38.

137. Cipolletta L, Zambelli A, Bianco MA, De Grazia F, Meucci C, Lupinacci G, et al. Acrylate glue injection for acutely bleeding oesophageal varices: a prospective cohort study. Dig Liver Dis. 2009;41(10):729–34.

138. Hernández Mondragón OV, Blancas Valencia JM, Blanco-Velasco G, Gonzalez Martinez MA, Solorzano Pineda OM, Hernandez Reyes ML. Tu1253 safety and efficacy of cyanoacrylate for the closure of the entry site during poem procedure. Gastrointest Endosc. 2017;85(5):AB602.

139. Hernández-Mondragón OV, Solórzano-Pineda OM, Blanco-Velasco G, Blancas-Valencia JM. Use of cyanoacrylate to treat mucosal perforations during or after peroral endoscopic myotomy. Endoscopy. 2016;48(S 01):E330-E1.

140. Khashab MA, El Zein M, Kumbhari V, Besharati S, Ngamruengphong S, Messallam A, et al. Comprehensive analysis of efficacy and safety of peroral endoscopic myotomy performed by a gastroenterologist in the endoscopy unit: a single-center experience. Gastrointest Endosc. 2016;83(1):117–25.

141. Avalos-Gonzalez J, Portilla-deBuen E, Leal-Cortes CA, Orozco-Mosqueda A, Estrada-Aguilar Mdel C, Velazquez-Ramirez GA, et al. Reduction of the closure time of postoperative enterocutaneous fistulas with fibrin sealant. World J Gastroenterol. 2010;16(22):2793–800.

142. Papavramidis TS, Kotzampassi K, Kotidis E, Eleftheriadis EE, Papavramidis ST. Endoscopic fibrin sealing of gastrocutaneous fistulas after sleeve gastrectomy and biliopancreatic diversion with duodenal switch. J Gastroenterol Hepatol. 2008;23(12):1802–5.

143. Rabago LR, Ventosa N, Castro JL, Marco J, Herrera N, Gea F. Endoscopic treatment of postoperative fistulas resistant to conservative management using biological fibrin glue. Endoscopy. 2002;34(8):632–8.

144. Lippert E, Klebl FH, Schweller F, Ott C, Gelbmann CM, Schölmerich J, et al. Fibrin glue in the endoscopic treatment of fistulae and anastomotic leakages of the gastrointestinal tract. Int J Color Dis. 2011;26(3):303–11.

145. Lippert E, Klebl FH, Schweller F, Ott C, Gelbmann CM, Scholmerich J, et al. Fibrin glue in the endoscopic treatment of fistulae and anastomotic leakages of the gastrointestinal tract. Int J Color Dis. 2011;26(3):303–11.

146. Lee YC, Na HG, Suh JH, Park IS, Chung KY, Kim NK. Three cases of fistulae arising from gastrointestinal tract treated with endoscopic injection of Histoacryl. Endoscopy. 2001;33(2):184–6.
147. Murakami M, Tono T, Okada K, Yano H, Monden T. Fibrin glue injection method with diluted thrombin for refractory postoperative digestive fistula. Am J Surg. 2009;198(5):715–9.
148. Shim CS, Cho YD, Kim JO, Bong HK, Kim YS, Lee JS, et al. A case of portal and splenic vein thrombosis after histoacryl injection therapy in gastric varices. Endoscopy. 1996;28(05):461.
149. See A, Florent C, Lamy P, Levy VG, Bouvry M. Cerebrovascular accidents after endoscopic obturation of esophageal varices with isobutyl-2-cyanoacrylate in 2 patients. Gastroenterol Clin Biol. 1986;10(8–9):604–7.
150. Hwang SS, Kim HH, Park SH, Kim SE, Jung JI, Ahn BY, et al. N-butyl-2-cyanoacrylate pulmonary embolism after endoscopic injection sclerotherapy for gastric variceal bleeding. J Comput Assist Tomogr. 2001;25(1):16–22.
151. Lee GH, Kim JH, Lee KJ, Yoo BM, Hahm KB, Cho SW, et al. Life-threatening intraabdominal arterial embolization after histoacryl injection for bleeding gastric ulcer. Endoscopy. 2000;32(5):422–4.
152. Jutabha R, Jensen DM, Egan J, Machicado GA, Hirabayashi K. Randomized, prospective study of cyanoacrylate injection, sclerotherapy, or rubber band ligation for endoscopic hemostasis of bleeding canine gastric varices. Gastrointest Endosc. 1995;41(3):201–5.

Vinay Dhir, Ankit Dalal, and Carmen Chu

Introduction

There has been a steady expansion in the indications of therapeutic EUS for pancreatic disorders over the past decade. This is supplemented by the evolution of EUS-specific accessories and stents. While PFC drainage remains the predominant indication for therapeutic EUS worldwide, a number of other procedures are under evaluation for ductal drainage, tumor therapy, or cancer pain relief. This chapter provides an overview of the current utilization of therapeutic EUS for pancreatic disorders.

Endoscopic-Ultrasound-Guided Peripancreatic Fluid Collection Drainage

Pancreatic fluid collections (PFCs) may occur as a result of acute or chronic pancreatitis, surgery, trauma, or neoplasia. These collections form as a consequence of either a disruption of the pancreatic duct or maturation of pancreatic necrosis. A pancreatic pseudocyst is defined as an encapsulated collection of fluid with a well-defined inflammatory wall usually outside the pancreas with minimal or no necrosis. This usually occurs more than 4 weeks after the onset of interstitial edematous pancreatitis. A walled-off pancreatic necrosis (WON) is a mature, encapsulated collection of pancreatic and/or peripancreatic necrosis that has developed a well-defined inflammatory wall. WON usually occurs more than 4 weeks after onset of necrotizing pancreatitis [1].

Acute PFCs generally do not warrant any intervention. They lack a well-defined wall, and undergo spontaneous regression within a few weeks after the onset of acute pancreatitis. Indications of drainage of a PFC include symptomatic pseudocysts causing pain, PFC causing mechanical obstruction of the gastric outlet or biliary system, and infected pseudocysts. Drainage is also indicated if the pseudocyst continues to increase in size without resolution

V. Dhir (✉) · C. Chu
Division of Pancreatic-biliary Endoscopy,
Institute of Digestive and Liver Care, SL Raheja Hospital,
Mumbai, India

A. Dalal
Division of Pancreatic-biliary Endoscopy,
Institute of Digestive and Liver Care,
SL Raheja Hospital, Mumbai, India

Division of Gastroenterology,
Baldota Institute of Digestive Sciences, Mumbai,
India

© Springer Nature Switzerland AG 2020
M. S. Wagh, S. B. Wani (eds.), *Gastrointestinal Interventional Endoscopy*,
https://doi.org/10.1007/978-3-030-21695-5_27

after 6 weeks. This is to avoid subsequent development of complications such as hemorrhage, perforation, or secondary infection.

The current therapeutic options include surgery, endoscopy, and percutaneous drainage. The advantages of endoscopic ultrasound (EUS)-guided drainage include the following: (1) it is minimally invasive; (2) it avoids local complications related to percutaneous drainage; and (3) it enables real-time visualization of PFCs and a decreased bleeding rate by avoiding the interposing blood vessels with the use of Doppler ultrasound [2, 3].

Prerequisites

Prior to EUS-guided PFC drainage, certain prerequisites are needed, which include (1) presence of a well-defined mature wall, (2) for pseudocysts, a timeframe of 4–6 weeks, (3) the fluid collection must be accessible endoscopically, such as being located within 1 cm of the duodenal or gastric walls, (4) paracolic collections cannot be accessed and would require adjunctive methods such as percutaneous drainage, and (5) correction of coagulopathy, if any [2].

Technique

Accessories for the procedure include the following:

1. Therapeutic linear echoendoscope with a working channel 3.7 or 3.8 mm
2. 19-G fine-needle aspiration (FNA) needle (lumen of the 22-G needle does not permit a 0.035-inch guidewire)
3. 0.025- or 0.035-inch guidewires
4. 4.5- or 5-Fr ERCP cannula or Soehendra dilators or an over-the-wire needle-knife catheter or cystotome catheter
5. Over-the-wire biliary balloon dilator
6. 7-, 8-, 8.5-, or 10-Fr double-pigtail plastic stents.
7. Self Expanding Metal Stents - AXIOS, (Xlumena Inc, Mountain View, California, USA), NAGI (Taewoong-Medical Co, Seoul, South Korea) (Fig. 27.1)

Stents for PFC Drainage: Plastic and SEMS

Double pigtail plastic stents (7F, 8.5F, and 10F) are traditionally used for PFC drainage. Single or multiple plastic stents can be placed during the procedure. Recently, SEMS specially designed for PFC drainage have been developed [4, 5]. The lumen-apposing stent (AXIOS, Xlumena Inc., Mountain View, California, USA) is a fully covered, 10-mm diameter, nitinol, braided stent with bilateral anchor flanges. When fully expanded, the flange diameter is twice that of the "saddle" section and is designed to hold tissue layers in apposition [4]. The stent is delivered constrained through a 10.5-Fr catheter that is inserted over the guidewire within the pseudocyst cavity. The "NAGI"-covered SEMS (Taewoong-Medical Co, Seoul, South Korea) is another specially designed SEMS with a 10-mm diameter in the center and 20-mm ends that can reduce the risk of migration [5]. The potential advantage of SEMS is a larger drainage orifice and the possibility of facilitating repeat entry into the cavity for endoscopic necrosectomy in the context of infected walled-off necrosis. Its potential utility is probably limited to the management of infected walled-off necrosis [6] (Fig. 27.2, Table 27.1).

Technical and Clinical Outcomes

EUS-guided PFC drainage has shown a technical success rate of more than 90% and a clinical success rate of 75–90% [7]. Depending on the type of collection, the treatment outcomes can vary. A recent study reported a treatment success rate of 93.5% for pseudocysts, but only 63.2% for WON with plastic stents [8]. This may be due to the small diameter of PS and the presence of solid debris in WON that is more difficult to drain through the fistula tract.

Consequently, straight biliary FcSEMS have been tried in patients with PFCs given theoretical advantages of improved drainage due to larger stent caliber. A study assessed the efficacy of these metal stents for pseudocyst drainage and the overall treatment success was excellent (85–95%) [6].

A randomized study failed to demonstrate superiority of FcSEMS over PS for pseudocyst

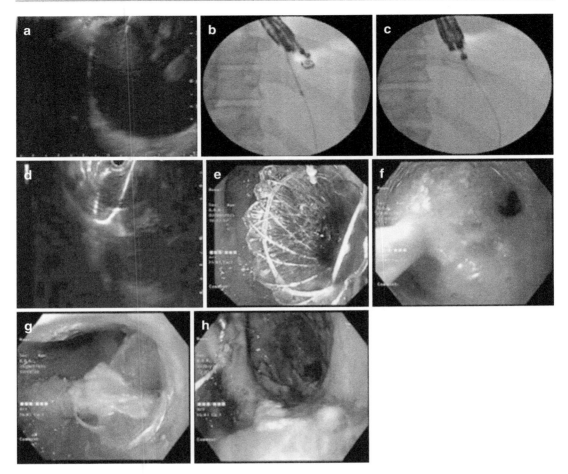

Fig. 27.1 Steps of EUS-guided PFC drainage and necrosectomy. (**a**) Needle puncture; (**b**) Track dilation with 6F cystotome. (**c**) CRE Balloon dilation till 8 mm; (**d**) Deployment of Nagi stent distal end; (**e**) Final deployment, endoscopic view; F) Necrotic debris blocking the stent; (**g**) Necrosectomy; (**h**) Clean cyst cavity after 4 sessions

drainage (clinical success 87% vs. 91%, $p = 0.97$) [9]. The only advantage of FcSEMS was shorter procedure time (15 min vs. 29.5 min).This was further confirmed in a meta-analysis that found no difference in overall treatment success rates between patients with pseudocysts treated with PS or with metal stents (85% vs. 83%, respectively) [10].

On the other hand, FcSEMS do seem to have superior rates of treatment success compared to PS when used to drain WON [11]. But the straight FCSEMS are prone to migration. Hence, LAMS with a unique "dumbbell" design that bring the walls of the lumen and the PFC close together were introduced. The early reported data have been impressive, with overall technical success rates exceeding 90% and clinical success rates of 85–91%, with many patients achieving complete resolution of WON without the need for DEN. Complications have been observed in 10–15% of patients, while very few patients have gone on to require surgery [12, 13]. Furthermore, migration of LAMS occurred in only 5% of patients,29 and their insertion required significantly shorter procedure times when compared to PS (25 min vs. 43 min, $p = 0.01$) [14]. A recent study found superior resolution rates of WON at 6-month follow-up when drainage had been performed with metal stents (both straight FcSEMS and LAMS) than with PS [12]. However, to date, no significant difference in efficacy has been shown between straight FcSEMS and the new LAMS, with long-term success rates of 95% vs. 90%, respectively [15].

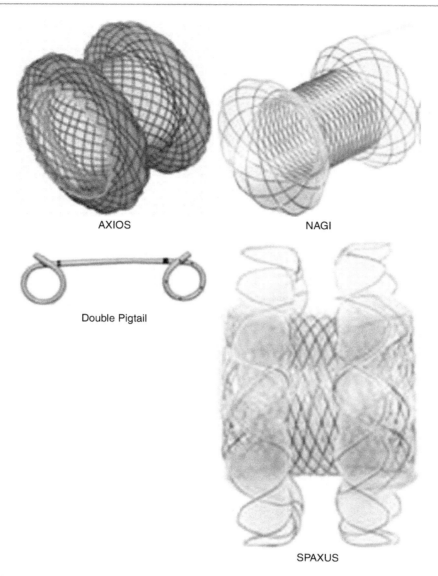

AXIOS   NAGI

Double Pigtail

SPAXUS

Fig. 27.2 Stents for PFC drainage

As with plastic stents, treatment outcomes for pancreatic pseudocysts and WON with LAMS also differ. A recent study evaluated the outcomes of PFC drainage with LAMS. It found that endoscopic therapy by using the LAMS was successful in 12 out of 12 patients (100%), with pancreatic pseudocysts compared with 60 of 68 patients (88.2%) with WON [16].

Two randomized trials that compared EUS-guided PPC drainage and conventional endoscopy-guided PPC drainage demonstrated that EUS-guided transmural approach is superior to conventional endoscopy-guided drainage in terms of technical success and complications [17, 18]. Several observational studies have investigated the efficacy of EUS-guided drainage of pseudocysts and abscesses. They all resulted in high technical and clinical success rates, ranging from 89% to 100% and 82% to 100%, respectively [19–21]. Ng et al [22] recently demonstrated that, although EUS-guided drainage of pseudocysts was technically successful in 93% of patients, the treatment success rate was 75% and the complication rate was

Table 27.1 Stents for PFC drainage: advantages and disadvantages

Stent type	Diameter	Advantage	Disadvantage
Double-pigtail plastic stent	7–10 Fr	Low risk of migration Easy to remove Inexpensive	More difficult to deploy Small diameter (increased risk of occlusion and secondary infection)
Straight biliary FcSEMS	6–10 mm	Easy to deploy Large diameter Ability to perform DEN through stent	Stent migration Possible increased risk of delayed bleeding Cost
LAMS AXIOSTM (Boston Scientific, Marlborough, MA, USA) NAGITM (Taewoong Medical, Gimpo, Korea) SPAXUSTM (Taewoong Medical, Gimpo, Korea) Aixstent® PPS (Leufen Medical, Berlin, Germany)	10,15 mm 10–16 mm 8,10,16 mm 10,14 mm	Easy to deploy Ability to deploy without need for wire exchange (AXIOS) Large diameter Ability to perform DEN through stent Lower risk of migration Reduced need for nasocystic drain Reduce need for fluoroscopy	Cost Lack of long-term safety

5%. Varadarajulu et al [18], in a comparison of the efficacy of EUS-guided and non-EUS-guided pseudocyst drainage, found that the technical success rate was 100% with EUS, but only 33% with the non-EUS-based approach. A recent randomized, controlled trial of EUS-guided versus surgical cystogastrostomy for pseudocyst drainage determined that there were no differences in terms of treatment success rate, complications, or recurrence, but there was a significantly shorter hospital stay (median, 2 d vs 6 d; $p < 0.001$) and lower costs in the endoscopic group [23]. An earlier randomized study by the same group yielded similar conclusions [24]. Therefore, the endoscopic approaches seem to be the preferred method for drainage of PFCs.

Adverse Events

A number of adverse events may occur when performing endoscopic management of PFCs including bleeding, perforation, secondary infection, and stent migration. The use of EUS may help to reduce the risk of bleeding by visualizing any intervening vessels. One prospective study reported a 13% rate of bleeding with conventional endoscopic drainage compared to no bleeding with EUS-guided interventions [18]. However, even with EUS guidance, bleeding remains an important adverse event, particularly

when metal stents are used [12]. Stent migration is a well-described complication for both PS and FcSEMS, which can occur externally into the GI tract or internally into the PFC. The risk of stent migration is in the range: 1–15% [8, 25]. Internal migration of a stent into the PFC cavity can result in bleeding if the stent erodes into a large blood vessel. Infection of PFCs after endoscopic intervention can occur in up to 20% of cases, often resulting in need for DEN or even surgical intervention. Indeed, a recent retrospective study showed a higher rate of adverse events with PS compared to FcSEMS (31% vs. 16%, $p = 0.006$), predominantly due to secondary infection that occurs when the stents become blocked and/or the drainage tract closes [26]. As a result, patients with PS were 2.9 times more likely to experience an adverse event compared to those with FcSEMS (odds ratio, 2.9; 95% confidence interval, 1.4–6.3) on multivariable analysis.

Duration of Stenting

Duration of stenting is an important, yet unresolved issue. PFCs have been shown to recur in 10–38% of patients [27, 28]. There are no data to confirm the long-term safety of leaving these stents in place. Prolonged stent placement (using PSs) was shown to be superior to protocolized stent removal by a prospective trial that randomized 28 patients to removal of the stents 2 weeks after PFC resolution or to keeping them in place. At 14 months, the recurrence rate was 38% in the stent-removal group compared to no recurrence in the long-term stent group, with no complications experienced by patients with prolonged stenting [28]. However, the patients who should benefit from prolonged transluminal stenting are those with a viable body or tail of the pancreas with a disrupted PD. In this "disconnected pancreatic duct syndrome (DPDS)," pancreatic secretions from the disconnected body and/or tail leak from the disrupted PD, resulting in persistence or recurrence of a pseudocyst. Long-term plastic stent has been demonstrated by multiple centers to be a safe and an effective solution in more than 90% of patients with DPDS [29–31]. A significant consideration when deciding upon the duration of transluminal stent placement is whether double pigtail PSs or a metal stent are in place. There are concerns about increased risks of delayed bleeding from a collapsed WON collection when a metal stent is in place, which is why stent removal is advised after the PFC resolves if an FcSEMS is in place, except for cases of DPDS.

Role of DEN

DEN consists of debridement of WON using a gastroscope that is inserted directly into the collection via the stomach or duodenum through the cystogastrostomy or cystoduodenostomy fistula tract. The tract is dilated to enable passage of the endoscope and then the necrotic debris is slowly removed from the WON and pulled back into the lumen using a variety of endoscopic tools.

The GEPARD trial evaluated outcomes with DEN [32]. It was a multicenter study of 93 patients with WON who underwent transluminal endoscopic debridement of peripancreatic and pancreatic necrosis, achieving an 80% success rate. Despite these encouraging results, complications were common, occurring in 26% of patients, with 7.5% mortality. Similar outcomes have been observed in subsequent studies

[33, 34] A recent meta-analysis found pooled rates of treatment success, adverse events, and mortality of 81%, 35%, and 6%, respectively [35] Reported adverse events include perforation, air embolism, and bleeding, which occurs in 3–21% of patients [32–35]. Therefore, despite the fact that DEN may contribute to accelerated patient recovery and clinical resolution of infected WON, the morbidity and mortality associated with the procedure should limit its use to circumstances in which patients have failed to improve after appropriate transluminal drainage, with a target treatment endpoint of clinical resolution of significant symptoms, not radiological resolution.

Conclusion

EUS-guided intervention is an important component of the treatment of PFCs and currently is the first-line approach for most patients. Recent advances have significantly improved the efficacy and safety of endoscopic PFC drainage procedures. The endoscopic management of pseudocysts has high rates of success regardless of what type of stent is used. On the other hand, WON remains a therapeutic challenge that poses significant morbidity and mortality. In these cases, EUS-guided placement of an FcSEMS, and in particular an LAMS, may provide clinical benefit over the use of double pigtail PSs.

EUS-Guided Pancreatic Duct Drainage

Introduction

Endoscopic retrograde pancreatography (ERP) is considered the first-line, standard treatment for treating main pancreatic duct (MPD) obstruction, stricture, or disruption. Endoscopic-ultrasound-guided pancreatic duct intervention (EUS-PDI) allows access and intervention to the MPD for patients with failed ERP or with surgically altered anatomy. It is technically demanding with a high risk for complications, but can serve as an alternative to surgical treatment. Proper patient selection is important, and indication and relative contraindications must be carefully assessed.

Indications

1. MPD hypertension due to PD stricture or stones in the MPD or IPMN
2. MPD disruption
3. Stenosis of the pancreatico-jejunal anastomosis
4. Failed ERCP

Contraindications

1. Unable to visualize PD on EUS
2. Multifocal PD stricture
3. Intervening blood vessels
4. Thrombocytopenia or coagulopathy

Technique

EUS-PDI can be divided into two main approaches: EUS-guided antegrade drainage and EUS-guided rendezvous technique.

EUS-Guided Antegrade Drainage

EUS-guided antegrade drainage is performed by accessing the MPD under EUS-guided puncture and creating a tract with subsequent antegrade placement of a stent across the pancreatic-gastric anastomosis, pancreatic-duodenal anastomosis, MPD stricture, papilla, or pancreatico-jejunal anastomosis (PJA) [36].

This approach can be subdivided into transluminal, transpapillary, or trans-anastomotic based on whether the stent traverses the site of ductal obstruction, papilla, or anastomosis.

EUS-Guided Rendezvous Technique

EUS-guided rendezvous achieves transpapillary or trans-anastomotic drainage using a rendezvous technique. This is achieved by retrograde stent placement from the papilla or anastomosis into the MPD via another endoscope. This procedure requires access to the papilla or anastomosis that has been traversed with a guidewire [37, 38].

EUS-PDI Procedure

The MPD is visualized and carefully assessed with a linear echoendoscope. Under combined fluoroscopic and EUS guidance, access into the MPD through the stomach or duodenum is achieved using a 19-gauge needle. Subsequentl, y a pancreatogram is performed and a guidewire can be passed into the MPD.

The rendezvous technique is performed after the guidewire is advanced across the papilla or anastomosis and coiled in the small intestine. The echoendoscope is removed leaving the guidewire in place. Depending on the anatomy, a standard therapeutic duodenoscope, colonoscope, or balloon-assisted enteroscope is then advanced to the papilla or the anastomosis, where the PD can be accessed with the guidance of the EUS placed wire to perform retrograde interventions.

For antegrade PD drainage, the echoendoscope is used throughout the procedure for placement of a stent into the MPD via the stomach or the duodenum. Once guidewire access is achieved into the MPD, dilation of the transmural tract is performed using tapered catheters, dilators, cystotomes or balloons. After tract dilatation, the stent can be deployed.

Outcomes

Although there are several studies reporting outcomes using EUS-PDI, overall the data are quite limited.

A systematic review of studies that focused only on EUS-guided PD access identified 222 patients who underwent EUS-PDI and demonstrated a 77% rate of technical success with a clinical success rate of 70% using either the antegrade or rendezvous technique. Adverse events developed in 19% of the patients, and included abdominal pain (7.7%), pancreatitis (3.1%), bleeding (1.8%), perforation (0.9%), peripancreatic abscess (0.9%), stripping of the guidewire coating (0.9%), and one patient each who developed fever, pneumoperitoneum, pseudocyst, pseudocyst with an aneurysm, and perigastric fluid collection (0.5%) [39].

An international, multicenter, retrospective study on the safety and efficacy of EUS-PDI after failed ERP showed a technical success rate of 89% and clinical success rate of 81%. The trans-papillary or trans-anastomotic approaches to stent placement via rendezvous wire access seemed to be the more successful technique. There was an increased likelihood of complete symptom resolution with the rendezvous technique but was not statistically significant. Immediate adverse events (AEs) (<24 hours) occurred in 20% of patients, with 15% experiencing major complications (6 patients with post-ERCP pancreatitis, 4 who developed pancreatic fluid collections, one with a MPD leak, and one with an intestinal perforation. Delayed AEs (>24 hours) occurred in 11% of patients (all of whom also had immediate AEs—2 pancreatitis, 1 MPD leak, and 4 abscesses treated with antibiotics). The method of approach (antegrade vs. rendezvous) was not a predictor of immediate or delayed AE [40].

A recent international, multicenter, retrospective study was performed to compare EUS PDI and ERP in terms of technical success, clinical success, and adverse event rates in patients with post-Whipple anatomy. A total of 66 patients underwent 75 procedures (40 EUS-PDI and 35 ERP). Technical success of EUS-PDI was 92.5% compared with 20% in the ERP group (odds ratio [OR], 49.3; $p < 0.001$). Clinical success was achieved in 87.5% of EUS-PDI procedures compared with 23.1% in the ERP group (OR, 23.3; $p < 0.001$). However, adverse events occurred more commonly in the EUS-PDI group (35% vs. 2.9%, $p < 0.001$) [41].

Potential contributing factors of treatment failure include small PD diameter, fibrotic pancreatic parenchyma, short length for guidewire insertion, lack of dedicated devices, lack of technical standard, and failure to navigate the guidewire through the site of obstruction, across the papilla or PJA [42].

It is difficult to determine the need for reintervention and to predict long-term clinical outcomes after initial successful intervention. Will et al. reported that 29% of patients having EUS-PDI ultimately required surgical intervention during a follow-up period of 4 weeks to 3 years [43].

Conclusions

Although the technical and clinical success rates of EUS-PDI are improving, it remains a challenging procedure with a high risk of adverse events. Considering the major limitations in alternative treatment options after failed ERP, EUS-PDI has the potential to become standard-of-care by avoiding more invasive and involved surgical interventions.

EUS Guided Pancreatic Cancer Therapy

Introduction

The availability of real-time assessment of anatomical details, precise needle advancement coupled with Doppler ultrasonography to avoid major vasculature has led EUS to leap from a diagnostic to the unparalleled era of therapeutic interventions. In recent years, EUS guided antitumor therapy has emerged as an exciting realm and has undergone various phases of experimentation in terms of its feasibility, safety, and efficacy. It can be broadly classified into direct and indirect methods. Direct methods include EUS-guided radio-frequency ablation, ethanol injection, photodynamic therapy, and brachytherapy. Indirect methods include EUS guide fine needle injection (FNI), fiducial placement. In indirect methods, EUS-guided intervention would allow determination of precise anatomical location, which is followed by a second process that has antitumor effects, for example, locally acting chemotherapeutic agents or external beam-guided stereotactic irradiation.

To date, majority of the above EUS-guided antitumor therapy has been targeting on pancreatic tumors. Adenocarcinoma of the pancreas carries a dismal prognosis, its deep seated anatomical location, aggressive tumor biology, and significant peritumoral desmoplastic reaction often entails suboptimal response to systemic chemotherapeutic agents, with an overall <7% survival despite optimal therapy. On the other end of the spectrum, the prevalence of pancreatic cystic lesion has been increasing, owing to the increase in availability and accuracy of cross-sectional imaging. Surgical resection remained the gold standard for lesions with malignant potential; however, curative resection is accompanied with significant morbidly and mortality, which might not be feasible among our aging patient population with significant comorbidities. This eloquently explained why pancreas has been the organ of interest in majority of the EUS-guided therapeutic interventions. Various direct and indirect EUS-guided therapeutic interventions have been attempted in both solid and cystic pancreatic tumors.

Treatment of Solid Pancreatic Tumor

EUS Guided Radio-Frequency Ablation (RFA)

The efficacy of radio-frequency ablation (RFA) is well established in the treatment of primary or metastatic liver tumors. It achieves the tumor-ablative effect by converting electromagnetic energy into thermal energy, inducing coagulative necrosis in the target tissue. Established method of delivery includes the following: percutaneous route under image guidance and operative approaches for deep-seated lesions have been widely used in treatment of hepatocellular carcinoma or liver secondaries; endoluminal approach has been used for inoperable cholangiocarcinoma. To date, four different types of EUS RFA probes are available for pancreatic tumors [44]: monopolar RF probes including the 19G EUS-FNA needle electrode (Radionics, Inc., Burlington, MA, USA), EUSRA RF electrode (STAR med, Koyang, Korea) and Habib™ (EMcision, London, UK). In monopolar RFA devices, a closed circuit is established between the RFA generator, the RFA needle, and the ground pad on the patient. Hybrid cryotherm probe (Hybrid-Therm; ERBE, Germany) is a bipolar RF probe coupled with internal cooling system. Energy flow is confined between the two electrodes of the RF probe and hence, a more focused area of heating is achieved with reduction in the associated heat sink effect. The delivery system comes either as through the needle device or the needle-type device. The needle-type device resembles an RFA needle that comes in variable caliber (14-19G); the whole device is insulated except for the tip of the needle where energy is delivered. It is recommended that the most challenging area should be ablated first in order to limit the visual artifacts that may hinder subsequent localization.

Intrinsic anatomical difference between the liver and pancreas means clinical application of RFA in pancreatic tumors is still in its infancy. Pancreas is a highly thermosensitive organ, with the lack of abundance of surrounding normal parenchyma; the close proximity to major vasculature and bile ducts entails that any thermal injury can lead to serious inflammatory consequences. In a recent review by Alvarez-Sanchez et al. [45], the current available data has been limited to a handful of small clinical series, total of 42 patients from seven published series received EUS-guided RFA for various pancreatic tumors including unresectable pancreatic cancer, PNET, IPMN and mucinous cyst, with a reported technical success rate of 86%. Favorable results were noted in a series of unresectable pancreatic tumors, with significant volume reduction in 16 out of 22 patients ($p = 0.07$), the median survival was 6 months (1–12 months). Complete ablation was reported in two patients with PNET and two had 50% reduction with vascular changes. In a case series by Lakhtakia et al. [46], three patients with insulinoma who refused operation remained asymptomatic up to 1 year after initial treatment. There was no procedure-related mortality, and most common adverse events are abdominal pain and mild pancreatitis.

Overall, current evidence suggests that EUS-guided radio-frequency ablation is safe and feasible; however, there are technical hurdles to overcome to promote its widespread use, the caliber of large bore RFA needle up to 14G may pose difficulty in penetrating pancreatic tumors with significant desmoplastic reaction, but the technique does provide an attractive option especially in patients who are not candidates to undergo pancreatic resection., We still await evidence on long-term efficacy prior to routine clinical application.

EUS-Guided Ethanol Injection

The first EUS-guided ethanol injection was done by Jürgensen C et al. [47] in 2006. A 78-year-old woman with repeated hypoglycemia was diagnosed to have insulinoma and she refused surgery. A total of 8-ml, 95% ethanol was injected into the pancreatic tumor with a 22G needle. She had a mild attack of pancreatitis, which settled with conservative treatment, but she remained symptom-free *for* up to 34 months after the procedure. Subsequent reports reported favorable results for the treatment of pancreatic neuroendocrine tumors [48]. The technique was later coupled with EUS-guided celiac plexus nerve block in the treatment of advanced pancreatic cancer. Facciorusso A et al. [49] reported a retrospective analysis of 123 patients with unresectable pancreatic tumor. Fifty-eight patients received EUS-guided CPN and 65 received the combined approach of EUS-CPN + EUS-ethanol injection. In the combined treatment group, a calculated volume of 95% ethanol equivalent to 75% of the pancreatic tumor volume was injected. The study showed that the combined treatment group had increased pain relief and complete pain response rate ($p = 0.005$ and $p = 0.003$, respectively). Moreover, there was a trend for longer median overall survival in the combined treatment group (8.3 months vs. 6.5 months, $p = 0.05$).

EUS Guided Fiducial Marker Placement

The advent of image-guided radiotherapy (IGRT) has been major advancement in the management of pancreatic cancer; the technique allows precise delivery of radiation to the target tissue with limited irradiation to the surrounding normal structures, eliminates the necessity of immobilization of the target tissue with quantification of respiratory-associated tumor motion. However, precise tumor location requires provision of several reference points. Fiducials are radiopaque coils or spheres placed into or adjacent to the tumor to guide the extent of irradiation. They are loaded into 19G needle after retracting the stylet and loaded in the tip of the needle, which is then sealed with bone wax. After tumor localization, three to four fiducially are deployed in the centre and periphery of the tumor, this can be done by pushing in the stylet or flushing with sterile water. Dhadham et al. [50] reported feasibility of fiducial deployment in 514 patients with GI malignancies; among them, 188 suffered from pancreatic cancer. Fiducials are deployed with either a 19G or 22G needle; the technical success was 99.5% and all the fiducial markers were inserted with no fluoroscopic guidance. Fiducial was not placed in one patient due to the intervening blood vessels; the overall migration rate was 0.4%, and complication was minimal.

The use of fiducial has also been investigated in preoperative localization small pancreatic neuroendocrine tumors. Law et al. [51] reported the successful localization of two patients with 7 mm and 9 mm PNET. The fiducials were identified with intraoperative ultrasound and the patients had successful parenchymal-sparing resection of the pancreatic tumor.

Treatment of Pancreatic Cystic Lesion

EUS-Guided Pancreatic Cystic Ablation

Pancreatic cystic neoplasm represents spectrum of disease entity that varies from benign to malignant lesions. The incidence of pancreatic cystic lesion increases with age and is in increasing trend owing to the improvement of cross-sectional imaging. The prevalence of pancreatic cystic lesion is estimated to be 2–16% on cross-sectional imaging. Common types of pancreatic cystic lesion include intraductal papillary neoplasm (IPMN), serous cystadenoma, and mucinous cystadenoma. Surgical resection remained the goldstandard in malignant or premalignant lesion; however, it is associated with significant morbidity and mortality.

EUS-guided ethanol ablation of pancreatic cystic lesion has first been shown to be safe and feasible by Gan et al. in 2005 [52]. A cohort of 25 patients (including 13 Mucinous Cystic neoplasm, 4 IPMN, 3 Serous cystadenoma, 3 pseudocysts, and 2 of unknown origin) with a median diameter of 19.4 mm were treated with ethanol. Cyst contents were aspirated with 22G needle, followed by ethanol injection of the volume equivalent *to* the volume of aspirate. Cyst resolution was observed in 35% of patients upon follow-up of 6–12 months. The value of EUS-guided ethanol lavage with paclitaxel injection was later investigated. Oh et al. [53] reported favorable results in a cohort of 47 patients who had pancreatic cystic lesion; upon follow-up at 12 months, pancreatic cysts disappeared in 75% of the patients.

Celiac Plexus Neurolysis

Introduction

Celiac plexus neurolysis (CPN) is the chemical ablation of the celiac ganglia and corresponding neural pathways. This is performed by injecting local anesthetic followed by absolute alcohol into the ganglia, resulting in moderate neuronal degeneration and fibrosis, hence inhibiting pain transmission from upper abdominal organs. The first percutaneous celiac plexus neurolysis was reported by Kappiset al [54] in 1914; since then, the procedure has been performed under fluoroscopic, ultrasound, and computed tomography (CT) guidance. The first endoscopic ultrasound-guided celiac plexus neurolysis (EUS-CPN) was reported in 1996 by Wiersema et al. [55] and Faigel et al. [56]; the technique has been popularized as it allows real-time, accurate assessment of the anatomical details. Safety profile of the procedure is further enhanced with the use of Doppler ultrasonography, which avoids puncturing the interposing vasculature.

The celiac plexus is the largest plexus of the sympathetic nervous system, located in the retroperitoneal space around the origin of the celiac axis and superior mesenteric artery. It comprises a dense network of ganglia with considerable variation in size (0.5–4.5 cm) and number [57]. The preganglionic sympathetic fibers of the celiac plexus constitute the greater (T5-10), lesser (T10-11), and the least (T12) splanchnic nerves, and the plexus also receives parasympathetic fibers from the celiac branch of the right vagus nerve. The left celiac plexus is located more caudally *than* its counterpart on the contralateral side. The celiac plexus innervates organs in the upper abdomen including stomach, pancreas, liver, spleen, adrenal glands, kidneys, abdominal aorta, mesentery, small bowel, and right colon.

Indication

Celiac plexus neurolysis provides an attractive adjunct in the management of intractable pain from the upper abdominal organs. Current pain management follows the stepwise approach suggested by the World Health Organisation [58], where we commence with the use of nonopioid analgesics and then gradually step up the use of opioids such as morphine. However, escalating dosage of opioid analgesics is often limited by its side effects: nausea, vomiting, constipation, drowsiness, confusion, addiction, and dependence. The use of CPN is particularly *pronounced* in the management of pancreatic cancer. The aggressive tumor biology and late manifestations entails that only 20% of the patient has resectable disease at the time of diagnosis, with a dismal 5% overall survival over 5 year. Moreover, up to 70–80% of the patients experience intractable pain over the course of the disease [57, 59]; hence, CPN becomes a promising adjunct in the course of tumor pain management.

Chronic pancreatitis is another disease entity where CPN plays an important role in pain management. Despite the benign nature of disease, the recurrent bouts of acute pancreatitis lead to progressive and irreversible destruction of pancreatic parenchyma, leading to gradual loss of endocrine and exocrine functions. The exact mechanism of pain is not understood; a postulated pathophysiological mechanism attributes to increase in pressure either within the pancreatic duct or in the pancreatic parenchyma, which leads to ischemia and the inflammation of pancreatic tissue. This process is further coupled with infiltration of neural inflammatory cells leading to alteration in the neural plasticity of the pancreas [60, 61], leading to the relentless bouts of deep, dull neuropathic pain, which is often opioid resistant.

Techniques of CPN

The two commonly used techniques for EUS CPN are, namely, the central technique and the bilateral technique. The central technique involves injection of neurolytic agent at the origin of the celiac artery. In bilateral technique, both sides of the celiac artery are injected.

Anesthetic agents, such as 0.25–0.75% bupivaciane, are usually injected prior to neurolytic agent to prevent transient exacerbation of pain. Ethanol is the most widely used neurolytic agent, while phenol could be used in patients with ethanol intolerance. It is generally considered that the transient pain exacerbation associated with ethanol injection does not occur with phenol, because it has an immediate local anesthetic effect. A retrospective case cohort by Ishiwateri et al. [62] showed no significant difference in the positive response rate (phenol 83% versus ethanol 69%) among the phenol group of six patients as compared to the ethanol group of 16 patients. Moreover, no significant difference was found in the frequencies of complication and duration of pain relief.

In central technique, the echoendoscope is advanced till the aorta is identified at the level of the diaphragm in the posterior wall of the gastric fundus; the celiac plexus was targeted at the point where the celiac artery (CA) originates from the aorta. The neurolytic agent is injected till the echogenic cloud is sufficiently widespread.

In the bilateral technique, the celiac artery is identified where it originates from the aorta, the echoendoscope is rotated clockwise until the celiac artery (CA) and superior mesenteric artery (SMA) is no longer seen, the needle is advanced to a point where SMA takes off from the aorta, half portion of the neuroleptic agent is injected, the echoendoscope is then rotated counterclockwise until both arteries are no longer seen, the needle is advanced to the right lateral base of the SMA, and the remaining portion of the agent is injected.

EUS-Guided Direct Ganglia Neurolysis (EUS-CGN)

EUS-guided direct ganglia neurolysis was first developed by Levi et al. [63] in 2008: the technique involves direct puncture of the celiac ganglion and followed by neurolytic agent injection. The ganglia usually appeared as small hypoechoic nodules with hyperechoic centre; sometimes, small neural interconnecting fibers may be visualized arising from the edges of large ganglia as thin hypoechoic lines. The rate of ganglia detection is 79–89%, and it may also vary among endosonographers (65–97%) [64]. The injection starts from the deepest part of the ganglia and is performed during withdrawal of the needle.

Efficacy

The initial report by Wiersema and Wiersema et al. [55] in 1996 showed significant improvement in pain control in 58 patients receiving EUS-CPN in up to 12 weeks following the procedure: among them, 45 patients (78%) experienced a decrease in pain score independently of narcotic use. In the systemic review by Nagels et al. [65], significant pain reduction was noted at weeks 2, 4, 8, and 12 with a mean difference in pain score of -4.26 [95%CI: -5.53-(-3.00)], -4.21 [95%CI: -5.29-(-3.13)], -4.13 [95%CI: -4.84-(-3.43)], -4.28 [95%CI: -5.63-(-2.94)], respectively. This is consistent with result from meta-analysis *by* Puli et al., [66] which showed a pain reduction in 80% [95%CI: 74.44–85.22] *of* the patients following EUS-CPN for pancreatic cancer and a 59% [95%CI: 54.51–64.30] of the patients receiving EUS-CPN for chronic pancreatitis. Despite the favorable effects in pain control, EUS-CPN is not associated with significant reduction in opioid use; many patients require same or less than baseline usage of narcotics.

According to a recent review by Yasuda and Wang et al. [67], the choice between central versus bilateral technique is still controversial: the meta-analysis by Puli et al. [66] showed superior result in pain relief among patients treated with bilateral procedure (84.54%; 95% CI = 72.15–93.77) as compared to those received central procedure(45.99%; 95% CI = 37.33–54.78). However, such result was not shown in subsequent RCT by Leblanc et al. [68], where there is no significant difference in pain relief between the central and bilateral techniques (central: 69%

vs bilateral: 81%; $p = 0.340$). Hence, the choice of central or bilateral technique is still a matter of debate.

Though the initial report by Levy et al. [63] showed promising result with regard to the use of EUS-CGN; the only RCT was a comparison between EUS-CGN versus EUS unilateral CPN, which showed substantial greater pain relief in the CGN group (73.5% vs 45.5%, $p = 0.026$) [69] with similar adverse events; however, conclusion with regards to superiority should await the availability of RCT comparing EUS-CGN with EUS bilateral CPN.

Adverse Events

Complications commonly associated with EUS-CPN are related to blockade of sympathetic efferent activity with parasympathetic overflow. Self-limiting diarrhea occurred in up to 23% of the patients, while transient hypotension is noted in 11–20% of the patients. About 29–34% of the patients may experience transient exacerbation of pain [59, 60, 64–67]. There *have* been reports of inebriation among Japanese patients [62], a phenomenon which may be due *to* high proportions of patients with aldehyde dehydrogenase (ALDH2) deficiency among Asian population.

Despite the theoretical enhancement in safety profile associated with better visualization and precision, there have been reports of major complications. Bacteremia and abscess formation *may be* induced as a needle is pierced through the gastrointestinal tract during the procedure; there *have* been reports of retroperitoneal abscess [70–72] in three patients receiving EUS-guided bilateral CPN for chronic pancreatitis. Therefore, antibiotic prophylaxis is recommended especially when steroid is used. Two cases of retroperitoneal bleeding [64, 67] have also been reported using the same technique. Three cases of paraplegia were noted, the postulated mechanism may be related to the high volume of alcohol injected to the celiac region, which diffused via intercostal artery toward the anterior spinal artery causing spinal infarction, another mechanism *may be* related to thrombosis or spasm of the artery of Adamkiewicz, which arises from the aorta at T7 to L4, anatomically in close relation to the celiac ganglion, it supplies the lower two-thirds of the anterior spinal artery.

Fatal ischemic complications have been reported. It is postulated that the sclerosing effect of alcohol led to acute thrombosis of the celiac trunk, resulting in pneumatosis of the stomach, duodenum, small bowel, and ascending colon in a patient receiving bilateral EUS-guided CPN for chronic pancreatitis. Vasospasm of the celiac artery as a result ethanol diffusion has resulted in infarction of liver, spleen, stomach, and small intestine in patients with pancreatic metastasis from lung cancer [73, 74].

References

1. Banks PA, Bollen TL, Dervenis C, et al. Classification of acute pancreatitis—2012: revision of the Atlanta classification and definitions by international consensus. Gut. 2013;62:102–11.
2. Seewald S, Ang TL, Teng KC, Soehendra N. EUS-guided drainage of pancreatic pseudocysts, abscesses and infected necrosis. Dig Endosc. 2009;21(Suppl 1):S61–5. [PMID: 19691738]. https://doi.org/10.1111/j.1443-1661.2009.00860.x.
3. Yoon WJ, Brugge WR. Endoscopic ultrasound and pancreatic cystic lesions-diagnostic and therapeutic applications. Endosc Ultrasound. 2012;1:75–9. [PMID: 24949341]. https://doi.org/10.7178/Eus.02.004.
4. Itoi T, Binmoeller KF, Shah J, et al. Clinical evaluation of a novel lumen-apposing metal stent for endosonography-guided pancreatic pseudocyst and gallbladder drainage (with videos). Gastrointest Endosc. 2012;75:870–6.
5. Itoi T, Nageshwar Reddy D, Yasuda I. New fully-covered self-expandable metal stent for endoscopic ultrasonography-guided intervention in infectious walled-off pancreatic necrosis (with video). J Hepatobiliary Pancreat Sci. 2013;20:403–6.
6. Fabbri C, Luigiano C, Cennamo V, et al. Endoscopic ultrasound-guided transmural drainage of infected pancreatic fluid collections with placement of covered self-expanding metal stents: a case series. Endoscopy. 2012;44:429–33.
7. Song TJ, Lee SS. Endoscopic drainage of pseudocysts. Clin Endosc. 2014;47:222–6. [PMID: 24944985]. https://doi.org/10.5946/ce.2014.47.3.222.
8. Varadarajulu S, Bang JY, Phadnis MA, Christein JD, Wilcox CM. Endoscopic transmural drainage of peripancreatic fluid collections: outcomes and predictors of treatment success in 211 consecutive patients. J Gastrointest Surg. 2011;15:2080–8. [PMID: 21786063]. https://doi.org/10.1007/s11605-011-1621-8.

9. Lee BU, Song TJ, Lee SS, et al. Newly designed, fully covered metal stents for endoscopic ultrasound (EUS)-guided transmural drainage of peripancreatic fluid collections: a prospective randomized study. Endoscopy. 2014;46:1078–84.

10. Bang JY, Hawes R, Bartolucci A, Varadarajulu S. Efficacy of metal and plastic stents for transmural drainage of pancreatic fluid collections: a systematic review. Dig Endosc. 2015;27:486–98.

11. Tarantino I, Barresi L, Fazio V, Di Pisa M, Traina M. EUS-guided self-expandable stent placement in 1 step: a new method to treat pancreatic abscess. Gastrointest Endosc. 2009;69:1401–3.

12. Siddiqui AA, Kowalski TE, Loren DE, et al. Fully covered self-expanding metal stents versus lumen-apposing fully covered self-expanding metal stent versus plastic stents for endoscopic drainage of pancreatic walled-off necrosis: clinical outcomes and success. Gastrointest Endosc. 2017;85:758–65.

13. Shah RJ, Shah JN, Waxman I, et al. Safety and efficacy of endoscopic ultrasound-guided drainage of pancreatic fluid collections with lumen-apposing covered self-expanding metal stents. Clin Gastroenterol Hepatol. 2015;13:747–52.

14. Gornals JB, De la Serna-Higuera C, Sánchez-Yague A, Loras C, Sánchez-Cantos AM, Pérez-Miranda M. Endosonography-guided drainage of pancreatic fluid collections with a novel lumen-apposing stent. Surg Endosc. 2013;27:1428–34.

15. Vazquez-Sequeiros E, Baron TH, Pérez-Miranda M, et al. Evaluation of the short- and long-term effectiveness and safety of fully covered self-expandable metal stents for drainage of pancreatic fluid collections: results of a Spanish nationwide registry. Gastrointest Endosc. 2016;84:450–7.. e2

16. Siddiqui AA, Adler DG, Nieto J, et al. EUS-guided drainage of peripancreatic fluid collections and necrosis by using a novel lumen-apposing stent: a large retrospective, multicenter U.S. experience. Gastrointest Endosc. 2016;83(4):699–707. https://doi.org/10.1016/j.gie.2015.10.020. Epub 2015 Oct 26

17. Park DH, Lee SS, Moon SH, Choi SY, Jung SW, Seo DW, Lee SK, Kim MH. Endoscopic ultrasound-guided versus conventional transmural drainage for pancreatic pseudocysts: a prospective randomized trial. Endoscopy. 2009;41:842–8. [PMID: 19798610]. https://doi.org/10.1055/s-0029-1215133.

18. Varadarajulu S, Christein JD, Tamhane A, Drelichman ER, Wilcox CM. Prospective randomized trial comparing EUS and EGD for transmural drainage of pancreatic pseudocysts (with videos). Gastrointest Endosc. 2008;68:1102–11. [PMID: 18640677]. https://doi.org/10.1016/j.gie.2008.04.028.

19. Ahn JY, Seo DW, Eum J, Song TJ, Moon SH, Park do H, Lee SS, Lee SK, Kim MH. Single-step EUS-guided transmural drainage of pancreatic pseudocysts: analysis of technical feasibility, efficacy, and safety. Gut Liver. 2010;4:524–9. [PMID: 21253303]. https://doi.org/10.5009/gnl.2010.4.4.524.

20. Lopes CV, Pesenti C, Bories E, Caillol F, Giovannini M. Endoscopic-ultrasound-guided endoscopic transmural drainage of pancreatic pseudocysts and abscesses. Scand J Gastroenterol. 2007;42:524–9. [PMID: 17454865]. https://doi.org/10.1080/00365520601065093.

21. Varadarajulu S, Tamhane A, Blakely J. Graded dilation technique for EUS-guided drainage of peripancreatic fluid collections: an assessment of outcomes and complications and technical proficiency (with video). Gastrointest Endosc. 2008;68:656–66. [PMID: 18599050]. https://doi.org/10.1016/j.gie.2008.03.1091.

22. Ng PY, Rasmussen DN, Vilmann P, Hassan H, Gheorman V, Burtea D, Surlin V, Săftoiu A. Endoscopic ultrasound-guided drainage of pancreatic pseudocysts: medium-term assessment of outcomes and complications. Endosc Ultrasound. 2013;2:199–203. [PMID: 24949396]. https://doi.org/10.4103/2303-9027.121245.

23. Varadarajulu S, Bang JY, Sutton BS, Trevino JM, Christein JD, Wilcox CM. Equal efficacy of endoscopic and surgical cystogastrostomy for pancreatic pseudocyst drainage in a randomized trial. Gastroenterology. 2013;145:583–90.e1. [PMID: 23732774]. https://doi.org/10.1053/j.gastro.2013.05.046.

24. Varadarajulu S, Trevino J, Wilcox CM, Sutton B, Christein JD. Randomized trial comparing EUS and surgery for pancreatic pseudocyst drainage. Gastrointest Endosc. 2010; 71: Ab116-Ab116.

25. Penn DE, Draganov PV, Wagh MS, Forsmark CE, Gupte AR, Chauhan SS. Prospective evaluation of the use of fully covered self-expanding metal stents for EUS-guided transmural drainage of pancreatic pseudocysts. Gastrointest Endosc. 2012;76:679–84.

26. Sharaiha RZ, DeFilippis EM, Kedia P, et al. Metal versus plastic for pancreatic pseudocyst drainage: clinical outcomes and success. Gastrointest Endosc. 2015;82:822–7.

27. Yang D, Amin S, Gonzalez S, et al. Transpapillary drainage has no added benefit on treatment outcomes in patients undergoing EUS-guided transmural drainage of pancreatic pseudocysts: a large multicenter study. Gastrointest Endosc. 2016;83:720–9.

28. Arvanitakis M, Delhaye M, Bali MA, et al. Pancreatic-fluid collections: a randomized controlled trial regarding stent removal after endoscopic transmural drainage. Gastrointest Endosc. 2007;65:609–19.

29. Devière J, Bueso H, Baize M, et al. Complete disruption of the main pancreatic duct: endoscopic management. Gastrointest Endosc. 1995;42:445–51.

30. Pelaez-Luna M, Vege SS, Petersen BT, et al. Disconnected pancreatic duct syndrome in severe acute pancreatitis: clinical and imaging characteristics and outcomes in a cohort of 31 cases. Gastrointest Endosc. 2008;68:91–7.

31. Varadarajulu S, Wilcox CM. Endoscopic placement of permanent indwelling transmural stents in disconnected pancreatic duct syndrome: does benefit outweigh the risks? Gastrointest Endosc. 2011;74:1408–12.

32. Seifert H, Biermer M, Schmitt W, et al. Transluminal endoscopic necrosectomy after acute pancreatitis:

a multicentre study with long-term follow-up (the GEPARD study). Gut. 2009;58:1260–6.

33. Yasuda I, Nakashima M, Iwai T, et al. Japanese multicenter experience of endoscopic necrosectomy for infected walled-off pancreatic necrosis: the JENIPaN study. Endoscopy. 2013;45:627–34.

34. Gardner TB, Chahal P, Papachristou GI, et al. A comparison of direct endoscopic necrosectomy with transmural endoscopic drainage for the treatment of walled-off pancreatic necrosis. Gastrointest Endosc. 2009;69:1085–94.

35. van Brunschot S, Fockens P, Bakker OJ, et al. Endoscopic transluminal necrosectomy in necrotising pancreatitis: a systematic review. Surg Endosc. 2014;28:1425–38.

36. Itoi T, Kasuya K, Sofuni A, et al. Endoscopic ultrasonography-guided pancreatic duct access: techniques and literature review of pancreatography, transmural drainage and rendezvous techniques. Dig Endosc. 2013;25:241–52.

37. Bataille L, Deprez P. A new application for therapeutic EUS: main pancreatic duct drainage with a "pancreatic rendezvous technique". Gastrointest Endosc. 2002;55:740–3.

38. Will U, Meyer F, Manger T, Wanzar I. Endoscopic ultrasound-assisted rendezvous maneuver to achieve pancreatic duct drainage in obstructive chronic pancreatitis. Endoscopy. 2005;37:171–3.

39. Fujii-Lau LL, Levy MJ. Endoscopic ultrasound-guided pancreatic duct drainage. J Hepatobiliary Pancreat Sci. 2015;22:51–7.

40. Tyberg A, Sharaiha RZ, Kedia P, et al. EUS-guided pancreatic drainage for pancreatic strictures after failed ERCP: a multicenter international collaborative study. Gastrointest Endosc. 2017;85:164–9.

41. Chen YI, Levy MJ, Moreels TG, et al. An international multicenter study comparing EUS-guided pancreatic duct drainage with enteroscopy-assisted endoscopic retrograde pancreatography after Whipple surgery. Gastrointest Endosc. 2017;85:170–7.

42. Dhir V, Isayama H, Itoi T, et al. EUS-guided biliary and pancreatic duct interventions. Dig Endosc. 2017;29:472. https://doi.org/10.1111/den.12818.

43. Will U, Fueldner F, Thieme AK, et al. Transgastric pancreatography and EUS-guided drainage of the pancreatic duct. J Hepato-Biliary-Pancreat Surg. 2007;14:377–82.

44. Lakhtakia S, Seo D-W, et al. Endoscopic ultrasonography-guided tumor ablation. Dig Endosc. 2017;29:486–94.

45. Alvarez-Sanchez M-V, Napoleon B, et al. Review of endoscopic radiofrequency in biliopancreatic tumours with emphasis on clinical benefits, controversies and safety. World J Gastroenterol. 2016;22:8257–70.

46. Lakhtakia S, Ramchandani M, Galasso D, et al. EUS-guided radiofrequency ablation for management of pancreatic insuli- noma by using a novel needle electrode (with videos). Gastrointest Endosc. 2016;83:234–9.

47. Jurgensen C, Schuppan D, Neser F, Ernstberger J, Junghans U. StolzelU.EUS-guidedalcohola

blationofaninsulinoma. Gastrointest Endosc. 2006;63:1059–62.

48. Signoretti M, Valente R, Repici A, Delle Fave G, Capurso G, Carrara S. Endoscopy-guided ablation of pancreatic lesions: technical possibilities and clinical outlook. World J Gastrointest Endosc. 2017;9(2):41–54.

49. Facciorusso A, Di Maso M, Serviddio G, Larghi A, Costamagna G, Muscatiello N. Echoendoscopic ethanol ablation of tumor combined with celiac plexus neurolysis in patients with pancreatic adenocacinoma. J Gastroenterol Hepatol. 2017;32:439–45.

50. Dhadham GC, Hoffe S, Harris CL, Klapman JB. Endoscopic ultra- sound-guided fiducial marker placement for image-guided radiation therapy without uoroscopy: safety and technical feasibility. Endosc Int Open. 2016;4:E378–82.

51. Law JK, Singh VK, Khashab MA, et al. Endoscopic ultrasound (EUS)-guided fiducial placement allows localization of small neuroendo- crine tumors during parenchymal-sparing pancreatic surgery. Surg Endosc. 2013;27:3921–6.

52. Gan SI, Thompson CC, Lauwers GY, Bounds BC, Brugge WR. Ethanol lavage of pancreatic cystic lesions: initial pilot study. Gastrointest Endosc. 2005;61:746–52.

53. Oh HC, Seo DW, Lee TY, et al. New treatment for cystic tumors of the pancreas: EUS-guided ethanol lavage with paclitaxel injection. Gastrointest Endosc. 2008;67:636–42.

54. Kappis M. Erfahrungen mit Lokalanasthesie bei Bauchoperationen. Verh Dtsch Gesellsch Chir. 1914;43:87–9.

55. Wiersema MJ, Wiersema LM, et al. Endosonography-guided celiac plexus neurolysis. Gastrointest Endosc. 1996;44:656–62.

56. Faigel DO, et al. Endosonography guided celiac plexus injection for abdominal pain dueto chronic pancreatitis. Am J Gastroenterol. 1996;91:1675.

57. Wong GY. Effect of neurolytic celiac plexus block on pain relief, quality of life, and survival in patients with unresectable pancreatic cancer: a randomized controlled trial. JAMA. 2004;291:1092–9.

58. World Health Organization. Cancer pain relief. 2nd ed. Geneva: WHO; 2006.

59. Wise JM, et al. Celiac plexus nerolysis in the management of unrepeatable pancreatic cancer. When and how? World J Gastroenterol. 2014;20(9):2186–92.

60. D'Haese JG, et al. Treatment options in painful chronic pancreatitis: a systematic review. HBP. 2014;16:512–21.

61. Santos D, et al. Clinical trial: a randomized trial comparing fluoroscopy guided percutaneous technique vs. endoscopic ultrasound guided technique of coeliac plexus block for treatment of painin chronic pancreatitis. Aliment Pharmacol Ther. 2009;29:979–84.

62. Ishiwatari H, et al. Phenol-based endoscopic ultrasound-guided celiac plexus neurolysis for East Asian alcohol-intolerant upper gastrointestinal cancer patients: a pilot study. World J Gastroenterol. 2014;20:10512–7.

63. Levy MJet al. Initial evaluation of the efficacy and safety of endoscopic ultrasound-guided direct Ganglia neurolysis and block. Am. J Gastroenterol. 2008;103:98–103.

64. Seicean A, et al. Celiac plexus neurolysis in pancreatic cancer: the endoscopic ultrasound approach. World J Gastroenterol. 2014;20(1):110–7.

65. Nagels W, et al. Celiac plexus neuroloysis for abdominal cancer pain: a systemic review. Pain Med. 2013;14:1140–63.

66. Puli S. Ret al. EUS-guided celiac plexus neurolysis for pain due to chronic pancreatitis or pancreatic cancer pain: a meta-analysis and systematic review. Dig Dis Sci. 2009;54:2330–7.

67. Yasuda I, Wang H-P, et al. Endoscopic ultrasound-guided celiac plexus block and neurolysis. Dig Endosc. 2017;29:455–62.

68. Leblanc JK, et al. A prospective, randomized study of EUS-guided celiac plexus neurolysis for pancreatic cancer: one injection or two? Gastrointest Endosc. 2011;74:1300–7.

69. Sahai AV, et al. Central vs. bilateral endoscopic ultrasound-guided celiac plexus block or neuroly- sis: a comparative study of short-term effectiveness. Am J Gastroenterol. 2009;104:326–9.

70. Gress F, et al. Endoscopic ultrasound (EUS) guided celiac plexus block (CB) for management of pain due to chronic pancreatitis (CP) a large single center experience. Gastrointest Endosc. 1997;45:AB173.

71. Muscatiello N, et al. Complication of endoscopic ultrasound-guided celiac plexus neurolysis. Endoscopy. 2006;38:858.

72. O'Toole TM, et al. Complication rates of EUS- guided celiac plexus blockade and neurolysis: results of a large case series. Endoscopy. 2009;41:593–7.

73. Loeve US, et al. Lethal necrosis and perforation of the stomach and the aorta after multiple EUS-guided celiac plexus neurolysis procedures in a patient with chronic pancreatitis. Gastrointest Endosc. 2013;77:151–2.

74. Jang HY, et al. Hepatic and splenic infarction and bowel ischemia following endoscopic ultrasound-guided celiac plexus neurolysis. Clin Endosc. 2013;46:306–9.

Interventional EUS: Bile Duct and Gallbladder

Anthony Yuen Bun Teoh, Kenjiro Yamamoto, and Takao Itoi

Introduction

Drainage of the bile ducts could be achieved by endoscopic, percutaneous, or surgical means [1]. Surgical bypass is the traditional method of obtaining biliary drainage. The approach is associated with low rates of recurrent biliary obstruction, but the invasive nature of the procedure causes more adverse events as compared to percutaneous and endoscopic drainage [2, 3]. Percutaneous biliary drainage avoids the need of surgery. It is associated with high success rates of 77–100% and an acceptable risk of adverse events (6–31%) [4, 5]. Nevertheless, the presence of an external tube is often cumbersome and external drainage of bile may cause fluid and electrolyte loss to the patient. As a result, endoscopic retrograde cholangiography (ERC) is currently the first-line approach for obtaining biliary drainage in patients with biliary obstruction. The procedure is associated with more

Electronic Supplementary Material The online version of this chapter (https://doi.org/10.1007/978-3-030-21695-5_28) contains supplementary material, which is available to authorized users.

A. Y. B. Teoh (✉)
Department of Surgery, Prince of Wales Hospital, The Chinese University of Hong Kong,
Shatin, Hong Kong SAR
e-mail: anthonyteoh@surgery.cuhk.edu.hk

K. Yamamoto · T. Itoi
Department of Gastroenterology, The University of Tokyo, Tokyo, Japan

than 90% success rates and avoids the problems associated with percutaneous tubes [6]. However, in less than 10% of the patients, deep cannulation of the bile ducts is not possible and percutaneous drainage may still be required. In the last decade, EUS-guided biliary drainage (EUS-BD) has emerged as an alternative approach for drainage of the bile ducts. The approach allows internal drainage of bile with either a transpapillary or transmural technique, depending on the etiology and level of obstruction. Furthermore, it could be performed at the same session of a failed ERC.

On the other hand, the gold standard for treatment of acute cholecystitis is laparoscopic cholecystectomy [7–11]. However, the procedure may not be suitable in patients who are at high-risk of surgery. Hence, percutaneous cholecystostomy is employed to provide a means of draining the gallbladder until the acute condition settles [12, 13]. Nevertheless, many of the cholecystostomies will become long-term and only 32.9% of the patients eventually received cholecystectomy in one study [14]. The continued caring of the external tube is again challenging to the patient. Recently, EUS-guided gallbladder drainage (EGBD) is gaining popularity and the approach provides an endoscopic alternative to percutaneous drainage of the gallbladder [15–31]. Furthermore, the gallstones can now be cleared by endoscopy after EGBD and this may potentially reduce the risk of recurrent cholecystitis [32].

In this chapter, we will provide an overview on the current developments in EUS-BD and

EGBD. The indications, techniques, outcomes, and risk of adverse events of both the techniques are discussed.

EUS-Guided Biliary Drainage

Types of EUS-Guided Biliary Drainage (EUS-BD)

EUS-BD comprises of a group of interventional EUS procedures aimed at achieving bile duct drainage [33, 34]. In the literature, there is no unified method in the nomenclature of these procedures and the same procedure may be named differently by different authors. Broadly, EUS-BD could be classified into the transpapillary or transmural techniques (Fig. 28.1). In transpapillary procedures, EUS-BD is performed with the eventual aim of obtaining transpapillary drainage. Transpapillary procedures include EUS-rendezvous ERCP (EUS-Rv) and EUS-guided antegrade stenting (EUS-AG). The concept of EUS-Rv is similar to percutaneous rendezvous ERCP. The use of EUS is to provide access to the proximal bile duct for introduction of a guidewire to pass across the papilla for subsequent cannulation by ERCP. In EUS-AG, the left intrahepatic is punctured to allow introduction of a guidewire and placement of stent in an antegrade fashion to achieve drainage.

Transmural procedures involve the creation of a neo-fistula and placement of stent between the bile duct and the stomach or the duodenum. In EUS-guided choledochoduodenostomies (EUS-CDS), a stent is placed between the common hepatic duct and the first part of the duodenum. In EUS-guided

hepaticogastrostomies (EUS-HGS), a stent is placed between the left intrahepatic ducts and the stomach. These are the most common types of transmural EUS-BD techniques. Other variations have also been described including hepaticoduodenostomies and choledochojejunostomy, but the performance of these procedures are much less common and feasibility of these techniques is dependent on the underlying anatomy [35, 36].

Indications of EUS-BD

The indication of EUS-BD is failed ERC due to failed deep biliary cannulation or an inaccessible papilla (Table 28.1) [37]. In the event of difficult biliary cannulation during ERC, advanced cannulation techniques including double guidewire technique and precut sphincterotomy should achieve cannulation in 73.4–100% of the patients

Table 28.1 Indications of EUS-guided biliary, pancreatic, and gallbladder drainage

Indications of EUS-guided biliary drainage
Failed deep biliary cannulation
Tumor obstruction
Tortuous common channel
Inaccessible papilla
Malignant duodenal obstruction
Altered GI anatomy
Prior duodenal metallic stenting
Unavailable or refusal of percutaneous drainage/ surgical procedures
Indications of EUS-guided gallbladder drainage
1. High-risk surgical candidate suffering from acute cholecystitis
2. Failure to wean from long-term cholecystostomy

Fig. 28.1 Nomenclature of EUS-BD

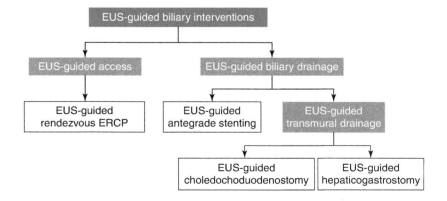

[37]. Thus, the use of EUS guidance to achieve biliary drainage should be uncommon and should not replace good ERC technique [38]. The decision to perform EUS-BD should also depend on the available expertise at the institution.

Technique of EUS-BD

EUS-Rv

EUS-Rv is usually performed when there is failed ERC due to a difficult papilla or malignant distal bile duct obstruction. The authors prefer to perform the procedure for benign conditions. The concept of EUS-Rv is similar to percutaneous rendezvous ERCP, but the procedure is performed under EUS guidance. It is a type of access procedure aimed at passage of the guidewire through the papilla to complete an ERC (Fig. 28.2). The bile duct can be punctured from the first or second part of the duodenum or from the stomach by a 19G needle. A guidewire is then passed through the papilla for retrieval by a duodenoscope. The retrieved wire is then used to guide bile duct cannulation, and the procedure is completed with ERC.

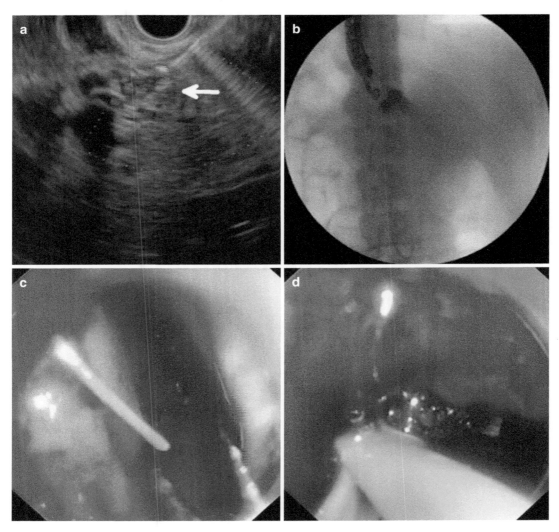

Fig. 28.2 EUS-Rv in patient with previous Billroth II gastrectomy and failed cannulation. (**a**) The left intrahepatic duct was punctured with a 19-gauge needle from the stomach. (**b**) After contrast injection, the guidewire was inserted across the papilla in an antegrade manner. (**c**) Retrieval of the guidewire with a gastroscope. (**d**) Cannulation of the bile duct on guidewire with insertion of a plastic stent

EUS-AG

EUS-AG is usually performed in the presence of an inaccessible papilla/anastomosis and a dilated intrahepatic duct. In EUS-AG, the aim is to place a stent in an antegrade manner across a stricture distal to the puncture site (Fig. 28.3 and Video 28.1). The left intrahepatic duct is first punctured by a 19G needle, followed by insertion of a guidewire. The guidewire is then manipulated across the stricture. The track is dilated with electrocautery. A covered or uncovered stent is then inserted in an antegrade manner and placed across the stricture.

EUS-CDS

EUS-CDS is usually performed when ERC fails due to a malignant distal common bile duct obstruction and when the first part of the duodenum is available for drainage. In EUS-CDS and –HGS, a neofistula is first created followed by placement of stent. In EUS-CDS, the common bile duct is punctured with a 19G

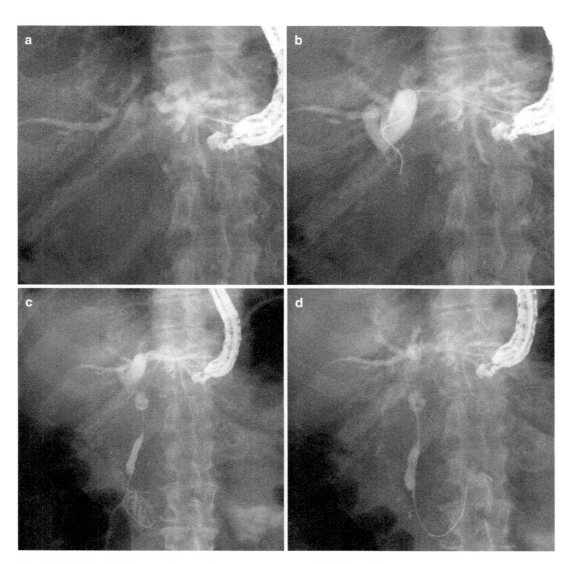

Fig. 28.3 EUS-guided antegrade stenting. (**a**) EUS-guided puncture of the left intrahepatic duct with a 19 gauge needle. (**b**) A guidewire was passed into the hepatic duct. (**c**) The guidewire was negotiated across the common bile duct stricture and through the papilla into the duodenum. (**d**) An uncovered biliary metallic stent was inserted across the stricture after track dilation

needle from the first part of the duodenum (Fig. 28.4). A guidewire is inserted through the needle and passed deeply into the biliary system. The track is then dilated with electrocautery and a 4 mm balloon. This is followed by insertion of a partially or fully covered biliary metal stent.

EUS-HGS

EUS-HGS can be performed when ERC fails due to a malignant bile duct obstruction, but the papilla is inaccessible or if the first of the duodenum is infiltrated by tumor (Fig. 28.5). The left intrahepatic duct is punctured with a 19G needle from the stomach. A guidewire is inserted through the needle deeply into the biliary system. The track is then dilated with electrocautery, and a partially or fully covered metallic stent is inserted bridging the left intrahepatic to the stomach.

Choice of the Technique

The advantages and disadvantages of each type of EUS-BD procedure are different, and applica-

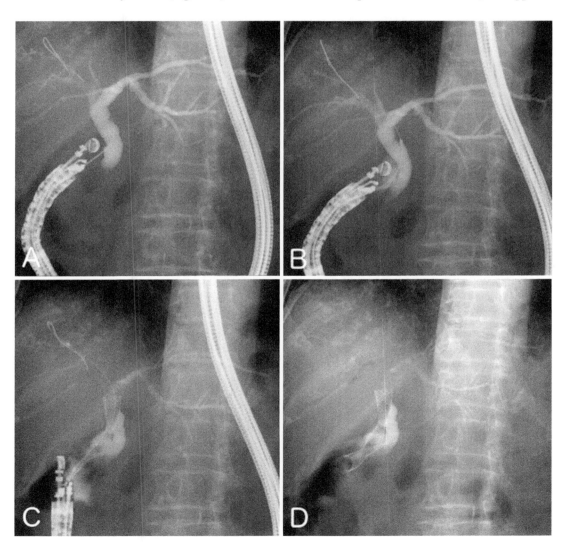

Fig. 28.4 EUS-guided choledochoduodenostomy. (**a**) EUS-guided puncture of the common hepatic duct with a 19 gauge needle. (**b**) The needle track was dilated with a co-axial diathermy was passage of the guidewire. (**c**) A fully or partially covered metallic stent was inserted. (**d**) Complete deployment of the CDS stent

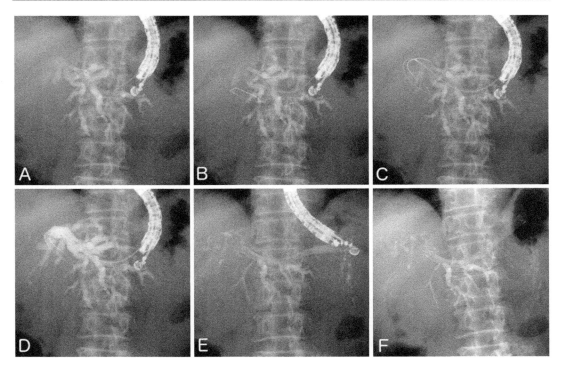

Fig. 28.5 EUS-guided hepaticogastrostomy. (**a**) EUS-guided puncture of the left intrahepatic duct with a 19-gauge needle. (**b**) A guidewire was passed into the hepatic duct. (**c**) The needle track was dilated with a coax-ial diathermy. (**d**) A full cholangiogram was performed with further contrast injection. (**e**) Deployment of a metal stent for HGS. (**f**) Complete deployment of the stent

bility is dependent on the underlying anatomy of the patient. In some patients, multiple techniques may be feasible and the choice depends on outcomes of the procedures, the underlying etiology, the availability of devices, and expertise.

As mentioned previously, EUS-Rv is mainly an access procedure and usually does not involve fistula dilation. The risk of the procedure is related to a prior difficult ERC and the additional risks from EUS-guided bile duct puncture are minimal. However, there are a number of obstacles to the procedure. Firstly, the difficulty of the procedure is related to guidewire manipulation across any existing stricture and through the papilla, and the reported success rate is 65–80% [39]. Thereafter, the echoendoscope needs to be exchanged with a duodenoscope for guidewire retrieval. The process is sometimes difficult, and there may be inadvertent displacement of the guidewire back into the bile duct during the process.

Similarly, the main difficulty of EUS-AG is manipulation of the guidewire across any stricture after bile duct puncture. The procedure also requires a dilated intrahepatic duct for puncture. In theory, there is a risk of bile leak from the puncture site, but if this occurs, it tends to be mild and self-limiting. The technique is suitable in patients where the papilla is inaccessible. However, if recurrent obstruction of the stent occurs, reintervention through the stent may not be possible and another EUS-BD procedure may be required.

EUS-CDS and –HGS are transmural EUS-BD techniques that require creation of a neofistula and creation of an anastomosis with placement of a stent. The potential advantages are that the procedures do not have risk of pancreatitis and the stents seldom suffer from tumor ingrowth as they are placed far away from the tumor. However, the integrity of the anastomosis is dependent on the properties of the stents placed and EUS-specific stents that encompass antimigratory properties are preferred [40]. In the event of stent misdeployment or migration, outcomes may be catastrophic. Potential adverse events from transmural procedures are higher and include pneumoperitoneum, bleeding, cholangitis, stent dislocation, free perforation, bile leak, and bile peritonitis. Rarer adverse events include hemobilia, acute cholecystitis, duodenal double puncture, mediastinitis, and mortality.

Outcomes of the EUS-BD Procedures

EUS-BD Versus Percutaneous Transhepatic Biliary Drainage (PTBD)

The main indication for EUS-BD is when ERC fails. Traditionally, biliary drainage is obtained by percutaneous drainage in this situation. Three retrospective and 2 randomized studies have compared EUS-BD with PTBD (Table 28.2) [41–45]. Among the retrospective studies, similar clinical success rates were reported in one study and higher clinical success rates in the EUS-BD group were reported in two studies. Outcomes from randomized studies have all shown equivalent success rates between the two groups. In all studies, the adverse events rates were significantly lower in the EUS-BD group and the need for reinterventions for EUS-BD was also lower in some studies.

A meta-analysis then included an additional 4 comparative studies published in abstract form and included 483 patients [46]. There were no differences in technical success between the two procedures (OR = 1.78; 95% CI, 0.69–4.59), but EUS-BD was associated with better clinical success (OR = 0.45, 95% CI: 0.23–0.89), fewer postprocedure adverse events (OR = 0.23, 95% CI: 0.12–0.47), and lower rates of reintervention (OR = 0.13, 95% CI: 0.07–0.24). There was no difference in length of hospital stay after the procedures. Thus, EUS-BD should be preferred over PTBD in the event of failed ERC.

EUS-BD Versus ERCP

Recently, three randomized studies have compared EUS-BD with ERC and metallic stenting (SEMS) as a primary means of obtaining biliary drainage in patients with malignant biliary obstruction (Table 28.3). The principle is that in EUS-BD, a stent is placed at a site that is away from the tumor. Thus, the chances of tumor ingrowth or overgrowth could be reduced and stent patency can be improved. Other potential benefits of EUS-BD over ERC include reduced procedural times and no risk of pancreatitis. However, this needs to be balanced against the need for dedicated expertise and devices, increased risks of bile leak, and stent migration. In two small randomized studies comparing EUS-CDS with ERC and SEMS, there were no differences in technical and clinical success rates, adverse events, and reinterventions [47, 48]. In the other study, EUS-CDS and -HGS using a dedicated device was compared with ERC with SEMS in unresectable malignant distal biliary obstruction [49]. The technical success rate of EUS-BD was not inferior to ERC with SEMS (93.8% vs 90.2%, $P = 0.003$), and clinical suc-

Table 28.2 Comparison of EUS-BD with PTBD

Author	Design	Year	Patients	Technical success (%)		Clinical success (%)		Adverse events (%)		Reinterventions (%)	
Bapaye [41]	Retrospective	2013	EUS 25	92	$P < 0.05$	92	$P < 0.05$	20	$P < 0.05$	–	
			PTBD 26	46		46		46			
Khashab [42]	Retrospective	2015	EUS 22	86.4	$P = 0.007$	100		18.2	$P = 0.08$	15.7	$P < 0.001$
			PTBD 51	100		92.2		39.2		80.4	
Sharaiha [43]	Retrospective	2016	EUS 47	91.6		62.2 25	$P = 0.03$	13	$P = NS$	1.3	$P < 0.001$
			PTBD 13	93.3				25		4.9	
Artifon [44]	RCT	2012	EUS 13	100		100		15.3	$P = NS$	–	
			PTBD 12	100		100		25			
Lee [45]	RCT	2015	EUS 34	94.1		87.5		8.8	$P = 0.022$	25	$P = 0.022$
			PTBD 32	96.9		87.1		31.2		54.8	

Table 28.3 Studies comparing EUS-BD with ERC and metallic stenting for primary biliary drainage

Author	Design	Year	Patients N	Type of procedure	Technical success (%)	Clinical success (%)	30-day adverse events (%)	Stent patency at 6 months (%)	Reintervention (%)
Park [47]	RCT	2018	14	EUS-CDS	93	100	31[a]	69[a]	–
			14	ERC	100	93	31	69	
Bang [48]	RCT	2018	34	EUS-CDS	90.9	97	14.7	–	3
			33	ERC	94.1	91.2	6.1		2.9
Paik [49]	RCT	2018	64	EUS-CDS or HGS	93.8	90.4	6.3	85.1	15.6
			61	ERC	90.2	94.5	19.7	48.9	42.6

RCT randomized controlled trial
[a]Only the overall number of patients with adverse events and stent dysfunction was provided in this study

Table 28.4 Outcomes of studies comparing EUS-BD procedures

Author	Design	Year	Patients N	Type of procedure	Clinical success (%)	30-day adverse events (%)	Mean duration of stent patency (days)
Dhir [50]	Retrospective	2012	58	EUS-Rv	98.3	3.4	–
			144	ERC	90.3	6.7	
Lee [51]	Retrospective	2017	50	EUS-Rv	93.3	–	–
			10	EUS-AG	100		
			1	EUS-HGS	100		
Bill [52]	Retrospective	2017	25	EUS-Rv	76	28	–
			25	PTBD	100	36	
Artifon [53]	RCT	2015	24	EUS-CDS	77	12.5	
			25	EUS-HGS	91%	20%	
Ogura [54]		2016	39	CDS 13	100	0	37
				HGS 26		0	133

cess rates were similar (90% vs 94.5%, $P = 0.49$). There were lower adverse events rates (6.3% vs. 19.7%, $P = 0.03$) and reintervention (15.6% vs. 42.6%) in the EUS-BD arm. Postprocedural pancreatitis was lower in the EUS-BD arm (0 vs. 14.8%, $P = 0.001$). A higher stent patency rate at 6 months (85.1% vs. 48.9%, $P = 0.001$) and longer mean patency time (208 days vs. 165 days) was also observed in EUS-BD.

The difference in results observed in the above three studies may be due to several reasons. Firstly, the first two studies are underpowered to detect any difference between the two drainage procedures. Moreover, in the third study by Paik et al., a dedicated single-step device was used for EUS-BD. The use of the device avoided the need for multiple instrumental exchange and lowers the risk of bile leak and stent migration.

Thus, based on these results, EUS-BD may have a potential to improve stent patency as compared to ERC with SEMS for patients with unresectable malignant biliary obstruction. However,

this is by no means a reason to replace good cannulation technique for ERC. Furthermore, the performance EUS-BD in surgical candidates may make subsequent surgery more difficult. Thus, ERC should still be the first-line approach for endoscopic biliary drainage in these patients.

Other Comparative Studies on EUS-BD

There are only a limited number of studies comparing the outcomes of different types of EUS-BD techniques and EUS-BD versus other methods of biliary drainage (Table 28.4). A retrospective study compared EUS-Rv with precut sphincterotomy after failed cannulation in benign and malignant conditions [50]. The overall rates of cannulation were similar between the two techniques, but EUS-Rv was associated with a higher 1st session cannulation rate. No differences in adverse events rates were observed, but precut sphincterotomy had more pancreatitis and bleeding, while periductal contrast leaks were seen in the EUS-Rv group. In another study, the outcomes of patients with failed ERCP were compared between two historical controls. One group included patients in which EUS-BD techniques were employed in patients with failed cannulation [51]. After the EUS-BD techniques were introduced, the rates of failed cannulation were significant reduced (3.6% vs. 1%, $P < 0.001$). When comparing EUS-BD and precut sphincterotomy alone, EUS-BD was associated with significantly higher success rate (95.1% vs. 75.3%, $P < 0.001$). EUS-Rv was also compared to percutaneous biliary drainage in patients with malignant distal biliary obstruction [52]. Although a poorer success rate was observed in the EUS-Rv group (76% vs. 100%, $P = 0.002$), the length of hospital stay was shorter ($P = 0.02$) and the need for repeated biliary interventions was lower ($P = 0.001$).

In comparing EUS-CDS and HGS, the results from a few comparative studies are available.

In a randomized trial, 49 patients with unresectable distal malignant biliary obstruction and failed ERCP received EUS-CDS or EUS-HGS [53]. The technical success rates were comparable among the procedures (91% vs. 96% respectively, $P = 0.61$). Clinical success was lower in the EUS-CDS group (77% vs. 91% respectively, $P = 0.23$) and HGS was associated with a numerically higher rate of adverse events (20% vs. 12.5%, $P = 0.729$), but observed differences in both parameters were not statistically significant, although this may be due to the presence of type 1 error. Ogura et al. also compared EUS-CDS and HGS in patients with concomitant duodenal and biliary obstruction in a randomized study [54]. No difference in technical success clinical success and adverse events rates were observed. Interestingly, EUS-CDS was associated with significantly shorter duration of stent patency in an obstructed duodenum (43 days vs. 133 days, $P = 0.05$).

Khan et al. conducted a systematic review and meta-analysis on studies reporting the outcomes of EUS-BD [55]. Seven studies were included, and overall, there was no difference in technical success between EUS-CDS and HGS (OR 1.32, $P = 0.56$). Six studies described postprocedure adverse events based on the method of drainage.

EUS-CDS appeared to be significantly safer to HGS with a pooled OR of 0.40 ($P = 0.02$). In 2 studies, the risk factors for developing adverse events were assessed. In 1 study, the use of non-coaxial electrocautery (needle knife) was independently associated with occurrence of adverse events (OR 12.4, $P = 0.01$). While in the other, both the use of plastic stenting (OR 4.95, 95%CI 1.41–17.38, $P = 0.01$) and the use of non-coaxial electrocautery (OR 3.95, 95%CI 1.16–13.40, $P = 0.03$) were independently associated with adverse events [56, 57].

Hence, EUS-CDS and HGS are both effective and safe techniques for drainage of distal biliary obstruction after failed ERC. Metallic stents should be placed when possible, and non-coaxial electrocautery should be avoided. Comparing the transmural techniques, EUS-CDS may be associated with shorter hospital stay and fewer adverse events. However, in the presence of duodenal obstruction, EUS-HGS may be the preferred procedure as it is associated with a longer stent patency, while, a CDS may be prone to restenosis due to tumor ingrowth or overgrowth.

EUS-Guided Gallbladder Drainage (EGBD)

EGBD is currently gaining popularity as an alternative to percutaneous drainage in patients who are unfit for cholecystectomy. The approach can be used to drain the gallbladder in patients suffering from acute cholecystitis or to convert patients that are on long-term cholecystostomy to endoscopic drainage (Table 28.1) [22]. Endoscopic gallbladder drainage could be achieved by the transpapillary or transmural approach [58–62]. The transpapillary approach is performed with a duodenoscope. It is technically more demanding as the cystic duct needs to be cannulated and stones that are obstructing the Hartman's pouch to be dislodged in order for successful drainage of the gallbladder to the duodenum with a plastic stent. Thus, the EUS-guided transmural approach may be more advantageous. The approach avoids the difficulties of the transpapillary approach and allows placement of a large diameter stent in the gallbladder. Furthermore, endoscopic gallbladder interventions could also be performed through the stent and it may potentially reduce the risk of recurrent cholecystitis.

EGBD involves creation of a cholecysto-gastric or duodenal fistula and placement of a stent for gallbladder drainage. There are a number of difficulties associated with the procedure. Firstly, the gallbladder is a freely mobile organ and the position may vary with different individuals. Furthermore, there is a risk of bile leak during the procedure during exchange of devices. Lastly, the integrity of the anastomosis is dependent on the stent. Premature migration of the stent can result in free perforation in two organs and result in catastrophic outcomes. Hence, a

reliable EUS-specific stent with high lumen apposing force that can reduce the number of device exchange is essential [63].

Technique of EGBD

There are two described techniques of EGBD (Fig. 28.6). The conventional method involves puncturing of the gallbladder under EUS-guidance, dilation of the needle track with a coaxial diathermy device, and balloons, followed by insertion of a lumen-apposing stent [17, 24, 64]. The direct puncture method involves single-step direct insertion of a cautery-tipped stent delivery system and deployment of the stent

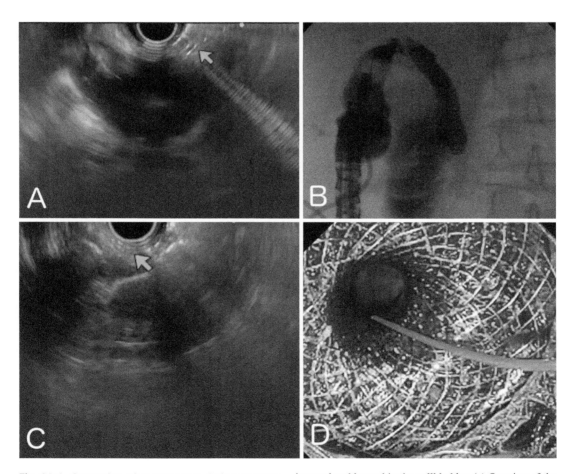

Fig. 28.6 Conversion of percutaneous cholecystostomy to EGBD. (**a**) The gallbladder punctured with a 19-gauge needle from the 1st part of the duodenum. (**b**) A guidewire inserted and looped in the gallbladder. (**c**) Opening of the distal flange of a lumen-apposing stent. (**d**) Opening of the proximal flange of a lumen-apposing stent

[65]. This method avoids the need of exchanging devices and reduces the risk of bile leak during the procedure. In situations where the endoscope position is stable with a large gallbladder, the direct method is preferred. However, in situations where the endoscope is at an unstable position or if the gallbladder is contracted, the conventional method is preferred.

How Does EGBD Compare to Percutaneous Drainage?

EGBD is associated with a high technical success of 90–98.7% and clinical success of 89–98.4% [21, 23, 25, 31]. Adverse events of 4.8–22%, including bleeding, recurrent cholecystitis, stent migration, and occlusion, have been reported. One randomized study compared EUS-guided placement of a naso-gallbladder drainage tube to percutaneous cholecystostomy as a temporarizing measure before cholecystectomy [17]. Similar technical (97% vs. 97%), clinical success rates (100% vs. 96%), and adverse events (7% vs. 3%) were reported. EGBD was associated with significantly lower postprocedure pain scores (1 vs. 5; $P < 0.001$). In terms of using EGBD as a definitive method for gallbladder drainage in patients suffering from acute cholecystitis, the results from four comparative studies are available [26–29]. Three studies used lumen-apposing stents, 1 study used regular fully covered metal stents. All studies reported comparable technical and clinical success rates between the two procedures. Teoh et al. reported significantly lower 1-year adverse events rates ($P < 0.001$) and readmission rates for reintervention ($P < 0.001$) in the EGBD group. The majority of these were due to tube-related problems in the PTC group. While the other 2 studies reported similar 30-day adverse events rate but a lower reintervention rate in the EGBD group. Irani et al. also reported lower postprocedural pain scores in the EGBD group. On the other hand, one study compared EGBD to PTC in patients with acute cholecystitis secondary to malignant cystic duct obstruction. No difference in success rates and adverse events were observed, but the EGBD group was associated with shorter hospital stay.

On the other hand, the large diameter stents used for EGBD can also act as a portal for advanced gallbladder interventions [32, 66]. After lithotripsy, stone clearance from the gallbladder could be achieved in 88% of the patients after a mean number of 1.25 sessions of per-oral cholecystoscopy. Image-enhanced mucosal imaging could also be performed, and gallbladder polyps could also be removed.

Conclusions

EUS-BD is gaining popularity as the procedure of choice in patients with failed ERC. Further comparative studies are required to demonstrate superiority of one type of EUS-BD procedure over the other. In EGBD, accumulating evidence supports the use of EGBD over percutaneous cholecystostomy for patients that are unfit for cholecystectomy. Future studies are also required to assess the optimal period of stent placement, the duration for stent exchange, and total duration of stent placement in EUS-guided transmural drainage. Excellent techniques with dedicated devices are essential to all procedures to produce optimal results and avoiding serious adverse events.

References

1. Moss AC, Morris E, Mac Mathuna P. Palliative biliary stents for obstructing pancreatic carcinoma. Cochrane Database Syst Rev. 2006:CD004200.
2. Lai EC, Mok FP, Tan ES, et al. Endoscopic biliary drainage for severe acute cholangitis. N Engl J Med. 1992;326:1582–6.
3. Speer AG, Cotton PB, Russell RC, et al. Randomised trial of endoscopic versus percutaneous stent insertion in malignant obstructive jaundice. Lancet. 1987;2:57–62.
4. van Delden OM, Lameris JS. Percutaneous drainage and stenting for palliation of malignant bile duct obstruction. Eur Radiol. 2008;18:448–56.
5. Zhao XQ, Dong JH, Jiang K, et al. Comparison of percutaneous transhepatic biliary drainage and endoscopic biliary drainage in the management of malignant biliary tract obstruction: a meta-analysis. Dig Endosc. 2015;27:137–45.
6. Baron TH, Petersen BT, Mergener K, et al. Quality indicators for endoscopic retrograde cholangiopancreatography. Am J Gastroenterol. 2006;101:892–7.

7. Kolla SB, Aggarwal S, Kumar A, et al. Early versus delayed laparoscopic cholecystectomy for acute cholecystitis: a prospective randomized trial. Surg Endosc. 2004;18:1323–7.

8. Lai PB, Kwong KH, Leung KL, et al. Randomized trial of early versus delayed laparoscopic cholecystectomy for acute cholecystitis. Br J Surg. 1998;85:764–7.

9. Lo CM, Liu CL, Fan ST, et al. Prospective randomized study of early versus delayed laparoscopic cholecystectomy for acute cholecystitis. Ann Surg. 1998;227:461–7.

10. Johansson M, Thune A, Nelvin L, et al. Randomized clinical trial of open versus laparoscopic cholecystectomy in the treatment of acute cholecystitis. Br J Surg. 2005;92:44–9.

11. Teoh AY, Chong CN, Wong J, et al. Routine early laparoscopic cholecystectomy for acute cholecystitis after conclusion of a randomized controlled trial. Br J Surg. 2007;94:1128–32.

12. Tsuyuguchi T, Itoi T, Takada T, et al. TG13 indications and techniques for gallbladder drainage in acute cholecystitis (with videos). J Hepatobiliary Pancreat Sci. 2013;20:81–8.

13. McKay A, Abulfaraj M, Lipschitz J. Short- and long-term outcomes following percutaneous cholecystostomy for acute cholecystitis in high-risk patients. Surg Endosc. 2012;26:1343–51.

14. Boules M, Haskins IN, Farias-Kovac M, et al. What is the fate of the cholecystostomy tube following percutaneous cholecystostomy? Surg Endosc. 2017;31:1707–12.

15. Lee SS, Park DH, Hwang CY, et al. EUS-guided transmural cholecystostomy as rescue management for acute cholecystitis in elderly or high-risk patients: a prospective feasibility study. Gastrointest Endosc. 2007;66:1008–12.

16. Jang JW, Lee SS, Park DH, et al. Feasibility and safety of EUS-guided transgastric/transduodenal gallbladder drainage with single-step placement of a modified covered self-expandable metal stent in patients unsuitable for cholecystectomy. Gastrointest Endosc. 2011;74:176–81.

17. Jang JW, Lee SS, Song TJ, et al. Endoscopic ultrasound-guided transmural and percutaneous transhepatic gallbladder drainage are comparable for acute cholecystitis. Gastroenterology. 2012;142:805–11.

18. Itoi T, Binmoeller KF, Shah J, et al. Clinical evaluation of a novel lumen-apposing metal stent for endosonography-guided pancreatic pseudocyst and gallbladder drainage (with videos). Gastrointest Endosc. 2012;75:870–6.

19. de la Serna-Higuera C, Perez-Miranda M, Gil-Simon P, et al. EUS-guided transenteric gallbladder drainage with a new fistula-forming, lumen-apposing metal stent. Gastrointest Endosc. 2013;77:303–8.

20. Moon JH, Choi HJ, Kim DC, et al. A newly designed fully covered metal stent for lumen apposition in EUS-guided drainage and access: a feasibility study (with videos). Gastrointest Endosc. 2014;79:990–5.

21. Choi JH, Lee SS, Choi JH, et al. Long-term outcomes after endoscopic ultrasonography-guided gallbladder drainage for acute cholecystitis. Endoscopy. 2014;46:656–61.

22. Law R, Grimm IS, Stavas JM, et al. Conversion of percutaneous cholecystostomy to internal transmural gallbladder drainage using an endoscopic ultrasound-guided, lumen-apposing metal stent. Clin Gastroenterol Hepatol. 2016;14:476–80.

23. Walter D, Teoh AY, Itoi T, et al. EUS-guided gall bladder drainage with a lumen-apposing metal stent: a prospective long-term evaluation. Gut. 2016;65:6–8.

24. Ge N, Sun S, Sun S, et al. Endoscopic ultrasound-assisted transmural cholecystoduodenostomy or cholecystogastrostomy as a bridge for per-oral cholecystoscopy therapy using double-flanged fully covered metal stent. BMC Gastroenterol. 2016;16:9.

25. Kahaleh M, Perez-Miranda M, Artifon EL, et al. International collaborative study on EUS-guided gallbladder drainage: are we ready for prime time? Dig Liver Dis. 2016;48:1054–7.

26. Teoh AY, Serna C, Penas I, et al. Endoscopic ultrasound-guided gallbladder drainage reduces adverse events compared with percutaneous cholecystostomy in patients who are unfit for cholecystectomy. Endoscopy. 2017;49:130–8.

27. Tyberg A, Saumoy M, Sequeiros EV, et al. EUS-guided versus percutaneous gallbladder drainage: isn't it time to convert? J Clin Gastroenterol. 2016;52:79.

28. Irani S, Ngamruengphong S, Teoh A, et al. Similar efficacies of endoscopic ultrasound gallbladder drainage with a lumen-apposing metal stent versus percutaneous transhepatic gallbladder drainage for acute cholecystitis. Clin Gastroenterol Hepatol. 2017;15:738–45.

29. Choi JH, Kim HW, Lee JC, et al. Percutaneous transhepatic versus EUS-guided gallbladder drainage for malignant cystic duct obstruction. Gastrointest Endosc. 2017;85:357–64.

30. Kamata K, Takenaka M, Kitano M, et al. Endoscopic ultrasound-guided gallbladder drainage for acute cholecystitis: long-term outcomes after removal of a self-expandable metal stent. World J Gastroenterol. 2017;23:661–7.

31. Dollhopf M, Larghi A, Will U, et al. Eus-guided gallbladder drainage in patients with acute cholecystitis and high surgical risk using an electrocautery-enhanced lumen-apposing metal stent device. Gastrointest Endosc. 2017;86:636.

32. Chan SM, Teoh AY, Yip HC, et al. Feasibility of per-oral cholecystoscopy and advanced gallbladder interventions after EUS-guided gallbladder stenting (with video). Gastrointest Endosc. 2016;85:1225.

33. Itoi T, Sofuni A, Itokawa F, et al. Endoscopic ultrasonography-guided biliary drainage. J Hepatobiliary Pancreat Sci. 2010;17:611–6.

34. Dhir V, Isayama H, Itoi T, et al. EUS-guided biliary and pancreatic duct interventions. Dig Endosc. 2017;29:472.

35. Park SJ, Choi JH, Park DH, et al. Expanding indication: EUS-guided hepaticoduodenostomy for isolated right intrahepatic duct obstruction (with video). Gastrointest Endosc. 2013;78:374–80.

36. Ogura T, Edogawa S, Imoto A, et al. EUS-guided hepaticojejunostomy combined with antegrade stent placement. Gastrointest Endosc. 2015;81:462–3.

37. Liao WC, Angsuwatcharakon P, Isayama H, et al. International consensus recommendations for difficult biliary access. Gastrointest Endosc. 2017;85:295–304.

38. Holt BA, Hawes R, Hasan M, et al. Biliary drainage: role of EUS guidance. Gastrointest Endosc. 2016;83:160–5.

39. Shah JN, Marson F, Weilert F, et al. Single-operator, single-session EUS-guided anterograde cholangiopancreatography in failed ERCP or inaccessible papilla. Gastrointest Endosc. 2012;75:56–64.

40. Park DH, Lee TH, Paik WH, et al. Feasibility and safety of a novel dedicated device for one-step EUS-guided biliary drainage: a randomized trial. J Gastroenterol Hepatol. 2015;30:1461–6.

41. Bapaye A, Dubale N, Aher A. Comparison of endosonography-guided vs. percutaneous biliary stenting when papilla is inaccessible for ERCP. United European Gastroenterol J. 2013;1:285–93.

42. Khashab MA, Valeshabad AK, Afghani E, et al. A comparative evaluation of EUS-guided biliary drainage and percutaneous drainage in patients with distal malignant biliary obstruction and failed ERCP. Dig Dis Sci. 2015;60:557–65.

43. Sharaiha RZ, Kumta NA, Desai AP, et al. Endoscopic ultrasound-guided biliary drainage versus percutaneous transhepatic biliary drainage: predictors of successful outcome in patients who fail endoscopic retrograde cholangiopancreatography. Surg Endosc. 2016;30:5500–5.

44. Artifon EL, Aparicio D, Paione JB, et al. Biliary drainage in patients with unresectable, malignant obstruction where ERCP fails: endoscopic ultrasonography-guided choledochoduodenostomy versus percutaneous drainage. J Clin Gastroenterol. 2012;46:768–74.

45. Lee TH, Choi JH, Park do H, et al. Similar efficacies of endoscopic ultrasound-guided transmural and percutaneous drainage for malignant distal biliary obstruction. Clin Gastroenterol Hepatol. 2016;14:1011–1019 e3.

46. Sharaiha RZ, Khan MA, Kamal F, et al. Efficacy and safety of EUS-guided biliary drainage in comparison with percutaneous biliary drainage when ERCP fails: a systematic review and meta-analysis. Gastrointest Endosc. 2017;85:904.

47. Park JK, Woo YS, Noh DH, et al. Efficacy of EUS-guided and ERCP-guided biliary drainage for malignant biliary obstruction: prospective randomized controlled study. Gastrointest Endosc. 2018;88:277–82.

48. Bang JY, Navaneethan U, Hasan M, et al. Stent placement by EUS or ERCP for primary biliary decompression in pancreatic cancer: a randomized trial (with videos). Gastrointest Endosc. 2018;88:9–17.

49. Paik WH, Lee TH, Park DH, et al. EUS-guided biliary drainage versus ERCP for the primary palliation of malignant biliary obstruction: a multicenter randomized clinical trial. Am J Gastroenterol. 2018;113:987–97.

50. Dhir V, Bhandari S, Bapat M, et al. Comparison of EUS-guided rendezvous and precut papillotomy techniques for biliary access (with videos). Gastrointest Endosc. 2012;75:354–9.

51. Lee A, Aditi A, Bhat YM, et al. Endoscopic ultrasound-guided biliary access versus precut papillotomy in patients with failed biliary cannulation: a retrospective study. Endoscopy. 2017;49:146–53.

52. Bill JG, Darcy M, Fujii-Lau LL, et al. A comparison between endoscopic ultrasound-guided rendezvous and percutaneous biliary drainage after failed ERCP for malignant distal biliary obstruction. Endosc Int Open. 2016;4:E980–5.

53. Artifon EL, Marson FP, Gaidhane M, et al. Hepaticogastrostomy or choledochoduodenostomy for distal malignant biliary obstruction after failed ERCP: is there any difference? Gastrointest Endosc. 2015;81:950–9.

54. Ogura T, Chiba Y, Masuda D, et al. Comparison of the clinical impact of endoscopic ultrasound-guided choledochoduodenostomy and hepaticogastrostomy for bile duct obstruction with duodenal obstruction. Endoscopy. 2016;48:156–63.

55. Khan MA, Akbar A, Baron TH, et al. Endoscopic ultrasound-guided biliary drainage: a systematic review and meta-analysis. Dig Dis Sci. 2016;61:684–703.

56. Khashab MA, Messallam AA, Penas I, et al. International multicenter comparative trial of transluminal EUS-guided biliary drainage via hepatogastrostomy vs. choledochoduodenostomy approaches. Endosc Int Open. 2016;4:E175–81.

57. Park DH, Jang JW, Lee SS, et al. EUS-guided biliary drainage with transluminal stenting after failed ERCP: predictors of adverse events and long-term results. Gastrointest Endosc. 2011;74:1276–84.

58. Toyota N, Takada T, Amano H, et al. Endoscopic naso-gallbladder drainage in the treatment of acute cholecystitis: alleviates inflammation and fixes operator's aim during early laparoscopic cholecystectomy. J Hepato-Biliary-Pancreat Surg. 2006;13:80–5.

59. Kjaer DW, Kruse A, Funch-Jensen P. Endoscopic gallbladder drainage of patients with acute cholecystitis. Endoscopy. 2007;39:304–8.

60. Itoi T, Sofuni A, Itokawa F, et al. Endoscopic transpapillary gallbladder drainage in patients with acute cholecystitis in whom percutaneous transhepatic approach is contraindicated or anatomically impossible (with video). Gastrointest Endosc. 2008;68:455–60.

61. Itoi T, Kawakami H, Katanuma A, et al. Endoscopic nasogallbladder tube or stent placement in acute

cholecystitis: a preliminary prospective randomized trial in Japan (with videos). Gastrointest Endosc. 2015;81:111–8.

62. Itoi T, Takada T, Hwang TL, et al. Percutaneous and endoscopic gallbladder drainage for the acute cholecystitis: international multicenter comparative study by a propensity score-matched analysis. J Hepatobiliary Pancreat Sci. 2017; 24:362.

63. Teoh AY, Ng EK, Chan SM, et al. Ex vivo comparison of the lumen-apposing properties of EUS-specific stents (with video). Gastrointest Endosc. 2016;84:62–8.

64. Itoi T, Coelho-Prabhu N, Baron TH. Endoscopic gallbladder drainage for management of acute cholecystitis. Gastrointest Endosc. 2010;71:1038–45.

65. Teoh AY, Binmoeller KF, Lau JY. Single-step EUS-guided puncture and delivery of a lumen-apposing stent for gallbladder drainage using a novel cautery-tipped stent delivery system. Gastrointest Endosc. 2014;80:1171.

66. Teoh AY, Chan AW, Chiu PW, et al. In vivo appearances of gallbladder carcinoma under magnifying endoscopy and probe-based confocal laser endomicroscopy after endosonographic gallbladder drainage. Endoscopy. 2014;46(Suppl 1 UCTN):E13–4.

Jason B. Samarasena, Kyle J. Fortinsky, and Kenneth J. Chang

Introduction

As new technologies are created, the field of interventional endoscopy and interventional EUS has widened its scope of practice [1]. From managing gastrointestinal bleeding, treating pancreaticobiliary diseases, and removing epithelial and subepithelial lesions, the possibilities of endoscopy are seemingly endless. EUS-guided procedures offer an entirely new approach to vascular access, especially those structures, which lie in close proximity to the gastrointestinal tract. Across medicine, there is a trend toward minimally invasive procedures, and EUS provides such an avenue to deal with both common and rare diseases and disorders. The chapter is organized into several sections that each highlights a separate procedure that can be performed under EUS guidance.

Electronic Supplementary Material The online version of this chapter (https://doi.org/10.1007/978-3-030-21695-5_29) contains supplementary material, which is available to authorized users.

J. B. Samarasena
Department of Medicine – Gastroenterology, University of California, Irvine Medical Center, Orange, CA, USA

K. J. Fortinsky · K. J. Chang (✉)
Department of Medicine, H.H. Chao Comprehensive Digestive Disease Center, University of California, Irvine Medical Center, Orange, CA, USA
e-mail: kchang@uci.edu

Esophageal Variceal Bleeding

Current AASLD guidelines suggest that patients with actively bleeding esophageal varices be treated with a combination of endoscopic variceal ligation (EVL) and medical management [2]. Although endoscopic sclerotherapy (ES) has been shown to be effective for management of acute bleeding episodes, it is associated with increased risks compared to EVL and is not recommended [3]. Up to 10–20% of patients may continue bleeding despite EVL and medical therapy. These patients require additional interventions, which may include temporary balloon tamponade or insertion of a transjugular intrahepatic portosystemic shunt (TIPS). Other emerging rescue procedures include fully covered esophageal stent insertion and hemostatic powders [4]. Some of the reported reasons for recurrent or refractory bleeding include dislodged bands, collateral blood flow, and postbanding ulceration [5].

Recent studies have suggested a possible role of EUS in the management of patients with esophageal varices. One study performed diagnostic EUS in patients after EVL for esophageal varices. Carneiro et al. found that there was a significant correlation between the diameter of paraesophageal varices and the risk of recurrent bleeding episodes [6]. Other groups have performed EUS-guided sclerotherapy for esophageal varices [7]. In one observational study of 5

M. S. Wagh, S. B. Wani (eds.), *Gastrointestinal Interventional Endoscopy*,
https://doi.org/10.1007/978-3-030-21695-5_29

patients, sodium morrhuate was injected into the esophageal varix until cessation of flow was noted by Doppler flow [7]. A mean of 2.2 sessions was required to eradicate the esophageal varices. None of the patients developed rebleeding after 15 months of follow-up and 1 patient developed an esophageal stricture requiring dilations. More recently, De Paulo et al randomized 50 patients with esophageal variceal bleeding to either EUS-guided sclerotherapy or endoscopic sclerotherapy [8]. There were no differences between the two groups in terms of number or procedures required to obliterate the vessels. Notably, rebleeding rates were associated with the presence of collateral vessels.

The potential use of EUS-guided therapy for esophageal variceal bleeding includes the identification of collateral blood vessels for targeted therapy. Whether EUS adds any benefit in terms of clinical outcomes remains to be seen. Further research is required to determine whether EUS-guided therapies are effective as salvage therapies and as a possible alternative to balloon tamponade, esophageal stenting, or TIPS.

Gastric Variceal Bleeding

Gastric varices occur in approximately 20% of patients with cirrhosis [9]. The Sarin classification is classically used to describe the location of these varices. Gastric varices that are contiguous with esophageal varices are described as either GOV-1 (extending along the lesser curve) or GOV-2 (extending into the fundus). Isolated gastric varices are separate from esophageal varices and are described as IGV1 (located in the fundus) or IGV-2 (located at the antrum or pylorus). Unlike esophageal varices, prophylactic endoscopic treatment for gastric varices is not recommended by current AASLD guidelines [10].

Current AASLD guidelines suggest either EVL or cyanoacrylate injection for management of GOV-1 gastric varices [2]. Both therapies are effective at initial hemostasis, although cyanoacrylate injection is associated with a lower risk of rebleeding [11]. The major risks associated with this injection include gastric ulceration, perfora-

tion, and embolization [12–15]. EVL can be challenging and is less effective than for esophageal varices [16]. Notably, cyanoacrylate injection is not approved for use in the US, although it is being performed in specialized centers within Canada and certain parts of Europe and Asia. The most widely accepted treatment for all other gastric varices (GOV-2 and IGV) includes TIPS and Balloon-occluded Retrograde Transvenous Obliteration (BRTO). Endoscopic CYA injection for GVs, first described in 1986, has become the treatment of choice for GVs [10, 17]. Hemostasis rates of 58–100% and rebleeding rates of 0–40% have been reported [18]. The major and most serious adverse event associated with CYA therapy is systemic embolization, including pulmonary embolism, cardiac embolism, splenic artery embolism, and paradoxical cerebral embolism in patients with a patent foramen ovale [19]. Additional complications include splenic vein thrombosis, renal vein thrombosis, entrapment of the needle in the varix by CYA, and damage to the endoscope [19]. One randomized trial of patients with GOV1 and GOV2 found that TIPS is more effective than glue injection in preventing rebleeding, but that TIPS did not have any mortality benefit and was associated with a higher rate of encephalopathy [20].

EUS offers certain opportunities to assist in the management of patients with gastric variceal bleeding. In some circumstances, EUS with Doppler can help identify the presence of gastric varices, which can sometimes be mistaken for thickened folds [21]. EUS assessment post treatment can also help identify ongoing flow, which warrants more aggressive treatment. Residual patency of gastric varices after treatment does correlate with subsequent bleeding risk [22]. Additionally, EUS-guided interventions can be useful in the event of poor visualization due to actively bleeding varices. Lastly, EUS-guided injection of sclerotherapy may permit enhanced visualization of the "feeder" vessel and ensuring the injection itself is placed directly within the vessel, which may reduce embolization risk when using CYA [23, 24]. Figure 29.1 depicts a case of identification of gastric varices by EUS followed by EUS-guided FNA injection of sclerosant.

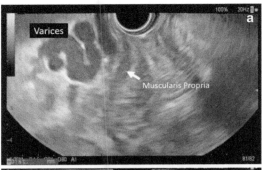

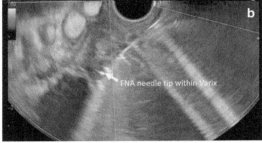

Fig. 29.1 (**a**) Identification by EUS of gastric varices. (**b**) EUS-guided FNA injection of sclerosant into gastric varix

Given the risks associated with cyanoacrylate injection, newer techniques have been developed, which utilize EUS-guided placement of metal coils. These coils, made of metal alloy and radially extending synthetic fibers, work to induce hemostasis through formation of clots. Different sizes of coils can be deployed through either a 19-gauge or 22-gauge needle depending on the size of the varix. The needle stylet is used to push and deploy the coil into the varix. Initial studies demonstrated efficacy of this technique in the management of gastric varices [25].

A retrospective trial compared 30 patients with gastric varices who received either EUS-guided glue injection or EUS-guided coil placement [26]. The rates of obliteration of varices were equivalent in both groups; however, the glue injection group had significantly more adverse events (58% vs. 9%, $p = 0.01$). The most common adverse event was asymptomatic pulmonary embolism as detected on routine CT scan.

Binmoeller et al. reported EUS-guided placement of coil combined with glue injection in 30 patients with large GVs who were poor candidates for TIPS [27]. The authors describe the

method of coil and glue injection of gastric varices, which was done under EUS-guidance through the esophagus. They explain that a transesophageal approach has the benefit of not puncturing the gastric mucosa directly and also avoiding any gastric contents. In their study, the vast majority of patients with follow-up EUS (23/24) had confirmed obliteration of their varices. No complications were reported. The same group published a study of 152 patients with a mean follow-up of 436 days [28]. Of 100 patients who had a follow-up EUS, 93% had confirmed obliteration of varices and recurrent bleeding occurred in only 10 patients.

Binmoeller et al. described their technique in great detail [27]. All patients are given broad-spectrum prophylactic intravenous antibiotics. The gastric fundus is filled with water to allow visualization and a curvilinear echoendoscope is positioned in the distal esophagus to visualize the gastric varices through the diaphragmatic crus. Color Doppler is used to visualize the gastric varices and to identify the feeder vessel. Next, a 19G or 22G straight FNA needle is used to puncture the varix through the esophageal wall and diaphragmatic crus. A 7-cm long, and 10- or 20-mm diameter coil is loaded into the FNA needle, and the stylet is used to push the coil into the varix. The coil diameter size is chosen based on the EUS-guided measurement of the short-axis diameter of the varix. A 0.035-inch coil can only be used with a 19G needle, while a 0.018-inch coil can be used with a 22G needle [29]. After coil placement, 1 mL of 2-octyl-CYA is injected into the varix over 30–45 seconds through the same needle using normal saline as a flush. A repeat EUS examination is performed 10 minutes later to note any persistent color Doppler flow, which may require additional management. Additional glue injections in 1 mL increments can be provided. Additional coils can also be delivered using a new FNA needle.

Two crucial aspects of the procedure to avoid damage to the echoendoscope are described. First, one should avoid using suction after glue injection to avoid damage to the suction channel of the echoendoscope. Second, after glue injection, the sheath of the needle is advanced 2–3 cm beyond the endoscope tip and the echoendoscope removed from the patient to avoid any contact of the glue with the working channel of the scope.

Postprocedure, the patient is closely monitored for 24–48 hours for signs of infection, bleeding, or embolization. Repeat upper endoscopy and EUS may be performed at 1-month postprocedure to ensure complete resolution of the varices. Additional endoscopic follow-up is guided by current AASLD guidelines.

Ectopic Variceal Bleeding

Patients with portal hypertension can develop ectopic varices, which occur most commonly around surgical stomas, duodenum, jejuno-ileum, and colon [30]. While rare, rates of bleeding from ectopic varices account for up to 5% of all variceal bleeding. Ectopic varices have a fourfold increased risk of bleeding compared to esophageal varices, and mortality rates have been reported up to 40% [31, 32].

Duodenal varices may be managed in a similar way to esophageal and gastric varices. One large review highlighted the use of TIPS, BRTO, band ligation, and sclerotherapy in these patients [33]. There are a few reports of successful obliteration of duodenal varices using EUS-guided coil placement with or without cyanoacrylate injection [34–36]. An additional report successfully obliterated a duodenal varix using EUS-guided thrombin injection [37].

Rectal varices arise from portosystemic collaterals that occur as a result of portal hypertension. These varices are commonly diagnosed on anoscopy [38]. The single largest study of rectal varices identified 96 cirrhotic patients, of which 51% had evidence of rectal varices on EUS [39]. Interestingly, only half of the patients identified on EUS to have varices actually had endoscopic evidence of varices. Massive bleeding from rectal varices has been reported in 0.5–3.6% of cases [40–42]. Sharma et al described a series of 5 patients with lower GI bleeding, 2 of whom required EUS to identify the rectal varices [43]. Several other groups have reported EUS-guided coiling and/or cyanoacrylate injection for rectal varices [44–48]. EUS-guided CYA injection has also been reported for use in the management of peristomal varices [49].

Nonvariceal Gastrointestinal Bleeding

Despite initial resuscitation, medical management, and endoscopic therapy, certain patients will have recurrent bleeding requiring additional interventions [50]. Endoscopic therapy for nonvariceal gastrointestinal bleeding may include one or a combination of the following: epinephrine injection, thermal coaptive therapy, clipping, and more recently hemostatic powders [51, 52]. Upon failing endoscopic therapy, the current standard of care would include either transcatheter arterial embolization (by interventional radiology) or surgical intervention. Ultrasound-guided techniques have allowed for some novel treatments for patients with nonvariceal gastrointestinal bleeding.

A Doppler endoscopic probe has been used to help characterize peptic ulcer rebleeding risk when compared to conventional measures such as the Forrest classification. While certain studies have shown no added benefit of the Doppler probe in the management of patients with ulcer-related bleeding [53, 54], one prospective study of 163 patients showed that the Doppler probe accurately predicted rebleeding rates based upon arterial blood flow at the base of the ulcer [55]. Importantly, the Doppler flow measured after endoscopic treatment correlated with rebleeding risk. This study was the first to highlight the role of Doppler in addition to the Forrest classification to determine a more accurate endpoint for endoscopic treatment. Future multicenter randomized controlled studies are needed to confirm these findings.

Endoscopic ultrasound–guided imaging has allowed for more precise interventions in the management of nonvariceal gastrointestinal bleeding. Fockens et al. were the first group to use a radial echoendoscope to aid in the management of 3 patients with Dieulafoy lesions [56]. Using EUS, they located a submucosal blood vessel, which was then injected with epinephrine/polidocanol as sclerotherapy.

Another reported case series used a curved linear echoendoscope to manage five patients with refractory gastrointestinal bleeding from GI stromal tumors, hemosuccus pancreaticus, and a duodenal ulcer [57]. These five patients had failed multiple prior endoscopic interventions requiring multiple transfusions. Each patient underwent a careful EUS examination to identify the culprit vessel, which was then injected with either alcohol or cyanoacrylate glue via a 22-gauge FNA needle. Postinjection imaging confirmed a lack of flow within the culprit vessel. Over a mean follow-up of 1-year, there were no complications or rebleeding events. A similar case series reported five patients with refractory GI bleeding secondary to a gastroduodenal artery aneurysm, fundal aneurysm, or Dieulafoy lesion. Using EUS guidance, the bleeding vessel was punctured with a 19-gauge FNA needle and injected with either cyanoacrylate glue or polidocanol. Over a mean follow-up of 9-months, only one patient rebled, requiring repeat EUS-guided injection. Several other case reports have used EUS-guided sclerotherapy to treat a variety of patients with bleeding from Dieulafoy's lesions [58, 59], a GIST [60], a splenic pseudoaneurysm after pseudocyst drainage [61], and arterial pseudoaneurysm s [62–64].

Law et al. examined the safety and efficacy of EUS-guided management of nonvariceal GI bleeding in 17 patients with refractory GI bleeding [65]. These patients included those with bleeding GIST, colorectal vascular malformations, duodenal masses or polyps, Dieulafoy lesions, peptic ulcers, rectally invasive prostate cancer, pseudoaneurysms, ulcerated esophageal cancer, and ulcer after Roux-en-Y gastric bypass. These patients had either failed endoscopic or radiologic procedures, or were not candidates for surgical intervention. Many of the patients had received multiple blood transfusions, failed multiple endoscopic attempts, and some even failed IR-guided interventions or surgical intervention. Various EUS-guided procedures were performed including sclerotherapy injection, coil embolization, and even band ligation, whereby EUS was used to create a subepithelial tattoo mark at the location of the vessel. After endoscopic treatment, Doppler confirmed eradication of the underlying blood vessel. Over a median follow-up of 1-year, only two patients had recurrent bleeding. One patient rebled 3 years later and required an additional EUS-guided intervention. Another patient with invasive prostate cancer continued to bleed despite endoscopic therapy.

While current international guidelines do not endorse a role for either Doppler assessment or EUS-guided therapy of nonvariceal GI bleeding [51, 52, 66], there are several case reports that suggest such treatments are both safe and effective for managing certain patients with refractory bleeding. Being able to target the culprit vessel directly and confirm complete eradication after endoscopic therapy may assist in the management of certain patients presenting with nonvariceal GI bleeding.

Pancreatic Pseudoaneurysms

Pancreatic pseudoaneurysms are a rare complication of pseudocyst formation in the context of chronic pancreatitis [67]. These pseudoaneurysms can result in life-threatening bleeding, especially in the context of EUS-guided cyst drainage [68]. While traditionally performed by IR-guided embolization [69], or surgery in severe circumstances [70], there is emerging data of an EUS-guided approach. There are several reports of successful treatment of pseudoaneurysms using a combination of EUS-guided coiling, thrombin injection, and glue injection [71–74].

Portal Pressure Gradient Measurement

Diagnosing and measuring portal hypertension is important in classifying and prognosticating patients with cirrhosis [75, 76]. Transcutaneous portal venography and pressure measurements are not performed in clinical practice due to technical difficulties and a high rate of complications [77]. The portal pressure gradient (PPG) can be measured as the difference between the portal vein pressure and the pressure within the hepatic vein. The most common approach to measuring portal pressure is the transjugular route by interventional radiologists [78]. In this approach, a catheter is placed into the jugular vein and advanced into the right hepatic vein under fluoroscopic guidance. Next, the hepatic vein pressure gradient (HVPG) is calculated by subtracting the free hepatic venous pressure from the wedged hepatic venous pressure [79]. A HVPG >5 mmHg is consistent with portal hypertension, while a HVPG >10 mmHg is consistent with clinically significant portal hypertension [80].

Lai and colleagues were the first to report EUS-guided portal vein pressure measurement in an animal study [81]. In a cohort of 21 pigs, a PH model was generated in 14 using polyvinyl alcohol injection and a coagulopathy model generated in 7 with heparin administration. The transduodenal approach was used to access the portal vein in 21 pigs with a 22G FNA needle and a transabdominal ultrasound (TAUS)-guided transhepatic approach in 14 of 21 pigs via a 22-gauge needle. PVP measurements were obtained in 18 of 21 swine. Minor complications found at necropsy included small subserosal hematomas at the EUS puncture site in all 21 pigs and a 25 mL blood collection between the liver and duodenum in 1 of 7 anticoagulated pigs. Failure to measure pressures in 3 subjects may have occurred due to thrombosis within the FNA needle. There was a strong correlation between EUS- and transhepatic-measured PVP ($r = 0.91$).

In 2007, Giday and colleagues used the transgastric approach with a 19G needle and modified ERCP catheter to obtain continuous PVP measurement without an echoendoscope in place [82]. Five pigs were successfully catheterized, and no hemorrhage or liver injury was noted on necropsy on all subjects despite use of a significantly larger caliber needle. Two of five pigs survived for 2 weeks and exhibited no signs of adverse events prior to and after necropsy. In 2008, the same group used the same methods to measure fluctuations in PVP and inferior vena cava (IVC) pressures in pigs that underwent common endoscopic procedures: esophagogastroduodenoscopy (EGD), colonoscopy, and ERCP. PV

and IVC were accessed using a 19G needle and modified ERCP catheter [83]. Access and pressure measurements of both vessels were achieved in all 5 pigs. Necropsy showed no evidence of injury in all subjects. A threefold increase in PVP was noted between baseline and during ERCP. Values of IVC pressure, as well as of PVP for EGD and colonoscopy, were similar between baseline and procedure time.

The first human case of EUS-guided PVP measurement was reported by Fujii-Lau and colleagues in 2014, in which a 22G FNA needle connected to an arterial pressure catheter was used to rule out portal hypertension in a 27-year-old man with arteriovenous malformations secondary to Noonan syndrome [84]. There was no evidence of bleeding or hemodynamic instability after the procedure.

Schulman et al. demonstrated a novel method of measuring PVP using an EUS-guided 22G needle, through which a wire with a digital pressure sensor was passed [85]. Conventional transjugular catheterization was performed as a control. Successful device placement and PVP measurement were achieved in 5 of 5 pigs with no hemorrhage or thrombosis noted on both EUS and postprocedural necropsy. Comparison of EUS-measured PVP with transjugular HVPG measurements showed a difference of within 1 mmHg for all pigs. The study endoscopists rated the procedure as having overall low subjective workload. The authors used the same device to perform PVP measurement in 5 other pigs that were then survived for 14 days before necropsy. PVP was again measured on day 14. No signs of complications were observed during the 2-week survival period, and necropsy again showed no abnormalities. PVP values on day 0 and day 14 were similar for all 5 pigs.

Our group demonstrated that EUS-guided PPG could be performed using a simple manometer setup without a wire [86]. The study was performed on 3 live pigs using a 25-gauge straight needle with a compact manometer. The portal vein, right hepatic vein, inferior vena cava, and aorta were punctured and pressures were measured. Simultaneously, an IR-guided approach was used to measure pressures in the aorta, inferior vena cava, and right hepatic vein

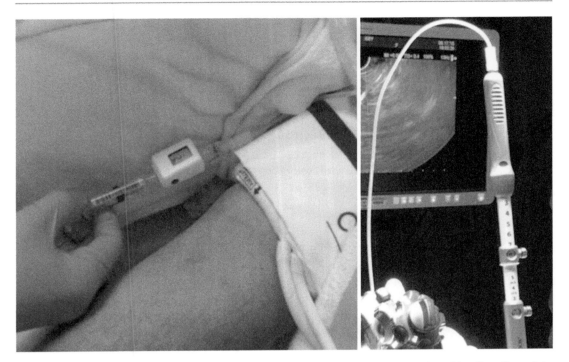

Fig. 29.2 Endoscopic Ultrasound–guided Portal Pressure Measurement apparatus showing noncompressible tubing attached to the FNA needle inlet (right pane) and compact manometer being placed at the mid-axillary line of the patient (left pane)

(wedged and free). The correlation coefficient was approximately 0.99 between EUS-guided and IR-guided approach. Similar results using slightly different devices have been reported by other groups in animal studies. The transhepatic route, which has been used in these animal studies, is thought to be protective against bleeding due to tamponade of the catheter track by the hepatic parenchyma. Furthermore, Doppler can be used to ensure there is no active bleeding during withdrawal of the needle.

Our group published the first study of EUS PPG measurements in a series of human patients [87]. All procedures were successful in obtaining a portal pressure gradient in 28 patients and there were no complications. The apparatus for PPG measurement includes a linear echoendoscope, a 25G FNA-needle, noncompressible tubing, a compact digital manometer, and heparinized saline. The tubing is connected by a luer lock to the distal port of the manometer, while the heparinized saline is connected to the proximal port of the manometer. The end of the tubing is connected via a Luer lock to the inlet of the 25G

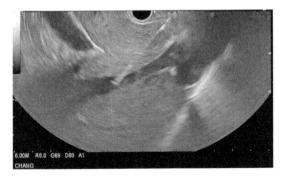

Fig. 29.3 EUS image of needle puncture of Middle Hepatic vein with 25G FNA needle

needle. Prior to echoendoscope insertion, the manometer is zeroed at the mid-axillary line. The patient remains supine during the EUS procedure, and the manometer is placed at the patient's mid-axillary line (Fig. 29.2).

The middle hepatic vein is targeted most commonly due to its larger caliber and better alignment with the needle trajectory on linear EUS (Fig. 29.3). Doppler flow is used to confirm the typical multiphasic waveform of hepatic venous

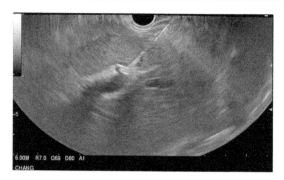

Fig. 29.4 EUS image of needle puncture of left portal vein with 25G FNA needle

flow. Using the 25G FNA needle, a transgastric transhepatic approach is used to puncture the hepatic vein. Approximately 1 cc of heparinized saline is used to flush the needle, which is visible on EUS, confirming good position within the vessel. Following the flush, the pressure reading on the manometer will immediately rise, fall, and equilibrate at a steady pressure, which is recorded. Repeat flushing and measurement is performed three times to ensure accuracy, and a mean hepatic vein pressure is recorded. The FNA needle is slowly withdrawn back into the needle sheath with Doppler flow to ensure there is no flow within the needle tract. If flow is noted within the needle track, the needle is kept in place to allow for tamponade and reduce risk of bleeding.

Next, the umbilical portion of the left portal vein is targeted (Fig. 29.4). Doppler flow is used to confirm the typical venous hum of portal venous flow. Using the 25G FNA needle, a transgastric transhepatic approach is used to puncture the portal vein. Three subsequent flushes and measurements are taken as above, which provides a mean portal vein pressure.

The portal pressure gradient is calculated by subtracting the mean portal vein pressure from the mean hepatic vein pressure. The patient is recovered in a similar manner to a routine diagnostic EUS with FNA. Postprocedural antibiotics are given for 5 days post procedure.

See Video 29.1 depicting a live case where PPG was measured in a human patient. The PPG

measurement correlated well to clinical and endoscopic parameters of cirrhosis including the presence of esophageal varices and portal hypertensive gastropathy. In a related study, our group showed the safety of combining EUS-guided liver biopsy and EUS PPG during the same endoscopy session [88]. These studies suggest that EUS-guided PPG measurements are both feasible and safe in cirrhotic patients. Furthermore, measuring portal pressure directly, as opposed to the commonly used HVPG provided by transjugular approach, may provide more accurate measurements, especially in the setting of presinusoidal portal hypertension.

Transjugular Intrahepatic Portosystemic Shunt (TIPS)

TIPS involves the creation of a low-resistance connection between the hepatic vein and intrahepatic portal vein using an expandable metal stent under angiographic and radiologic guidance. TIPS is indicated in patients with refractory ascites, variceal bleeding, and may be considered in patients with hepatorenal syndrome [89–92]. The first EUS-guided placement of an intrahepatic portosystemic shunt was performed in a live porcine model [93]. Under EUS-guidance, a 19-gauge FNA needle was passed through the hepatic vein into the portal vein, and after contrast confirmed adequate needle placement, a metal stent was placed over a 0.035-inch guidewire that bridged the hepatic and portal veins. The procedure was performed in 2 separate live pigs, and during 2-week follow-up, there were no complications. Two other groups utilized a similar procedural technique using instead a fully covered lumen-apposing metal stent (LAMS) to minimize the risk of possible stent migration. Both of these subsequent studies were performed in porcine models with no apparent complications [85, 94].

A recent editorial, however, highlights the danger of immediately concluding that EUS-guided placement of an intrahepatic is both safe and effective [95]. First, the procedure may be associated with a higher risk of bleeding when performed in cirrhotic patients with elevated portal pressures and poor coagulation. Second, there may be a higher risk of infection compared to traditionally placed TIPS due to the transgastric puncture. Third, a key component of TIPS is to choose the correct hepatic vein so as to minimize the angulation of the stent. Lastly, since the risks of TIPS are fairly low already, it is unclear whether EUS-guided procedure would have any significant benefits.

Intravascular Thrombi and Venous Sampling

Portal vein thrombosis may occur in the context of cirrhosis, hepatocellular carcinoma, pancreaticobiliary malignancy, and hematologic disorders including thrombophilias [96–98]. Staging of hepatocellular carcinoma and pancreaticobiliary malignancies rely on the accurate differentiation of a tumor thrombus from a benign portal vein thrombus [99–102]. Although contrast-enhanced ultrasound, CT, and MR have been shown to be helpful, occasionally imaging is nondiagnostic. In certain cases, targeted biopsies of the portal vein may be helpful for staging. Several reports have shown that EUS-guided FNA of a portal vein thrombus is both safe and helpful in differentiating a benign from a malignant thrombus. Importantly, FNA of the extrahepatic portal vein can be performed using a transduodenal approach, thus avoiding any liver tissue. EUS-guided FNA has also been useful in sampling a splenic artery thrombus, pulmonary artery thrombus, and an IVC thrombus in suspected hepatocellular carcinoma, lung cancer, and adrenal cancer, respectively [103–105].

One study examined the role of EUS-guided FNA of remote malignant thrombi in a retrospective cohort of 17 patients [106]. Of these patients, 12/17 (70.5%) patients had positive cytology. Most importantly, of the 8 patients with pancreatic cancer, 2/8 (25%) patients who were previously deemed resectable were now considered unresectable. Other studies have confirmed this finding, noting that circulating tumor cells in the context of pancreaticobiliary malignancy are found more frequently from portal vein blood than peripheral blood [107, 108].

Access to the Heart

Given the proximity of the esophagus to the heart and the widespread use of transesophageal echocardiography, some endoscopists have postulated a possible role for EUS-guided therapies of the heart. Fritscher-Ravens et al performed the first reported EUS-guided puncture of the heart using 19-gauge and 22-gauge needles [109]. Using this technique, they were able to access the left atrium, left ventricle, coronary arteries, and aortic valve. In the study, they successfully injected contrast agents, sampled pericardial fluid, biopsied a left atrial mass, performed radio-frequency ablation of the aortic valve, and inserted pacing wires. There were no complications during the procedures. There are 3 reports of EUS-guided cardiac access performed in human patients. One group described an EUS-guided drainage of a pericardial cyst [110], while two other groups described FNA of a pericardial tumor [111], and FNA of a right atrial tumor [112]. All three of these procedures had no significant adverse events.

Chemotherapeutics

Systemic chemotherapy is the mainstay of treatment for many types of cancer and is commonly associated with dose-limiting side effects. Furthermore, certain patients may not be candidates for systemic chemotherapy due to underlying comorbidities. Newer techniques, including transarterial chemoembolization (TACE), have provided certain patients with alternatives to traditional chemotherapy or surgical resection [113, 114]. TACE allows for microbead injection into the hepatic artery and affords higher hepatic drug levels with lower systemic levels, but major risks include decompensation of underlying liver disease and ischemic biliary strictures, since the hepatic artery is the sole provider of biliary duct blood supply [115, 116]. Newer techniques have attempted to inject chemotherapy in the portal vein in order to reduce the risk of ischemic biliary strictures. EUS-guided portal vein injection of chemotherapy (EPIC) has been performed successfully in animal models [117, 118]. EPIC allows for placement of drug-eluting microbeads or nanoparticles that results in lower systemic drug levels, but higher liver drug levels when compared to systemic injection. No direct comparisons between EPIC and TACE have been performed. Emerging evidence has suggested a role of direct portal vein injection of iodine-125 seeds into patients with HCC complicated by portal vein tumor thrombosis [119]. While these procedures were performed under CT guidance and results were promising, an EUS-guided approach may be equally efficacious and perhaps safer.

The Future of EUS-Guided Vascular Therapy

EUS-guided vascular procedures are an exciting field that bridges gastroenterology with interventional radiology. As equipment and techniques continue to develop, it is likely that more patients will be able to benefit from these less-invasive procedures. Given the specialized equipment and expertise required to perform many of these procedures, they will likely continue to be confined to high-volume tertiary care centers. Large multicenter prospective randomized controlled trials, which compare EUS-guided procedures with the current standard of care, are required to better delineate the effectiveness and safety of these procedures. While many of the procedures outlined in this chapter are innovative and exciting, few have been able to prove clinical benefit above and beyond the current standards of care.

Conclusion

EUS-guided vascular interventions are a promising new field that requires high-quality evidence in order to be incorporated into current guidelines. These less-invasive procedures offer alternatives to traditional endoscopy and interventional radiology, especially in patients in whom other options are limited or not feasible.

References

1. Chang KJ, Wiersema MJ. Endoscopic ultrasound-guided fine-needle aspiration biopsy and interventional endoscopic ultrasonography. Emerging technologies. Gastrointest Endosc Clin N Am. 1997;7(2):221–35.
2. Garcia-Tsao G, Abraldes JG, Berzigotti A, Bosch J. Portal hypertensive bleeding in cirrhosis: risk stratification, diagnosis, and management: 2016 practice guidance by the American Association for the study of liver diseases. Hepatology. 2017;65(1):310–35.
3. Laine L, Cook D. Endoscopic ligation compared with sclerotherapy for treatment of esophageal variceal bleeding. A meta-analysis. Ann Intern Med. 1995;123(4):280–7.
4. Escorsell A, Pavel O, Cardenas A, et al. Esophageal balloon tamponade versus esophageal stent in controlling acute refractory variceal bleeding: a multicenter randomized, controlled trial. Hepatology. 2016;63(6):1957–67.
5. Irisawa A, Saito A, Obara K, et al. Endoscopic recurrence of esophageal varices is associated with the specific EUS abnormalities: severe periesophageal collateral veins and large perforating veins. Gastrointest Endosc. 2001;53(1):77–84.
6. Carneiro FO, Retes FA, Matuguma SE, et al. Role of EUS evaluation after endoscopic eradication of esophageal varices with band ligation. Gastrointest Endosc. 2016;84(3):400–7.
7. Lahoti S, Catalano MF, Alcocer E, Hogan WJ, Geenen JE. Obliteration of esophageal varices using EUS-guided sclerotherapy with color Doppler. Gastrointest Endosc. 2000;51(3):331–3.
8. de Paulo GA, Ardengh JC, Nakao FS, Ferrari AP. Treatment of esophageal varices: a randomized controlled trial comparing endoscopic sclerotherapy and EUS-guided sclerotherapy of esophageal collateral veins. Gastrointest Endosc. 2006;63(3):396–402.. quiz 63
9. Sarin SK, Lahoti D, Saxena SP, Murthy NS, Makwana UK. Prevalence, classification and natural history of gastric varices: a long-term follow-up study in 568 portal hypertension patients. Hepatology. 1992;16(6):1343–9.
10. Garcia-Tsao G, Sanyal AJ, Grace ND, Carey W, Practice Guidelines Committee of the American Association for the Study of Liver D, Practice Parameters Committee of the American College of G. Prevention and management of gastroesophageal varices and variceal hemorrhage in cirrhosis. Hepatology. 2007;46(3):922–38.

11. Rios Castellanos E, Seron P, Gisbert JP, Bonfill CX. Endoscopic injection of cyanoacrylate glue versus other endoscopic procedures for acute bleeding gastric varices in people with portal hypertension. Cochrane Database Syst Rev. 2015;5:CD010180.

12. Singh V, Singh R, Bhalla A, Sharma N. Cyanoacrylate therapy for the treatment of gastric varices: a new method. J Dig Dis. 2016;17(6):392–8.

13. Marquez-Galisteo C, Giraldez-Gallego A, Nacarino-Mejias V, Rincon-Gatica A, Lopez-Ruiz T. Portal vein thrombosis following endoscopic treatment for gastric varices with N-butyl-2-cyanoacrylate: management with TIPS. Rev Esp Enferm Dig. 2015;107(4):246–7.

14. Oh SH, Kim SJ, Rhee KW, Kim KM. Endoscopic cyanoacrylate injection for the treatment of gastric varices in children. World J Gastroenterol. 2015;21(9):2719–24.

15. Robaina G, Albertini R, Carranza M, Herrena Najum P. Pulmonary embolism after endoscopic injection with N-butyl-2-cyanoacrylate for gastric varices. Medicina (B Aires). 2016;76(6):373–5.

16. Mishra SR, Sharma BC, Kumar A, Sarin SK. Primary prophylaxis of gastric variceal bleeding comparing cyanoacrylate injection and beta-blockers: a randomized controlled trial. J Hepatol. 2011;54(6):1161–7.

17. Soehendra N, Nam VC, Grimm H, Kempeneers I. Endoscopic obliteration of large esophagogastric varices with bucrylate. Endoscopy. 1986;18(1):25–6.

18. de Franchis R, Primignani M. Endoscopic treatments for portal hypertension. Semin Liver Dis. 1999;19(4):439–55.

19. Seewald S, Ang TL, Imazu H, et al. A standardized injection technique and regimen ensures success and safety of N-butyl-2-cyanoacrylate injection for the treatment of gastric fundal varices (with videos). Gastrointest Endosc. 2008;68(3):447–54.

20. Lo GH, Liang HL, Chen WC, et al. A prospective, randomized controlled trial of transjugular intrahepatic portosystemic shunt versus cyanoacrylate injection in the prevention of gastric variceal rebleeding. Endoscopy. 2007;39(8):679–85.

21. Boustiere C, Dumas O, Jouffre C, et al. Endoscopic ultrasonography classification of gastric varices in patients with cirrhosis. Comparison with endoscopic findings. J Hepatol. 1993;19(2):268–72.

22. Iwase H, Suga S, Morise K, Kuroiwa A, Yamaguchi T, Horiuchi Y. Color Doppler endoscopic ultrasonography for the evaluation of gastric varices and endoscopic obliteration with cyanoacrylate glue. Gastrointest Endosc. 1995;41(2):150–4.

23. Sarin SK, Kumar A. Sclerosants for variceal sclerotherapy: a critical appraisal. Am J Gastroenterol. 1990;85(6):641–9.

24. Romero-Castro R, Pellicer-Bautista FJ, Jimenez-Saenz M, et al. EUS-guided injection of cyanoacrylate in perforating feeding veins in gastric varices: results in 5 cases. Gastrointest Endosc. 2007;66(2):402–7.

25. Romero-Castro R, Pellicer-Bautista F, Giovannini M, et al. Endoscopic ultrasound (EUS)-guided coil embolization therapy in gastric varices. Endoscopy. 2010;42(Suppl 2):E35–6.

26. Romero-Castro R, Ellrichmann M, Ortiz-Moyano C, et al. EUS-guided coil versus cyanoacrylate therapy for the treatment of gastric varices: a multicenter study (with videos). Gastrointest Endosc. 2013;78(5):711–21.

27. Binmoeller KF, Weilert F, Shah JN, Kim J. EUS-guided transesophageal treatment of gastric fundal varices with combined coiling and cyanoacrylate glue injection (with videos). Gastrointest Endosc. 2011;74(5):1019–25.

28. Bhat YM, Weilert F, Fredrick RT, et al. EUS-guided treatment of gastric fundal varices with combined injection of coils and cyanoacrylate glue: a large U.S. experience over 6 years (with video). Gastrointest Endosc. 2016;83(6):1164–72.

29. Hall PS, Teshima C, May GR, Mosko JD. Endoscopic ultrasound-guided vascular therapy: the present and the future. Clin Endosc. 2017;50(2):138–42.

30. Helmy A, Al Kahtani K, Al Fadda M. Updates in the pathogenesis, diagnosis and management of ectopic varices. Hepatol Int. 2008;2(3):322–34.

31. Rana SS, Bhasin DK, Rao C, Singh K. Endoscopic ultrasound-guided treatment of bleeding duodenal varix. Indian J Gastroenterol. 2011;30(6):280–1.

32. Saad WE, Lippert A, Saad NE, Caldwell S. Ectopic varices: anatomical classification, hemodynamic classification, and hemodynamic-based management. Tech Vasc Interv Radiol. 2013;16(2):158–75.

33. Kinzel J, Pichetshote N, Dredar S, Aslanian H, Nagar A. Bleeding from a duodenal varix: a unique case of variceal hemostasis achieved using EUS-guided placement of an embolization coil and cyanoacrylate. J Clin Gastroenterol. 2014;48(4):362–4.

34. Fujii-Lau LL, Law R, Wong Kee Song LM, Gostout CJ, Kamath PS, Levy MJ. Endoscopic ultrasound (EUS)-guided coil injection therapy of esophagogastric and ectopic varices. Surg Endosc. 2016;30(4):1396–404.

35. Mukkada RJ, Chooracken MJ, Antony R, Augustine P. EUS-guided coiling for bleeding duodenal collateral vessel. Gastrointest Endosc. 2016;84(6):1057–8.

36. So H, Park do H, Jung K, Ko HK. Successful endoscopic ultrasound-guided coil embolization for severe duodenal bleeding. Am J Gastroenterol. 2016;111(7):925.

37. Krystallis C, McAvoy NC, Wilson J, Hayes PC, Plevris JN. EUS-assisted thrombin injection for ectopic bleeding varices--a case report and review of the literature. QJM. 2012;105(4):355–8.

38. Al Khalloufi K, Laiyemo AO. Management of rectal varices in portal hypertension. World J Hepatol. 2015;7(30):2992–8.

39. Wiechowska-Kozlowska A, Bialek A, Milkiewicz P. Prevalence of 'deep' rectal varices in patients with cirrhosis: an EUS-based study. Liver Int. 2009;29(8):1202–5.

40. McCormack TT, Bailey HR, Simms JM, Johnson AG. Rectal varices are not piles. Br J Surg. 1984;71(2):163.

41. Johansen K, Bardin J, Orloff MJ. Massive bleeding from hemorrhoidal varices in portal hypertension. JAMA. 1980;244(18):2084–5.

42. Wilson SE, Stone RT, Christie JP, Passaro E Jr. Massive lower gastrointestinal bleeding from intestinal varices. Arch Surg. 1979;114(10):1158–61.

43. Sharma M, Rai P, Bansal R. EUS-assisted evaluation of rectal varices before banding. Gastroenterol Res Pract. 2013;2013:619187.

44. Philips CA, Augustine P. Endoscopic ultrasound-guided management of bleeding rectal varices. ACG Case Rep J. 2017;4:e101.

45. Jana T, Mistry T, Singhal S. Endoscopic ultrasound-guided hemostasis of rectal varices. Endoscopy. 2017;49(S 01):E136–E7.

46. Weilert F, Shah JN, Marson FP, Binmoeller KF. EUS-guided coil and glue for bleeding rectal varix. Gastrointest Endosc. 2012;76(4):915–6.

47. Connor EK, Duran-Castro OL, Attam R. Therapy for recurrent bleeding from rectal varices by EUS-guided sclerosis. Gastrointest Endosc. 2015;81(5):1280–1.

48. Storm AC, Kumbhari V, Saxena P, et al. EUS-guided angiotherapy. Gastrointest Endosc. 2014;80(1):164–5.

49. Tsynman DN, DeCross AJ, Maliakkal B, Ciufo N, Ullah A, Kaul V. Novel use of EUS to successfully treat bleeding parastomal varices with N-butyl-2-cyanoacrylate. Gastrointest Endosc. 2014;79(6):1007–8.. discussion 8

50. Lu Y, Loffroy R, Lau JY, Barkun A. Multidisciplinary management strategies for acute non-variceal upper gastrointestinal bleeding. Br J Surg. 2014;101(1):e34–50.

51. Barkun AN, Bardou M, Kuipers EJ, et al. International consensus recommendations on the management of patients with nonvariceal upper gastrointestinal bleeding. Ann Intern Med. 2010;152(2):101–13.

52. Laine L, Jensen DM. Management of patients with ulcer bleeding. Am J Gastroenterol. 2012;107(3):345–60.. quiz 61

53. Jakobs R, Zoepf T, Schilling D, Siegel EG, Riemann JF. Endoscopic Doppler ultrasound after injection therapy for peptic ulcer hemorrhage. Hepato-Gastroenterology. 2004;51(58):1206–9.

54. van Leerdam ME, Rauws EA, Geraedts AA, Tijssen JG, Tytgat GN. The role of endoscopic Doppler US in patients with peptic ulcer bleeding. Gastrointest Endosc. 2003;58(5):677–84.

55. Jensen DM, Ohning GV, Kovacs TO, et al. Doppler endoscopic probe as a guide to risk stratification and definitive hemostasis of peptic ulcer bleeding. Gastrointest Endosc. 2016;83(1):129–36.

56. Fockens P, Meenan J, van Dullemen HM, Bolwerk CJ, Tytgat GN. Dieulafoy's disease: endosonographic detection and endosonography-guided treatment. Gastrointest Endosc. 1996;44(4):437–42.

57. Levy MJ, Wong Kee Song LM, Farnell MB, Misra S, Sarr MG, Gostout CJ. Endoscopic ultrasound (EUS)-guided angiotherapy of refractory gastrointestinal bleeding. Am J Gastroenterol. 2008;103(2):352–9.

58. Folvik G, Nesje LB, Berstad A, Odegaard S. Endosonography-guided endoscopic band ligation of Dieulafoy's malformation: a case report. Endoscopy. 2001;33(7):636–8.

59. Ribeiro A, Vazquez-Sequeiros E, Wiersema MJ. Doppler EUS-guided treatment of gastric Dieulafoy's lesion. Gastrointest Endosc. 2001;53(7):807–9.

60. Kumbhari V, Gondal B, Okolo Iii PI, et al. Endoscopic ultrasound-guided angiotherapy of a large bleeding gastrointestinal stromal tumor. Endoscopy. 2013;45(Suppl 2 UCTN):E326–7.

61. Gonzalez JM, Ezzedine S, Vitton V, Grimaud JC, Barthet M. Endoscopic ultrasound treatment of vascular complications in acute pancreatitis. Endoscopy. 2009;41(8):721–4.

62. Chaves DM, Costa FF, Matuguma S, et al. Splenic artery pseudoaneurysm treated with thrombin injection guided by endoscopic ultrasound. Endoscopy. 2012;44. Suppl 2 UCTN:E99–100.

63. Lameris R, du Plessis J, Nieuwoudt M, Scheepers A, van der Merwe SW. A visceral pseudoaneurysm: management by EUS-guided thrombin injection. Gastrointest Endosc. 2011;73(2):392–5.

64. Roach H, Roberts SA, Salter R, Williams IM, Wood AM. Endoscopic ultrasound-guided thrombin injection for the treatment of pancreatic pseudoaneurysm. Endoscopy. 2005;37(9):876–8.

65. Law R, Fujii-Lau L, Wong Kee Song LM, et al. Efficacy of endoscopic ultrasound-guided hemostatic interventions for resistant nonvariceal bleeding. Clin Gastroenterol Hepatol. 2015;13(4):808–12 e1.

66. Gralnek IM, Dumonceau JM, Kuipers EJ, et al. Diagnosis and management of nonvariceal upper gastrointestinal hemorrhage: European Society of Gastrointestinal Endoscopy (ESGE) guideline. Endoscopy. 2015;47(10):a1–46.

67. Mathew G, Bhimji SS. Aneurysm, pancreatic pseudoaneurysm. Treasure Island: StatPearls; 2017.

68. Bhasin DK, Rana SS, Sharma V, et al. Non-surgical management of pancreatic pseudocysts associated with arterial pseudoaneurysm. Pancreatology. 2013;13(3):250–3.

69. Beattie GC, Hardman JG, Redhead D, Siriwardena AK. Evidence for a central role for selective mesenteric angiography in the management of the major vascular complications of pancreatitis. Am J Surg. 2003;185(2):96–102.

70. Arnaud JP, Bergamaschi R, Serra-Maudet V, Casa C. Pancreatoduodenectomy for hemosuccus pancreaticus in silent chronic pancreatitis. Arch Surg. 1994;129(3):333–4.

71. Jeffers K, Majumder S, Vege SS, Levy M. EUS-guided pancreatic pseudoaneurysm therapy: bet-

ter to be lucky than good. Gastrointest Endosc. 2018;87(4):1155.

72. Roberts KJ, Jones RG, Forde C, Marudanayagam R. Endoscopic ultrasound-guided treatment of visceral artery pseudoaneurysm. HPB (Oxford). 2012;14(7):489–90.

73. Robb PM, Yeaton P, Bishop T, Wessinger J. Endoscopic ultrasound guided embolization of a pancreatic pseudoaneurysm. Gastroenterology Res. 2012;5(6):239–41.

74. Robinson M, Richards D, Carr N. Treatment of a splenic artery pseudoaneurysm by endoscopic ultrasound-guided thrombin injection. Cardiovasc Intervent Radiol. 2007;30(3):515–7.

75. Sanyal AJ, Bosch J, Blei A, Arroyo V. Portal hypertension and its complications. Gastroenterology. 2008;134(6):1715–28.

76. Frye JW, Perri RE. Perioperative risk assessment for patients with cirrhosis and liver disease. Expert Rev Gastroenterol Hepatol. 2009;3(1):65–75.

77. Armonis A, Patch D, Burroughs A. Hepatic venous pressure measurement: an old test as a new prognostic marker in cirrhosis? Hepatology. 1997;25(1):245–8.

78. Groszmann RJ, Wongcharatrawee S. The hepatic venous pressure gradient: anything worth doing should be done right. Hepatology. 2004;39(2):280–2.

79. Chelliah ST, Keshava SN, Moses V, Surendrababu NR, Zachariah UG, Eapen C. Measurement of hepatic venous pressure gradient revisited: catheter wedge vs balloon wedge techniques. Indian J Radiol Imaging. 2011;21(4):291–3.

80. Feu F, Garcia-Pagan JC, Bosch J, et al. Relation between portal pressure response to pharmacotherapy and risk of recurrent variceal haemorrhage in patients with cirrhosis. Lancet. 1995;346(8982):1056–9.

81. Lai L, Poneros J, Santilli J, Brugge W. EUS-guided portal vein catheterization and pressure measurement in an animal model: a pilot study of feasibility. Gastrointest Endosc. 2004;59(2):280–3.

82. Giday SA, Ko CW, Clarke JO, et al. EUS-guided portal vein carbon dioxide angiography: a pilot study in a porcine model. Gastrointest Endosc. 2007;66(4):814–9.

83. Giday SA, Clarke JO, Buscaglia JM, et al. EUS-guided portal vein catheterization: a promising novel approach for portal angiography and portal vein pressure measurements. Gastrointest Endosc. 2008;67(2):338–42.

84. Fujii-Lau LL, Leise MD, Kamath PS, Gleeson FC, Levy MJ. Endoscopic ultrasound-guided portal-systemic pressure gradient measurement. Endoscopy. 2014;46(Suppl 1 UCTN):E654–6.

85. Schulman AR, Ryou M, Aihara H, et al. EUS-guided intrahepatic portosystemic shunt with direct portal pressure measurements: a novel alternative to transjugular intrahepatic portosystemic shunting. Gastrointest Endosc. 2017;85(1):243–7.

86. Huang JY, Samarasena JB, Tsujino T, Chang KJ. EUS-guided portal pressure gradient measurement with a novel 25-gauge needle device versus standard transjugular approach: a comparison animal study. Gastrointest Endosc. 2016;84(2):358–62.

87. Huang JY, Samarasena JB, Tsujino T, et al. EUS-guided portal pressure gradient measurement with a simple novel device: a human pilot study. Gastrointest Endosc. 2017;85(5):996–1001.

88. Tsujino T, Huang JY, Samarasena JB, et al. Safety and feasibility of combination EUS-guided portal pressure gradient measurement and liver biopsy: the realization of endo-hepatology. Gastrointest Endosc. 2016;83(5):AB415–AB6.

89. D'Amico G, Pagliaro L, Bosch J. The treatment of portal hypertension: a meta-analytic review. Hepatology. 1995;22(1):332–54.

90. Colombato L. The role of transjugular intrahepatic portosystemic shunt (TIPS) in the management of portal hypertension. J Clin Gastroenterol. 2007;41(Suppl 3):S344–51.

91. Ochs A, Rossle M, Haag K, et al. The transjugular intrahepatic portosystemic stent-shunt procedure for refractory ascites. N Engl J Med. 1995;332(18):1192–7.

92. Gines P, Uriz J, Calahorra B, et al. Transjugular intrahepatic portosystemic shunting versus paracentesis plus albumin for refractory ascites in cirrhosis. Gastroenterology. 2002;123(6):1839–47.

93. Buscaglia JM, Dray X, Shin EJ, et al. A new alternative for a transjugular intrahepatic portosystemic shunt: EUS-guided creation of an intrahepatic portosystemic shunt (with video). Gastrointest Endosc. 2009;69(4):941–7.

94. Binmoeller KF, Shah JN. Sa1428 EUS-guided transgastric intrahepatic portosystemic shunt using the axios stent. Gastrointest Endosc. 2011;73(4):AB167.

95. Bosch J. EUS-guided intrahepatic portosystemic shunt: a real alternative to transjugular intrahepatic portalsystemic shunt? Gastrointest Endosc. 2017;85(1):248–9.

96. de Suray N, Pranger D, Brenard R. Portal vein thrombosis as the first sign of a primary myeloproliferative disorder: diagnostic interest of the V617F JAK-2 mutation. A report of 2 cases. Acta Gastroenterol Belg. 2008;71(1):39–41.

97. Regnault H, Emambux S, Lecomte T, et al. Clinical outcome of portal vein thrombosis in patients with digestive cancers: a large AGEO multicenter study. Dig Liver Dis. 2018;50(3):285.

98. Fujiyama S, Saitoh S, Kawamura Y, et al. Portal vein thrombosis in liver cirrhosis: incidence, management, and outcome. BMC Gastroenterol. 2017;17(1):112.

99. Lai R, Stephens V, Bardales R. Diagnosis and staging of hepatocellular carcinoma by EUS-FNA of a portal vein thrombus. Gastrointest Endosc. 2004;59(4):574–7.

100. Michael H, Lenza C, Gupta M, Katz DS. Endoscopic ultrasound -guided fine-needle aspiration of a portal vein thrombus to aid in the diagnosis and staging of hepatocellular carcinoma. Gastroenterol Hepatol (N Y). 2011;7(2):124–9.

101. Moreno M, Gimeno-Garcia AZ, Corriente MM, et al. EUS-FNA of a portal vein thrombosis in a patient with a hidden hepatocellular carcinoma: confirmation technique after contrast-enhanced ultrasound. Endoscopy. 2014;46(Suppl 1 UCTN):E590–1.

102. Kayar Y, Turkdogan KA, Baysal B, Unver N, Danalioglu A, Senturk H. EUS-guided FNA of a portal vein thrombus in hepatocellular carcinoma. Pan Afr Med J. 2015;21:86.

103. Delconte G, Bhoori S, Milione M, et al. Endoscopic ultrasound-guided fine needle aspiration of splenic vein thrombosis: a novel approach to the portal venous system. Endoscopy. 2016;48(Suppl 1 UCTN):E40–1.

104. Sisman G, Erzin YZ, Senturk H. Diagnosis of adrenocortical carcinoma via endosonography-assisted fine-needle aspiration of inferior vena cava thrombosis: first case in the literature. Dig Endosc. 2013;25(3):338–9.

105. Gincul R, Gomez V, Kerr SE, Zhang J, Levy MJ. Endoscopic ultrasound-guided fine-needle aspiration of a pulmonary artery malignant thrombus. Endoscopy. 2015;47 Suppl(1):E547–9.

106. Rustagi T, Gleeson FC, Chari ST, et al. Remote malignant intravascular thrombi: EUS-guided FNA diagnosis and impact on cancer staging. Gastrointest Endosc. 2017;86(1):150–5.

107. Allard WJ, Matera J, Miller MC, et al. Tumor cells circulate in the peripheral blood of all major carcinomas but not in healthy subjects or patients with nonmalignant diseases. Clin Cancer Res. 2004;10(20):6897–904.

108. Catenacci DV, Chapman CG, Xu P, et al. Acquisition of portal venous circulating tumor cells from patients with pancreaticobiliary cancers by endoscopic ultrasound. Gastroenterology. 2015;149(7):1794–803 e4.

109. Fritscher-Ravens A, Ganbari A, Mosse CA, Swain P, Koehler P, Patel K. Transesophageal endoscopic ultrasound-guided access to the heart. Endoscopy. 2007;39(5):385–9.

110. Larghi A, Stobinski M, Galasso D, Amato A, Familiari P, Costamagna G. EUS-guided drainage of a pericardial cyst: closer to the heart (with video). Gastrointest Endosc. 2009;70(6):1273–4.

111. Romero-Castro R, Rios-Martin JJ, Gallego-Garcia de Vinuesa P, et al. Pericardial tumor diagnosed by EUS-guided FNA (with video). Gastrointest Endosc. 2009;69(3 Pt 1):562–3.

112. Gornals JB, de la Hera M, de Albert M, Claver E, Catala I. EUS cardiac puncture-guided right atrial tumor. Gastrointest Endosc. 2015;82(1):165.

113. Zhang X, Wang K, Wang M, et al. Transarterial chemoembolization (TACE) combined with sorafenib versus TACE for hepatocellular carcinoma with portal vein tumor thrombus: a systematic review and meta-analysis. Oncotarget. 2017;8(17):29416–27.

114. Chen J, Huang J, Chen M, et al. Transcatheter arterial chemoembolization (TACE) versus hepatectomy in hepatocellular carcinoma with macrovascular invasion: a meta-analysis of 1683 patients. J Cancer. 2017;8(15):2984–91.

115. Kim W, Clark TW, Baum RA, Soulen MC. Risk factors for liver abscess formation after hepatic chemoembolization. J Vasc Interv Radiol. 2001;12(8):965–8.

116. Kim HK, Chung YH, Song BC, et al. Ischemic bile duct injury as a serious complication after transarterial chemoembolization in patients with hepatocellular carcinoma. J Clin Gastroenterol. 2001;32(5):423–7.

117. Faigel DO, Lake DF, Landreth TL, Kelman CC, Marler RJ. EUS-guided portal injection chemotherapy for treatment of hepatic metastases: feasibility in the acute porcine model. Gastrointest Endosc. 2016;83(2):444–6.

118. Faigel D, Lake D, Landreth T, Kelman C, Marler R. Endoscopic ultrasonography-guided portal injection chemotherapy for hepatic metastases. Endosc Ultrasound. 2014;3(Suppl 1):S1.

119. Zhang FJ, Li CX, Jiao DC, et al. CT guided 125iodine seed implantation for portal vein tumor thrombus in primary hepatocellular carcinoma. Chin Med J. 2008;121(23):2410–4.

Index

© Springer Nature Switzerland AG 2020
M. S. Wagh, S. B. Wani (eds.), *Gastrointestinal Interventional Endoscopy*,
https://doi.org/10.1007/978-3-030-21695-5